CORPVS MEDICORVM GRAECORVM

EDIDERVNT

ACADEMIAE BEROLINENSIS HAVNIENSIS LIPSIENSIS

XI 1, 3, 1

STEPHANI ATHENIENSIS

IN HIPPOCRATIS APHORISMOS COMMENTARIA I–II

EDIDIT ET IN LINGVAM ANGLICAM VERTIT

LEENDERT G. WESTERINK

BEROLINI IN AEDIBVS ACADEMIAE SCIENTIARVM MCMLXXXV

STEPHANUS OF ATHENS

COMMENTARY ON HIPPOCRATES' APHORISMS

SECTIONS I–II

TEXT AND TRANSLATION
BY

LEENDERT G. WESTERINK

AKADEMIE-VERLAG · BERLIN 1985

Erschienen im Akademie-Verlag, DDR - 1086 Berlin, Leipziger Str. 3–4

Lizenznummer: 202 · 100/114/85
Printed in the German Democratic Republic
Gesamtherstellung: IV/2/14 VEB Druckerei »Gottfried Wilhelm Leibniz«,
4450 Gräfenhainichen · 6133
LSV 0886
Bestellnummer: 754 034 6 (2028/26/I)
07000

TO JULIE, M. D.

VORWORT

Ebenso wie bei dem Prognostikon-Kommentar des Stephanos (s. CMG XI 1,2) handelt es sich auch bei seinem Kommentarwerk zu den hippokratischen Aphorismen um Vorlesungsnachschriften. Die Vorlesung des Stephanos über die Aphorismen des Hippokrates gliedert sich in sechs Abschnitte, die in unterschiedlichen Fassungen in drei voneinander unabhängigen Überlieferungssträngen auf uns gekommen sind. Lediglich der dritte und vierte Abschnitt sowie einige wenige Zeilen von der Einleitung zum fünften Abschnitt sind in der Originalfassung erhalten geblieben. Der erste und zweite Abschnitt und ein Teil des dritten Abschnitts liegen in einer von einem späteren Redaktor gekürzten und bearbeiteten Fassung vor, während der fünfte und sechste Abschnitt demgegenüber verhältnismäßig geringfügige Kürzungen aufweisen, so daß hier nicht zu entscheiden ist, ob diese Veränderungen ebenfalls zu Lasten einer späteren Bearbeitung gehen oder ob sie darauf zurückzuführen sind, daß die erhaltenen Nachschriften der Vorlesungsabschnitte V und VI von einer anderen Person und zu einem anderen Zeitpunkt angefertigt wurden als die der Vorlesungsabschnitte III–IV.

Es ist das Verdienst von L. G. Westerink, die komplizierte Überlieferungssituation des vorliegenden Textes, der bisher nur in Auszügen in der Edition von F. R. Dietz aus dem Jahre 1834 zu benutzen war, aufgeklärt und damit eine zuverlässige Grundlage für die erste vollständige Ausgabe des Aphorismenkommentars geschaffen zu haben. Als Hilfsmittel zur Textgestaltung wurden die unter dem Namen des Theophilos überlieferten Scholien zu den hippokratischen Aphorismen herangezogen, die im wesentlichen nichts anderes sind als eine Kompilation von Exzerpten aus den Aphorismenkommentaren des Galen und des Stephanos. Eine Pionierleistung stellt auch die dem griechischen Text beigegebene englische Übersetzung dar, die auch dem philologisch nicht vorgebildeten Benutzer den Zugang zu diesem Zeugnis spätantiker Hippokratesexegese ermöglicht.

Da Stephanos sich in seinen Vorlesungen über die hippokratischen Aphorismen nicht auf die eigentliche Texterklärung beschränkt hat, sondern vielmehr gleichzeitig darum bemüht war, seinen Hörern medizinische Theorien von allgemeinerer Bedeutung nahezubringen, weist das Kommentarwerk insgesamt einen beträchtlichen Umfang auf. Dieser Umstand macht es erforderlich, den Kommentar in drei gesonderten Bänden zu publizieren, die der in der Überlieferung vorgegebenen Einteilung entsprechend jeweils den Text von zwei Vorlesungsabschnitten enthalten werden.

Die Redaktion
des Corpus Medicorum Graecorum
Jutta Kollesch

CONTENTS

BIBLIOGRAPHY

Agnellus of Ravenna, Lectures on Galen's De sectis, Latin Text and Translation by Seminar Classics 609, Buffalo 1981 (Ambros. G 108 inf., fol. 22r–48r)

–, In Galeni artem, Ambros. G 108 inf., fol. 48v–91r

–, In Galeni libellum De pulsibus ad tirones, Ambros. G 108 inf., fol. 92r–114v

–, In Galeni libros Ad Glauconem, Ambros. G 108 inf., fol. 114v–130r

B. Alexanderson, Die hippokratische Schrift Prognostikon. Überlieferung und Text, Göteborg [1963] (Studia Graeca et Latina Gothoburgensia 17)

Anonymus Latinus, In Aphorismos, MS. Karlsruhe, Aug. 120, fol. 120r–204v

G. Baffioni, Inediti di Archelao da un codice Bolognese, Boll. del Comit. per la prep. dell'Ed. Naz. dei Classici Gr. e Lat., N. S. 3, 1955, p. 17–36

–, Scolii inediti di Palladio al De sectis di Galeno, Boll. del Comit. per la prep. dell'Ed. Naz. dei Classici Gr. e Lat., N. S. 6, 1958, p. 61–78

–, Il codex Vindobonensis med. Graec. 16, foll. 325v–328v, Jahrb. d. österr. byz. Ges. 9, 1960, p. 41–46

–, Il Trattato „De Febrium Differentia" nei Codici Greci Vindobonensi, s. l. [1961]

A. Beccaria, Sulle tracce di un antico canone latino di Ippocrate e di Galeno I, Italia medioev. e umanistica 2, 1959, p. 1–56; II, ibid. 4, 1961, p. 1–75; III, ibid. 14, 1971, p. 1–23

W. Bräutigam, De Hippocratis Epidemiarum libri sexti commentatoribus, Diss. Königsberg 1908

U. C. Bussemaker, Traité d'Etienne sur les urines, Revue de philol., de litt. et d'hist. anc. 1, 1845, pp. 415–438; 543–560

CAG = Commentaria in Aristotelem Graeca, Berlin 1882–1909

CMG = Corpus Medicorum Graecorum

CPG = Corpus Paroemiographorum Graecorum, edd. E. L. Leutsch, F. G. Schneidewin, 2 vols., Göttingen 1839–1861 (repr. Hildesheim 1958)

K. Deichgräber, Art. "Theophilos" (No. 16) in: RE V A, 1934, col. 2148–2149

F. R. Dietz, Apollonii Citiensis, Stephani, Palladii, Theophili, Meletii, Damascii, Ioannis, aliorum Scholia in Hippocratem et Galenum, 2 vols., Königsberg 1834 (repr. Amsterdam 1966)

F. Z. Ermerins, Anecdota medica Graeca, Leiden 1840 (repr. Amsterdam 1963)

H. Flashar, Beiträge zur spätantiken Hippokratesdeutung, Hermes 90, 1962, p. 402–418

Claudius Galenus, Opera omnia, ed. C. G. Kühn, 20 vols., Leipzig 1821–1833 (= K.)

Claudius Galenus Pergamenus, Scripta minora, edd. J. Marquardt, I. Müller, G. Helmreich, 3 vols., Leipzig 1884–1893

Galenus, De temperamentis libri III, ed. G. Helmreich, Leipzig 1904

–, De usu partium libri XVII, ed. G. Helmreich, 2 vols., Leipzig 1907/1909

–, De sanitate tuenda, ed. K. Koch, in: CMG V 4,2, Leipzig and Berlin 1923

–, In Hippocratis De natura hominis commentaria III, ed. J. Mewaldt, in: CMG V 9,1, Leipzig and Berlin 1914

–, In Hippocratis Epidemiarum librum VI commentaria I–VI, ed. E. Wenkebach, commentaria VI–VIII, transl. F. Pfaff, CMG V 10,2,2, 2nd ed., Berlin 1956

–, On the Parts of Medicine; On Cohesive Causes; On Regimen in Acute Diseases in Accordance with the Theories of Hippocrates, ed. and transl. M. Lyons, CMG Suppl. Or. II, Berlin 1969

Œuvres complètes d'Hippocrate, ed. and transl. E. Littré, 10 vols., Paris 1839–1861 (= L.)

Hippocrates, Opera quae feruntur omnia, ed. H. Kühlewein, 2 vols., Leipzig 1894/1902 (= Kw.)

–, ed. and transl. W. H. S. Jones, vol. IV, London and Cambridge, Mass. 1953 (Loeb Classical Library)

–, De alimento; De flatibus, ed. J. L. Heiberg, in: CMG I 1, Leipzig and Berlin 1927
–, Prognostikon see Alexanderson
J. L. Ideler, Physici et medici Graeci minores, 2 vols., Berlin 1841/1842 (repr. Amsterdam 1963)
Io(h)annes, In Hippocratis librum De natura pueri, Dietz II 205–235
–, Commentaria in sextum librum Hippocratis Epidemiarum, ed. C. D. Pritchet, Leiden 1975
–, Commentaria in librum De sectis Galeni, ed. C. D. Pritchet, Leiden 1982
F. E. Kind, Art. "Leon" (No. 26) in: RE XII, 1925, col. 2014
–, Art. "Stephanos" (No. 20) in: RE III A, 1929, col. 2404–2405
A. Kousis, The Apotherapeutica of Theophilus according to the Laurentian Codex Plut. 75,19, Πρακτικὰ 'Ακαδημίας 'Αθηνῶν 19, 1944, p. 35–45
Leo, Synopsis, Ermerins 79–221
M. Meyerhof, Von Alexandrien nach Bagdad, Sitzungsber. Preuß. Akad., Phil.-hist. Kl. 23, 1930
–, Johannes Grammatikos (Philoponos) von Alexandrien und die arabische Medizin, Mitt. des Deutschen Instituts für ägypt. Altertumsk. in Kairo 2, 1931, p. 1–21
–, La fin de l'école d'Alexandrie, d'après quelques auteurs arabes, Archeion 16, 1933, p. 1–15
E. Nachmanson, Ein neuplatonischer Galenkommentar auf Papyrus, Minnesskr. utgiven av filol. Samfundet in Göteborg, 1925, p. 201–217
Palladius, In Hippocratis Epidemiarum librum VI, Dietz II 1–204
–, In Galeni librum De sectis, ed. G. Baffioni, Scolii inediti
–, Kommentar zu Hippokrates 'De fracturis' und seine Parallelversion unter dem Namen des Stephanus von Alexandria, ed. D. Irmer, Hamburg 1977
Psellus, De omnifaria doctrina, ed. L. G. Westerink, Nijmegen and Utrecht 1948
RE = Paulys Real-Encyclopädie der classischen Altertumswissenschaft, edd. G. Wissowa, W. Kroll, K. Mittelhaus, K. Ziegler, Stuttgart/Munich 1893–1974
A. Revilla, Catálogo de los códices griegos de la Biblioteca de el Escorial, vol. I, Madrid 1936
M. Richard, 'Απὸ φωνῆς, Byzantion 20, 1950, p. 191–222
V. Rose, Ion's Reisebilder und Ioannes Alexandrinus der Arzt, Hermes 5, 1871, p. 205–215
F. Sezgin, Geschichte des arabischen Schrifttums, vol. III, Leiden 1970
H. E. Sigerist, The Medical Literature of the early Middle Ages, Bull. of the Inst. of the Hist. of Med. 2, 1934, p. 26–50
P. Speck, Die kaiserliche Universität von Konstantinopel (Byz. Archiv, H. 14) 1974, pp. 65–66; 76–77
Stephanus the Philosopher, A Commentary on the Prognosticon of Hippocrates, ed. and transl. J. M. Duffy, CMG XI 1,2, Berlin 1983
–, In Galeni librum I Ad Glauconem, Dietz I 233–344
–, Commentary on Hippocrates De fracturis: see Palladius
O. Temkin, Geschichte des Hippokratismus im ausgehenden Altertum, Kyklos 4, 1932, p. 1–80
–, Studies on Late Alexandrian Medicine I (Alexandrian commentaries on Galen's De sectis ad introducendos), Bull. of the Inst. of the Hist. of Med. 3, 1935, p. 405–430
–, Byzantine Medicine: Tradition and Empiricism, Dumbarton Oaks Papers 16, 1962, p. 95–115
–, Galenism. Rise and Decline of a Medical Philosophy, Ithaca and London [1973]
Theophilus, In Aphorismos, Dietz II 245–544
–, De hominis fabrica, ed. W. A. Greenhill, Oxford 1842
–, De pulsibus, Ermerins 1–77
–, De excrementis, Ideler I 397–408
–, De urinis, Ideler I 261–283
M. Wellmann, Die Fragmente der sikelischen Ärzte Akron, Philistion und des Diokles von Karystos, Fragmentsammlung der griechischen Ärzte, vol. I, Berlin 1901

INTRODUCTION

A. The manuscript tradition

What is extant of Stephanus' lectures on the Aphorisms has come down to us in three independent volumes, each representing a different version of the original, namely:

(I) an abridged and revised version of sect. I 1–III 25, preserved in Ambrosianus S 19 sup., Paris Gr. 2222 and 2223 (formerly also in St.-Remi 549, now lost, but of which a Latin translation is extant in Paris Lat. 6854) and, partly, in Vatican Gr. 279;

(II) the complete text of sect. III–IV, plus a few lines of the introduction to sect. V, in the first part of Escorial Σ. II. 10;

(III) the "Asclepius" version of sect. V 1–VI 55 in the second part of Escorial Σ. II. 10.

Finally, we have (IV) the Theophilus scholia, which to a great extent depend on Stephanus and can sometimes help to correct the text.

The first few pages of (I) (p. 28,4–32,17), selected extracts from (I)–(III), and the full text of (IV) were published by Dietz, II, p. 236–544.

I. The abridged version of I 1–III 25

Ambrosianus S 19 sup. (= A) (Ae. Martini-D. Bassi, Catalogus codicum Graecorum Bibliothecae Ambrosianae, Milan 1906, II, p. 846–847). Paper, a. 1348, foll. 189. **A**

fol. 2^r–188^v Σχόλεα σὺν θεῶ τῶν ἀφορισμῶν ἱπποκράτους· ἐξήγησις στεφάνου ἀθηναίου τοῦ φιλοσόφου [καὶ θεοφίλ(ου) add. al. m.]. fol. 2^r–124^r line 26: Stephanus I 1–III 25; fol. 124^r line 26–fol. 188^v line 20: Theophilus III 26–VII 60. A later hand (= A^2), besides making some incidental emendations in the text, has systematically corrected and completed the lemmata from a codex of the Aphorisms. **A^2**

fol. 188^v colophon:

τριὰς φύλαττε τοῖν δυοῖν θεοδώροιν
οἷν ἐπωνύμοιν, καμπανῶ παγωμένω·
τιμῆ ἀγγέλω λευΐτη γεγραφότι·
ἀκέστωρι τε σοφῶ τῶ κεκτημένω.
δώρησαι δ' αὐτοῖς καὶ πταισμάτων τὴν λύσιν.

ἐτελειώθ(η) ἐν ἔτει ἑξακισχιλιωστ(ῷ)· ὀκτακοσιωστῷ· πεντηκοστῷ ἕκτω· ἰνδ(ικτιῶνι) α'· μηνὶ μαρτ(ίω) δεκάτ(η) ἡμέρ(α) δευτ(έ)ρα[1].

fol. 189^{r} the following poem in Byzantine trimeters[2]:

Τοὺς Ἀφορισμοὺς ἀγαπῶν Ἱπποκράτους
ὡς ὠφελείας οὐ βραχείας πραχθέντας
θέλων τε τούτους ἐντρύφημα κατέχειν
πάντων ἐνύλων κρεῖττον ἐντρυφημάτων,
πρὸ μὲν χρόνων σφᾶς ἠρξάμην πολλῶν γράφειν,
τέλος δ' ἔθηκα τῇ γραφῇ ταύτῃ μόλις.
ὀψιτέλεστος δ' ἡ γραφή μοι συνέβη
οὐκ ἐξ ὀλίγων, ἀλλὰ πολλῶν αἰτίων,
νοσημάτων τε χαλεπῶν καὶ ποικίλων
καὶ παντοδαπῶν ἐν βίῳ μελημάτων
καὶ συνεχόντων ἅμα δυστυχημάτων.
εἴπω τἀληθές; – οὐ γὰρ ἄλλο δεῖ λέγειν –
τούτοις συνῆν ἅπασι καὶ ῥαθυμία,
ἥτις με καὶ πρίν, ἀλλὰ νῦν σφοδρῶς ἔχει.
ἔοικε δ' αὕτη μὴ συνεῖναί μοι φύσει,
ἀλλ' ἐντήκεσθαι πρός γε τῆς ἀ⟨θυ⟩μίας.
δυοῖν δὲ τούτους ἐκ βίβλων ἐγεγράφειν,
τῆς τε Στεφάνου τοῦ λίαν σοφωτάτου
καὶ Θεοφίλου τοῦ βραχυλογωτάτου,
πηγῶν ὕδωρ ἀντλήσας ἐξ ἀλλοτρίων,
ὅπερ σύνηθές ἐστι τοῖς παναπόροις.
πλὴν ἀλλὰ τέλος τῇ γραφῇ θείς, ὡς ἔφην,
τῷ παντελείῳ τοῦ θεοῦ πατρὸς λόγῳ
Χριστῷ προσάγω πάλιν εὐχαριστίαν.

P Paris Gr. 2222 (= P) (H. Omont, Inventaire sommaire des manuscrits grecs de la Bibliothèque Nationale, II, Paris 1888, p. 216). Paper, 14th cent., foll. 104.

fol. 1^{r}–104^{v} Μελετίου ἰατροῦ καὶ φιλοσόφου ἐξήγησις εἰς τοὺς ἀφορισμούς. fol. 1^{r}–69^{r} line 20: Stephanus I 1–III 25; fol. 69^{r} line 30 – fol. 104^{v}: Theophilus III 26–VII 60.

A direct copy of P is Paris Gr. 2223 (Omont, ibid.), 16th cent., from the Baluze collection, which was purchased for the Royal Library in 1719.

[1] Monday, March 10, 1348. It is not easy to make sense of the jumble of datives and duals in the "verse". According to M. Vogel-V. Gardthausen, Die griechischen Schreiber des Mittelalters und der Renaissance, Leipzig 1909 (repr. Heidelberg 1966), p. 7, the scribe Angelos the "levite" (deacon) wrote the book for Theodore Kampanos and Theodore Pagomenos. This, however, leaves the "learned physician and owner" in line 4 unexplained. Perhaps only two persons are involved: Theodore Angelos Kampanos, deacon and scribe, and Theodore Pagomenos (= Pepagomenos), physician and owner of the book.

[2] The ends of the even lines, written in the right hand column, are blurred, and the underlined words have been retouched by a later hand. At line 2 read προξένους for πραχθέντας.

Another copy was (apparently) the lost codex of St.-Remi in Reims, described by B. Montfaucon (Bibliotheca manuscriptorum nova, II, Paris 1739, p. 1289): "Cod. 549. bomb. saec. 16. Meletii et Medici et Philosophi commentarium in Aphorismos Hippocratis." The St.-Remi MSS. belonged to the collection of Charles, cardinal de Lorraine (1524–1574), most of which was destroyed by a fire in 1774. The Meletius MS. was translated into Latin not long before 1629 by a nephew of Gentien Hervet; he dedicated his work to the cardinal's great-grandnephew Henri de Lorraine (1614–1664), later fifth duc de Guise, then abbot of St.-Remi, but not yet archbishop of Reims, to which office he was designated in 1629. The translation is Paris Lat. 6854; the dedication and the introductory part of the text were published by Dietz, II, p. 240–244.

Vatican Gr. 279 (= Z) (J. Mercati-P. Franchi de' Cavalieri, Codices Vati- Z
cani Graeci, I, Rome 1923, p. 372–378). Paper, 14th cent., part I, foll. 218.

fol. 1^r–24^r ⟨Theophilus⟩ In aphorismos I 1–II 36 (p. 329,11 Dietz).

fol. 25^r–29^r ⟨Psellus, Omnifaria Doctrina⟩ 18–31.

fol. 30^r–209^r Τῶν ἀφορισμῶν ἱππο(κράτ)ους ἡ βίβλος.

Aphorisms with commentary by Stephanus, Galen and Theophilus, as follows: fol. 30^r–54^r line 21: Stephanus I 1–11 (infra, p. 28,4–88,26 λόγον); fol. 54^r line 22–fol. 189^v line 3: Galen I 11–V 72 (XVII 2, p. 380,8 φυλάττεσθαι – 887,15 K.); fol. 189^v line 4–fol. 209^r: Theophilus VI 1–VII 60 (p. 486,15–543,4 Dietz).

fol. 209^v colophon in verse (no name or date).

fol. 210^r–217^v miscellaneous medical texts.

The three MSS. derive from an archetype (= ω) in which errors and omis- ω
sions were already numerous. It seems that its first page was in a slightly damaged
condition when the common hyparchetype of A and P (= α) was written, and α
considerably more so when Z (or its ancestor) was copied. At least, this can be inferred from the size of the lacuna at p. 30,12, where, however, coincidence cannot be excluded: the numerous gaps in the first pages of Z may have been caused independently. Thus much is certain, that the two complete MSS. present a more faithful picture of the archetype; the scribe of Z permitted himself some freedom with the wording, dropping in an occasional γε, δηλαδή, or οὑτοσί, to improve the Greek, while his understanding of the medical content was not too clear. The consensus of A and P must therefore serve as the basis of the text throughout[1].

The origin of the abridged version can be reconstructed with a fair degree of certainty from the information contained in the redactor's poem, combined with the condition of the text. The initial project must have been to rewrite the entire commentary of Stephanus, as far as extant at the time; the copy used

[1] Common errors in APZ: e. g. pp. 30,9. 15. 21. 26; 32,10; 36,13; 64,14; 68,13; 70,15; connective errors in AP against Z: pp. 36,13; 38,4. 9; 46,17; 50,14; separative errors in Z against AP: pp. 28,5–7 (lac.); 32,5 (lac.); 34,18; 36,7–8; 38,25–26; 42,27; 44,4; 52,2 (lac.). 7 etc. The rare cases of agreement between A^2 and Z are accidental; at p. 32,14 A^2 correctly inserts σύντομος, but then the definition in question was widely known; μετανάστασις at p. 34,9 is an obvious *lectio facilior*. – The spelling of all the three MSS. is on the whole good; all write consistently ἀδδηφάγος, and often ἀφημερινός (or -ηνός). Mistakes of the usual type (confusion between homophonous vowels and between double and single consonants) have been ignored in the apparatus, except in special cases, such as rare words.

was similar to, but not identical with, the first part of the Escorial MS. before its beginning was lost. The clumsy Greek was improved somewhat, the original lecture form[1] reduced to that of a regular commentary, and some of the references and digressions omitted. This plan was actually executed for sections I–II and the beginning of III. Though in the Escorialensis sections I and II are lost, the number of missing leaves is known, and assuming that the writing was the same, we can calculate that less than a quarter of the text was left out in the process of abridging[2]. Then, however, discouraged by worries, misfortunes and illness, the redactor decided to reduce his task by more drastic cutting, so that less than one third is left of III 4–18 and only about one half of III 19–25. At that point, realizing that at this rate of abridging his work would have no *raison d'être* beside the existing commentary of Theophilus (itself essentially a summary of Stephanus), he completed the project by simply transcribing the remainder from his copy of Theophilus, which, as most others do, ended at VII 60. An alternative possibility would be that his copy of Stephanus did not go beyond III 25, but it is a less likely one, first because the original title as preserved in A mentions Stephanus only, while in the poem at the end both sources are named; secondly because the impatience shown in the treatment of III 4–25 is difficult to understand if the end was already in sight.

The time of the revision cannot be determined more precisely than between ca. 900 (the earliest date for Theophilus is ca. 850, see below, p. 18) and ca. 1300 (the latest probable date for the archetype). The prosody of the poem provides no workable criterion: the freedom in the handling of the dichrona and even occasional mistakes in visible quantities (long ε, short η) are features already appearing about 900; much here depends on the individual poet.

II. The complete version of III–IV

E Escorial Σ. II. 10 (= E), first part (Revilla, I, p. 312–316). Vellum, 10th cent., foll. 149.

The MS. originally consisted of 30 quaternions (numbered Α–Λ) plus one binion (numbered ΛΑ) and one separate leaf; at present, 14 quaternions are lost at the beginning, which must have contained the commentary on sections I and II with the author's name and the title. Section IV ends in the middle of fol. 149ᵛ; a different hand has added the beginning of the introduction to section V (only 12 lines). The two blank lines at the end of the page and the fact that no complete quaternion was used, prove that the exemplar also ended at this point.

This part of the commentary is preserved in its authentic form, that of a student's notebook. The division into the original lectures is marked, not only by a heading at the beginning but also by a standard formula, which is part of the text, at the end of each, according to the practice of Olympiodorus and his

[1] Traces are left at pp. 58,15; 70,10; 118,31 (θεωρία), and 136,29 (πρᾶξις).
[2] From the Escorial MS. the first 112 foll. are missing; the extant text in AP is equivalent to 86 foll.

school (from ca. 540 onward)[1]. There is no trace of any abridging; on the contrary, the report is so circumstantial and repetitious that it sometimes looks as if the teacher's own words were taken down in shorthand. The shapeless, ungrammatical Greek is no doubt the notetaker's own, and the same may hold for the poor spelling, though on the other hand it is obvious that the scribe who wrote the MS. was not a highly-educated man.

III. The "Asclepius" version of V 1–VI 55

Escorial Σ. II. 10 (= E), second part (Revilla, I, p. 312–316). Vellum, 10th–11th cent., fol. 150–270. E

The second part of the Escorial MS. was a separate volume, written a little later in a more elegant and also somewhat more correct hand. It may have been commissioned to complement the first part, but this is not certain. In its present form, it consists of fifteen numbered quaternions, ending at VI 55; but since the last quaternion is filled to the last line, it may originally have contained the complete commentary either on V–VI or on V–VII. There was a lacuna in the exemplar after V 48; the copyist left most of fol. 208^v blank and proceeded with V 52 at the top of fol. 210^r. Not much later, somebody else filled the gap by inserting the Theophilus scholia on V 49, 49 A, 50 and 51, marked εξ αλλ(ου) αντιγρα(φου), which probably means that his copy, as many others, was anonymous; his text differs not inconsiderably from Dietz's. As the space left blank on fol. 208^v was not nearly sufficient, he added another leaf of coarser vellum (now fol. 209).

The text of what (for reasons to be explained below, p. 20–23) I call the "Asclepius" version, is still recognizable as consisting also of lecture notes, but the only trace left of this are the headings of lectures 3 and 4 in section V (foll. 178^v and 188^v); the rest are lost and, what is more important, the Olympiodorean practice of marking the end of each lecture in the text itself is not followed. The beginning is different from the fragment of the "complete" version preserved on fol. 149^v; here, as well as at the beginning of section VI, the "Asclepius" version omits the general observations on the section as a whole which characterize Stephanus I–IV. Since the codex provides no author's name, it follows either that the lecturer is not Stephanus, or that his lectures were taken down by a different *reportator*, who permitted himself some more abridging. I shall presently return to this question.

IV. The Theophilus scholia

It is perhaps more prudent to speak of the "Theophilus scholia" than of "the scholia of Theophilus", as long as his exact role (author or revisor?) has not been cleared up.

Provisionally, the evidence is the following. There are four main types of the text:

[1] Eight lectures in sect. III, six in sect. IV, where, however, the division is dropped after fol. 94^v. On the Olympiodorean form of the commentary see M. Richard; some additional examples in L. G. Westerink, Ein astrologisches Kolleg aus dem Jahre 564, Byz. Zeitschr. 64, 1971, p. 6–21 (at p. 7, Stephanus Ad Glauconem is included wrongly).

(i) The unrevised version of Urbinas Gr. 64 (10th–11th cent.), under the title 'Αφορισμοὶ τοῦ 'Ιπποκράτου (sic) γραφέντες παρὰ Θεοφίλου πρωτοσπαθαρίου καὶ ἐπὶ τοῦ χρόνου τρίτου μετὰ τῶν σχολίων αὐτῶν, and with the subscription (al. m.) Τέλος τῶν σχολίων Θεοφίλου φιλοσόφου εἰς τοὺς 'Αφορισμοὺς 'Ιπποκράτους. Other MSS. belonging to this group, but independent of the Urbinas, are: Paris Gr. 2228 (14th/11th cent.), Berlin Gr. 120 (15th cent.), Ambrosianus L 110 sup. (15th cent.), Karlsruhe 449 (15th–16th cent.), Paris Gr. 2149 (16th cent.). The Paris and Berlin MSS. have the title Θεοφίλου φιλοσόφου ἐξήγησις, the other two are anonymous (the Karlsruhe MS. is *initio mutilus*). Paris Gr. 2296, and its copy Göttingen Hist. nat. 5, though they also have this title, belong to type iii.

(ii) The Urbinas revised and expanded (especially in the latter half) by a 13th cent. hand; direct or indirect copies are Escorial y. I. 8, Vatican Gr. 1062, Laurentianus 86,9, Vienna Phil. Gr. 74, Ambrosianus B 113 sup. and A 95 sup. They all show the same title as the Urbinas, except for the last, which has no author's name. The origin of the supplements is unknown; there are several samples in Dietz, II (from Ambr. B 113 sup.), e.g. p. 514–515, n. 3.

(iii) An anonymous group headed by Vatican Gr. 2254 (10th–11th cent.): Σχόλια εἰς τοὺς 'Ιπποκράτους 'Αφορισμοὺς κατὰ σύνοψιν (so, too, Vienna Med. Gr. 16 and Turin B. III. 37); an insertion characteristic of this type is to be found e.g. in Dietz, II, p. 386–387, n. 3. Though, with the exception of Paris Gr. 2296 (and its Göttingen copy) no extant MS. mentions an author's name, it should be noted that the redactor of the Stephanus-Theophilus text used a copy of this type and that to him the author is Theophilus.

(iv) The text of V 49–51 inserted in Escorial Σ. II. 10 fol. 208v–209v. It is a good deal longer than the current version and was apparently anonymous ("from another MS.").

Though the testimony of the MSS. is thus fairly strong in support of Theophilus, it seems to be invalidated by the (no doubt authentic) title as preserved in the Urbinas: "The Aphorisms of Hippocrates, written by Theophilus ... with their scholia." Here, the role claimed by Theophilus himself is apparently little more than that of a copyist, or at best an editor. This impression is confirmed by the early fragment of a longer version in the Escorial MS. (iv).

There is other useful information to be found in the heading of the Urbinas: it also solves the controversial problem of the chronology of Theophilus. The corrupt ἐπὶ τοῦ χρόνου τρίτου can hardly be anything but a mistaken attempt to complete an abbreviated court title, and the correction suggested to me by Prof. Ihor Ševčenko, ἐπὶ τοῦ χρ(υσο)τρι(κλίνου), carries immediate conviction. The πρωτοσπαθάριοι τοῦ χρυσοτρικλίνου (i. e. those who received their insignia in the Golden Hall) can be dated, on the ground of ample evidence, between the middle of the ninth century and the end of the eleventh[1]. In the present case, however, the *terminus ad quem* is the tenth century, the date of Paris Suppl. Gr. 446, which contains the De febrium differentia.

[1] I owe the following details to the kindness of N. Oikonomides: not yet in the Taktikon Uspenskij (middle of the ninth cent.); current in Philotheus, Cletorologion (A. D. 899), pp. 150,5–6; 176,26–27; 176,38–177,2 Bury (J. B. Bury, The Imperial Administrative System in the Ninth Century, London 1911) and in Constantine Porphyrogennetus, De cerimoniis, pp. 8;

The medical writer Theophilus[1] may consequently be the protospatharios to whom Photius wrote his Letters 123 and 192 (Laourdas-Westerink), but there is no evidence to decide this and it is not relevant to the present question. The physician Theophilus mentioned in Leo's Synopsis (p. 161 Ermerins) as a victim of asthma, is probably not a contemporary of Leo's, but the result of a confusion between the physician Theophilus whose curious delirium symptoms are described by Galen, De sympt. diff. 3 (VII, p. 60,11–61,9 K.), and another of Galen's colleagues, Antipater, mentioned De loc. aff. IV 11 (VIII, p. 293,8–296,6 K.) in the context of "asthma"; Leo refers to the second passage in the immediately preceding lines.

The procedure followed by the author of the scholia, whether Theophilus or an anonym, is clear: his compilation consists of excerpts, partly from Galen's commentary, partly from Stephanus, with some additions which may come from a third written source, or, more probably, from his own stock of medical knowledge. The most important point for the present purpose is that there is no perceptible difference in his handling of the "Stephanus" and the "Asclepius" versions.

B. The authorship

The only authority for the attribution to Stephanus of the commentary on sections I–III 25 is the Milan MS., but it is borne out by the redactor's own testimony (the iambic poem) and by a strong family resemblance with the two other commentaries by Stephanus, those on the Prognostic and on Galen's Ad Glauconem, so that there can be no reasonable doubt on this score.

As regards Meletius, who appears as the author in the Parisinus, I have considered the possibility that he might be the redactor of the abridged version, which would explain the title in P. However, as Prof. R. Renehan pointed out to me, Meletius seems to have risen to the status of a classic in medical literature, so that (at a very late time, it is true) some anonymous pieces were added to his literary property. The main difficulty is, of course, that the common hyparchetype of A and P can hardly have presented both titles jointly, so that, if the one in A is genuine, that in P, despite its authentic ring, must be either a wild conjecture

9; 20; 23; 30; 33; 123; 521; 546; 568; 570; 587; 692 (partly time of Leo VI, partly later). Outside these technical treatises, the first known occurrence is in Nicholas I, Letter 53,53–54, ed. R. J. H. Jenkins and L. G. Westerink, Washington 1973 (A. D. 921; here already the formula πρωτοσπαθάριος καὶ ἐπὶ τοῦ χρυσοτρικλίνου, which is strictly speaking incorrect). Last mention on record A. D. 1071 (Codice Diplomatico Barese IV, Le pergamene di S. Nicola di Bari, ed. F. Nitti di Vito, Bari 1900, p. 92). On the rank of protospatharios generally see R. Guilland, Recherches sur les institutions byzantines, II, Berlin – Amsterdam 1967, p. 99–131 (esp. p. 113; the name Theophilus pp. 101 and 103–104).

[1] There is no reason to assume more than one (see Speck, p. 76, n. 7); not only the commentary on the Aphorisms and the De hominis fabrica, but also the treatises De pulsibus and De excrementis (Laurentianus 74,31) and De urinis (Richard, p. 208) are formally attributed to the protospatharios. In Marc. App. Gr. V 12, fol. 118r (De pulsibus), he is called βα(σιλικὸς) πρωτοσπαθάριος καὶ ἀρχιατρός.

or a deliberate forgery, occasioned by the loss of the original title, presumably owing to a rubricator's carelessness.

The complete commentary on sections III and IV, because of the overlapping between versions (I) and (II), automatically also goes to Stephanus of Athens, who taught in the second half of the 6th century, or, at the very latest, in the seventh. It should be emphasized that this date is entirely independent of the question of his identity with Stephanus of Alexandria the philosopher, author of two commentaries on Aristotle (CAG XV, book III, and XVIII 3), as well as of an astronomical work. It rests firmly on Richard's argument that the "Olympiodorean" type of commentary, of which we have about a dozen examples datable to that period, cannot be shown by one single instance to have continued to exist after it.

The moot point of the relationship between the two namesakes[1] must remain in abeyance until the evidence of the minor works is completely available. The most important clue is still, for the moment, the story about Gesius (below, p. 256,3–8), to which attention was already drawn by Bussemaker[2]. Classroom anecdotes of this type for obvious reasons do not survive long outside their original context, and if Stephanus was among those who heard Gesius make this little joke at his own expense (about 530 or 540 at the latest), he cannot have been the philosopher who went to Constantinople under Heraclius. If, on the other hand, he knew it only indirectly through Asclepius, who may still have been teaching about 560/570, the possibility remains open. This brings us to the complicated problem of the "Asclepius" version of sections V and VI.

Asclepius' name occurs twice in the second part of the Escorial MS.: once at fol. 187^r in the sentence, ὁ μέντοι Ἀσκληπιὸς ὁ ὑπομνηματιστὴς τοῦ Ἱπποκράτους ἐκ τῶν Ἱπποκράτους τὰ Ἱπποκράτους ἐξηγούμενος τὴν δέουσαν αὐτῷ ἐξήγησιν ἐπεντέθεικεν (as opposed to Galen, who deleted the passage). This looks like a mere reference by the lecturer to his predecessor Asclepius. The situation is somewhat different at fol. 208^r, where the formula used is Ὁ δὲ Ἀσκληπιός, ⟨ὁ⟩ τοῦ παρόντος βιβλίου ἐξηγητής, and in a number of similar cases in which the same formula occurs without the proper name: foll. 156^v; 221^v; 263^r ὁ μέντοι ἐξηγητὴς τοῦ παρόντος βιβλίου, and fol. 245^v ὁ δὲ ἐξηγητὴς τοῦ βιβλίου (in all four cases, the "commentator's" interpretation is contrasted with Galen's). Though nothing prevents us from understanding these references in the same way as the first, they leave the alternative possibility that the "commentator" may be the lecturer himself; this is, without any doubt, the case in Stephanus, De interpretatione: CAG XVIII 3, p. 61,33 φησὶ δὲ τοῦ βιβλίου ὁ ἐξηγητής. Generally speaking, in the Alexandrian commentaries ὁ ἐξηγητής denotes either the commentator *par excellence* (in the commentaries on Aristotle, Alexander of Aphrodisias) or the lecturing teacher[3]. The plural, οἱ ἐξηγηταί, may designate the older commentators in general, but it may also serve as a kind of courtesy plural to

[1] Cf. Anonymous Prolegomena to Platonic Philosophy, ed. L. G. Westerink, Amsterdam 1962, p. XXV, n. 94; Speck, p. 65, n. 52.

[2] Traité d'Etienne, p. 421–422.

[3] Also in Olympiodorus, In meteora: CAG XII 2, pp. 51,27 and 53,13, in spite of Stüve's statement to the contrary (praef., p. IX).

refer to the lecturer himself (e. g. Olympiod., In Alcib.: p. 9,23 Westerink [Amsterdam 1956], referring back to p. 5,17sqq.).

In Stephanus, sections III–IV, we are faced with a very similar difficulty. There, too, the ἐξηγητὴς τοῦ παρόντος βιβλίου is opposed to Galen at fol. 34ᵛ; we have ὁ ἐξηγητής (against Galen) at fol. 22ʳ and οἱ ἐξηγηταί in the same sense at fol. 120ᵛ (probably also at fol. 88ᵛ). Dietz (II, p. X) is inclined to think that in all these cases Asclepius may be meant, and there is some support for this in the expression (fol. 69ᵛ) ὁ μέντοι νεώτερος ἐξηγητής, ὃν ἡμεῖς ἐξηγούμεθα (Asclepius as reported by Stephanus), though even this will admit of the explanation "the present lecturer (Stephanus), whose comments I am taking down", since the verb ἐξηγεῖσθαι is used at fol. 1ᵛ in the sense of reporting somebody's teaching. A few lines farther down the νεώτερος ἐξηγητής is referred to as αὐτὸς ὁ ἐξηγητής, so that it is advisable to assume that the same person (whether Stephanus or Asclepius) is intended throughout. The same ambiguity prevails in Stephanus' commentary on the Prognostic, where the νέος ἐξηγητής (CMG XI 1,2, pp. 126,1 and 256,32) may be either Asclepius (Dietz, II, p. X) or Stephanus.

Apart from the different formal characteristics already mentioned in the description of the two parts of the Escorial MS., the "Stephanus" and the "Asclepius" version are strikingly close in almost every other respect: the use made of Galen's commentary; references to Hippocrates and Galen and to courses past or prospective dealing with their writings; in the definition, classification and aetiology of diseases; in a great many typical phrases and turns of speech which occur over and over again in both. To be more specific: while in both versions much of the material ultimately derives from Galen's commentary, it is manifest that the lecturer usually did not bother to consult it directly: several statements allegedly taken from it are either not found in Galen at all, or in a different work; quite often, when the lecturer's "own" interpretation is contrasted with Galen's, both are actually taken from Galen. As regards references to earlier and forthcoming courses: Stephanus refers back to Εἰσαγωγαί (i.e. Galen, De sectis and Ad Glauconem), Φυσική (Galen, De temperamentis and De naturalibus facultatibus), Ἀνατομαί, and separately to Galen's Ars (probably included in the Εἰσαγωγαί); the "Asclepius" version to Εἰσαγωγαί, Φυσική, Ἀνατομή and separately to De sectis and Ad Glauconem. As future courses Stephanus mentions Περὶ αἰτίας (= De differentia morborum, De morborum causis, De symptomatum differentia, De causis symptomatum), De differentia febrium, De diebus decretoriis and Διαγνωστική (= De locis affectis), the "Asclepius" version only De crisibus[1]. Besides the overall correspondence in form and content, an even more significant point is that almost all the cross-references in the "Asclepius" version to subjects already discussed in sect. I–IV, are found back, often *verbatim*, in Stephanus.

The sole chronological indication in the "Asclepius" version, a remark on the Persians' concern for dynastic continuity (fol. 216ʳ), places it at least before the middle of the seventh century.

[1] Such references are to the course, not necessarily to the text discussed in it; see e.g. infra, p. 32,4–5.

A final relevant fact, already pointed out before, is that in the Theophilus scholia there is no perceptible difference between sections I–IV on the one hand and V–VI on the other; in both, we find that the Stephanus/Asclepius commentary, sometimes rendered freely, sometimes word for word, is the principal source besides Galen. Since the combination of the two as we have it in the Escorial MS. appears to be accidental, and since the Theophilus text does not depend directly on this MS., the only possibility (except for sheer coincidence) is that the author of the scholia used a continuous commentary which was not materially different from Escorial parts I + II.

Combining these data, we are left with two possible conclusions:

(1) The entire commentary as published here represents Stephanus' lectures on the Aphorisms. Owing to the loss of sect. I–II in the Escorial MS., we have this part only in the shortened version of AP; the rest, III–IV and V–VI, have survived in the form of the original lecture notes, but those notes were taken by two different *reportators* and very probably in different years. The second notetaker was less strict in using the Olympiodorean formulas than most of his contemporaries, or else his work was slightly revised and abridged at a later time. Stephanus repeatedly acknowledges his indebtedness to Asclepius, who is the ἐξηγητής in III–IV as well as in V–VI.

(2) Sections I–IV (in their complete form) were a classroom report of Stephanus' lectures, while V–VI are a similar report of Asclepius' lectures and should by rights be published under his name. In this case the ἐξηγητής is Stephanus in sect. III–IV and Asclepius in V–VI.

This Asclepius is mentioned by his namesake Asclepius of Tralles (CAG VI 2, p. 143,31–32) as ὁ τῆς ἰατρικῆς διδάσκαλος who with him attended Ammonius' course on the Metaphysics; however, the wording does not entirely preclude the interpretation that the two were identical. The editor of the commentary on the Metaphysics also edited Ammonius' course on Nicomachus[1]. Finally we have a rhetorician, Asclepius the "sophist", cited in the scholia on Demosthenes[2], who might qualify for identification with either one or both of the two, though this chance is extremely remote. If the commentary on V–VI is the work of Asclepius the pupil of Ammonius, neither the story about Gesius nor the pre-Olympiodorean form of the commentary would require further explanation. Olympiodorus must have been among the very latest of Ammonius' students.

The second assumption would imply that Stephanus was content to repeat Asclepius' lectures practically unchanged. Such a proceeding is so common among the Alexandrian professors of the sixth century that it may be said to have been the rule rather than the exception. Unfortunately, this very fact makes it next to impossible to decide questions of authorship on other than external evidence[3], which in this case is lacking. For the purpose of the present edition it makes little difference which of the two possibilities applies: the corpus as a whole forms so

[1] Ed. L. Tarán, Transactions of the American Philosophical Society 59,4, Philadelphia 1969.

[2] Demosthenes, ed. W. Dindorf, vol. VIII, Oxford 1851, pp. 141,10; 341,2; 392,8; 397,11.

[3] As a warning example: Olympiodorus has been credited, on the grounds of general resemblance and specific parallels, with the authorship of (1) a commentary on Porphyry, (2) one on the De interpretatione, (3) one on the Analytics, and (4) prolegomena to Plato.

obviously a unity that a joint publication (with an index covering both parts) may be considered justified.

C. The text of Hippocrates

As long as no accurate and detailed information on the text of the Aphorisms is available, it is difficult to determine the relationship between the Hippocrates text in Stephanus and the rest of the tradition. As usual, the matter is further complicated by discrepancies between (a) lemmata, (b) direct references to them in the same context, and (c) stray quotations elsewhere.

For the moment, on the ground of the data in Littré, Jones, and the principal Theophilus MSS., the following tentative conclusions can be formulated:

(1) The basic type of the Hippocrates text, as well as its variations, are of essentially the same kind throughout the entire commentary. This is borne out by some cross-references and especially by the readings in III 1–25, where the abridged and complete versions overlap.

(2) On the whole, the Hippocrates text of the commentary agrees with the branch of the tradition represented by C′ (Paris Suppl. Gr. 446) and Theophilus: cf. pp. 70,2; 80,14; 90,6–7; 134,14; 154,19; 156,6; 202,25; 220,1. 30; 230,14. Where the two separate, Stephanus sometimes joins C′ (pp. 76,22; 100,2; 210,28; 248,12), sometimes Theophilus (pp. 150,37; 164,19; 190,9; 234,24). It should be added that the correspondence is by no means complete and that the three Theophilus MSS. which I have consulted very frequently part company.

The resemblance is nevertheless close enough to suggest a personal link between Theophilus and C′, which happens to be also the oldest MS. containing a work of Theophilus (De febrium differentia), as well as the Synopsis of his (near) contemporary Leo.

Though obviously part of the variants in Stephanus and of the conflicting readings within the work itself are simply copyists' errors, I have deliberately abstained from interfering with the Hippocrates text, in order not to confuse the issue. A few insertions, immediately recognizable as such, are mainly intended to serve the reader's convenience.

Acknowledgments are due to the Netherlands Organization for the Advancement of Pure Research and to the Graduate School of the State University of New York at Buffalo, both of which provided funds for the purchase of microfilms and other photographical material, as well as to the American Philosophical Society, which enabled me to examine originals at Paris, San Lorenzo, Milan and Rome. My thanks go also to the Zentralinstitut für Alte Geschichte und Archäologie of the Akademie der Wissenschaften der DDR for the decision to include this edition in the series of the Corpus Medicorum Graecorum, and to Dr. sc. Jutta Kollesch and Dr. Diethard Nickel, who carefully revised the typescript, eliminating some serious errors and contributing many marked improvements.

A number of suggestions by J. M. Duffy, both for the text and the translation, have been gratefully adopted.

The translation of the lemmata owes much to W. H. S. Jones' Loeb edition (1953). If in spite of this it is not better than it is, this may be partly excused by the necessity of adapting it as far as possible to the various, often wayward, interpretations proposed in Stephanus' commentary.

Buffalo, December 1977 L. G. Westerink

ΣΧΟΛΙΑ ΣΥΝ ΘΕΩΙ
ΤΩΝ ΑΦΟΡΙΣΜΩΝ ΙΠΠΟΚΡΑΤΟΥΣ,
ΕΞΗΓΗΣΙΣ ΣΤΕΦΑΝΟΥ ΑΘΗΝΑΙΟΥ ΤΟΥ ΦΙΛΟΣΟΦΟΥ

A COMMENTARY WITH GOD'S HELP
ON THE APHORISMS OF HIPPOCRATES:
LECTURES BY STEPHANUS OF ATHENS THE PHILOSOPHER

CONSPECTVS SIGLORVM

A = Ambrosianus S 19 sup.; a. 1348
  A^2 = eiusdem codicis corrector
P = Parisinus Gr. 2222; s. XIV
  P^2 = eiusdem codicis corrector
Z = Vaticanus Gr. 279; s. XIV
  Z^2 = eiusdem codicis corrector

ω = consensus codicum APZ
α = consensus codicum AP

Hipp. = Hippocratis codices (sec. Littré et Jones)
  C′ = Parisinus Suppl. Gr. 446; s. X
  M = Marcianus Gr. 269; s. XI
  V = Vaticanus Gr. 276; s. XII

Theoph. = Theophili codices
  S = Parisinus Gr. 2228; s. XIV/XI
  U″ = Urbinas Gr. 64; s. X–XI
  V″ = Vaticanus Gr. 2254; s. X–XI

Dietz = F. R. Dietz, Scholia in Hippocratem et Galenum, Regimontii a. 1834, vol. II, p. 236–544

ΣΧΟΛΙΑ ΣΥΝ ΘΕΩΙ
ΤΩΝ ΑΦΟΡΙΣΜΩΝ ΙΠΠΟΚΡΑΤΟΥΣ,
ΕΞΗΓΗΣΙΣ ΣΤΕΦΑΝΟΥ ΑΘΗΝΑΙΟΥ ΤΟΥ ΦΙΛΟΣΟΦΟΥ

Σκοπός ἐστι τῷ συγγραφεῖ πάντα τὰ τῆς τέχνης ἡμῖν παρέχειν κεφάλαια καὶ φύσεως ἔργα. σκοπεῖ τοίνυν τὴν φύσιν, θεμέλιον ἔχουσαν τὰ στοιχεῖα, συναγομένην δὲ καὶ συνιζάνουσαν κράσεσι, μεριζομένην δὲ εἰς χυμούς, ἐλλαμπομένην δὲ δυνάμεσι, μόρια διαπλάττουσαν πρὸς τὴν τοῦ παντὸς σώματος ἐναρμόνιον σύνθεσιν διαφόρου χρείας τε καὶ ἐνεργείας ἕνεκεν. καὶ ταῦτα μὲν περὶ φύσεως πραγματεύεται. ἐπεὶ δὲ καὶ τῶν παρὰ φύσιν ἡ τριμερὴς κακία πέφυκεν ἐπηρεάζειν τοῖς σώμασιν ἡμῶν, νοσήματα, συμπτώματα, αἴτια, τοῖς μὲν νοσήμασιν ἀμετρίᾳ λυμαινομένοις τὰς ἐναντίας ἀντεισάγει ἀμετρίας, ὡς αὐτὸς προϊὼν λέγει· «τὰ ἐναντία τῶν ἐναντίων ἰάματα». ἐνίσταται δὲ καὶ πρὸς τὰ συμπτώματα παρηγορῶν τε καὶ καταπραΰνων τὸ θρασὺ τούτων καὶ ἀνήμερον ἢ καὶ ἰώμενος, ὥσπερ αὐτὸς προϊὼν λέγει· «νάρκη ὀλίγη ὀδύνης ληκτική». ἀλλὰ καὶ τῶν αἰτίων ἐκκόπτων τε καὶ ἀναστέλλων τὰς ἐπιδρομὰς πανταχόθεν ἀκηλίδωτον τὴν σωτηρίαν ἐργάζεται. λόγῳ τε ἅμα καὶ πείρᾳ χρώμενος

4–32,13] *cf.* Ammon. In isag.: CAG IV 3, p. 21,5–23,24 In categ.: CAG IV 4, p. 8,20–15,2 In interpret.: CAG IV 5, p. 1,12–8,23 In analyt. priora: CAG IV 6, p. 1,3–7,25 Simplic. In categ.: CAG VIII, p. 8,9–20,12 In physica: CAG IX, p. 1,3–6,3 Olympiod. In categ.: CAG XII 1, p. 12,18–14,11 In meteora: CAG XII 2, p. 1,18–6,18 Philop. In categ.: CAG XIII 1, p. 8, 23–13,32 In analyt. priora: CAG XIII 2, p. 1,5–6,18 Eliae In isag.: CAG XVIII 1, p. 35,1–39, 33 In categ.: ibid., p. 127,2–134,11 In analyt. priora: Mnemosyne, S. IV, 14, 1961, p. 138, 15–139,35 David. In isag.: CAG XVIII 2, p. 80,5–83,6 Proleg. Vossiana in Dionys. Thrac.: Grammatici Graeci I 3, ed. A. Hilgard, Lipsiae 1911 (Hildesheim 1965), p. 3,27–4,19 Proleg. Vaticana: ibid., pp. 123,25–124,12; 159,16–161,26 Proleg. in Aphthonium: Prolegomenon Sylloge, ed. H. Rabe, Lipsiae 1931, pp. 74,9–79,24; 127,22–141,7; 166,23–170,25 Proleg. in Hermog. De stat.: ibid., pp. 202,13–205,13; 244,9–254,19; 288,12–293,13; 302,5–303,26; 304, 4–317,11; 336,15–338,22 De invent.: ibid., p. 362,4–373,23 De ideis: ibid., pp. 384,7–388,14; 401,23–409,25; 420,7–426,26 Steph. In Progn. I prooem.: CMG XI 1,2, p. 26,6–34,11 Pallad. In Epid. VI: II 1,5–4,26 Dietz In fract.: p. 16,2–22,6 (= Steph. p. 17,3–23,7) Irmer Ioann. In nat. pueri: II 205,5–208,6 Dietz In Epid.: 120 a 3–b 38 Pritchet In sect.: 2 ra 52–2 rb 25 Pritchet Agnell. In sect.: p. 30,9–34,18 ed. Buffal. In artem: fol. 48^v–49^r In puls. ad tir.: fol. 92^r–93^r Anon. Lat. In Aphor.: fol. 121^v–122^v (Beccaria II, p. 39–41) 9sq.] *cf.* Gal. De sympt. diff. 1: VII 42,6–8 K. 11 τὰ – ἰάματα] Hipp. Flat. 1: CMG I 1, p. 92,8 *cf.* Aphor. II 22: IV 476,6–8 L. 13sq. νάρκη – ληκτική] Hipp. Aphor. V 25: IV 540,17 L. 15 λόγῳ – 30,2 λόγου] *cf.* Steph. In Progn. III 30: CMG XI 1,2, p. 290,23–28

1 ΣΧΟΛΙΑ – 3 ΦΙΛΟΣΟΦΟΥ] μελετίου ἰατροῦ καὶ φιλοσόφου ἐξήγησις εἰς τοὺς ἀφορισμούς P: τῶν ἀφορισμῶν ἱπποκράτους ἡ βίβλος Z Σχόλεα A 3 *post* ΦΙΛΟΣΟΦΟΥ *add.* καὶ θεοφίλ(ου) A^2 4 παρέχειν] παραδηλῶσαι Z 5 θεμέλιον] *spat. 12 litt. in* Z 6 κράσεσι] *spat. 10 litt. in* Z 7 μόρια] *spat. 12 litt. in* Z *ante* διαφόρου *add.* ἐκ A, *spat. 9 litt. praeb.* Z: *fort.* ἐκ⟨πονηθέντα⟩ *supplendum est* 8 πράγματ *(ambig.)* Z 9 τῶν παρὰ] τὴν A: διὰ τῶν παρὰ Z τριημερὴς Z 10 μὲν *om.* Z 11 ὡς αὐτὸς] ὥσπερ Z 13 ὀδύνης] *spat. 8 litt. in* Z 15 χρώμενος *om.* Z

A COMMENTARY WITH GOD'S HELP ON THE APHORISMS OF HIPPOCRATES: LECTURES BY STEPHANUS OF ATHENS THE PHILOSOPHER

The author's intention is to instruct us in all the essentials of the art and in the works of Nature. To this end he studies Nature, with the elements as its basic material, the temperaments as its uniting and stabilizing forces, the humors as its parts, the faculties as the light that permeates it, and the parts of the body as shaped by it for the harmonious construction of the whole in view of various needs and functions. These are the subjects he discusses with reference to Nature. On the other hand, there is also the abnormal, which afflicts our bodies with the threefold evil of diseases, symptoms and causes; as for diseases, since the harm they cause is due to disproportion, he fights them by the contrary kind of disproportion, as he himself puts it farther down: "opposites cure opposites". But he also treats the symptoms, soothing and assuaging their harsh, painful effects, and sometimes even curing them, as he says later on: "a light numbness suppresses pain". Finally, by eliminating the causes and preventing their onslaught he protects our health from harm on every side. The weapons he uses in fighting the

καθάπερ τισὶν ὅπλοις κατὰ τῶν παρὰ φύσιν ὁπλίζεται, τῷ μὲν λόγῳ τὴν μέθοδον ἐξευρίσκων, τῇ δὲ πείρᾳ ταύτην ἐκκαλούμενος, ᾗ καὶ τὸ βέβαιον παρεγγυᾷ τοῦ λόγου. ἐπάνεισι δ' οὖν καὶ ἐπὶ μετέωρα καὶ μείζονα· σκοπεῖ[ν] γὰρ ἀέρων ἀλλαγάς, ἀνέμων ἐμπνεύσεις, ὑδάτων διαφοράς, ταῖς τῶν ἄστρων ἐπιτολαῖς τε καὶ κρύψεσι ποικιλλόμενος. ταῦτα πάντα ὁ σκοπὸς τοῦ παρόντος ἐπαγγέλλεται συγγράμματος.

Χρησιμεύει δὲ καὶ τελείοις καὶ ἀτελέσιν, ὀψιμαθέσι καὶ ἐκ νηπίας ἡλικίας φοιτῶσιν, ὁδοιποροῦσι καὶ ἐν πόλεσι διατρίβουσιν, εὐφυέσι καὶ ἀφυέσι, προθύμοις τε καὶ ῥαθύμοις· τελείοις μὲν καὶ εὐφυέσι τῶν προεγνωσμένων ἑαυτοὺς ἐν κεφαλαίῳ ἀναμιμνῄσκειν, ἀτελέσι δὲ καὶ ὁδοιποροῦσιν, ὅτι τὰ ἐν πολλοῖς κατ' ἀποτάδην εἰρημένα, ταῦτα ἐν ὀλίγοις περικλείεται.

Ὅτι δὲ γνήσιον Ἱπποκράτους τὸ σύγγραμμα, ἐμαρτύρησαν Ῥοῦφός τε καὶ Σαβῖνος καὶ Σωρανὸς καὶ Πέλοψ καὶ Γαληνός· καὶ τοσοῦτόν ἐστι γνήσιον, ὥστε γνώμονι τούτῳ κεχρημένοι οἱ ἐξηγηταὶ ⟨ἐκ⟩ τούτου τῶν ἄλλων συγγραμμάτων, εἴτε γνήσια εἶεν εἴτε νόθα, ἐποιήσαντο τὴν κρίσιν. οὐ μὴν ἀλλὰ καὶ τὸ εἶδος τῆς ἀπαγγελίας καὶ ἡ ἀγχίνοια τῶν λεγομένων καὶ τὸ ἡδὺ τῆς φράσεως τῆς Ἱπποκράτου⟨ς⟩ μεγαλονοίας ἀποδεικνύει τὸ σύγγραμμα.

Ζητείσθω δὲ καὶ ἡ αἰτία τῆς ἐπιγραφῆς. ἰστέον οὖν, ὅτι ἐκ τοῦ τρόπου τῆς διδασκαλίας τὴν ἐπιγραφὴν ἐποιήσατο Ἀφορισμοὺς τὸ βιβλίον ἐπιγράψας.

Ἡ δὲ τάξις διττή ἐστιν, ἡ μὲν πρὸς τὴν φύσιν, ἡ δὲ πρὸς τὸν λόγον ἀποβλέπουσα. καὶ τῇ πρὸς τὴν φύσιν ἐξακολουθοῦντες τάξει τὸ Περὶ ἀνθρώπου φύσεως ⟨πρῶτον⟩ ἀναλεγόμεθα ἐν τοῖς Ἱπποκρατείοις· ⟨. . .⟩ ἐκεῖσε γὰρ μανθάνομεν τὴν προσεχῆ ὕλην τῆς γενέσεως καὶ τὴν σύμπηξιν τοῦ ἡμετέρου σώματος· καὶ ἐνταῦθα ἐν τρίτῃ τάξει ἀναγνωσθέντος τοῦ παρόντος βιβλίου. ἡ δὲ τοῦ λόγου τάξις πρότερον τοὺς Ἀφορισμοὺς παρακελεύεται ἀναλέγεσθαι διὰ τὸ καθολικὸν καὶ κεφαλαιῶδες καὶ σύντομον τῶν ἐνταῦθα παραδιδομένων. καλὸν δὲ τοῖς εἰσαγομένοις εἰς τὴν Ἱπποκράτους ἰατρικὴν πρὸ παντὸς τὸν Ὅρκον καὶ τὸν Νόμον ἐκμανθάνειν.

Ἕκτον ἐστὶ κεφάλαιον ἡ εἰς τὰ μόρια διαίρεσις. καὶ ἰστέον, ὅτι ὁ μὲν Σωρανὸς εἰς τρία τμήματα διεῖλε τοῦτο τὸ βιβλίον, ὁ δὲ Ῥοῦφος εἰς τέσσαρα, ὁ δὲ Γαληνὸς εἰς ἑπτά, ᾧπερ καὶ πειθόμεθα.

11–12 Γαληνός] *cf.* Anon. Lat. In Aphor.: fol. 122r (Beccaria II, p. 40,17–20) Gal. De ord. libr. suor. 3: Scr. min. II 86,23–87,2 Müller = XIX 57,7–10 K. 19–26] *cf.* Steph. In Progn. I prooem.: CMG XI 1,2, p. 30,31–32,27 Pallad. In Epid. VI: II 4,1–11 Dietz Ioann. In nat. pueri: II 207,6–15 Dietz Anon. Lat. In Aphor.: fol. 122r (Beccaria II, p. 40,29–35) 27–29] *cf.* Anon. Lat. In Aphor.: fol. 122v (Beccaria II, p. 41,42–44) Gal. De libr. propr. 6: Scr. min. II 112,27–113,1 Müller = XIX 35,16–17 K.

2 ᾗ] ἢ A: ᾗ *ex* ἢ *corr.* Z βέβαιον] *spat. 13 litt. in* Z 3 μείζων Z σκοπεῖν α: *om.* Z: *corr. Dietz, II, p. 238,23* γὰρ ἀέρων] ὡρῶν γὰρ Z 4 ἀστέρων A 6 ἀτεχνέσιν Z *post* καὶ[III] *add.* τοῖς Z 7 ἐν πόλεσι διατρίβουσιν] ἐν πόλεσι τρίβουσιν P: ἐμπορεύουσιν Z *ante* καὶ[II] *add.* τε Z 8 ἀφυέσι P ἀναμιμνήσκοντες Z 9 ἀτελέσι] ἐμπορεύουσι Z κατ' ἀποτάδην *scripsi*: καταλογάδην ω 11 Ὅτι] ἔτι Z δὲ *om.* A ἱπποκράτου A ἐμαρτύρησε Z 12 Σαβῖνος] ῥουφῖνος A πέλωψ α καὶ Γαληνός *om.* Z καὶ τοσοῦτόν *scripsi*: καθὼ τὸν A: *spat. 7 litt. et* σόν P: *spat. 18 litt. in* Z 13 ἐκ *addidi* τούτου – 14 κρίσιν] *spat. 8 litt. in* Z τούτων A 15 ἐπαγγελίας ω: *correxi* ἱπποκράτου AZ: *corr.* P 16 ἀποδείκνυσι Z 21 πρῶτον *addidi* *lac. indicavi, supple fere* ἔπειτα τὸ Περὶ παιδίου φύσεως,; *cf. Ioann.* 23 ἀναγνωσθέντες Z 25 δὲ *om.* A ἱπποκράτου Z 26 Ὅρκον *scripsi*: ὅρον ω 27 μόρια] μέρ(η) Z καὶ *om.* A 28 *ante* τρία *add.* τὰ Z 29 ὅπερ Z

abnormal are both reason and trial: by reason he discovers the method, by trial he brings it out into the open, at the same time confirming the soundness of his reasoning. Meanwhile he also relates this to greater, cosmic influences: he considers changes of air, directions of winds, various properties of waters, taking into account also the manifold changes brought about by the heliacal rising and the occultation of constellations. All this is included in the program of the present work.

Its usefulness extends to the accomplished as well as to the imperfect, to late learners as well as to those whose training has begun in childhood, to traveling physicians and to those practicing in cities, to the talented and the untalented, the eager and the indolent; to the accomplished and talented it is helpful as a concise reminder of material already mastered; for the imperfect and those on the road it has the advantage of reducing to a few words what would need a long exposition if stated in full.

That it is a genuine work of Hippocrates is affirmed by Rufus, Sabinus, Soranus, Pelops and Galen; it is so evidently genuine that the commentators have used it as a standard to decide the genuineness or spuriousness of the other writings. Besides, the form of the presentation, the acuteness of the contents and the attractive style prove that it is a work of the master mind of Hippocrates.

Let us also explain the title. (Hippocrates) derives it from the form of presentation, calling the book Aphorisms.

Its place (in the curriculum) can be determined in two ways, either from the natural or from the logical point of view. Following the natural arrangement we read On the Nature of Man first of the Hippocratic writings; +next comes On the Nature of the Child,+[1] because in it we learn about the immediate material of our formation and about the shaping of our own bodies; then, in the third place, the present book is read. The logical order prescribes that we read the Aphorisms first because of the universal, summary and concise character of its content. It is good, though, for those who are introduced to Hippocratic medicine, to memorize the Oath and the Law first of all.

The sixth point is the division into parts. Soranus divided the book into three sections, Rufus into four, Galen into seven; we follow the last.

[1] +next – Child+: see the app. crit.

ʼΑνάγεται δὲ τὸ παρὸν σύγγραμμα οὐχ ὑπὸ ἓν μέρος τῆς Ἱπποκρατικῆς, ἀλλʼ ὑπὸ πάντα τὰ μέρη ὥσπερ καὶ ἡ Τέχνη Γαληνοῦ. ἐπειδὴ γὰρ περὶ πάντων τῶν μερῶν τῆς ἰατρικῆς ἐνταῦθα διαλέγεται κεφαλαιώδη καὶ σύντομον διδασκαλίαν ποιούμενος, εἰκότως καὶ ὑπὸ τὸ θεωρητικὸν καὶ ὑπὸ τὸ πρακτικὸν καὶ τὰ καθʼ ἕκαστον πάντα [τὰ] μόρια τῆς διαιρέσεως, ἅτινα ἐν Εἰσαγωγαῖς μεμαθήκαμεν, τὸ παρὸν ἀναχθήσεται σύγγραμμα.

Τρόπῳ δὲ διδασκαλικῷ χρῆται ἀφοριστικῷ, ὅπερ δῆλον γέγονε τὴν αἰτίαν τῆς ἐπιγραφῆς ζητούντων ἡμῶν. ἕτεροι γὰρ παρὰ τοὺς Γαληνείους διδασκαλικοὶ τρόποι παρʼ αὐτῷ τρεῖς, ἀφοριστικός, ὑφηγηματικός, καὶ μικτός. καὶ ἀφοριστικὸς μέν ἐστιν ὁ ἐν ὀλίγαις λέξεσι πολλὰ περικλείων νοήματα· ὑφηγηματικὸς δέ ἐστιν ὁ κατὰ διέξοδον πλατικῶς τῶν νοουμένων τὴν διδασκαλίαν ποιούμενος· μικτὸς δὲ ὁ ἐξ ἀμφοῖν συγκείμενος καὶ μήτε ἄγαν ἐσταλμένος ὡς ὁ ἀφοριστικὸς μήτε ἐν πλάτει διεξερχόμενος τὴν ἔννοιαν καθάπερ ὁ ὑφηγηματικός.

ʼΑφορισμὸς δέ ἐστι λόγος σύντομος αὐτοτελῆ διάνοιαν ἀπαρτίζων. ἢ καὶ οὕτως· λόγος πενόμενος μὲν κατὰ τὴν λέξιν, πλουτῶν δὲ τοῖς ἐνθυμήμασιν. εἴρηται δὲ ἀφορισμὸς διὰ τὸ καθʼ ἕκαστα περιορίζεσθαι μὲν τὰ νοούμενα, ἀφορίζεσθαι δὲ καὶ ἀποδιίστασθαι ἀπὸ τῶν πρὸ αὐτῶν καὶ ἀπὸ τῶν μετʼ αὐτά.

I 1 [I 1: IV 458,1–2 L.] Ὁ βίος βραχύς, ἡ δὲ τέχνη μακρή, ὁ δὲ καιρὸς ὀξύς, ἡ δὲ πεῖρα σφαλερή, ἡ δὲ κρίσις χαλεπή.

Νῦν ἐπὶ τὴν ἐξέτασιν ἥκομεν τοῦ κειμένου, συνθήκαις τισὶ πρότερον ἑαυτοὺς κατασφαλιζόμενοι ὥστε ἐπὶ ἑκάστου τῶν ἀφορισμῶν, ἢ καὶ ἐπὶ τῶν πλείστων, τέσσαρά τινα ζητεῖσθαι κεφάλαια· πρῶτον τὴν σαφήνειαν τῆς λέξεως, εἴπερ ταύτης ἐστὶ δεόμενος, δεύτερον τὴν διάνοιαν τοῦ ἀρχαίου, τρίτον τὸ χρήσιμον τῆς ἐννοίας, καὶ τέταρτον τὴν διάκρισιν τῶν ἀληθῶν καὶ ψευδῶν ἐξηγήσεων. ἐπὶ τούτοις συμφωνηθεῖσιν ἀρξώμεθα τῆς λέξεως.

ʼΙστέον οὖν, ὅτι προοιμίῳ κεκόσμηται ὁ λόγος καὶ ἑνὶ καὶ δυσί· καὶ τὸ μὲν πρῶτον προοίμιον ἀποφαντικὸν εἶναι δοκεῖ, τὸ δὲ δεύτερον συμβουλευτικόν. ἔχει δὲ ἑκάτερον οὕτως· τὸ μὲν πρῶτον ὁ βίος βραχύς, ἡ δὲ τέχνη μακρή, ὁ δὲ καιρὸς ὀξὺς καὶ τὰ ἑξῆς· τοῦτο ἀποφαντικόν· τὸ δὲ δεύτερον ἔχει οὕτως· [I 1: IV 458,2–3 L.]

1–6] *cf.* Anon. Lat. In Aphor.: fol. 122r (Beccaria II, p. 40,23–27) 3–6] *i. e. Steph. in prolegomenis ad* Gal. De sect. *librum (ut apud* Pallad., In sect.: 75,15–77,22 Baffioni *et* Ioann., In sect.: 1 vb 13–59 Pritchet*)* 7–13] *cf.* Steph. In Progn. I prooem.: CMG XI 1,2, p. 32,33–34,6 Pallad. In Epid. VI: II 4,19–26 Dietz Ioann. In nat. pueri: II 207,33–208,6 Dietz Anon. Lat. In Aphor.: fol. 22r–v (Beccaria II, p. 41,36–42) 8sq. ἕτεροι – μικτός] *v.* Gal. Ars med. prooem.: I 305,2–6 K. 14–17] *v.* Theoph. In Aphor.: II 245,30–246,1 Dietz 14–15 ἐνθυμήμασιν] *v.* [Gal.] Def. med. 5: XIX 349,14–17 K. ʼΑφορισμὸς – ἀπαρτίζων] *cf.* Anon. Lat. In Aphor.: fol. 122v (Beccaria II, p. 41,45–46) 26–34,2 συμβουλευτικόν] *cf.* Gal. In Aphor. I 1: XVII B 347,9–14 K.

1 *post* Ἱπποκρατικῆς *add.* διδασκαλίας P 3 κεφάλαιον δὴ A *ante* διδασκαλίαν *add.* τὴν Z 5 τὰ *delevi* ἅτινα] *spat. 6 litt. in* Z 6 ἀναθήσεται A 7 κέχρηται Z γέγονε] γέγονεν εἶναι Z 9 ἀφηγηματικὸς P 10 δʼ^{I} *om.* α παρακλείων Z νοήματα *scripsi*: ῥήματα ω ἀφηγηματικὸς P ἐστιν^{II} *om.* Z 11 τὴν *scripsi*: καὶ α: *om.* Z 12 ἐστενωμένος Z 13 ἀφηγηματικὸς P 14 σύντομος *om.* α, *inser.* A^{2} 15 τὴν λέξιν] τὴν τέχνην A: τὰς συλλαβὰς Z πλουτῶν δὲ] πλοῦτον δὲ παρέχων Z 16 καθʼ ἕκαστα] καθάπερ Z 19 σφαλερὰ A 20 ἑαυτῷ Z 23 ἐστὶ δεόμενος *scripsi*: *spat. 4 litt. et* τί δεόμενος α: δεόμενος εἴ Z 24 τούτοις *scripsi*: δὲ τοῖς α: τούτοις τοῖς Z 25 ἀρξόμεθα A 28 μακρὰ Z 29 οὕτως ἔχει Z

As regards the division of Hippocratic medicine under which this work falls, it does not belong to one specific part, but rather to all, as also does Galen's Art. He deals here with all the parts of medicine in a summary and concise form; therefore obviously this book will be found to belong both to the theoretical and to the practical branch (of medicine) and to each of their several subdivisions, which we have learned in the Introduction.

The form of presentation is aphoristic, as we have seen when explaining the title. (Hippocrates) has three forms of presentation different from Galen's: the aphoristic, the expository and the mixed form. The aphoristic form comprises in few words a wealth of ideas; the expository form presents the ideas discursively and diffusely; the mixed form, which is composed of both, neither has the excessive compactness of the aphoristic style nor does it develop the thought as diffusely as the expository style does.

An aphorism is a concise statement containing a complete thought. Or otherwise: a statement sparing of words, but rich in ideas. It is called aphorism ("a demarcation") because each thought is self-contained, and is demarcated and separated from the preceding and the following ones.

I 1. Life is short, the art is long, the moment is swift, trial is risky, judgment is difficult.

We are now coming to the study of the text; but before we do so, we will commit ourselves to consider for each aphorism — or, at least, for most — the following four points: first, the clarification of the wording, if needed; secondly, the ancient author's meaning; thirdly, the usefulness of the idea; fourthly, the decision between true and false interpretations. Having agreed upon this, let us begin to study the text.

The work, instead of one, has two prefaces, the first of which presents itself as a statement, the second as advice. The two run as follows: the first, Life is short, the art is long, the moment is swift, etc.; this is a statement; the

δεῖ δὲ οὐ μόνον ἑαυτὸν παρέχειν τὰ δέοντα ποιέοντα καὶ τὰ ἑξῆς· τοῦτο δὲ συμβουλευτικόν. ἀλλ' εἰ δοκεῖ, ταῖς ὑποσχεθείσαις συνθήκαις ἀκολουθοῦντες ἐπὶ τὴν σαφήνειαν πρῶτον τραπῶμεν τῶν λέξεων· καὶ ἀρκτέον ἀπὸ τοῦ πρώτου.

Ἰστέον τοιγαροῦν, ὅτι τὸ τοῦ βίου ὄνομα πολλὰ σημαίνει. λέγεται γὰρ βίος ὁ τόπος, ἐν ᾧ τις διατρίβει· οὕτω γὰρ Σωκράτην μὲν Ἀκαδημαϊκὸν βίον μετιέναι φαμέν, Πλάτωνα δὲ Στωϊκόν· ἀλλὰ καὶ ἀμφίβια ζῷα κατὰ τοῦτο τὸ σημαινόμενον λέγομεν. λέγεται βίος καὶ τὸ ἐπιτήδευμα, ὅ τις μετέρχεται· οὕτω γοῦν φαμεν τόνδε μὲν τὸν ἄνθρωπον ἰατρικὸν βίον μετιέναι, τόνδε δὲ γραμματικόν. λέγεται βίος καὶ ἡ ἐνθένδε τῆς ψυχῆς μετανάστευσις· οὕτω γὰρ τὸ ἀποβιῶναί φαμεν καὶ τῷ τέλει τοῦ βίου χρήσασθαι. λέγεται βίος καὶ τὸ εἶδος τῆς ζωῆς· καθ' ὃ λέγομεν τόνδε σεμνὸν καὶ κόσμιον βίον ἑλέσθαι ἢ φιλόσοφον ἢ σώφρονα. λέγεται βίος καὶ ὁ χρόνος τῆς ζωῆς· καθ' ὅ φαμεν τῶν ζῴων τὰ μὲν μακρόβια, τὰ δὲ ὀλιγόβια. λέγεται βίος καὶ ὁ χρόνος τῆς ζωῆς ἑκάστου, ἀλλ' οὐ πᾶς, ἀλλ' ἐκεῖνος, ἐν ᾧ ἐπιτηδείως πρὸς μάθησιν διακείμεθα. τοσαυταχῶς οὖν τοῦ βίου λεγομένου ἢ κατὰ τοῦ τελευταίου σημαινομένου ἢ κατὰ τοῦ προτελευταίου ἐστὶν ὁ λόγος τῷ Ἱπποκράτει. βραχὺ δὲ εἶπε δηλονότι τὸ ὀλίγον.

Ἡ δὲ τέχνη μακρή. ὅτι δὲ μακρά ἐστιν ἡ τέχνη καὶ σχεδὸν ἄπειρος, τριχῶς ἔστι παραστῆσαι· ἐκ τῆς διαιρέσεως, ἐκ τῆς δοκιμασίας καὶ χρήσεως, καὶ ἐκ τῆς τελειώσεως. καὶ ἔξεστιν ἀναμνῆσαι τῆς διαιρέσεως. διαιρεῖται γοῦν ἡ ἰατρικὴ εἰς θεωρητικὸν καὶ πρακτικόν· τὸ δὲ θεωρητικὸν εἰς φυσιολογικόν, ⟨αἰτιολογικὸν⟩ καὶ σημειωτικόν· τὸ φυσιολογικὸν εἰς στοιχεῖα, κράσεις, χυμούς, μόρια, δυνάμεις καὶ ἐνεργείας, καὶ ἐφ' ἑκάστου τούτων ζητοῦμεν ποσόν, ποιὸν καὶ ὀνόματα. ἐπὶ μὲν στοιχείων ποσόν, ὅτι τέσσαρα· ἀλλὰ καὶ ποιόν, ὅτι τὸ μὲν θερμόν, τὸ δὲ ξηρόν, τὸ δὲ ψυχρόν, τὸ δὲ ὑγρόν· ἀλλὰ καὶ ὀνόματα, λέγεται γὰρ τὸ μὲν θερμὸν πῦρ, τὸ δὲ ψυχρὸν ὕδωρ, τὸ δὲ ξηρὸν γῆ, τὸ δὲ ὑγρὸν ἀήρ. ἀλλὰ καὶ τῶν κράσεων τὸ ποσόν, ὅτι ἐννέα· καὶ τὸ ποιόν, ὅτι τέσσαρες ἁπλαῖ καὶ τέσσαρες σύνθετοι καὶ μία τις ἐξ ἰσομοιρίας κεκραμένη, ἥτις καὶ εὔκρατος ὠνόμασται. ὁμοίως καὶ περὶ τῶν χυμῶν τὸ ποσόν, ὅτι τέσσαρες· τὸ ποιόν, ὅτι ὁ μὲν θερμὸς καὶ ξηρός, ὁ δὲ θερμὸς καὶ ὑγρός, ὁ δὲ ψυχρὸς καὶ ὑγρός, ὁ δὲ ψυχρὸς καὶ ξηρός· τὰ δὲ ὀνόματα, ὅτι ὁ μὲν καλεῖται χολή,

4–16] *v.* Theoph. In Aphor.: II 246,11–23 Dietz 19 διαιρεῖται – 38,13 μυῶν] *cf.* Pallad. In sect.: 75,15–76,24 Baffioni Ioann. In sect.: 1 vb 13–59 Pritchet Agnell. In sect.: p. 24,4–30,8 ed. Buffal. Epit. anon. Vindob. med. Gr. 35, fol. 329^{r} (Temkin, Studies, p. 412) Epit. arab. Mus. Brit. Addit. 23407, fol. 2^{v} (ibid., p. 412–413) διαιρεῖται – 21 ἐνεργείας] *v.* Theoph. In Aphor.: II 246,25–30 Dietz 21 τὸ – ἐνεργείας] *cf.* Steph. Ad Glauc.: I 241,11–12 Dietz 23sq. ὅτι^{I} – ὑγρόν] *cf.* Steph. Ad Glauc.: I 241,14–15 Dietz 25 ἀλλὰ – 27 ὠνόμασται] *cf.* Gal. De temp. I 8: p. 31,27–32,4 Helmr. = I 559,2–9 K. Steph. Ad Glauc.: I 241,16–17 Dietz 27 ὁμοίως – 36,1 φλέγμα] *cf.* [Gal.] Def. med. 65: XIX 363,14–364,3 K. Steph. Ad Glauc.: I 241,17–19 Dietz

2 ἀκολουθεῖν Z 4 πολλὰ σημαίνει] πολυσήμαντον Z 8 τόνδε^{II}] τὸν Z 9 ἐνθάδε P μετανάστασις A^{2}Z τῷ] τὸ Z 10 ἐχρήσατο Z τῆς ζωῆς εἶδος Z 11 βίον ἑλέσθαι] ἐξελέξατο βίον Z 11sq. τῆς ζωῆς χρόνος Z 12 καθ' ὅ] καὶ Z 13 ὁ – ἑκάστου] ὁ *et spat. 8 litt.* A: ὁο *et spat. 6 litt.* P 14 διακείμεθα] ἔρχεταί τις. λέγεται βίος καὶ ἡ τῶν τεσσάρων ὡρῶν συλλογή Z 15 προτελευταίου] πρὸ τοῦ τελευταίου P βραχὺς Z 16 τὸ ὀλίγον] διὰ τὸ ὀλίγον τῆς ἀνθρώπου ζωῆς Z 17 ὅτι] Ετι A: ἐπεὶ Z μακρά] μακρή α τρία Z 18 τῆς διαιρέσεως] ταύτης κεφάλαια Z ἐκ^{II}] ἔκ τε Z καὶ^{I}] ἐκ τῆς Z 19 ἀναμνῆσαι *coni. Dietz, II, p. 249, n. 2*: ἀνακινῆσαι Z: ἀνα *et spat. 7 vel 5 litt.* AP εἰς] εἴς τε τὸ Z 20 *post* καὶ^{I} *add.* τὸ Z δὲ *om.* Z αἰτιολογικὸν *add. Duffy (cf. infra, p. 36,25–28)* 22 ἀφ' Z 24sq. τὸ^{III} – γῆ] τὸ δὲ ξηρόν, γῆ· τὸ δὲ ψυχρόν, ὕδωρ Z 29 ὑγρός] ξηρὸς Z ξηρός] ὑγρὸς Z

second, (The physician) must not only be prepared to do his own duty, etc.; this is advice. If you agree, we will adhere to the commitment we made, and begin with the clarification of the wording, taking the first preface first.

The word life, then, has a variety of meanings. "Life" can be the place where one stays; thus we say that Socrates spends his life in the Academy, Plato in the Stoa; in this sense we also speak of "amphibious" animals (i. e. "living a double life"). "Life" is also a person's occupation; thus we say that this man makes a living as a doctor, that one as a schoolmaster. Then the word "life" is used with reference to the departure of the soul; e.g., in the phrases "departing this life" and "ending one's life". "Life" is further used for conduct, as we say that a person leads a decent and respectable life, or a philosopher's life, or a life of abstention. "Life" also denotes the duration of life; in this sense we describe some animals as long-lived, others as short-lived. Instead of the entire lifetime of the individual, "life" may also mean that part of it during which we are capable of learning. Of all these different meanings of "life", Hippocrates refers either to the last or to the last but one. By short he means, of course, little.

The art is long. There are three ways to show that the art (of medicine) is long and indeed almost infinite: from the number of branches into which it is divided, from the time needed to test and practice it, from the time needed to become perfect. Let us recapitulate the division. Medicine is divided into a theoretical and a practical part; the theoretical part into physiology, aetiology, and semiology; physiology into elements, temperaments, humors, parts, faculties and functions, and with regard to each of these we raise the questions of number, quality, and names. In the case of the elements, their number is four; qualities are hot, dry, cold, moist; the names are: fire for the hot, water for the cold, earth for the dry, air for the moist. As for the temperaments, their number is nine; from the point of view of quality, four are simple, four are composite, and one is a mixture of equal parts, which is accordingly called well-tempered. Similarly as regards humors: their number is four; their qualities, hot and dry, hot and moist, cold and moist, cold and dry; as for the names, one is called bile, one blood, one

ὁ δὲ αἷμα, ὁ δὲ μέλας, ὁ δὲ φλέγμα. καὶ οὗτοι μὲν οἱ στοιχειώδεις· πολλοὶ δὲ καὶ ἕτεροί εἰσιν ἐν ἡμῖν χυμοὶ παρὰ τούτους, χολὴ ἡ λεκιθώδης καὶ ἰσατώδης καὶ ἰώδης καὶ ἡ ὠχρά· ὥσπερ οὖν καὶ τοῦ φλέγματος διαφοραὶ τρεῖς, τὸ μὲν γάρ ἐστι γλυκύ, τὸ δὲ ἁλυκόν, τὸ δὲ ἄποιον· ὁμοίως τριττός τίς ἐστι καὶ ὁ μελαγχολικὸς χυμός, ὁ ἐξ ὑπεροπτήσεως τῆς ξανθῆς χολῆς γινόμενος, ὅντινα καὶ ἀσφαλτώδη ὀνομάζουσι διὰ τὸ στίλβειν ἀσφάλτου δίκην, καὶ ὁ κατὰ ἀπόσβεσιν καὶ ὁ ἐκ τοῦ ἀπογεωθέντος φλέγματος γινόμενος. ὡσαύτως καὶ περὶ τῶν μορίων τὸ ποσὸν διάφορον ὂν κατὰ ἀριθμὸν καὶ αἱ Ἀνατομικαὶ παραδιδόασιν ἐγχειρήσεις· τὰ μὲν γὰρ εἰρήκαμεν ὁμοιομερῆ εἶναι, τὰ δὲ ὀργανικά, καὶ τῶν ὁμοιομερῶν τὰ μὲν ἁπλᾶ, ὥσπερ νεῦρον καὶ ὀστοῦν καὶ χόνδρος καὶ σύνδεσμος καὶ ὑμὴν καὶ σάρξ, τὰ δὲ σύνθετα, ὥσπερ φλέβες καὶ ἀρτηρίαι καὶ μύες· τῶν δὲ ὀργανικῶν ὀνόματα γαστὴρ καὶ ἧπαρ καὶ ἐγκέφαλος καὶ πνεύμων καὶ καρδία καὶ νεφροὶ καὶ κύστις καὶ ὄρχεις καὶ τὰ τοιαῦτα. καὶ τὸ π⟨οιὸν τῶν⟩ μορίων, ὅτι τὰ μέν εἰσιν ἀρχαί, τὰ δὲ ἄρχεται, τὰ δὲ συμφύτους ἔχει τὰς δυνάμεις, τὰ δὲ ἐπικτήτους, τὰ δὲ συμφύτους ἅμα καὶ ἐπικτήτους, τὰ δὲ ἐνεργά, τὰ δὲ χρειώδη. ὅσον δὲ περὶ τὴν τούτων θεωρίαν τὸ περισπούδαστον, αἱ Ἀνατομικαὶ ἡμᾶς ἐκδιδάσκουσι βίβλοι. εἴρηται δὲ τὸ ποσὸν τῶν δυνάμεων, ὅτι τρεῖς αὗται, ψυχικαί, ζωτικαί, φυσικαί. καὶ τῶν μὲν ψυχικῶν εἰσι φαντασία λογισμὸς μνήμη νοῦς διάνοια δόξα αἵ τε κατὰ μέρος αἰσθήσεις καὶ αἱ κατὰ προαίρεσιν κινήσεις, αἱ ζωτικαὶ δὲ εἰς ἀναπνευστικὴν καὶ σφυγμικήν, αἱ φυσικαὶ δὲ εἰς γεννητικήν, αὐξητικὴν καὶ θρεπτικήν, καὶ αἱ τούτων ὑπηρέτιδες, ἑλκτική, καθεκτική, ἀλλοιωτικὴ καὶ ἀποκριτική. ὁμοίως καὶ περὶ τῶν ἐνεργειῶν, ὅτι κατά τινα παραγωγὴν παρονομάζεται, οἷον φανταστικὴ μὲν ἡ δύναμις, φαντασία δὲ ἡ ἐνέργεια, λογιστικὴ μὲν ἡ δύναμις, λογισμὸς δὲ ἡ ἐνέργεια, καὶ μνημονευτικὴ μὲν ἡ δύναμις, μνήμη δὲ ἡ ἐνέργεια· ὡσαύτως καὶ ἐπὶ τῆς σφυγμικῆς, ὅτι σφυγμός, καὶ ἐπὶ τῆς θρεπτικῆς, ὅτι θρέψις. εἴρηται δὲ καὶ περὶ τῶν αἰτίων κατὰ διαίρεσιν, ὅτι τὰ μὲν αὐτῶν εἰσι προκαταρκτικά, τὰ δὲ προηγούμενα, τὰ δὲ συνεκτικά· πάλιν τὰ μὲν αὐτῶν εἰσι καθ' αὑτά, τὰ δὲ πρός τι, καὶ τὰ μὲν πόρρω, τὰ δὲ προσεχῆ, καὶ τὰ μὲν φυλακτικά, τὰ δὲ ἐπανορθωτικά, καὶ τὰ μὲν ὑγιεινά, τὰ δὲ νοσερά, τὰ δὲ οὐδέτερα. τὸ δὲ σημειωτικὸν διαιρεῖται εἰς διαγνωστικὸν προγνωστικὸν ἀναμνηστικόν. καὶ ταῦτα μὲν περὶ τοῦ

1 καὶ[I] – 7 γινόμενος] *cf.* [Gal.] Def. med. 70: XIX 364,16–365,5 K. *infra*, vol. II, foll. 26[v]; 40[r] 7 ὡσαύτως – 12] *i. e. Stephanus* Gal. De anat. administr. *libros explicans, desideratur apud Galenum; cf.* Gal. In Hipp. De nat. hom. comm. I prooem.: CMG V 9,1, p. 6,11–26 8 τὰ μὲν – 15 χρειώδη] *cf.* Steph. Ad Glauc.: I 241,19–24 Dietz 16 εἴρηται – 25 θρέψις] *cf.* Steph. Ad Glauc.: I 241,25–242,7 Dietz 19 αἱ – 21 ἀποκριτική] *cf.* Gal. De fac. nat. I–III: Scr. min. III 101–257 Helmr. = II 1–214 K. 25sq. εἴρηται – συνεκτικά] *cf.* Steph. Ad Glauc.: I 242,22–23 Dietz [Gal.] Def. med. 154–157: XIX 392,7–393,10 K. Theoph. In Aphor.: II 246,31–32 Dietz 28sq. τὸ δὲ – ἀναμνηστικόν] *v.* Theoph. In Aphor.: II 247,1–3 Dietz

2 ἰσατώδης *sec. [Gal.] scripsi*: σατώδης α: σαπώδ(ης) Z 3 γάρ *om.* α 4 ἄπιον α *(*οι *sscr.* A*)* 6 ἀπογαιωθέντος A 7sq. καὶ – καὶ *om.* Z 8 εὑρήκαμεν Z 9sq. νεῦρα καὶ ὀστᾶ καὶ χόνδροι καὶ σύνδεσμοι Z 11 μύες] νεῦρα A: πιμελὴ Z καὶ[III *et* IV] *om.* Z 12 καὶ[I] *om.* Z πνεύμων] σπλὴν P: *spat. 5 litt. in* A καὶ[II, III, IV, V] *om.* Z ὄρχις A 12sq. τὸ ποιὸν τῶν *scripsi*: τὸ π *et spat. 4 litt.* P: τὸ περὶ A: τόποι Z 13sq. τὰς δυνάμεις, τὰ δὲ ἐπικτήτους *scripsi (cf. Steph. Ad Glauc.: I, p. 241,20–21 Dietz)*: τὰς ἀρχάς, τὰ δὲ ἐπικτήτους Z: καὶ A: *om.* P 14 ἐπικτήτους[II]] γρ. ἐπιρρύτους *in mg.* A *(cf. Steph. Ad Glauc.: I, p. 241,21–22 Dietz)* 15 περὶ] παρὰ Z 16 *ante* ἡμᾶς *add.* καὶ α 17 *ante* φυσικαί *add.* καὶ Z 20 ἑλκτική – καὶ[III]] οἷον ἡ ἑλκτική· ἡ καθεκτική· ἡ ἀλλοιωτική· καὶ ἡ Z 25 *ante* ὅτι *add.* καὶ Z 27 ἑαυτὰ Z 27sq. φυλακτικά – μὲν *post* μὲν *(lin. 26) trsp.* Z 28 σημειωματικὸν Z

black humor, one phlegm. These are the elementary humors; but we have many other humors besides, the yolklike, the woad-colored, the verdigris-colored and the pale-yellow bile; similarly, there are three varieties of phlegm, one kind being sweet, one salty, one tasteless; in the same way, we have three kinds of black bile, one produced by over-heating of the yellow bile – called asphaltlike because it has the glitter of asphalt –, one resulting from a process of quenching, one produced by the hardening of phlegm. So, too, the sum of the parts of the body, which is the total of various numbers, is discussed in the Practical Anatomy; we said, there, that some are homogeneous, others organic, and of the homogeneous some are simple, such as nerve, bone, cartilage, ligament, membrane and flesh, others composite, such as veins, arteries and muscles; names of organic parts are stomach, liver, brain, lungs, heart, kidneys, bladder, testicles and so forth. As regards the qualities of the parts, some are vital organs, others are subordinate; in the case of some, their faculties are connatural, in others adventitious, in others, again, both connatural and adventitious; some are active, some are dependent. The importance of the theory of this is made clear by the Books on Anatomy. We have already discussed the number of the faculties, distinguishing three kinds, the psychic, the vital, the natural. To the psychic faculties belong imagination, ratiocination, recollection, intellect, thought, opinion, the individual senses and voluntary motions; the vital faculties are the respiratory and the pulsatory; the natural faculties are the reproductive, the growth-producing and the nutritive faculty, and those subsidiary to them, the attractive, retentive, transformative and secretory faculties. We also dealt with functions, observing that they are in a derivative relation (to faculties), e.g. the faculty is imaginative, the function imagination, the faculty is ratiocinative, the function ratiocination, the faculty is recollective, the function is recollection; similarly with the pulsatory faculty and the pulse, the nutritive faculty and nutrition. We have further classified causes as immediate, antecedent, or sustaining; or otherwise, as absolute or relative; as remote or proximate; as preservative or corrective; as wholesome, unwholesome, or neutral. Semiology is subdivided into diagnosis, prognosis and anamnesis. So

θεωρητικοῦ· ἐπεξέλθωμεν δέ, εἰ δοκεῖ, καὶ τῇ τοῦ πρακτικοῦ διαιρέσει. διαιρεῖται τοίνυν τὸ πρακτικὸν εἰς ὑγιεινὸν νοσερὸν οὐδέτερον· τὸ ὑγιεινὸν εἰς φυλακτικὸν προφυλακτικὸν εὐεκτικόν· ἔτι μέντοι καὶ τοῦτο ἐν τῇ τοῦ †πρακτικοῦ† διαιρέσει ζητήσωμεν, ὅτι διαιρεῖται πάλιν εἰς παιδοκομικὸν γηροκομικόν, εἰς φυλακτικὸν προφυλακτικόν· τὸ δὲ νοσερὸν εἰς διαιτητικὸν φαρμακευτικὸν χειρουργικόν. καὶ ἐπὶ μὲν τοῦ διαιτητικοῦ ζητοῦμεν τὰ εἴδη τῶν τροφῶν καὶ τὰς ποιότητας αὐτῶν καὶ τὰς δυνάμεις, ποῖαι τυχὸν εὔχυμοι ποῖαι κακόχυμοι, ποῖαι εὐστόμαχοι καὶ ποῖαι κακοστόμαχοι. ἐπὶ δὲ τοῦ φαρμακευτικοῦ ζητοῦμεν τὴν κατὰ μέρος ὕλην, πολλὴ δὲ αὕτη· ἢ γὰρ ἐν πρέμνοις θεωρεῖται ἢ ἐν θάμνοις ἢ ἐν ῥίζαις ἢ ἐν φλοιοῖς ἢ ἐν βοτάναις ἢ ἐν ὀποῖς ἢ ἐν δάκρυσιν ἢ ἐν χυλοῖς καὶ τοῖς τοιούτοις. πρὸς τούτοις ἀσκεῖν δεῖ καὶ τὸ χειρουργικόν, πῶς δεῖ μεταχειρίζεσθαι τὰ ὄργανα· ὅτι δεῖ κεχρῆσθαι εἴτε εὐθείαις εἴτε ἐγκαρσίοις εἴτε λοξαῖς εἴτε σκολιαῖς ταῖς χειρουργίαις, καὶ πρὸς τὴν θέσιν τῶν μυῶν. καὶ τούτων μὲν κεφαλαιωδῶς καὶ συντόμως τὴν μνήμην ἐποιησάμεθα· πόσον δὲ καὶ ποῖον οἴει ἕκαστον τῶν ἐνταῦθα παρειλημμένων τὸ πλάτος ἔχειν; οὐκ οἶμαι γοῦν οὐδαμῶς ἔτι ἀμφιβάλλειν σε περὶ τοῦ μακρὰν εἶναι τὴν τέχνην· πρῶτον γὰρ ἄν τις εὑρήσειε ταῦτα, εἶτα χρήσαιτο, εἶτα πεῖραν λήψαιτο, καὶ τότε τέλειος ἐν τούτοις γένοιτ' ἄν.

Ὁ δὲ καιρὸς ὀξύς. καιρὸν τὸν χρόνον λέγει, ὀξὺ δὲ τὸ ἀκμαῖον καὶ σύντομον. ὀξὺν τοίνυν τὸν καιρὸν λέγει ἢ διὰ τὴν χρῆσιν τῶν βοηθημάτων, ἐπειδὴ τῶν δυσχερῶν ἐστι τὸ διαγνωσθῆναι αὐτόν, ὥστε κατὰ τὸν δέοντα καιρὸν προσαγαγεῖν τὰ βοηθήματα. οὐ γὰρ πᾶς καιρὸς τῶν αὐτῶν δεῖται βοηθημάτων, ἀλλ' ἕτερα μὲν ἀρχῆς βοηθήματα, ἕτερα δὲ ἀναβάσεως, καὶ ἄλλα πάλιν ἀκμῆς καὶ ἕτερα παρακμῆς. δεῖ γὰρ εἰδέναι ὅτι «αἱ ψυχαὶ τῶν βοηθημάτων οἱ καιροί εἰσι», καὶ τοῦτο διχῶς· ἢ γὰρ πρὸς τὴν ⟨κατα⟩σκευὴν τοῦ βοηθήματος παραλαμβάνεται ὁ καιρὸς ἢ πρὸς τὸν καιρὸν τοῦ νοσήματος τὸ βοήθημα. οὐ μὴν ἀλλὰ καὶ διὰ τὸ ῥευστὸν τῆς ὕλης ἔτι μᾶλλον ὀξὺς ἀποδείκνυται ὁ καιρός· πολλάκις γὰρ δεῖται τροφῆς ὁ ἄρρωστος, καὶ μελλόντων ἡμῶν δοῦναι περὶ τὴν ἐπίδοσιν εἰσέβαλε παροξυσμὸς ἢ σύμπτωμά τι περιστατικὸν καὶ ἐκώλυσεν ἡμᾶς θρέψαι. ταῦτα τῆς ὀξύτητος τοῦ καιροῦ τὰ συμπτώματα· διὰ ταῦτα τοίνυν καὶ οἱ γραφεῖς ὀπισθόψιλον τὸν Καιρὸν γράφειν εἰώθασι μηδὲν ἕτερον διὰ τούτου ἐνδεικνύμενοι ἢ ὅτι παρῳχηκότα τοῦτον ἀδύνατόν ἐστι κατόπιν λαμβανόμενον αὖθις ὀπίσω ἀγαγεῖν.

1 διαιρεῖται – 5 χειρουργικόν] *cf.* Theoph. In Aphor.: II 247,3–6 Dietz 14 οὐκ – 17] *v.* Theoph. In Aphor.: II 247,6–10 Dietz 18–28 θρέψαι] *v.* Theoph. In Aphor.: II 247,13–24 Dietz 21sq. ἀλλ' – παρακμῆς] *cf.* Gal. De crisib. I 2: IX 551,1–2 K. Thrasyb. 32. 35: I 193,2–4; 195,14–15 K. [Gal.] Def. med. 136: XIX 388,4–5 K. Steph. Ad Glauc.: I 342,21–23 Dietz 23 αἱ – εἰσι] *v.* Hipp. Morb. I 5: VI 146,21–148,2 L. Procl. In Alcib.: p. 120,14–15 Westerink (Amstelodami 1954) Decem dubit.: p. 51,5–6 Boese (Berolini 1960) Olympiod. In Alcib.: p. 39,7 Westerink (Amstelodami 1956) In Phaed.: 9 § 9,10–11 Westerink (Amstelodami 1976) 25sq. οὐ – καιρός] *v.* Gal. In Aphor. I 1: XVII B 346,16–347,1; 353,10–12 *cf.* Steph. Ad Glauc.: I 237,1–4 Dietz

3 πρακτικοῦ] ὑγιεινοῦ *Agnell., recte, ut vid.*: διαιτητικοῦ *Theoph.* 4 ὅτι] ἐπεὶ Z *ante* πάλιν *add.* τοῦτο Z γηροκομικόν] προκομικὸν α εἰς[II] *om.* Z φυλακτικὸν] ἀναληπτικὸν *Theoph., Agnell.* 6 καὶ[I] *om.* Z 7 ποῖα τυχὸν εὔχυμα· καὶ ποῖα κακόχυμα· ποῖα εὐστόμαχα· καὶ ποῖα κακοστόμαχα Z 9 πρέμνοις] θέμνοις α: δένδροις P[2] 12 ἐγκαρσίαις Z 15 μακρὴν P 16 ταύτην Z εἶτα χρήσαιτο *om.* Z 22 ἕτερα[II]] ἄλλα Z 24 σκευὴν ω: *supplevi* 25sq. ἀλλὰ – καιρός *om.* Z 27 εἰσέβαλλε A 29 ὀπισθόψολον Z

much for the theoretical part; let us now go through the division of the practical part. The practical part, then, is subdivided into the care of the healthy body, the sick body, and that which is neither; the care of the healthy body into preservative and preventive medicine and condition training; again, we must look at the care of the healthy body[1] in this way, too, that it in its turn is subdivided into pediatrics and geriatrics, preservative and preventive care; and so is the care of the sick body into dietetics, pharmaceutics and surgery. In dietetics we study the kinds of nutriment, their qualities and their powers: which foods have a beneficial, and which a harmful effect on the humors, which are good for the stomach and which are bad. In pharmaceutics we examine the details of the *materia medica*, a comprehensive subject, since it is found in trees, in shrubs, in roots, in bark, in herbs, in sap, in resin, in juices, etc. In addition to these, one has to study surgery: how we are to handle the tools; that incisions must be straight or athwart or oblique or crooked, depending on the position of the muscles. We have only mentioned these points summarily and briefly, leaving it to you to imagine the extent and difficulty of a study in depth of each of the subjects enumerated here. I think you will have no doubt whatever left as to whether the art is long: first a man has to become acquainted with this material, then apply it, then acquire experience, and only thus can he hope to become perfect.

The moment is swift. The moment means time, swift means critical and soon gone. (Hippocrates) calls the moment swift, either in view of the application of remedies – since it is a difficult thing to discern one's opportunity, so as to administer the remedies at the right moment. Not every moment requires the same remedies: some are suited to the beginning (of a disease), others when it is on the increase, others again during the acme, others during the decrease. It is very true that "opportunity is the soul of treatment", and this in two different ways: either we wait for the right moment to prepare the medicine, or we choose the medicine with a view to the momentary state of the disease. Besides, the moment proves even more swift owing to the fluctuating nature of the matter; often the patient needs food, and when we intend to give it to him, just at the moment when it should be administered, a paroxysm sets in, or an accidental symptom appears and prevents us from feeding him. Such incidents are part of the swiftness of the moment; and this is why painters traditionally represent Time as bald from behind, indicating precisely this fact, that once it is past, it is impossible to grasp it from behind and bring it back.

[1] See the app. crit.

Ἡ δὲ πεῖρα σφαλερή. πεῖραν λέγει τὴν διὰ χειρῶν τριβήν· σφαλερὰν δὲ αὐτὴν ἐκάλεσεν, ἐπειδὴ πάντα τὰ βοηθήματα τῶν πρός τί εἰσι, καὶ ὃ βοήθημα τόνδε ὠφέλησεν, ἕτερον ἔβλαψε, καίτοι τοῦ αὐτοῦ εἴδους τοῦ νοσήματος ὑποκειμένου, ὅπερ γίνεται διά τινα ἰδιοτροπίαν στομάχου ἢ γαστρὸς ἢ κεφαλῆς ἢ ἑτέρου μορίου.

Ἡ δὲ κρίσις χαλεπή. κρίσιν λέγει τὸν λόγον, χαλεπὸν δὲ τὸ δυσκατάληπτον. καὶ ἔστι τοῦτο †οὐ πρός τι† ὁμολογούμενον, ὅτι χαλεπὸν εἰς κατάληψιν ὁ λόγος· πᾶσαι γοῦν αἱ τῶν ἀρχαίων βίβλοι καὶ μέχρι τοῦ παρόντος διαφωνίας μεσταὶ τυγχάνουσιν. οἱ δὲ ἐμπειρικοὶ ἑτέραν ἐξήγησιν τούτου λέγουσιν, ὅτι κρίσιν ὁ Ἱπποκράτης ἐνταῦθα ὀνομάζει τὴν ἐπίκρισιν. καὶ ἵνα ἐξ ὑποθέσεως νοηθῇ τὸ λεγόμενον, ὑποκείσθω πλευριτικὸς ἄρρωστος· τοῦτον λαβὼν ὁ ἰατρὸς ὑπέκλυσε τὴν γαστέρα, εἶτα ἐφλεβοτόμησεν, ἐχρήσατο δὲ καὶ πυρίαις διαφόροις, πρὸς τούτοις καὶ ἐκάθηρεν, εἶτα καταπλάσματα καὶ ἀνακόμματα καὶ ἀποζέματα ἥρμοσε τῷ πάθει· ἐφ' οἷς ῥᾳστώνη γέγονε τῶν ὀδυνῶν καὶ εἰς κρείττονα τάξιν ὁ ἄνθρωπος προέκοψε. λοιπὸν ζητεῖ ὁ ἐμπειρικός, πολλῶν γενομένων, ποῖόν ἐστι τὸ ὠφελῆσαν, δυσχερὲς δὲ τοῦτο καταλαβεῖν φησιν. ἀπόβλητος δέ ἐστιν ἡ δόξα καὶ τῆς Ἱπποκράτους ἀξίας ἀλλότρια τὰ λεγόμενα· οὐδὲ γάρ ἐστι χαλεπὸν δογματικῷ ἰατρῷ τὸ ἐρευνῆσαι καὶ γνῶναι ἐπὶ τῶν τοιούτων τοὺς λόγους καὶ τὰς αἰτίας τῶν ἐκβάσεων. ὥστε κρίσιν νῦν τὴν κατὰ λόγον αἰτίαν ἀκουστέον.

Καὶ μέχρι τῶν ἐνταῦθα πᾶσα ἡμῖν ἐσαφηνίσθη ἡ τοῦ πρώτου προοιμίου λέξις· λοιπόν, εἰ δοκεῖ, ἐρευνήσωμεν καὶ τὴν ἔννοιαν τῶν λεγομένων. φησὶν ὁ Ἱπποκράτης· ὁ βίος βραχύς· καὶ ἴσως ἀπορήσει τις πρὸς αὐτὸν ὅτι «Πῶς, ὦ Ἱππόκρατες, τὸν βίον τῶν ἀνθρώπων βραχὺν ἀποφαίνῃ; καὶ μὴν ὁρῶμεν, ὅτι μέχρις ἑκατὸν ἢ καὶ ἑκατὸν εἴκοσιν ἐνιαυτῶν διαρκεῖ τὸ ζῷον τοῦτο· εἰ δὲ καὶ πρὸς ἕτερα ζῷα τοῦτο παραβαλὼν ἔφης, ὁρῶμεν, ὅτι τινὰ τῶν ζῴων μέχρις εἴκοσιν ἐτῶν ζῇ, τινὰ δὲ ὀλιγοβιώτερα τυγχάνει, ἔνια δὲ τούτων ἐφήμερον ἔχει τὴν ζωήν, ὡς τὰ ἐν Ἰορδάνῃ γινόμενα, ἅ φησιν ὁ Ἀριστοτέλης ἀνίσχοντος μὲν ἡλίου ἀναβιοῦν, θνῄσκειν δὲ δύνοντος. τούτων οὖν πάντων μακροβιωτέρας οὔσης τῆς τῶν ἀνθρώπων ζωῆς πῶς σὺ βραχὺν τὸν βίον αὐτῶν ἐκάλεσας;» λέγει δὲ πρὸς ταῦτα ὁ Ἱπποκράτης ὅτι «Οὐ πρὸς ἕτερα ζῷα παραβαλὼν τὴν τῶν ἀνθρώπων ζωὴν βραχύβιον τὸ ζῷον τοῦτο ὠνόμασα, ὁπότε καὶ τοῦτ' ἐξῆν, εἴ γε τὴν πρὸς τὰ μακρόβια ζῷα, ἐλέφαντά φημι τυχὸν ἢ κορώνην, ἐποιούμεθα σύγκρισιν· ἀλλὰ πρὸς τὴν τέχνην τὸν χρόνον τῆς ζωῆς παραμετρήσας, ἐπειδήπερ εὗρον ταύτην πολλῷ τῷ μέτρῳ ὑπερβάλλουσαν, βραχυχρόνιον ἔφην τὸν ἄνθρωπον.»

6–19] *v.* Gal. In Aphor. I 1: XVII B 347,1–9; 354,4–355,4 K. 6–9 τυγχάνουσιν] *v.* Theoph. In Aphor.: II 247,33–248,4 Dietz 26 ἔνια – 28 δύνοντος] *v.* Aristot. Hist. anim. V 19: 552 b 17–23

1 *post* πεῖραν *add.* ἐνταῦθα Z *post* διὰ *add.* τῶν Z 3 εἴδους τοῦ] εἶδον Z 4 ἢ κεφαλῆς ἢ γαστρὸς A 7 ἔστι] ἔτι A οὐ πρός τι] ὡς ἱπποκράτ(ης) λέγει Z: *cruces posui* 8 βίβλοι καὶ] βιβλιωθῆκαι Z 9 ἐτύγχανον Z δὲ] γὰρ Z 10 τὴν ἐπίκρισιν ὀνομάζει Z 11 ὁ ἰητρὸς λαβὼν Z ἀπέκλισε Z 12 καὶ[II] *om.* A 14 τῶν ὀδυνῶν ἐγεγόνει Z 15 γιγνομένων Z 16 ἱπποκράτας P: ἱπποκράτου AZ: *correxi* 20 πᾶσιν Z 21 ὁ *om.* Z 22 ἀπορήσει] ἀπορήσειε δ' ἄν Z ὅτι] τὸ Z ὁ ἱπποκράτ(ης) Z 23 ἀποφαίνει Z, 24 ἑκατὸν[I] – εἴκοσιν] εἴκοσι καὶ ἑκατὸν Z 25 ἔφης] εὕροις Z ὅτι *om.* Z *post* τινὰ *add.* μὲν P εἴκοσιν ἐτῶν ζῇ] αἰτῶν εἴκοσι καὶ μόνων ζῆν Z 26 τυγχάνοι Z 27 ὁ *om.* Z ἀναβιοῦντα Z 28 δύναντος Z 29 λέγει δὲ] καὶ φησὶ Z ὁ Ἱπποκράτης] οὗτος Z 31 ὠνόμασται α 32 φησι Z σύγκρασιν P 33 ἐπειδὴ Z 34 ἔφην] ἔχειν Z

Trial is risky. By trial he means practical routine; he called it risky, because all remedies are relative, and a remedy that is beneficial to one patient is detrimental to another, even if it is a case of the same disease; this is due to a peculiarity of the stomach, the belly, the head or some other part.

Judgment is difficult. By judgment he means the reason, and by difficult hard to grasp. This, indeed, is a matter of unqualified (?) agreement, that the reason (of things) is difficult to apprehend; certainly all the books of the ancients and down to our own time are full of controversy. The empiricists have a different interpretation: they say that Hippocrates uses judgment here in the sense of an evaluation afterwards. To explain this by means of a hypothetical case, let us take a pleurisy patient; the doctor has given him an enema, then bled him, he has also applied heat in various forms, further he has purged him, then treated the complaint with plasters and poultices and decoctions; after which the pain has abated and the patient's condition has improved. The empiricist now wonders which of all these measures is the one that has been beneficial, and he says that this is difficult to determine. However, this doctrine is to be rejected and the interpretation is unworthy of Hippocrates; as a matter of fact, for a physician of the dogmatic school it is not difficult in cases such as this to investigate the reasons and causes of the events. Judgment must therefore be understood here as rational explanation.

Thus far we have elucidated the first preface word for word; let us now also examine the meaning of the text. Hippocrates says Life is short; and perhaps somebody will object: "My dear Hippocrates, how can you maintain that human life is short? Actually, we see that this animal lasts as many as a hundred or a hundred and twenty years; if you meant in comparison with other animals, we see that some of them live up to twenty years, others have shorter lives, and some of them have a lifespan of only one day, as those animals bred in the river Jordan, of which Aristotle says that they start life at sunrise and die at sunset. As man outlives them all, how can you call his life short?" Hippocrates' answer to this is: "It was not on the ground of a comparison between man's life and that of other animals that I described this animal as short-lived – though even this would be possible, if we compared ourselves with long-lived animals, such as the elephant or the crow –; but I measured our lifetime by the standard of the art, and because I found that the art exceeds it by far, I said that human life is short."

Ὁ βίος οὖν βραχύς, ἐπειδὴ ἡ τέχνη μακρή· καὶ ἀντιστρέφει· ἡ τέχνη μακρή, ἐπειδὴ ὁ βίος βραχύς· μακρὰ δὲ ἡ τέχνη διὰ τὸ τὸν καιρὸν ὀξὺν εἶναι καὶ ταχέως παρατρέχειν· ὁ δὲ καιρὸς ὀξὺς διὰ τὸ τὴν πεῖραν σφαλερὰν εἶναι, τοῦ μὲν μὴ ἀναμένοντος, τῆς δὲ ἐν τριβῇ πλείονι κατορθουμένης· ἀνάγκη οὖν τῷ μὲν τὴν ὀξύτητα ἐπιτείνεσθαι, τῇ δὲ τὸ σφάλμα. σφαλερὰ δὲ καὶ ἄλλως ἡ πεῖρα, ὅτι ἡ κρίσις χαλεπὴ καὶ ἀκατάληπτος ὁ λόγος. ἰστέον γάρ, ὅτι δυσὶν ὀργάνοις χρωμένη βεβαιοῦται ἡ ἡμετέρα τέχνη, λόγῳ τε καὶ πράξει· καὶ ὁ μὲν λόγος τοῦ θεωρητικοῦ ἐστιν, ἡ δὲ πρᾶξις τοῦ πρακτικοῦ· τούτων τῶν δύο τὸ μὲν ἀκατάληπτον ὑπάρχει ἢ δυσκατάληπτον, ὁ λόγος φημί, τὸ δὲ ἕτερον σφαλερόν, τουτέστιν ἡ πεῖρα.

12 [I 1: IV 458,2–4 L.] Δεῖ δὲ οὐ μόνον ἑωυτὸν παρέχειν τὰ δέοντα ποιέοντα, ἀλλὰ καὶ τὸν νοσέοντα καὶ τοὺς παρεόντας καὶ τὰ ἔξωθεν.

Τοῦτο προτρεπτικὸν εἶναι δοκεῖ τὸ προοίμιον· πρὸς δὲ τὸν ἰατρὸν διαλέγεται ὅτι «Δεῖ σε ἑτοιμότατα τοῖς χρῄζουσιν ἑαυτὸν διδόναι.» τὸ δὲ τὰ δέοντα ποιέοντα δεῖται ζητήσεως· χρεὼν γὰρ εἰπεῖν, τί δεῖ τὸν ἰατρὸν μεταστελλόμενον διαπράττεσθαι. ταῦτα τοίνυν, ὡς ἐν ἕκτῃ λέγεται Ἐπιδημίᾳ, πολλά εἰσι καὶ διάφορα. πρῶτον μὲν γὰρ δεῖ αὐτὸν ἄνθρωπον ἀνεπίληπτον καὶ αἰδέσιμον εἶναι, τηρεῖν τε τὸ εὔσχημον κατά τε κουρὰν καὶ ὄνυχας καὶ ὀσμὴν καὶ ἐσθῆτα καὶ ἦθος. κατὰ μὲν κουράν, ὥστε μήτε κομᾶν μήτε περιέργως κείρεσθαι, ἑκάτερον γὰρ ἄλογον. τοὺς δὲ ὄνυχας μὴ ἄγαν ηὐξημένους ἔχειν, ἐκτὸς μέντοι τῶν χειρουργῶν, οὗτοι γὰρ χρείαν αὐτῶν ἔχουσιν, ἐν ταῖς χειρουργίαις κεχρημένοι τούτοις δίκην σαρκολάβων· ἐπὶ δὲ τοῦ διαιτητικοῦ οὐ δέον ἐστὶν ηὐξημένους εἶναι τοὺς ὄνυχας, πρῶτον μέν, ὅτι ῥύπος αὐτοῖς ἐγγίνεται, ὅπερ βδελυκτόν ἐστι, λοιπὸν δέ, ὅτι ἐν τῇ σημειώσει τοῦ τε σφυγμοῦ καὶ τῶν σπλάγχνων ἢ καὶ ἑτέρου τινὸς μορίου τῇ πιλήσει τῆς ἀφῆς πλήττεται ὁ ἄρρωστος καὶ ἀνιᾶται. δεῖ δὲ αὐτὸν μήτε δυσῶδες ὄζειν μήτε μύροις τισὶν ὑπαλείφεσθαι, τοῦτο γὰρ καλλωπισμοῦ ἕνεκεν τοῖς ἀνθρώποις σπουδάζεται. κατὰ δὲ τὴν ἐσθῆτα οὐ δεῖ αὐτὸν ῥυπαροφόρον εἶναι, ἀλλ' οὐδὲ μὴν ἐστιβασμένον ὥστε σηρικά τινα ἀμφιέννυσθαι. κατὰ δὲ τὸ ἦθος τῆς ψυχῆς δεῖ αὐτὸν ἐπιεικὲς καὶ κόσμιον ἔχειν τοῦτο, καὶ οὐ μόνον ὡς ἄνθρωπον, ἀλλὰ καὶ ὡς ἰατρόν, καὶ μὴ θρασύν τινα καὶ αὐθάδη καὶ περίεργον εἶναι, τοῦτο γὰρ σοβαρότητός ἐστι· μήτε αὖ κατηφῆ τε καὶ σκυθρωπόν, τοῦτο γὰρ δειλίας ἐστί.

Ταῦτα πάντα δεῖ ἀσκεῖν τὸν ἰατρόν, μᾶλλον μὲν ὡς ἄνθρωπον, ἧττον δὲ ὡς

1–2 βραχύς] *cf.* Theoph. In Aphor.: II 246,23 Dietz 2 μακρὰ – 4 κατορθουμένης] Gal. In Aphor. I 1: XVII B 346,6–8 K. 5sq. σφαλερὰ – λόγος] *v.* Theoph. In Aphor.: II 247,32–33 Dietz 13–14 διδόναι] *cf.* Theoph. In Aphor.: II 250,10–12 Dietz 16 ταῦτα – 28 ἀμφιέννυσθαι] *v.* Hipp. Epid. VI 4,7: V 308,15–16 L. *cf.* Gal. In Hipp. Epid. VI comm. IV 10: CMG V 10,2,2, p. 206,12–207,21 Pallad. In Epid. VI: II 112,21–114,5 Dietz 28 κατὰ – 31] *cf.* Gal. In Hipp. Epid. VI comm. IV 10: CMG V 10,2,2, p. 205,11–20 32–44,10 προσέρχεσθαι] *cf.* Gal. In Hipp. Epid. VI comm. IV 10: CMG V 10,2,2, p. 203,8–16 Pallad. In Epid. VI: II 111,21–112,1 Dietz

1 ἀντιστρόφως Z *post* τέχνη^{II} *add.* δὲ Z 2 μακρὴ Z 3 μήτ' Z 4 τῷ] τὸν A 5 ὅτι] ἐπειδὴ Z 7 *post* δὲ *add.* γε Z 8 *post* τούτων *add.* οὖν Z 9 ὁ – φημί] ὅπέρ ἐστιν ὁ λόγος Z τουτέστιν] ὅπέρ ἐστιν Z 16 *post* ἐν *add.* τ(ῇ) A 17 τε] δὲ A 20 χρείας A 23 *post* δέ *add.* καὶ Z 27 ἐστιβασμένον] ἑτοιμασμένον Z 29 καὶ^{I} *om.* Z τινα] καὶ ἰταμὸν Z 30 αὖ] οὖν A 32 *post* Ταῦτα *add.* γὰρ α

Life, then, is short because the art is long; the statement can be reversed: the art is long because life is short. The reason why the art is long is that the moment is swift and passes quickly; the reason why the moment is swift is that trial is risky, since the moment does not wait, while trial, to be successful, requires considerable routine, so that inevitably, as the swiftness of the moment increases, so does the risk of the experiment. Trial is risky also because judgment is difficult, i.e. the reason (of things) is inapprehensible. We must be aware that our art is based on the use of two instruments, reason and practice, reason belonging to the theoretical part (of medicine), practice to the practical part; now of these two, the one, reason, is inapprehensible or at least difficult to apprehend, and the other, trial, is fallible.

I 2. Not only (the physician) himself must be prepared to do what is necessary, but the patient, those around him, and external circumstances must also co-operate.

This preface has a hortatory character; addressing the doctor, it tells him to be always ready for those who need him. But the words to do what is necessary require closer inspection: we must specify what the doctor should do when he is summoned. This, as described in the sixth book of the Epidemics, is a great variety of things. To begin with, he should be a person of blameless respectability, and observe the decencies as regards haircut, nails, odor, apparel and character. As for the hair, he should wear it neither long nor excessively short, since both are absurd. His nails should not be too long, except in the case of the surgeon, who needs them, for he uses them in surgery as a kind of forceps; the dietitian, however, should not have long nails, in the first place because they become dirty, which is offensive, and further because in feeling the pulse, the intestines or any other part of the body, the pressure of the touch hurts and troubles the patient. He should neither smell bad nor use perfumed oils, for this is a habit of people who want to attract attention. In his dress he should be neither dirty nor overly refined, to the extent of wearing silk, for instance. In respect of character he should be modest and controlled, not only as a man, but also as a physician; he should not be overbearing, conceited and meddlesome, which are the results of excessive self-confidence, nor, on the other hand, subdued and sullen, which comes from lack of confidence.

The doctor should cultivate all these habits, in the first place as a man, and

ἰατρόν. ἃ δὲ μᾶλλον αὐτὸν ὡς ἰατρὸν δεῖ διαπράττεσθαι, εἴτε ἐν εἰσόδοις εἴτε ἐν ἐξόδοις ἤγουν περιόδοις, θεωρεῖται κατά τε τὸν τρόπον τῶν εἰσόδων καὶ τὸ ποσὸν αὐτῶν. κατὰ μὲν τὸν τρόπον δεῖ αὐτὸν ἐπίστασθαι, ὁπηνίκα χρὴ ἀνθηρῶς εἰσιέναι μετὰ φωνῆς καὶ φθέγματος τρανοτέρου, ὁπηνίκα δὲ μεθ' ἡσυχίας, ἠρέμα καὶ πραέως, καὶ αὐτῷ δὲ τῷ βήματι τοιῶσδε ἢ τοιῶσδε χρώμενον, ὅπερ πρὸς τὴν τῶν νοσημάτων ποιότητα μεθαρμόζεται. ἔνθα μὲν οὖν ὀξὺ ὑπόκειται νόσημα καὶ πυρετὸς διακαὴς καὶ πολλὰ δεινὰ συμπτώματα μετ' ἀγρυπνίας συνεδρεύει, τότε δεῖ τὸν ἰατρὸν ἠρέμα εἰσέρχεσθαι ἐννοοῦντα, μή τι ἄρα ὁ ἄνθρωπος φύσεως δῶρον ηὐτύχησε καὶ εἰς ὕπνον ἐτράπη· ἔνθα δὲ καταφορικὸν ἢ ληθαργικὸν ἢ κωματῶδες ὑπόκειται νόσημα, τότε δεῖ μετὰ φθέγματος τρανοτέρου τὸν ἰατρὸν προσέρχεσθαι. ἐν γοῦν τῇ Μεγάλῃ θεραπευτικῇ ὁ Γαληνὸς ὑπέθετο εὑρεθῆναι αὐτῷ τινα καθεύδοντα, εἶθ' ἑαυτὸν ὑποχωρήσαντα καὶ αὖθις ἐπανελθόντα καὶ τὸν ἄρρωστον ὁμοίως ὕπνῳ κατεχόμενον· εἶτα λοιπόν, ἐπειδὴ τροφῆς ἐδεῖτο κατὰ τὸν καιρὸν ἐκεῖνον διὰ τὸ ἐξασθενεῖν τὴν δύναμιν, μετὰ βοῆς χρησάμενον τῇ εἰσόδῳ διαναστῆσαι τοῦ ὕπνου τὸν ἄνθρωπον, ὥστε μεταλαβεῖν τῆς δεούσης τροφῆς. δεῖ δὲ αὐτὸν καὶ ἀπεριέργως ποιεῖσθαι τὰς περιόδους· οὐ γὰρ εἰκὸς ἀνερχόμενον πρὸς τὸν ἄρρωστον ἀποφαίνεσθαι· «Τοῦτο τὸ σκεῦος τί ποιεῖ;» οὐδέ· «Μετάθες αὐτὸ ἐκεῖ κἀκεῖνο μετένεγκε ὧδε», ἀλλὰ δεῖ σπεύδειν αὐτὸν περὶ τὴν διάγνωσιν καὶ τὴν θεραπείαν τοῦ νοσήματος. ἀλλὰ μὴν οὐδὲ πολλάκις αὐτὸν εἰσιέναι προσήκει, ἵνα μὴ δόξειε προσκορής, τῇ μέσῃ δὲ κεχρῆσθαι τάξει. τοῦτο δὲ τὸ εἶδος διατυποῖ τοῦ νοσήματος· εἰ μὲν γὰρ κάτοξυ τὸ νόσημα καὶ πολλὰ καὶ μεγάλα συμπτώματα, πλείοσι περιόδοις δεῖ κεχρῆσθαι τὸν ἰατρόν, ἵνα τὰ ὄντα μὲν παρηγορήσῃ, τὰ μέλλοντα δὲ προαναστείλῃ· εἰ δέ γε χρόνιόν ἐστι τὸ νόσημα καὶ νωθρὸν καὶ δυσκίνητον, οἷον ἕλκος μὴ κακόηθες, ἀρκετὸν καὶ ἅπαξ τῆς ἡμέρας τὴν ἐπίσκεψιν ποιήσασθαι. δεῖ δέ σε καὶ τυραννικὸν εἶναι πρὸς τὰ νοσήματα καὶ μὴ προσώποις μηδὲ ἀξίᾳ καθυπείκειν τὴν τέχνην, μηδὲ εἰ βασιλεῖς εἶεν ἢ ἄρχοντες, τούτων αὐτὴν δευτέραν ἀποφαίνου. δεῖ δὲ πρὸς τούτοις καὶ τῶν αἰτίων πάντων ἀνιχνεύειν τὰς ἐφόδους καὶ τὴν φύσιν, καὶ μάλιστα τῶν προκαταρκτικῶν αἰτίων, ἅτινα ἔστιν ὅτε τῷ ἀδήλῳ τῆς αἰσθήσεως λανθάνοντα σφάλλει τὸν τεχνίτην. ἐν γὰρ τούτοις πᾶσι παρασκευαζόμενος ὁ ἰατρὸς ῥᾷστα τοῦ τέλους τύχοι. τοῦτο γάρ ἐστι τὸ τὰ δέοντα ποιέοντα.

Ἔστι δὲ ἃ καὶ τὸν νοσέοντα χρὴ συνεισάγειν· χρὴ γὰρ τὸν νοσοῦντα πειθήνιον εἶναι τῷ ἰατρῷ καὶ πάντα εὐμενῶς δέχεσθαι τὰ προστασσόμενα. οὕτως γάρ φησιν ὁ ἰατρὸς ἐν Ἐπιδημίαις, ὅτι ἡ τέχνη διὰ τρία ἐστίν· ἔστι γὰρ ὁ ἰατρός, ἡ νόσος καὶ τὰ αἴτια κατὰ διάμετρον, καὶ μέσος ὁ ἄρρωστος. καὶ τὰ ἐναντία οὐδέποτε εἰς ὁμόνοιαν ἔρχονται, ἡ νόσος φημὶ καὶ ἡ τέχνη, ἀλλὰ διὰ πάντων ἀντιστρατεύονται ἀλλήλοις· ὁ δὲ νοσῶν ἑκατέρῳ συννεῦσαι δύναται. εἰ μὲν οὖν μετὰ τῆς τέχνης γένηται καὶ τῷ

10 ἐν – 15 τροφῆς] Gal. Meth. med.: X K.; *locum non inveni* 31–46,4] *cf.* Gal. In Hipp. Epid. VI comm. IV 10: CMG V 10,2,2, p. 204,14–205,2 31–32 προστασσόμενα] *v.* Theoph. In Aphor.: II 250,14–15 Dietz 32 οὕτως – 34 ἄρρωστος] Hipp. Epid. I 11 (5): I 190,3–4 Kw. = II 636,1–2 L.

2 ἤγουν] ἢ ἐν Z 3 χρὴ] δεῖ A 4 μετὰ – τρανοτέρου *om.* Z 5 *ante* ὅπερ *add.* καὶ Z 9 καταφορικῷ ἢ ληθαργικῷ P νοσήματι α 10 εἰσέρχεσθαι A 11 τινὰ καθεύδοντα αὐτῷ A 12 αὖθις] πάλιν A 13 λοιπόν *om.* A 16 πρὸς τὸν ἄρρωστον ἀνερχόμενον A 17 αὐτῷ A 19 πολλὰ α προσῆκεν α δόξῃ A 20 διατυπεῖ A 21 δεῖ *om.* α 22 προαναστέλλῃ Z 23 μὴ *om.* Z 26 πρὸ A 27 προκαταρκτικῶν] πρακτιῶν Z 28 *ante* τὸν *add.* τὲ α 34 ὁ *om.* Z 35 *post* διὰ *add.* τῶν Z 36 τῆς *om.* α

only in the second as a physician. The behavior that may be expected from him more specifically as a physician, whether in his home calls or when he leaves to go on a tour, has to do with the manner of his visits and with their frequency. As regards the manner, he must know when it is best to come in briskly, speaking in a loud and clear voice, and when (it is better to enter) in silence, quietly and calmly, also adapting his footstep to either one of these approaches; this varies with the character of the disease. When there is a case of acute illness, burning fever and many disquieting symptoms attended with sleeplessness, the doctor should make his entrance quietly, bearing in mind that perhaps Nature has been kind to the patient and he may have gone to sleep; but when he has to do with a torpid, lethargic or comatose disease, the doctor will raise his voice as he comes to the bedside. Thus Galen in the Great Therapeutics takes the case of a man he finds asleep; he retreats, and when he comes back the patient is still sleeping; then, because the man at that point needed food in view of his weakened condition, he woke him up by a boisterous entrance, so that he could partake of the necessary food. (The physician) should further mind his own business when visiting; it is bad manners to come to a patient and remark "What is that piece of furniture doing here?" or "Better move it over there and put that one in its place"; he should give his entire attention to diagnosing and treating the illness. Nor should he come too often, to avoid seeming obtrusive, but keep the happy mean. This is determined by the type of the disease: if the disease is very acute and the symptoms are many and severe, the physician must make repeated visits, so as to alleviate the present evils and check the forthcoming ones; if, on the other hand, the disease is chronic, sluggish and slow in its progress, as for instance a non-malignant ulcer, one visit a day will suffice. You must be a tyrant, (if necessary,) in the face of disease and not allow the art to yield to person or rank; even if your patients are emperors or lords, never admit that medicine has to take orders from them. Finally, you must investigate the inroads and the nature of all the causes, but especially the immediate ones, which sometimes owing to the weakness of our perception escape attention and lead the trained physician into error. If the physician is prepared for all this, he will have the best chance of attaining his end. This is what is meant by doing what is necessary.

The patient, too, must make his contribution: the patient must obey the doctor and submit willingly to all his directions. The physician (Hippocrates) in the Epidemics puts it in this way, that the art of medicine depends on three factors: first there is the physician, then the disease and the causes at the opposite end, and between them the patient. The opposites, i.e. the disease and the art, can never agree, but are involved in everlasting warfare; the patient, however, can join either of the two. If he sides with medicine and follows the doctor's

ἰατρῷ ὁμονοήσῃ, καταπαλαίεται τὸ νόσημα· εἰ δὲ ἀπειθήσῃ τοῖς ὑπὸ τοῦ ἰατροῦ λεγομένοις καὶ συννεύσῃ τῇ νόσῳ, ἀνάγκη πᾶσα τὴν τέχνην νικηθῆναι, δύο γὰρ ἑνὶ καθ' ἑκάτερον λόγον εὑρίσκονται ἀντικαθιστάμενα. καὶ τοῦτό ἐστι τὸ τὰ δέοντα ποιέοντα.

Παρόντα⟨ς⟩ δὲ δεῖ νοῆσαι τούς τε ὑπηρετοῦντας τῷ ἀρρώστῳ καὶ τοὺς ὁπωσοῦν ἄλλως ἢ διὰ φιλίαν ἢ διὰ συγγένειαν προσεδρεύοντας αὐτῷ ἐν τῇ νόσῳ. καὶ δεῖ τοὺς μὲν ὑπηρετοῦντας μηδαμῶς ὑπόπτους εἶναι τῷ νοσοῦντι, ἀνίαν γὰρ ἐμποιεῖ τοῖς νοσοῦσι τῶν μισουμένων ἡ θέα· ἀλλὰ δεῖ αὐτοὺς εὐμεταχειρίστως καὶ καθαρῶς μετιέναι τὰ ἐπιτασσόμενα ὀργάνου τάξιν ἐπέχοντας. τεσσάρων γὰρ ὄντων τῶν θεραπευτικῶν σκοπῶν, τοῦ τε ἀπὸ τοῦ ποσοῦ καὶ τοῦ ἀπὸ τοῦ ποιοῦ καὶ τοῦ καιροῦ καὶ τοῦ τρόπου τῆς χρήσεως, οἱ μὲν τρεῖς μάλιστα ὑπὸ τοῦ ἰατροῦ τυποῦνται, ὁ δὲ τρόπος τῆς χρήσεως ἐπίκοινός πώς ἐστι, καὶ ἐν τῷ ἰατρῷ καὶ ἐν τοῖς ἐξυπηρετοῦσι θεωρούμενος. φέρε γάρ, εἰ οὕτως ἔτυχεν, ὑποτυπῶσαι τὸν ἰατρὸν τό τε ποσὸν καὶ τὸ ποιὸν καὶ τὸν καιρὸν τῆς τροφῆς, ὥστε ἐπιδοθῆναι ποτήριον χυλοῦ τῷ ἀρρώστῳ ὥρᾳ δευτέρᾳ, καὶ ταῦτα εἰπόντα ἀπαλλαγῆναι, τοῦτο τοίνυν εὐσχημόνως καὶ καθαρῶς χρὴ μεταχειρίσασθαι τοὺς ὑπηρετοῦντας τὸ ἐπιταχθέν· ὅπερ τοῦ τρόπου τῆς χρήσεως τῶν συνόντων τῷ ἀρρώστῳ ἐστὶ καὶ πρὸς ὑπουργίαν τεταγμένων. τὰ δὲ τῶν ἑτέρως ὁπωσοῦν προσεδρευόντων δεῖ ἔχειν οὕτως, ἵνα μηδὲν ἀνιαρὸν μηνύωσιν αὐτῷ τῶν ὡς εἰκὸς συμβαινόντων, μὴ περὶ ἀποβολῆς χρημάτων ἢ φίλων ἢ συγγενῶν, μηδ' ἀκαταθύμιον καὶ ἀνάρμοστον ἔντευξιν ἐπ' αὐτῷ ποιῶνται, ἀλλ' ἐκείνας κινῶσι τὰς ὁμιλίας, αἷς ἐπίστανται ἡδόμενον τὸν ἄρρωστον. ταῦτά τοι χρεὼν καὶ τοὺς παρεόντας πράττειν.

Καὶ τὰ ἔξωθεν. ἔξωθεν ὀνομάζει τὴν τοῦ περιέχοντος ἡμᾶς ἀέρος φύσιν καὶ τὰ κατά τινα τύχην ἀπροόπτως συμβαίνοντα, ὥστε εἰ μὴ καὶ ταῦτα κατὰ τὸν προκείμενον σκοπὸν ἐπιγένωνται, πολλὴν ἔχειν δύναμιν τοῦ διακόψαι τὸ ἐλπιζόμενον τέλος. καὶ ἵνα σαφὲς γένηται τὸ λεγόμενον, ὑποκείσθω τις πυρέττων· τοῦτον ὁ παρακολουθῶν ἰατρὸς σημειωσάμενος προέγνω, ὡς μέλλει κρίνεσθαι ὁ πυρετὸς δι' ἱδρώτων τῇ ἑβδόμῃ τῶν ἡμερῶν, καὶ ταῦτα εἰπὼν ἀνεχώρησεν· εἶτα ἐλθὼν τῇ ὑστεραίᾳ καὶ προσδοκήσας πρὸς τὴν πρόρρησιν τὴν ἀπόβασιν καὶ ἰσόθεος νομισθῆναι, οὐ μόνον τούτου ἐστέρηται, ἀλλὰ τοὐναντίον διαγελᾶται μὴ γενομένης τῆς δι' ἱδρώτων κρίσεως. δεῖ οὖν τὸ τηνικαῦτα, εἴπερ μήτε ἐξ αὐτοῦ τι προημελήθη περὶ τὴν σημείωσιν μήτε ἐκ τοῦ νοσοῦντος ἡμάρτηταί τι ἢ ἐκ τῶν παρεόντων, ἐπὶ τὰ ἔξωθεν ἀναδραμεῖν καὶ θεωρῆσαι, μή τι ἄρα κατὰ τὸν ἀέρα συμβέβηκεν ἐναντιούμενον τῇ τοιαύτῃ κρίσει· ἴσως γὰρ ψυχροῦ γεγονότος αὐτοῦ στεγάνωσίν τινα γενέσθαι καὶ σύμπτυξιν τῶν πόρων καὶ πύκνωσιν, ὥστε τῆς ἐπὶ τὰ ἔξω κωλυομένης

5–9 ἐπέχοντας] *cf.* Theoph. In Aphor.: II 250,15–16 Dietz 9 τεσσάρων – 11 χρήσεως] *v.* Gal. Ad Glauc. I 1: XI 2,1–4 K. *cf. infra*, p. 66,16–18 18 τὰ δὲ – 21 ἄρρωστον] *cf.* Theoph. In Aphor.: II 250,16–17 Dietz 23–48,10] *cf.* Gal. De dieb. decr. I 11: IX 823,16–825,5 K. 23–24 συμβαίνοντα] *cf.* Theoph. In Aphor.: II 250,18–19 Dietz

1sq. ὁμονοήσει . . . ἀπειθήσει . . . συννεύσει ω: *correxi* 2 ἑνὶ] ἕνια Z 5 παρόντα ω: *correxi* 6 φελίαν P: ὠφέλειαν P[2] 7 τῶν νοσούντων Z 8 εὐμεταχειρίστους PZ καθαροὺς P 9 ἐπίχοντας Z 10 ἀπὸ[I]] ἐπὶ Z 13 φέρεται AZ 17 τῶ τρόπω Z: τοῦτο α: *correxi* 18 οὕτως ἔχειν A 19 *post* εἰκὸς *add.* γε Z 20 οὐ καταθύμιον P 24 τὰ *om.* Z 25 ἐπιγένονται ω: *correxi* ἔχει Z 28 τῇ ἑβδόμῃ τῶν ἡμερῶν δι' ἱδρώτων Z 30 *post* ἀλλὰ *add.* καὶ Z 31 τὸ *om.* Z 32 παρόντων Z 34 αὐτῶ Z 35 γενέσθαι] γεννᾶ *ex* γενᾶ *mut.* Z σύμπτηξιν A[2]P: σύμπυξιν Z

opinion, the disease will be overcome; but if he disobeys the doctor's orders and takes the side of the disease, medicine will inevitably lose, for in both cases we have a fight of two against one. This is meant by (the patient) doing what is necessary.

By those around him we must understand those who attend the patient as well as those who are present in the sickroom in any other capacity, e.g. as friends or relatives. The attendants should not be in any way objectionable to the patient, for it is irritating to sick people to look at faces they dislike; they should follow up directions promptly and strictly, since they serve as instruments only. Of the four points to be considered in therapeutics, viz., the quantity, the quality, the moment, and the application, the other three are mainly determined by the physician, while the application is somehow common ground, being the business both of the doctor and of the attendants. Suppose that the doctor has prescribed the quantity and the quality of the food and the time to take it, for instance, a cup of gruel to be served to the patient at the second hour, after which he has gone away; it is now the duty of the attendants to execute these orders properly and strictly; this is part of the application of the treatment by those who attend to the patient and minister to his needs. As for those who are in the sickroom for other reasons, their concern should be not to inform him of any unpleasant things such as are apt to occur, the loss of money, friends or relatives, and to avoid subjects of conversation that are distasteful and uncongenial to him; rather, they should bring round the conversation to topics they know the patient will enjoy. So much for the duties of those around him.

And external circumstances. By external he means the nature of the surrounding air and certain unforeseen accidental events of such a kind that, if they do not also turn out in accordance with the treatment as planned, they have a strong chance of thwarting the expected outcome. To make the meaning of this clear, let us take a case of fever: the physician in charge, after observing the patient, arrives at the prognosis of a crisis through sweating on the seventh day, makes a statement to this effect and leaves; the next day he returns, expecting that the outcome must have been in accordance with his prediction and that people will look upon him as a divine being; as it is, he is not only denied this satisfaction, but actually becomes a laughingstock, for the crisis through sweating does not take place. Under these circumstances – assuming that there has been no negligence on his part in the observation of the symptoms and that the patient or those in attendance have made no mistake either – we must take external factors into account and consider the possibility that there may have been a change in the air which was unfavorable to such a crisis; perhaps it has turned cold, with, as a result, tightening and contraction and closing of the pores, so that the diseased

τῇ ὕλῃ ἐκβάσεως ταύτην ἀντικαταρρεῦσαι τῷ βάθει. πολλάκις δὲ οὐ τοῦτο, ἀλλὰ βοή τις ἐξαίφνης φοβερά, οἷον ἀπὸ βροντῆς, ἐπιστᾶσα κατέπληξε τὸν ἄνθρωπον, καὶ συννεύσασα ἡ φύσις οὐκ ἴσχυσεν ἐφαπλῶσαι ἑαυτὴν καὶ τῇ οἰκείᾳ χρήσασθαι ἀποκριτικῇ δυνάμει πρὸς ἔκκρισιν τῶν λυπούντων· ἔστι δ' ὅτε καὶ ῥαγδαίας βροχῆς γενομένης τοῦτο συμβέβηκεν. οὐ δεῖ δὲ ἀποφαυλίζειν τὰ τοιαῦτα, ἐπειδὴ πάντα συμβαίνει ἐν τοῖς πράγμασιν. καὶ θυρίδος δέ τινος πλησίον τῆς κλίνης οὔσης εἰ τύχοι δι' αὐτῆς εἰσρεῦσαι ὕδωρ καὶ καταβρέξαι τὴν τοῦ ἀρρώστου στρωμνήν, ὡς ἐντεῦθεν μετακομισθῆναι τοῦτον μετὰ θορύβου τινὸς καὶ ταραχῆς, ἀνακοπῆναι συμβαίνει τὴν ὁρμὴν τῆς φύσεως καὶ τὸν ἱδρῶτα ἐπισχεθῆναι. τοῦτο οὖν ἐστιν ἀκουστέον καὶ τὰ ἔξωθεν.

Αὕτη ἐστὶν ἡ τοῦ δευτέρου προοιμίου σαφήνεια· ἐφεξῆς δὲ εἴπωμεν καὶ τὴν ἔννοιαν τοῦ ἀρχαίου. διὰ τούτου τοῦ προοιμίου βούλεται ὁ Ἱπποκράτης ἅπασαν σπουδὴν καὶ ἐπιμέλειαν καὶ φροντίδα καὶ ἀγρυπνίαν τὸν ἰατρὸν καταβάλλεσθαι, εἰ μέλλει τοῦ τέλους τῆς τέχνης, φημὶ δὴ τῆς ὑγείας, δημιουργὸς ἔσεσθαι. καὶ οὐ μόνον τὸν ἰατρὸν δεῖ τούτου τυχεῖν βουλόμενον τὰ δέοντα συνεισαγαγεῖν, ἀλλὰ καὶ τὸν νοσοῦντα καὶ τοὺς παρόντας καὶ τὰ ἔξωθεν εἰς μίαν συμφωνίαν συνεῖναι. σπουδαιότατον δέ φημι χρῆναι τοῦτον εἶναι διὰ τὸ ἀξίωμα τῆς ὕλης, διὰ τὸ τίμιον τοῦ ὑποκειμένου· ἄνθρωπος γὰρ τοῦτο, πάντων τῶν ἐπὶ γῆς τὸ τιμιώτατον· ὥστε ἡ περὶ τὸ ὑποκείμενον τοῦ ἰατροῦ ἀτυχία μεγάλων κακῶν γίνεται πρόφασις, θάνατον γὰρ ἀπεργάζεται.

Δεῖ δὲ καὶ τοῦτο εἰδέναι κατὰ τοῦτο τὸ προοίμιον, ὅτι δύο τινῶν ὄντων, τοῦ μὲν ἀμφιβαλλομένου, τοῦ δὲ ὁμολογουμένου, τὸ μὲν ἀκατασκεύαστον εἴασε, τὸ ὁμολογούμενον, λέγω δὴ τὸ δεῖν τὸν ἰατρὸν μετὰ πολλῆς σπουδῆς διδόναι ἑαυτὸν τὰ δέοντα ποιέοντα, ὡς ἂν τούτου πάντως γενησομένου, τὸ δὲ ἕτερον κατεσκεύασεν, ἀμφίβολον ὑπάρχον, φήσας ὅτι ἀλλὰ καὶ τοὺς νοσοῦντας καὶ τοὺς παρόντας καὶ τὰ ἔξωθεν. οἴεται γὰρ ὁ πολὺς ἄνθρωπος ἐν μόνῳ τῷ ἰατρῷ τὸ πᾶν τοῦ ἀποτελέσματος κεῖσθαι, οὐχ οὕτως δὲ ἔχει, ὡς ἡ παροῦσα ἔδειξεν ἔννοια.

Ἐπίστησον δὲ ἐν τούτῳ τῷ προοιμίῳ καὶ θαύμασον τὴν τέχνην τοῦ Ἱπποκράτους καὶ τὸ τούτου ἐνθύμημα. παντὸς γινομένου πράγματος τέσσαρά ἐστι γενεσιουργικὰ αἴτια, ποιητικὸν ὀργανικὸν ὑλικὸν τελικόν, ἔστι πρὸς τούτοις καὶ τὰ ὧν οὐκ ἄνευ λόγον ἔχοντα, τόπος φημὶ καὶ χρόνος. ταῦτα οὖν διὰ μιᾶς λέξεως ὁ Ἱπποκράτης ἐδήλωσε· διὰ μὲν γὰρ τοῦ εἰπεῖν δεῖ δὲ οὐ μόνον ἑωυτὸν παρέχειν πρὸς τὸν ἰατρὸν ἀποτεινόμενος τὸ ποιητικὸν τῆς ὑγείας ἐδήλωσεν αἴτιον· ἐπαγαγὼν δὲ τὰ δέοντα ποιέοντα τὸ τελικὸν εἰσήγαγεν, ἡ γὰρ τῶν δεόντων ποίησις ὑγείαν ἐργάζεται, ἥτις τέλος ἐστὶ τῆς ἰατρικῆς· εἶτα προσθεὶς καὶ τὸν νοσέοντα τὸ ὑλικὸν τέθηκε· διὰ δὲ τοῦ εἰπεῖν καὶ τοὺς παρεόντας τὸ ὀργανικὸν ἐσήμανεν· ἐπαγαγὼν δὲ καὶ τὰ ἔξωθεν τὰ ὧν οὐκ ἄνευ ἐπεκήρυξε, χρόνον φημὶ καὶ τόπον.

Ἐν οἷς εὕρηται ἡμῖν ἥ τε σαφήνεια τῶν λέξεων ἑκατέρου προοιμίου καὶ αὐτὴ ἡ

16 σπουδαιότατον – 18 τιμιώτατον] *cf.* Gal. In Aphor. I 1: XVII B 353,12–354,4 K.

3 *post* οἰκείᾳ *add.* φύσει Z 4 γιγνομένης Z 5 συμβέβηκεν] συννεύει γενέσθαι Z 7 ὕδωρ εἰσρεῦσαι Z εἰσρεῦσαν P καὶ *om.* P 8 καὶ] ἢ Z 9 τὴν *om.* Z ἐστιν *om.* P 11 εἴπομεν α 12 *post* τούτου *add.* τοίνυν Z 14 μέλλ *(ambig.)* A: μέλλοι Z 15 συναγαγεῖν Z 16 *post* συμφωνίαν *add.* πάντας Z 17 ἐχρῆν Z 18 *ante* γῆς *add.* τῆς Z 19 τοῦ ὑποκειμένου Z ἀποτυχία P 22 *ante* τὸ[I] *add.* καὶ Z 25 ὑπάρχον] εἶναι Z παρεόντας Z 29 *post* παντὸς *add.* γοῦν Z 30 *ante* τελικόν *add.* καὶ Z 32 γὰρ *om.* A 34 *post* τελικὸν *add.* αὖ Z 35 *post* εἶτα *add.* τούτοις Z 36 τέθηκε] πέφηνε Z ἀπεσήμηνεν Z

matter, finding the way out barred, flows back inward. Often there is another cause: there has been a sudden frightening noise, for instance of thunder, which has upset the patient; nature shrinks together and does not have the force to expand again and to use its own secretory faculty in order to excrete the harmful substances; this has also happened after a violent rainstorm. One should not make light of such things, for they all occur in actual fact. Again, if there is a window near the bed, and the rain comes in and makes the patient's bedclothes wet, so that he has to be removed from there with a certain amount of confusion and turmoil, the result may be that the impulse of nature is checked and the sweating suppressed. This is what we must understand by external circumstances.

So much to elucidate the wording of the second preface; let us next consider the ancient author's intention. What Hippocrates wants to say in this preface is that the physician must make every effort, apply all his care and attention, and be always on the alert, if he is to achieve the goal of the art, that is, health. And not only the physician must contribute his share to accomplish this, but the patient, the attendants and external factors should co-operate with him in complete harmony. Total commitment, in my opinion, is demanded of him because of the worth of his material, the value of the substance with which he deals: this is man, the most precious thing on earth; so that the physician's failure in handling his material is disastrous, its outcome being death.

Another point to be noticed with regard to this preface is that it consists of two statements, one controversial, the other generally admitted; he does not trouble to substantiate the one which we all admit, namely, that the physician should make every effort to do what is necessary – this he considers a matter of course –; but he does argue the other, questionable, point, when he says: but the patient, those around him, and external circumstances (must) also (co-operate). This is because most people believe that the result depends entirely on the doctor; wrongly, as the present observation proves.

Also worthy of notice and admiration in this preface is Hippocrates' technique and his way of reasoning. Everything in process of becoming has four generating causes, an efficient, an instrumental, a material and a final cause, and besides these there are the necessary concomitants, to wit, place and time. Hippocrates denoted each of these by one phrase: when he said, with reference to the physician, that not only he himself must be prepared, he indicated the efficient cause of health; when he added to do what is necessary, he introduced the final cause, since doing the necessary leads to health, which is the final goal of medicine; next, when he went on and the patient, he established the material cause; the words and those around him signify the instrumental cause; finally, by adding and external circumstances, he formally posits the necessary concomitants, time and place.

Thus far our clarification of the wording of the two prefaces, as well as of the

τοῦ συγγραφέως διάνοια· ἐφ' οἷς ἀκόλουθόν ἐστι τὴν αἰτίαν παραδοῦναι. ὁ βίος βραχὺς εἶπεν, ἡ δὲ τέχνη μακρή, ἢ ὅτι προτροπῆς χάριν τῷ λόγῳ ἐχρήσατο, ἵνα σπουδαίως τὴν τέχνην ἀναλεξώμεθα, μακρὰν οὖσαν, ἢ ὅτι «Ἐπειδὴ ὁ βίος βραχύς, ἡ δὲ τέχνη μακρή, ὁ δὲ καιρὸς ὀξὺς καὶ διὰ ταῦτα ταχέως ἀποδιδράσκει, δεῖ σε ἄγρυπνον εἶναι καὶ φροντιστικὸν καὶ πρόθυμον, οὐ γὰρ ἐνδέχεται τὸν βραδύνοντα κερδῆσαί τι.»

I 3 [I 2: IV 458,5–7 L.] Ἐν τῇσι ταραχῇσι τῆς κοιλίης καὶ τοῖσιν ἐμέτοισι τοῖσιν αὐτομάτως γιγνομένοισιν, εἰ μὲν οἷα δεῖ κενοῦσθαι κενοῦται, ξυμφέρει τε καὶ εὐφόρως φέρουσιν· ἢν δὲ μή, τοὐναντίον.

Ἄξιον ἐπιζητῆσαι, τίνος χάριν ἀπὸ γαστρὸς ἄρχεται· κοιλίαν γὰρ τὴν σιτοδόχον ἀκουστέον γαστέρα. καὶ λέγομεν πρὸς τοῦτο πρώτην μὲν αἰτίαν τοιαύτην· ἴσμεν, ὅτι ἡ πρώτη τῆς τροφῆς πέψις ἐν τῷ μορίῳ τούτῳ γίνεται· πάντα γὰρ τὰ καταπινόμενα εἰς αὐτὴν παραγίνονται πρῶτον κἀκεῖσε τὴν τῆς χυλοποιήσεως πέψιν ὑφίσταται· εἰκότως οὖν ἔδει αὐτὴν καὶ ἐν τῇ διδασκαλίᾳ πρώτην ἀπειληφέναι τάξιν. ἔστι δὲ καὶ ἄλλην αἰτίαν εἰπεῖν· τὰ τῆς γαστρὸς πάθη καὶ συνήθη ἡμῖν εἰσι καὶ διὰ τὴν συνήθειαν ἧττον λυποῦσιν. οὕτω γοῦν ἀκουστέον τῶν ἀνθρώπων ὁσημέραι λεγόντων «ἠπέπτησα», «ἐμπεπνευμάτωμαι», «κλυδωνισμοί μοι ἐγένοντο» ἢ «βορβορυγμοὶ» ἢ «στρόφοι» ἢ ὅσα τοιαῦτα, ἅτινα οὐδὲ ἰατρεύεσθαι φιλεῖ ἑτοίμως τῇ ἐντελεῖ πέψει ἀποκαθιστάμενα. ἐπεὶ οὖν συνήθη ἡμῖν ἐστι τὰ τοιαῦτα τῆς γαστρὸς πάθη, εἰκότως ἀπὸ γαστρὸς ἤρξατο. ἔστι δὲ καὶ ἄλλην αἰτίαν εἰπεῖν· οὐχ ἁπλῶς ἀπὸ γαστρὸς καὶ κατὰ πρῶτον λόγον ἄρχεται, ἀλλὰ περὶ κενώσεως ἤτοι καθάρσεως τεχνικῆς διαλαβεῖν προθέμενος, φημὶ δὴ τῆς δι' ὑπηλάτου φαρμάκου γιγνομένης, ἐπειδὴ ταύτην εὑρίσκει διὰ τῶν φυσικῶν ὑπονόμων ἀπαντῶσαν – φυσικοὶ δὲ ὑπόνομοι τῆς τοιαύτης ἐκκρίσεως αὐτή τε ἡ γαστήρ, τὰ τοῦ παντὸς σώματος τηνικαῦτα ὑποδεχομένη ῥεύματα, καὶ μετ' αὐτὴν ἔντερα λεπτὰ καὶ παχέα καὶ τὸ ἀπευθυσμένον –, εἰκότως ἠναγκάσθη ὑπὸ τῆς ἀκολουθίας τοῦ λόγου τῆς γαστρὸς μνημονεῦσαι ὡς ὄργανον τῆς τοιαύτης ἐκκρίσεως ὑπαρχούσης. ἔστι δὲ καὶ ἄλλην καλλίστην αἰτίαν εἰπεῖν· πάνυ τεχνικῶς ὁ συγγραφεὺς ἀπὸ γαστρὸς ἤρξατο, ἐπιστάμενος, ὅτι δύναται αὕτη κακῶς πάσχουσα τὰς τρεῖς ἀρχὰς τὰς πρωτίστας τοῦ ἡμετέρου σώματος εἰς συμπάθειαν ἀγαγεῖν, ἐγκέφαλόν φημι καὶ καρδίαν καὶ ἧπαρ. τὸν μὲν τῇ τῶν νεύρων συγγενείᾳ· πολλῶν γὰρ αἰσθητικῶν νεύρων μετέσχεν ἡ γαστήρ, καὶ μάλιστα κατὰ τὸ αὐτῆς στόμα, ὥστε ἑτοιμότατα τῆς ἐνδείας τοῦ παντὸς σώματος ἐπαισθάνεσθαι, ὡς μὴ λιμῷ διαφθαρῆναι λεληθότως τὸ ζῷον. τὴν δὲ καρδίαν τῇ γειτνιάσει· ἐπίκειται γὰρ ὁ στόμαχος τῇ ἀορτῇ καλουμένῃ ἀρτηρίᾳ, ἥτις

10–12 γίνεται] *v.* Theoph. In Aphor.: II 253,9–11 Dietz 15 ἔστι – 27 ὑπαρχούσης] *v.* Theoph. In Aphor.: II 253,7–9 Dietz 29sq. τὰς^{I} – ἧπαρ] *cf.* Gal. De loc. aff. V 1: VIII 298, 10–14 K. Steph. Ad Glauc.: I 246,8–9 Dietz

1 ὑφ' P οἷς] ἧς Z 2 μακρὰ Z 4 μακρὰ Z 8 εἰ] ἢν A^{2}Z *Hipp.*, *cf. infra, p. 54,35* 8sq. κενοῦσθαι κενοῦται] καθαίρεσθαι καθαίρωνται *Hipp.*, *cf. infra, p. 54,35* 9 κενοῦται] κενοῦνται Z φορέουσιν Z 10 *post* ἄρχεται *add.* καὶ φημὶ Z 13 κἀκεῖ γε Z 14 ὑφίσταται] πεπίστευται α 15 εἰσι] ἐστι Z 16 λυποῦσα Z 17 ἐμπνευμάτωμαι P βορβορισμοὶ Z 18 ἰατρεῦσαι Z 19 πέψει] ἀποπέψει Z 21 καὶ *om.* Z ἄρχεται λόγον Z 22 γενομένης α 25 ἔντερα] ἕτερα Z 26 ἠναγκάσθη] καὶ ἀνεγκάσθη Z *post* τῆς^{I} *add.* αὐτῆς Z 28 ἀπὸ γαστρὸς *om.* Z 32 ἑτοιμότατον P: ἑτοιμότ^{T} A 33 τῇ . . . καρδίᾳ Z

author's own meaning; it remains to explain the reason. Either Hippocrates intends the words Life is short, the art is long as an admonition to study the art of medicine diligently because of the length of the task; or else what he wants to say is: "Since life is short and the art long, and since the moment is swift and thus escapes us quickly, you must be watchful, alert and eager, for the tardy man can never gain anything."

I 3. In cases of disturbance of the belly and spontaneous vomiting, if the matter purged out is of the right kind, this is beneficial and easily tolerated; if not, the contrary.

A relevant question is why his first subject is the stomach; for belly here is to be understood as the stomach, the receptacle of food. The first reason we can mention is the following: as we know, the first digestion of food takes place in this part; whatever is swallowed reaches the stomach first and there undergoes the digestive process of conversion into chyle; it is therefore logical that it should have the first place also in instruction. Another reason one can give is that stomach complaints are familiar to us and thanks to that familiarity trouble us less. It is an everyday thing to hear people say: "I had an indigestion", "I have gas on the stomach", "I had splashings", "rumblings", "cramps", etc., things for which people usually do not even see a doctor, as they are set right by complete digestion. Thus our familiarity with such stomach troubles makes it natural for him to start with the stomach. A third reason we can mention is that (Hippocrates) does not begin with the stomach simply for its own sake; his object is to discuss artificial evacuation or purging, that is, by means of a suppository; and finding that it takes place through the natural channels – the natural channels for this form of excretion being the stomach itself, which at that time receives influxes from the entire body, and after it the small and the large intestine and the rectum – he was naturally forced by the course of his disquisition to refer to the stomach as an organ of this excretion. Another explanation, and the most satisfactory, is this: by beginning with the stomach the author shows his expertise, for he is aware that when the stomach is affected it can pass on this affection to the three first principles of our body, i.e. the brain, the heart and the liver. It affects the brain through the kindred nature of the nerves; for the stomach has many sensory nerves, especially at its upper orifice, so that it may readily perceive a deficiency in any part of the body, otherwise the organism could die of starvation without being aware of it. The stomach can affect the heart by its proximity, being situated next to the so-called aorta, which is the first of our arteries, springing from the

ἡμῖν ἐστιν ἡ πρώτη τῶν ἀρτηριῶν, ἀπὸ καρδίας βλαστάνουσα· ἔνθεν στομάχου πάσχοντος αἱ καλούμεναι καρδιακαὶ γίνονται συγκοπαί τε καὶ λιποψυχίαι διὰ τὸ τὴν καρδίαν διὰ μέσης τῆς ἀορτῆς εἰς συμπάθειαν ἄγεσθαι. ὅτι δὲ καὶ τὸ ἧπαρ κακῶς πασχούσῃ τῇ γαστρὶ συνδιατίθεται, οὐδένα οἶμαι ἀμφιβάλλειν τῶν νοῦν ἐχόντων, τῇ ὁμοιότητι τῆς ἐνεργείας εἰς συμπάθειαν ἀγόμενον. ἄμφω γὰρ κοινοεργεῖ· τῆς μὲν γὰρ ὕλης ἡ γαστὴρ τὴν χυλοποίησιν πεπίστευται, ἀπὸ δὲ ταύτης τὸ ἧπαρ τὴν ἀπὸ χυλοῦ εἰς αἷμα μεταβολὴν ἀπεργάζεται· ἀνάγκη οὖν πᾶσα κακῶς πασχούσης τῆς γαστρὸς ἀναγγελθῆναι τὸ πάθος τῷ ἥπατι διὰ μέσου τοῦ ἐν τῷ χυλῷ ὑπ' αὐτῆς πλημμεληθέντος, καὶ οὕτως αὐτὸ[ν] εἰς συμπάθειαν ἑλκυσθῆναι. ἀπὸ γαστρὸς οὖν ἄρχεται καὶ βούλεται περὶ τεχνικῆς καθάρσεως διαλεχθῆναι.

Ἰστέον δέ, ὅτι οἱ βλάπτοντες χυμοὶ τὸ ἡμέτερον σῶμα ἢ ποιότητι παρατρεπόμενοι ἀνιῶσιν ἢ ποσότητι εἰς ἀμετρίαν ἐκφερόμενοι. καθ' ἑκάτερον γὰρ ἡ βλάβη συνίσταται· καὶ ἧττον κακὸν καθ' ἑκάτερον βλαβῆναι τὸ σῶμα ἢ κατ' ἄμφω· διχῶς γὰρ ἐν ταῖς τοιαύταις βλάβαις πάσχει καὶ καταπίπτει ἡ δύναμις, καὶ τῇ ποιότητι τῆς ὕλης ἀνιωμένη καὶ δακνομένη καὶ τῇ ποσότητι βαρυνομένη καὶ καταβαπτιζομένη. πρόκειται δὲ νῦν τῷ Ἱπποκράτει τῆς κατὰ ποιότητα βλάβης τῶν χυμῶν ἀπαλλάξαι τὸ σῶμα. καὶ πῶς τοῦτο γίνεται; ἡνίκα καθάρωμεν τὸν ἐκτραπέντα χυμόν· καθαίρεται δὲ διὰ τῶν ὑπηλάτων καὶ καθαρτικῶν καλουμένων φαρμάκων. «Καὶ ποῖα ταῦτά ἐστιν;» ἴσως ἐρεῖς· οὔτε γὰρ πάντα ἕνα ἄγει χυμὸν οὔτε ἓν πάντας, ἀλλ' ἕκαστον ἰδίαν ἀντιπάθειαν καὶ ἐναντίωσιν πρὸς τόνδε ἢ τόνδε τὸν χυμὸν κέκτηται. χολαγωγὰ τοίνυν ἐστὶ καθαρτήρια τό τε τῆς ἀσκαμωνίας δάκρυον καὶ τὸ ἀψίνθιον καὶ ἡ ἀλόη καὶ τὰ παραπλήσια· φλεγμαγωγὰ δὲ ἀγαρικόν τε καὶ κολοκυνθὶς καὶ εὐφόρβιον καὶ λευκὸς ἐλλέβορος καὶ τὰ ὅμοια· μελαγχολικὸν δὲ κενοῖ λίθος Ἀρμένιος, ἐπίθυμον, χαμαίδρυον, μέλας ἐλλέβορος· τινὰ δὲ ὑδραγωγά ἐστι καὶ πνευμάτων καταρρηκτικά, οἷον πέπλιον, ὑδραγωγὸς λίθος, λαθυρίς, Κνίδιος κόκκος, ἡ λεπὶς τοῦ κεκαυμένου χαλκοῦ καὶ τὰ τούτοις παραπλήσια, ὧν ἐστι καὶ τὸ ἐλατήριον. ταῦτα εἴρηται ὥστε τῆς ὕλης ἡμᾶς τῶν καθαιρόντων στοιχείωσιν ἔχειν, κἀπειδὰν τοῦ λυποῦντος χυμοῦ κάθαρσιν παραλαβεῖν βουληθείημεν, τῷ οἰκείῳ καὶ ἁρμοδίῳ φαρμάκῳ χρήσασθαι.

Ἀλλ' ἴσως ἐρεῖς· «Καὶ πόθεν ἔχω τὸν τοιοῦτον χυμὸν διαγνῶναι;» διαγινώσκομεν οὖν τὸν καθάρσεως ἐπιδεόμενον χυμὸν ἀπὸ τριῶν τινων· ἀπὸ τοῦ εἴδους τοῦ νοσήματος, ἀπὸ τῶν συνόντων αὐτῷ συμπτωμάτων καὶ ἀπὸ τῶν συστοίχων. καὶ ἀπὸ μὲν τοῦ εἴδους τοῦ νοσήματος οὕτως· πρό⟨σ⟩σχες, εἰ τριταῖός ἐστιν ὁ πυρετὸς ἢ καῦσος ἢ ἴκτερος, ταῦτα γὰρ πάντα χολὴν ἔχει τὸ ὑλικὸν αἴτιον, καὶ δεῖ σε χολαγωγὸν ἐπιδοῦναι βοήθημα. εἰ δὲ ἀμφημερινός ἐστιν ὁ πυρετὸς ἢ κῶμα ἢ λήθαργος

1 ἔνθεν – 3 ἄγεσθαι] *cf.* Gal. De loc. aff. V 2: VIII 302,10–14 K. 16sq. πρόκειται – σῶμα] *v.* Gal. In Aphor. I 2: XVII B 357,6–8 K. 21 χολαγωγὰ – 26 ἐλατήριον] *cf.* Steph. Ad Glauc.: I 303,14–15 Dietz 33 πρόσσχες – 54,3 ὑπήλατον] *cf.* Gal. In Aphor. I 2: XVII B 360,7–13 K.

2 καρδιακαὶ] *spat. 16 litt. et* καὶ Z 4 τῶν] τὸν P 5 ἀγομένην A κοινοεργῆ A 6 τὴν[II]] τὸν Z 7 μεταβολὴν] χυλὸν Z 9 αὐτὸν AZ: *corr.* P 11 δέ *om.* A ποιότ(η)τα A 12 ποσότ(η)τα A: ποσότιτος P 17 καθαίρωμεν Z 21 ἀσκαμωνίας] ἀ- *eras. in* P 22 *post* παραπλήσια *add.* τούτοις Z ἀγαρικόν τε καὶ] τό τε ἀγαρικὸν καὶ ἡ Z *post* καὶ[IV] *add.* τὸ Z 24 *post* δὲ *add.* καὶ Z ἐστι] εἰσι A 26 τὸ κεκαυμένον χαλκοῦν Z *post* ταῦτα *add.* δὲ A 27 στοιχείωσιν ἔχειν] στοιχείων συνέχει Z 29 *ante* χρήσασθαι *add.* δεῖ Z 30 *post* διαγνῶναι *add.* καὶ φαμὲν Z 31 οὖν] τοίνυν Z *post* ἀπὸ[II] *add.* τε Z 32 συστοίχων] στοιχείων A 33 πρόσχες α: *om.* Z: *correxi* 34 ἴκτερος] ἕτερόν τι Z 35 *post* ἐπιδοῦναι *add.* τούτω Z

heart; hence, stomach complaints lead to so-called cardiac syncopes and fainting-fits, because through the intermediary of the aorta the heart is also affected. Finally, that a bad condition of the stomach communicates itself also to the liver, is a fact which, I believe, no sensible person will doubt; it is passed on to the liver as a result of the similarity of their functions. The two, indeed, work as a team: while the stomach has the task of converting the matter into chyle, the liver then takes over and brings about the change from chyle into blood; thus inevitably, when the stomach is affected, the disorder communicates itself to the liver through the defect in the chyle produced by the stomach, and so the liver is affected in turn. (Hippocrates') starting-point, then, is the stomach, and his subject is artificial purgation.

It should be remarked that humors which cause damage to our bodies do so either by qualitative deterioration or by quantitative excess. The damage may be done by either of the two; and it is a lesser evil for the body to be exposed to one only than to both; for in such cases our power (of resistance) suffers and collapses for two reasons, when it is not only tormented and stung by the quality of the matter, but also burdened and stifled by its quantity. Here, Hippocrates aims at freeing the body from the harm due to the quality of the humors. How is this brought about? By purging out the deteriorated humor by means of so-called suppositories and purgatives. You may well ask, which kind; for neither do all (purgatives) expel one particular humor nor does one and the same expel all; rather, each has a counteraction of its own and opposes this or that specific humor. Purges for bile, for instance, are resin of scammony, absinthe, aloe and the like; for phlegm, agaric, colocynth, spurge, white hellebore, etc.; atrabiliar humor is purged by Armenian limestone, epithymum, germander, black hellebore; some medicines discharge water and gases, such as wild purslane, water-purging stone, caper spurge, the Cnidian berry, flakes of burnt copper and similar drugs, one of which is elaterium. This list is meant to give us an elementary notion of the matter of purgatives, so that, when we want to proceed to purging out a harmful humor, we can use the proper and suitable drug.

Perhaps you will ask: "How can I diagnose such a humor?" There are three criteria by means of which we determine the humor that needs purging: the character of the disease, the symptoms that attend it, and correlative factors. The character of the disease can guide you as follows: observe whether the fever is a tertian, or a causus, or jaundice; if so, since all these have bile as their material cause, you must administer a purge for bile. If, on the other hand, it is a quotidian

ἤ τι τῶν τοιούτων, φλέγμα ἐστὶ τὸ βλάπτον, καὶ δεῖ σε φλεγμαγωγὸν δοῦναι φάρμακον. εἰ δέ γε τεταρταῖός ἐστιν ἢ μέλας ἢ ἴκτερος ἢ μελαγχολία, μελαγχολικός ἐστιν ὁ ἐνοχλῶν χυμὸς τῷ σώματι, καὶ κατὰ τοῦτο δεῖ σε ἁρμόσαι καὶ τὸ φάρμακον ὑπήλατον· ὥσπερ οὖν ἐπὶ τῶν ὑδεριώντων τὸν ἀσκίτην ὕδερον, ἐπειδὴ ὑγροῦ ἐστι περιουσία, ὑδραγωγοῖς χρώμεθα τοῖς καθαρσίοις. ἀπὸ δὲ τῶν συμπτωμάτων οὕτως· ἐὰν εὕρῃς ἐν τῷ ἀνθρώπῳ δίψαν ἀφόρητον καὶ ἀγρυπνίαν πολλὴν καὶ ζέσεως αἴσθησιν καὶ βρασμόν τινα περὶ τὰ ὑποχόνδρια γινόμενον, χολώδη ἐστὶ τὰ τοιαῦτα συμπτώματα, καὶ δεῖ σε τοῖς χολὴν κενοῦσι χρήσασθαι. εἰ δὲ μηδὲν τούτων ἐνοχλεῖ τῷ σώματι, ἄδιψος δὲ πάντῃ ἐστὶν ὁ ἄνθρωπος καὶ πλαδῶντα ἔχει τὸν στόμαχον καὶ σίελον πολὺ ἀποπτύει καὶ κενεμεσίας ὑφίσταται καταφορικός τε καὶ κωματώδης καὶ ὑπνηλός ἐστι, φλέγμα ἐνοχλεῖ τῷ τοιούτῳ, καὶ δεῖ σε τοῖς φλέγμα κενοῦσι χρήσασθαι. ἀπὸ δὲ τῶν συστοίχων οὕτως· ἐπισκοπήσεις γὰρ ὥρας καὶ χώρας καὶ ἡλικίας καὶ κράσεις καὶ βίους καὶ τὰ λοιπά. εἰ μὲν γὰρ ἀκμαστικός ἐστι τὴν ἡλικίαν ὁ κάμνων καὶ ἡ ὥρα θερινὴ καὶ τὸ κατάστημα θερμὸν καὶ τὸ χωρίον ὁμοίως καὶ ὁ βίος ὑπόκειται ἄγρυπνος καὶ φροντιστικὸς καὶ ταλαίπωρος καὶ δίαιτα ἐνδεὴς καὶ ἐδεσμάτων προσφορὰ θερμοτέρων καὶ τὰ τοιαῦτα, δῆλον, ὅτι χολή ἐστιν ἡ πλεονάζουσα καὶ ταύτην δεῖ σε καθᾶραι. εἰ δ' ἀνάπαλιν ὥρα μὲν ὑπόκειται χειμερία, χώρα δὲ ψυχρὰ καὶ τὸ κατάστημα τοιοῦτον καὶ ἡλικία γεροντικὴ ἢ παρακμαστικὴ καὶ ὁ βίος ἀνειμένος καὶ ἀργὸς καὶ ἀφρόντιστος καὶ ἀταλαίπωρος καὶ δίαιτα ἐν πλησμοναῖς καὶ μέθαις καὶ λουτρῶν χρῆσις μετὰ κόρον πρὸ πέψεως καὶ τὰ τοιαῦτα, δῆλον, ὅτι φλέγματος ὑπόκειται περιουσία καὶ δεῖ σε τοῦτο κενῶσαι.

Χρὴ μέντοι καὶ τοῦτο εἰδέναι, ὅτι πρὸς τὴν κατὰ ποιότητα ἐκτροπὴν τῶν χυμῶν ἐνιστάμενοι καὶ ταύτης τὸ σῶμα δι' ὑπαγωγῆς λυτρούμενοι, καθαίρειν λεγόμεθα· πρὸς δὲ τὴν κατὰ ποσότητα ἀμετρίαν ἐνιστάμενοι καὶ τοῦ ταύτης βάρους τὸ κάμνον σῶμα κουφίζοντες, κενοῦν λεγόμεθα. τὰ μὲν οὖν τὸ πρῶτον ποιοῦντα φάρμακα καθαρτικὰ λέγονται, ἀποκαθαίρουσι γὰρ τὸ σῶμα τῆς διοχλούσης αὐτὸ κακοχυμίας· τὰ δὲ τὸ δεύτερον ποιοῦντα κενωτικὰ λέγονται.

Ἀλλὰ ταῦτα μὲν ἡ τέχνη ἐργάζεται· ἡ δέ γε φύσις προθεμένη κάθαρσιν ποιῆσαι οὐδενὶ τούτων ἐνδιατρίβει οὐδὲ δεῖται ζητῆσαι εἶδος νοσήματος ἢ διαφορὰν συμπτωμάτων ἢ συνδρομὴν συστοίχων πρὸς τὸ γνῶναι τὸν παραληπτέον χυμόν, ἀλλ' αὐτοδίδακτος οὖσα καὶ ἑαυτὴν γινώσκουσα δεόντως οἰκονομεῖ τὰ οἰκεῖα ἔργα καὶ ἐπανίσταται κατὰ τοῦ λυποῦντος χυμοῦ καὶ τοῦτον ἐκκαθαίρει τοῦ σώματος.

Εἰ δὲ εἴπῃς· «Καὶ πόθεν δῆλον αὐτομάτου καθάρσεως γενομένης, εἴτε φυσικῶς αὕτη ἀπήντησεν εἴτε βίᾳ συμπτώματος γέγονε;» πρὸς τοῦτό σοι ὁ Ἱ π π ο κ ρ ά τ η ς φησίν· ἢ ν μ ὲ ν ο ἷ α δ ε ῖ κ α θ α ί ρ ε σ θ α ι κ α θ α ί ρ ο ν τ α ι, ξ υ μ φ έ ρ ε ι τ ε κ α ὶ ε ὐ φ ό ρ ω ς φ έ ρ ο υ σ ι ν· ἢ ν δ ὲ μ ή, τ ο ὐ ν α ν τ ί ο ν, τουτέστιν ἐκ τῆς ἑπομένης εὐφορίας τοῦτο

11 ἀπὸ – 21] *cf.* Gal. In Aphor. I 2: XVII B 359,10–360,7 K. 22–25 λεγόμεθα] *v.* Gal. In Aphor. I 2: XVII B 357,14–358,2 K. Theoph. In Aphor.: II 253,12–14 Dietz 28–32] *cf.* Gal. In Aphor. I 2: XVII B 358,8–14 K.

2 ἢ^{I} – ἐστιν^{II} *om.* P ἢ^{II} *om.* A 5 ἐὰν] ἤνπερ Z 9 τὸν στόμαχον ἔχει Z πολὺ *om.* Z 11 τοιούτῳ] ζώω Z φλέγμα κενοῦσι] φλεγμαγωγοῖς φαρμάκοις Z 16 *post* πλεονάζουσα *add.* τῶ σώματι Z 17 καθαίρειν Z 18 *post* ἢ *add.* καὶ Z 20 χρήσεις A κόρου Z 25 κάμνον *om.* Z τὸ] τὰ Z 26 *post* καθαρτικὰ *add.* ταῦτα Z λέγ(ε)ται A διενοχλούσης Z αὐτῶ Z 28 καθάρσιον A 31 αὐτὴν Z δέοντος P 33 Εἰ δὲ εἴπῃς *deest in* A: εἰ δ' ἴσως εἴποις Z γενομένης *om.* Z 34 συμπτώματα α 35 δή A καθαίρωνται Z^{2}

fever, a coma, lethargy or something similar, phlegm is the cause of the trouble, and you must prescribe a drug that purges out phlegm. If it is quartan fever, black fever, jaundice or an atrabiliar condition, it is the atrabiliar humor which afflicts the body, and you must give a medicine adapted to this, in the form of a suppository; similarly, in cases of the dropsy called ascites, which is an excess of moisture, we apply medicines that discharge water. The symptoms can be used (for the purpose of diagnosis) in cases such as these: if in a patient you find intolerable thirst, a great lack of sleep, and a sensation of burning heat, a kind of boiling around the hypochondrium, those are bilious symptoms and you must use cures to evacuate bile. If there are in the body no troubles of this kind at all, but the patient is entirely without thirst, has a splashy stomach, spits out a great deal of saliva, has fits of vomiturition and is torpid, comatose and sleepy, this man is bothered by phlegm and you have to use a drug to drain it off. As regards correlative factors, you will consider the season, the region, the age, the temperament, the occupation, and so forth. For example, if the patient is in his prime, the season is summer, the weather hot, the region also hot, and if the man's life is one of little sleep, much worry, hard work, while his diet is spare and the food he takes is on the hot side, etc., it is obvious that there is a surplus of bile and that this has to be purged. If, conversely, the season is winter, the region cold and the weather too, if the patient is old or past his prime and his life is an easy and idle one, free from worry and toil, and if further he has a habit of excessive food, heavy drinking, and bathing after an abundant meal before it is digested, and so on, then of course you have to do with an excess of phlegm, and this is what you must evacuate.

It should further be observed that, when we oppose the qualitative deterioration of the humors and rid the body of it by clearing them out downwards, we are said to "purge"; but when we oppose excess in quantity and relieve the ailing body of its burden, the word is "evacuate". Drugs that do the former are called "purgatives", because they purify the body of the unwholesome humors that disturb it, while those that bring about the latter are called "evacuants".

These, however, are things with which medicine is occupied; as for nature, when it sets itself to effect a purge, it does not bother with any of these and has no need to study the character of the disease, the diversity of the symptoms, or the concurrence of correlative factors to decide which humor has to be dealt with, but being self-taught and knowing itself, it arranges its own affairs in the proper way, fights its battle against the troublesome humor and clears it out of the body.

Now if you ask, "How does it become clear, when a spontaneous purge takes place, whether it has come about naturally or forcibly, as the result of one of the symptoms?" Hippocrates' answer is: If the matter purged out is of the right kind, this is beneficial and easily tolerated; if not, the contrary, in other words, you can infer it from the resulting feeling of well-being. If such a

γνώσῃ. ταύτης γὰρ ἐπακολουθούσης ἀβίαστος πάντως ἡ κάθαρσις γίνεται· εἰ δὲ βίᾳ συμπτώματος ἀπαντήσει, οὐ μόνον εὐφορία οὐχ ἕψεται, ἀλλὰ καὶ πολλῶν κακῶν αὔξησίς τε καὶ ἐπίδοσις ἔσται. τί οὖν φαμεν; ἐπὶ πάσῃ φυσικῇ κενώσει πάντως εὐφορία ἕπεται, οὐχ ὁμοίως δέ, ἀλλ' ἢ παραχρῆμα ἢ μετ' οὐ πολὺ ὕστερον, ὅπερ γίνεται διὰ δύο αἰτίας· ἢ γὰρ δι' ἔκλυτον καὶ βλα⟨κι⟩κὸν καὶ πλαδαρὸν ἦθος ψυχῆς ἀνεπαίσθητος πρὸς τὸ παρὸν ἡ εὐφορία καὶ ἀπαλλαγὴ τῶν κακῶν εἶναι δοκεῖ, ἢ διὰ τὸν κενούμενον χυμὸν τοῦτο συμβαίνει, καὶ τοῦτο διχῶς, ἢ διὰ τὴν σύστασιν αὐτοῦ ἢ διὰ τὴν ποιότητα. διὰ μὲν τὴν σύστασιν, ἡνίκα πάχος ὑπόκειται· ἐπὶ γὰρ τῶν ἐκκρίσεων τῶν παχέων χυμῶν μὴ ὑφ' ἓν καὶ ἀθρόως γινομένης τῆς καθάρσεως, ἀλλὰ καταμεριζομένης κομματικῶς ἤτοι κατ' ὀλίγον προβαινούσης ἡ γινομένη ἀπαλλαγὴ λανθάνει τὴν αἴσθησιν, ἄχρις ὅτου τὸ πᾶν ὑπαντήσει κεφάλαιον ἀθροιζόμενον καὶ τῷ κοινῷ πέρατι τὰ τῆς εὐφορίας παρακολουθήσει. διὰ δὲ τὴν ποιότητα τοῦ κενουμένου ὑπαντᾷ ὕστερον ἡ εὐφορία τρόπῳ τοιῷδε· ἔσθ' ὅτε δριμὺς ἐσχάτως ἐστὶ χυμὸς ὁ κενούμενος, καὶ τῇ παρόδῳ δάκνων καὶ ἀνιῶν τὰ μόρια, δι' ὧν ἐκκρίνεται, ὀδύνης τινὸς καὶ ἀνίας τούτοις ἐγκαταλείπει διάθεσιν. ἀνάγκη γὰρ ἐπὶ τῶν τοιούτων χυμῶν πρότερον τὴν ἐντεθεῖσαν ὀδύνην τοῖς μορίοις παύσασθαι καὶ οὕτω τὴν τῆς εὐφορίας ἐπακολουθῆσαι συναίσθησιν. καθαίρει δὲ ἡ φύσις τοὺς ἐν ἡμῖν χυμοὺς τῇ ἀποκριτικῇ χρωμένη δυνάμει· ταύτῃ γὰρ ἐπεγειρομένῃ χρῆται καὶ τὴν τῶν λυπούντων ἀποτρίβεται βλάβην. δεῖ τοίνυν τὸν ἰατρὸν μιμητὴν τῆς φύσεως ὑπάρχοντα τεχνικὴν κάθαρσιν παραλαβεῖν προθέμενον εἰς εὐφορίαν ἀγαγεῖν τὸν κάμνοντα. πῶς δὲ ποιήσεις εὐφορίαν; δηλονότι τοῦ λυποῦντος χυμοῦ τὴν κάθαρσιν ποιούμενος.

Ἐν τῇσι ταραχῇσι τῆς κοιλίης. ταραχὴν κοιλίας ἐνταῦθα καλεῖ τὴν εἰς γαστέρα γινομένην ἀθρόαν τῶν χυμῶν συνδρομὴν ἀπὸ παντὸς τοῦ σώματος· κοιλίαν δὲ τὴν σιτοδόχον ὀνομάζει. ἔστι δὲ τροπικὴ ἡ λέξις ἀπὸ τῆς ἐν θαλάσσῃ ταραχῆς τῶν ὑδάτων ληφθεῖσα.

Καὶ τοῖσιν ἐμέτοισι τοῖσιν αὐτομάτως γινομένοισιν. τοῦτο δυνατὸν καὶ πρὸς τὸ ἄνω συνάψαι καὶ καθ' ἑαυτὸ ἐξηγήσασθαι. πρὸς μὲν τὸ ἀνωτέρω οὕτως· διὰ τοῦ ταραχὴν ἐν τῇ γαστρὶ γενέσθαι καὶ συγκίνησιν τῶν χυμῶν παρεδήλωσε τῶν ἐκ τοῦ παντὸς σώματος εἰς αὐτὴν εἰσρεόντων διὰ τὴν εὐπάθειαν τοῦ στομάχου· ἐνέφηνε δὲ τὴν τοιαύτην τοῦ στομάχου εὐπάθειαν ἐμέτου μνημονεύσας, τοῦ στομάχου γὰρ τοῦτο σύμπτωμα. ἰδία δὲ αὐτοῦ ἐξήγησις λεγέσθω τοιαύτη· ἐπὶ πάσης μὲν κενώσεως διὰ γαστρὸς γινομένης ταραχὴ προηγεῖται, κατ' ἐξαίρετον δὲ ἐπὶ τῶν ἐμέτων διὰ τὸ πλούσιον τῶν ἐν τῷ στομάχῳ καταφυομένων αἰσθητικῶν νεύρων. μήποτε δὲ καὶ ἑτέρως ἔστιν ἐξηγήσασθαι τὸ χωρίον, καὶ ταραχὴν μὲν γαστρὸς ἐννοῆσαι οὐ μόνον τὴν εἰς αὐτὴν συνδρομὴν τῶν χυμῶν, ἀλλὰ καὶ τὴν δι' αὐτῆς ἔκκρισιν· τὰς γὰρ τοιαύτας κενώσεις ταραχὰς εἰώθαμεν ὀνομάζειν. ἐπεὶ δὲ τῶν εἰς αὐτὴν ἀθροιζομένων χυμῶν διττή ἐστιν ἡ ἔκκρισις, ἡ μὲν δι' ἐντέρων, ἡ δὲ διὰ στομάχου καὶ στόματος, ἑκατέραν τούτων προθέμενος διαλαβεῖν ὁ Ἱπποκράτης διὰ μὲν τῆς ταραχῆς τὴν κάτω γινομένην ἐδήλωσεν ἔκκρισιν, διὰ δὲ τῶν ἐμέτων τὴν

1 διαγνώσῃ Z 5 βλακὸν ω: *correxi* ἀναπαίσθητος Z 6 *post* καὶ *add.* ἡ Z 8 *ante* διὰ *add.* καὶ Z τὴν *om.* Z 9 καταμεριζομένην α 10 κομματικὸς Z γενομένη P λανθάνη P 11 ὑπαντῆσαι A 12 κενωμένου Z 14 *ante* ὀδύνης *add.* καὶ α 17 καθαίρει] ἀνάγκη Z 18sq. τῇ . . . βλάβη Z 20 προϊέμενον ω: *correxi* 22 κοιλίας] κοιλίης Z 24 ἡ λέξις, τροπικὴ Z 25 ὑδάτων] κυμάτων Z 27 καὶ πρὸς τὸ] τῷ Z *ante* πρὸς^{II} *add.* καὶ Z τὸ^{II}] τῷ AZ: *corr.* Z^2 ἀνωτέρω] ἄνω Z 28 *ante* τοῦ *add.* τὴν Z 29 εἰσιόντων Z 30 δὲ] γὰρ Z τὴν *om.* Z 32 γενομένης P

feeling follows, the purge is definitely unconstrained; but if it is due to the forcible action of a symptom, not only will euphoria fail to appear, but many evils will develop and increase. What we mean is that any natural evacuation is necessarily followed by euphoria, not always, however, at the same time, but either immediately or a little later; this can have two causes: either it is due to weakness, dullness and lack of resilience in the patient's psyche that the well-being and the deliverance from his troubles remain unnoticed for the moment, or else the humor that is evacuated is responsible; here again, there are two possibilities: the cause is either its consistency or its quality. Its consistency, in cases of a thick humor, because in the excretion of thick humors, when purgation does not occur all at once and simultaneously, but comes by fits and starts or proceeds gradually, the resulting relief remains unperceived, until all the matter has gathered and come out, and the feeling of euphoria follows at the end of the entire process. The quality of the evacuated matter, on the other hand, may delay the sensation of well-being under circumstances such as these: sometimes the evacuated humor is extremely acrid, and in passing through it stings and irritates the parts through which it is excreted, leaving in them a feeling of pain and irritation. When humors are of this kind, the pain caused to those parts must cease first and only then can the awareness of euphoria follow. Nature purges the humors in us by using its secretory faculty; when this is activated, it makes use of it to get rid of the harmful effects of noxious matter. Therefore the physician as an imitator of Nature must resort to artificial purgation, in order to give the patient that sense of well-being. How can you achieve this? Obviously by purging out the troublesome humor.

In cases of disturbance of the belly. What is here called a disturbance of the belly is a simultaneous inflow into the stomach of humors from the entire body; by belly he means the receptacle of food. The word (disturbance) is metaphorical, being transferred from the disturbed waters of the sea.

And spontaneous vomiting. These words can be both linked with the preceding ones and explained by themselves. With the preceding words they are linked as follows: by referring to a disturbance of the stomach (Hippocrates) implied a concentrated motion of humors from the entire body into the stomach, due to its sensitivity; and he indicated this sensitivity of the stomach by mentioning vomition, a symptom which belongs to the stomach. By themselves they can be interpreted thus: any evacuation through the belly is preceded by a disturbance, but especially so in the case of vomition because of the great number of sensory nerves that are implanted in the stomach. Perhaps another explanation of the passage is possible: by disturbance of the belly we can understand, not only the gathering in it of the humors, but also their excretion through it; it is indeed customary to call this kind of evacuation a disturbance. Now since there are two ways in which the humors collected there can be secreted, one through the intestines, the other through the stomach and the mouth, Hippocrates intended to deal with both of these and therefore he used the term "disturbance" for excretion downwards and "vomiting" for excretion upwards, it being understood that

ἄνω, ὡς ἂν τοῦ ἑπομένου, φημὶ δὴ τῆς εὐφορίας, καθ' ἑκάτερον τρόπον κενώσεως ἐπακολουθοῦντος ὁμοίως.

Αὐτόματον δὲ δηλοῖ οὐ τὸ ὑφ' ἑαυτοῦ καὶ ἀναιτίως γινόμενον, ἀλλὰ τὸ ἄδηλον πρὸς τὴν αἴσθησιν ἔχον τὴν ποιήσασαν αἰτίαν, ὅπερ ἐστὶ τὴν φυσικήν. αὐτόματον οὖν κάθαρσιν ἐνταῦθα καλεῖ ὁ Ἱπποκράτης τὴν ὑπὸ τῆς φύσεως γινομένην πρὸς ἀντιδιαστολὴν τῆς τεχνικῆς. κέχρηται ⟨δὲ⟩ καὶ ἡ τέχνη οὐ μόνον ὑπηλάτοις καθαρσίοις, ἀλλὰ καὶ ἐμετικοῖς.

[I 2: IV 458,7–8 L.] Οὕτω καὶ κενεαγγείη εἰ μὲν οἷα δεῖ κενοῦσθαι κενοῦται, ξυμφέρει. ἰστέον, ὅτι κενεάγγειά ἐστιν ἡ τῶν ἀγγείων κένωσις, ἥτινι εὐθέως ἕπεται σύμπτωσις. γίνεται δὲ διχῶς· ἢ γὰρ ὑπὸ ἀμέτρου κενώσεως συμβαίνει ἢ ὑπὸ λιμαγχονίας. φαίνεται δὲ κἀνταῦθα περὶ καθάρσεως διαλεγόμενος, ἀλλ' οὐ φυσικῆς, ὡς ἀνωτέρω ἐδήλωσεν ἅτε δὴ τοῦ αὐτομάτου μνημονεύσας, ἀλλὰ περὶ τεχνικῆς, ὡς δείκνυται διὰ τῶν ἑπομένων. ἐπιφέρει γάρ· [I 2: IV 458,9–10 L.] ἐπιβλέπειν οὖν δεῖ καὶ ὥρην καὶ χώρην καὶ ἡλικίην καὶ νούσους, ἐν ᾗσι δεῖ ἢ οὔ. τούτων ἡ τέχνη δεῖται, ὡς ἐν τῇ θεωρίᾳ εἰρήκαμεν, πρὸς τὸ διαγνῶναι τὸν ἐκτραπέντα κατὰ ποιότητα χυμόν. ταῦτα δέ ἐστιν ἡ τῶν συστοίχων σειρά· τῶν γὰρ κυριωτέρων μνημονεύσας πάντα συμπεριέλαβε, καὶ τὴν τῶν νοσημάτων καὶ τῶν συμπτωμάτων φύσιν, ἀφ' ὧν τὴν ἔνδειξιν τῆς καθάρσεως ποιεῖσθαι ὑπεθέμεθα. τοῦτο οὖν ἐστιν, ὃ λέγει ὁ Ἱπποκράτης, ὅτι ἐπιβλέπων εἰς τὰ νοσήματα καὶ τὰ συμπτώματα καὶ τὰ αἴτια καὶ τὰ σύστοιχα δυνήσῃ διαγνῶναι τὸν δεόμενον καθάρσεως χυμόν.

Ἐν ᾗσι δεῖ ἢ οὔ. λέγει, ὅτι δεῖ σε διαγνῶναι τὸν λυποῦντα χυμὸν καὶ κατὰ τοῦτον δοῦναι τὸ φάρμακον· τοῦτο δὲ διαγινώσκεις ἐκ τοῦ εἴδους τοῦ νοσήματος καὶ ἐκ τῶν συστοίχων καὶ ἐκ τῶν συμπτωμάτων. ἐν ᾗσι δεῖ ἢ οὔ, τουτέστιν ἐν αἷς ἡλικίαις καὶ χώραις καὶ ὥραις καὶ ἐν οἷς συμπτώμασι καὶ ἐν αἷς νόσοις δεῖ σε καθᾶραι χολὴν ἢ οὔ.

I 4 [I 3: IV 458,11–12 L.] Ἐν τοῖσι γυμναστικοῖσιν αἱ ἐς ἄκρον εὐεξίαι σφαλεραί, ἢν ἐν τῷ ἐσχάτῳ ἔωσιν.

Διαλεχθεὶς περὶ καθάρσεως τῆς ἐν ποιότητι ἀνιώσης τὸ σῶμα λέγει νῦν καὶ περὶ τῆς κατὰ ποσότητα τὸ σῶμα ἀνιώσης τῶν χυμῶν ἀμετρίας· καὶ λαμβάνει ἐν τῷ λόγῳ ὑπόθεσιν πληθώραν τὴν ἐν αἱματικῷ χυμῷ πλεονάζοντι γινομένην καὶ τῇ ποσότητι βλάπτουσαν, ἣν καὶ διὰ κενώσεως ἤτοι φλεβοτομίας θεραπεύει. καὶ μὴ εἴπῃς ὅτι «Τὸ αἷμα φίλιον ὂν καὶ οἰκεῖον καὶ προσηνὲς καὶ τὴν ζωὴν ἡμῶν συντηροῦν πῶς βλάπτον ὑπόκειται;» ἀλλ' ἐννόησον, ὅτι καὶ τὸ ἔλαιον, τροφὴ τῆς φλογὸς ὑπάρχον, πολὺ κατ' αὐτῆς ἐπιχεόμενον καταπνίγει ταύτην καὶ ἀποσβέννυσιν. οὕτως οὖν καὶ τὸ αἷμα ἐντὸς μὲν τῶν ὅρων τῆς συμμετρίας περιγραφόμενον φίλιον τῇ φύσει

4 αὐτόματον – 6 τεχνικῆς] *v.* Theoph. In Aphor.: II 253,18–19 Dietz 11sq. φαίνεται – τεχνικῆς] *v.* Theoph. In Aphor.: II 254,13–14. 17–19 Dietz 13sq. ἐπιβλέπειν – οὔ] *v.* Theoph. In Aphor.: II 255,3–5 Dietz 15 ὡς – εἰρήκαμεν] *v. supra*, p. 52,30–54,21 28–29 ἀμετρίας] *v.* Gal. In Aphor. I 3: XVII B 362,5–7 K. Theoph. In Aphor.: II 258,10–12 Dietz

1 δὴ] δὲ Z 4 *ante* αἰτίαν *add.* τὴν Z 6 δὲ *add.* P 8 *ante* καὶ *add.* δὴ Z εἰ] ἢν Z *Hipp.* κενοῦσθαι κενοῦται] γίνεσθαι γίνηται *Hipp.* κενοῦται] κενοῦνται Z 11 φέρεται Z 14 νόσους P 16 συστοίχων] στοιχείων α 18 ὑποθώμεθα Z 21 λυποῦντα] δεόμενον Z 22 τοῦτον] τοῦτο A 26 εἰς α: ἐπ' *Hipp., item infra, pp. 62,20. 31; 170,11* 29 λαμβάνειν Z 34 *ante* πολὺ *add.* ὅταν Z

the attendant phenomenon of euphoria presents itself equally in both forms of evacuation.

Spontaneous is not what happens of its own accord and without cause, but anything of which the efficient cause – that is to say, the natural one – escapes our perception. What Hippocrates calls here a spontaneous purge is therefore a purge effectuated by nature, as opposed to an artificial one. The art, too, uses not only suppositories as purgatives, but emetics as well.

Similarly with emptying of the vessels: if the matter evacuated is of the right kind, it is beneficial. Note that "emptying of the vessels" means evacuation of the vessels, which is immediately followed by a collapse. It has a twofold origin: it is brought about either by immoderate evacuation or by excessive dieting. Once more (Hippocrates') subject seems to be purgation, not, however, the natural process, which he must have referred to above, since he spoke of spontaneous, but the artificial kind, as the sequel proves. For he continues: One must therefore consider the season, the place, the age and the disease, in which to act or not to act. These are the criteria the art needs, as we said in the general discussion, to determine the humor that has deteriorated as regards its quality. It is the list of correlative factors; by mentioning the principal ones he included everything, also the character of the diseases and of the symptoms, from which we instructed you to take your indication in purging. What Hippocrates means, then, is this: By considering the diseases, the symptoms, the causes and the correlative factors you will be able to diagnose the humor that needs purging.

In which to act or not to act. I.e., you must diagnose the noxious humor and administer your purgative accordingly; and the way to diagnose it is on the ground of the character of the disease, the correlative factors and the symptoms. In which to act or not to act, that is to say, in what age groups and regions and seasons and with what symptoms and for what diseases you should purge out bile or not.

I 4. In athletes a top condition is dangerous, when it has reached the extreme limit.

After discussing purgation of humors which by their quality trouble the body, he now passes on to the excess of humors which does so by quantity; as a case in point he takes plethora, which consists in a superabundance of the sanguine humor and which causes harm through quantity; he treats it by evacuation, i.e. bleeding. Do not say: "How can blood, which is benign, natural and beneficial to us, which maintains our lives, be thought of as something harmful?" Think of oil, which feeds the flame; yet, if too much is poured on the flame, it chokes it and quenches it. Similarly blood, if kept within the limits of right proportion, is benign

καθίσταται, ἐκτρεπόμενον δὲ καὶ εἰς ἀμετρίαν περιγενόμενον πολέμιον καὶ βλαπτικὸν αὐτῇ εὑρίσκεται. πάσας γὰρ τὰς ἐν ἡμῖν δυνάμεις βλάψαι δύναται, ψυχικάς, φυσικάς, ζωτικάς. καὶ τῶν ψυχικῶν τὰς ἡγεμονικάς, αἰσθητικὰς δηλαδὴ καὶ κινητικάς. οὕτω γοῦν οἱ πλήθει αἵματος περιρρεόμενοι τὸ σῶμα, εἰς ὄγκον ἄμετρον αὐτοῦ ἐκτρεπομένου, δυσκίνητοι γίνονται μηδὲ τὸ τοῦ σώματος ἄχθος φέρειν δυνάμενοι· τὸ γὰρ ἡμέτερον σῶμα ἐξ ὀχοῦντος καὶ ὀχουμένου σύγκειται, καὶ ὀχοῦσι μὲν αἱ δυνάμεις αἱ κινητικαί, ὀχεῖται δὲ τὸ σῶμα. οὐ μὴν ἀλλὰ καὶ τὰς αἰσθητικὰς βλάπτει δυνάμεις τὸ πλῆθος τοῦ αἵματος, παροράσεις ἐμποιοῦν ποιοτήτων, ἀτμῶν ἀναθυμιάσεις καὶ βαρυηκοΐας καὶ ναρκώσεις ἀλλοκότους τε γεύσεις. μεθαρμόζει δὲ καὶ τὰς λογικὰς πρὸς τὸ χεῖρον· οὔτε γὰρ λογίζεσθαι δεόντως οὔτε μὴν μνημονεύειν ἢ φαντάζεσθαι ἀμέμπτως δύνανται κατακλυζομένου τοῦ ψυχικοῦ πνεύματος καὶ παχυνομένου τῷ πλήθει τοῦ αἵματος. ἀδικεῖ δὲ τὰς ζωτικὰς τῇ πληρώσει τῶν ἀρτηριῶν διαστέλλεσθαι καὶ συστέλλεσθαι ἀμέμπτως μὴ δυναμένων· πνιγμὸς οὖν τὸ τηνικαῦτα ἀπειλεῖται, καὶ τοῦτο γὰρ καλῶς ἐν ἑτέρῳ ὑπ' αὐτοῦ εἴρηται· «καὶ φλεβῶν ἀπολήψεις πνιγμὸν ἐμποιέουσιν»· εἴωθε γὰρ ὁ Ἱπποκράτης ὁμωνύμως καὶ τὰς ἀρτηρίας φλέβας ὀνομάζειν. καταλύει δὲ καὶ τὰς φυσικὰς δυνάμεις τὸ πλῆθος τοῦ αἵματος· πεπληρωμένων γὰρ τῶν ἀρτηριῶν, πνιγομένου τοῦ ἐμφύτου θερμοῦ ἅτε μὴ ῥιπιζομένου, συμβαίνει παχυμερὲς τοῦτο κατεψυγμένον χωρεῖν τῇ γαστρὶ καὶ βλάπτειν αὐτὴν εἰς πέψιν· ἧστινος ἀποτυγχανούσης βλάπτεται τὰ λοιπὰ ἐξ ἀνάγκης πάντα, ἐξαιμάτωσις, ἀνάδοσις, πρόσθεσις, θρέψις καὶ τὰ λοιπά· ἀτροφούντων δὲ τῶν μορίων καταβάλλονται αὐτῶν αἱ φυσικαὶ δυνάμεις, ἑλκτικὴ δηλαδή, καθεκτική, ἀλλοιωτικὴ καὶ ἀποκριτική. ἄλλως τε πεπληρωμένων πάντων τῶν ἀγγείων ἀδιάπνευστα γίνεται τὰ ἐν αὐτοῖς, ἀδιάπνευστα δὲ ὄντα σηπεδόνος αἴτια γίνεται, ἐπὶ δὲ σηπεδόνος πυρετοὶ ἐξάπτονται, κἀντεῦθεν πάλιν καταλύονται αἱ φυσικαὶ δυνάμεις. ἡ ῥῆξις πολλάκις ἐπακολουθεῖ τῇ ἀμετρίᾳ τοῦ αἵματος, καὶ τοῦτο τυχὸν περὶ τὸν θώρακα· ἐπὶ δὲ τῇ ῥήξει τοῦ ἀγγείου αἵματος ἀναγωγὴ καὶ ἕλκος γίνεται· ἐπὶ δὲ τῷ ἕλκει φθίσις, τουτέστιν ἴσχνανσις καὶ ἀτροφία· ἐπὶ δὲ τούτοις πᾶσιν ἀπειλεῖται θάνατος.

Καὶ ταῦτα μὲν ἐπὶ τῶν ἀγυμνάστων σωμάτων περιουσίᾳ τροφῶν τοιούτων καὶ ἀργίᾳ τὸ αἷμα ἀθροισάντων. παράδειγμα δὲ εἰ δοκεῖ τοῦ λόγου ἀθλητικὴ γενέσθω εὐεξία, οὕστινας ὁρῶμεν τῇ γυμνασίᾳ καὶ τῇ κινήσει τοῦ σώματος τὴν εὐεξίαν καὶ πολυαιμίαν κεκτημένους· ὁπότε γὰρ τούτοις εἰς πλῆθος ἐκτραπῇ τὸ αἷμα, εὐθέως βλάπτονται πάσας τὰς εἰρημένας βλάβας, ἔτι γε μὴν καὶ ἀνορεξίαις περιπίπτουσι καὶ τῷ τῇ γυμνασίᾳ μὴ σχολάζειν ἀνίσχυροι γίνονται. εἰ οὖν ἐπὶ τούτων ἐν ἄκρᾳ ὑγείᾳ εἶναι δοκούντων τὸ πλῆθος τοῦ αἵματος τοσούτων κακῶν αἴτιον καθίσταται, πολλῷ μᾶλλον ἐπὶ τῶν ἀγυμνάστων ἢ νενοσηκότων πλεονάζον τὸ αἷμα μείζονα ἂν δεινὰ ἀπεργάσηται.

Ὥστε οὖν ἐπειδὴ βλαπτικόν ἐστι τὸ πλῆθος τοῦ αἵματος, ὁρμητέον ἐπὶ τὴν θεραπείαν αὐτοῦ. ἔστιν οὖν ἡ ἴασις αὐτοῦ κένωσις διὰ φλεβὸς γινομένη τεχνικῶς,

14sq. καὶ[II] – ἐμποιέουσιν] Hipp. Acut., app. 6 (4): I 148,23–149,1 Kw. = II 402,10–404,1 L. *cf. infra*, vol. II, fol. 23[v]

1 παραγινόμενον P 4 γοῦν] γὰρ Z ἀμέτρου A 5 γένονται P 6 ἠχομένου Z 11 ἀπέμπτως P 12 τὰς] καὶ Z 15 γὰρ *om.* Z 16 δὲ *om.* Z ψυχικὰς A 17 πνιγομένου] καὶ καταπνιγομένου Z 20 πρόθεσις α, *post* θρέψις *trsp.* A 27 ἴσχνοσις Z 31 καὶ *om.* α 33 πάσαις ταῖς εἰρημέναις βλάβαις Z ἀνορεξία A 34 τῷ *om.* Z 35 *ante* ἐν *add.* τῶν Z τοσοῦτον Z 36 πλεονάζειν Z 39 τεχνικῶς γιγνομένη Z

to our nature, but when it deviates from them and increases to the point of excess, it is found to be noxious and harmful to nature. It can, indeed, damage all our faculties, the psychic, the natural and the vital ones. Of the psychic faculties it affects the governing, i. e. the sensory and motor, powers. Thus people who have an overflowing surplus of blood in their bodies, owing to the disproportionate bulk it assumes, move with difficulty and cannot even bear the weight of their own bodies; for our body consists of a carrying and a carried part, the carrying part being the motor faculties, the carried part the body. But a superabundance of blood also damages the sensory faculties, causing faulty perceptions of visual qualities, exhalation of fumes, hardness of hearing, fits of numbness and abnormal taste perceptions. It also brings about a change for the worse in the rational faculties, since these people can neither reason properly nor remember nor imagine things faultlessly, because the psychic pneuma is overwhelmed and coarsened by the surplus of blood. Secondly, it causes harm to the vital faculties, because the congested arteries cannot expand and contract normally, so that the danger of suffocation then arises, as he has observed rightly in another work: "And clogged veins cause suffocation"; for Hippocrates has this habit of indicating arteries by the generic name of "veins". Finally, the abundance of blood breaks down the natural faculties also: when the arteries are congested, the innate heat is smothered because it is no longer fanned, and as a result it reaches the stomach in a coarse and chilled condition and impedes its digestive function; when this fails, all the rest is necessarily affected: conversion into blood, distribution, absorption, nutrition, etc.; then, as the parts are atrophied, their natural faculties fail, to wit, the attractive, the retentive, the transformative and the secretory faculty. Besides, when all the vessels are full, their content is no longer ventilated, and being unventilated it causes putrefaction, on the basis of the putrefaction fevers are kindled, and the upshot is once more that the natural faculties break down. Or again, often the excessive quantity of blood leads to the rupture (of a vessel), for example in the chest; the rupture of the vessel causes spitting of blood and a festering wound; the festering wound, consumption, i. e. emaciation and wasting; the end of all this is the menace of death.

This happens in the case of unexercised bodies, which by a surfeit of a particular kind of food and by idleness have collected a surplus of blood. To illustrate our point, however, let us take the healthy condition of athletes, who obviously owe their perfect condition and their fullness of blood to exercise and motion of the body: when their fullbloodedness becomes excessive, not only do all the troubles we mentioned appear immediately, but in addition they suffer from a lack of appetite, and being unable to spend their usual time training, they lose their strength. Now if excess of blood can cause such havoc in those reputed to be in perfect health, all the greater must be the harm done by a surplus of blood to people who lack exercise or are ill.

Having thus established that excess of blood is detrimental, we must proceed to treatment. The cure is artificial evacuation through a vein, i.e., bleeding. How

τουτέστι διὰ φλεβοτομίας. τὸ δὲ μέχρι πόσου δεῖ παραλαβεῖν τὴν κένωσιν, ἐπιφέρει θαυμασίως· [I 3: IV 460,4 L.] «ὁκοία ἂν ἡ φύσις ᾖ τοῦ μέλλοντος ὑπομένειν», τυχὸν ὅπως ἂν ἡ δύναμις τοῦ κάμνοντος ὑπαγορεύσειε καὶ τὰ λοιπὰ σύστοιχα. εἰ μὲν γὰρ ἔρρωται ἡ δύναμις, ὅσον ἡ χρεία ἀπαιτεῖ, κένωσον· εἰ δὲ ἀσθενεῖ μετρίως, μετρίαν καὶ τὴν κένωσιν παραληπτέον, τὸ ἐγκαταλιμπανόμενον γὰρ διὰ τῆς ἀσιτίας καὶ τρίψεως ἀποκενοίημεν ἄν· εἰ δὲ πάνυ ἄρρωστός ἐστιν ἡ δύναμις, ἀρνούμεθα τὴν κένωσιν, ὑπόγυιος γὰρ ἐπ' αὐτῶν ὁ θάνατος.

Καλὸν δὲ ἡμᾶς καὶ τοῦτο εἰδέναι, ὅτι, ὅπερ ἐν τῷ Περὶ διαίτης ὀξέων πεποίηκε καὶ ἐν τῷ Περὶ ἀγμῶν καὶ ἄρθρων, τούτῳ καὶ νῦν τῷ τρόπῳ παρηκολούθησεν. ὡς γὰρ ἐν τῷ Περὶ διαίτης ὀξέων βουλόμενος δεῖξαι, ὅτι ἡ ἐναλλαγὴ τοῦ ἔθους βλάβην ἐν τῷ σώματι δύναται ποιεῖν, ἔλεγεν, ὅτι οἱ εἰθισμένοι δὶς σιτεύεσθαι ἅπαξ τρεφόμενοι βλάπτονται μεγάλα καὶ ἀνάπαλιν, καὶ οἱ εἰθισμένοι ἀριστᾶν μὴ δειπνεῖν δέ, μὴ ἀριστήσαντες ἀλλὰ δειπνήσαντες βλάπτονται καὶ ἀνάπαλιν – συμπτώματα γὰρ αὐτοῖς ἐπιγίνεται τοιάδε καὶ τοιάδε, ὧν ἐκεῖσε τὸν κατάλογον ποιεῖται –, καὶ ἐπὶ τούτοις εὐθέως καὶ τὰς θεραπείας ἐπήγαγεν, οὕτως καὶ ἐνταῦθα πεποίηκεν· εἰπὼν γὰρ τὸ παράδειγμα τῆς ἀθλητικῆς εὐεξίας οὐκ ἦλθεν εὐθὺς ἐπὶ τὸ πρᾶγμα, ἀλλ' ἐπὶ τὴν θεραπείαν αὐτοῦ μεταξυλαβήσας αὐτὴν ὑπό τε τοῦ παραδείγματος καὶ τοῦ πράγματος· καὶ τίς ἡ θεραπεία; δηλονότι ἡ κένωσις. τοῦτο δὲ ὑπὸ πολλῆς προθυμίας ἐποίησε τοῦ τέλους τῶν ὑπισχνουμένων ὑπὸ τῆς θεραπείας ἀγαθῶν ἐφιέμενος.

Ἐν τοῖσι γυμναστικοῖσιν αἱ ἐς ἄκρον εὐεξίαι σφαλεραί, ἢν ἐν τῷ ἐσχάτῳ ἔωσιν. ἰστέον, ὅτι γυμναστικοὺς καλεῖ τοὺς ἀθλητὰς τοὺς τὸν βίον τῆς γυμνασίας μετερχομένους καὶ ἐπιτηδεύοντας καταπαλαίειν ἑτέρους. εὐθὺς γὰρ οἱ οὕτως γυμναζόμενοι βούλονται μὴ τῇ τέχνῃ μόνον ἢ τῇ δυνάμει, ἀλλὰ καὶ τῷ βάρει τοῦ σώματος καταγωνίζεσθαι τὸν ἀντίπαλον. μηδὲ γὰρ ἐκεῖνο γυμναστικὸν ἀκουστέον τὸ σῶμα τὸ σπανιάκις ἱππασίᾳ χρώμενον ἢ τοξείᾳ ἢ δρόμῳ ἢ σειρομάστῃ ἀφαιρέσεως μετρίας ἕνεκεν τῶν ἀθροιζομένων ὑγρῶν καὶ πνευμάτων ἐλλειποῦς τῆς πέψεως γενομένης ἢ δι' ἀγρυπνίαν ἢ δι' ἀδηφαγίαν ἢ δι' ἀσθένειαν φυσικὴν τοῦ ἐμφύτου θερμοῦ· ἰστέον δέ, ὅτι οἱ παλαιοὶ γυμναστικὰ σώματα ἐκάλουν τὰ τὸν πένταθλον ἀγῶνα ἀγωνιζόμενα, πάλην πυγμὴν παγκράτιον δρόμον καὶ δίσκου βολήν.

Αἱ ἐς ἄκρον εὐεξίαι. ἰστέον, ὅτι τὸ ἄκρον δύο σημαίνει· δηλοῖ γὰρ καὶ τὸ κάλλιστον, ὥσπερ φαμὲν ἄκρον εἶναι εὐγενῆ, δηλοῖ δὲ καὶ τὴν εἰς ἔσχατον πέρας ἄφιξιν, οὗ τι οὐκ ἔστιν ἐπέκεινα. κατὰ τὸ δεύτερον οὖν σημαινόμενον τὸ ἄκρον φησὶν ὁ Ἱπποκράτης, τὸ δηλοῦν τὸ ἔσχατον πέρας τῆς εὐεξίας, οὐ μὴν τὴν σύμμετρον εὐεξίαν καὶ ἀρίστην, ὡς δηλοῖ τὸ λύειν αὐτὴν παρακελεύεσθαι ὡς σφαλεράν. ἵνα γὰρ

2sq. ὁκοία – σύστοιχα] *v.* Gal. In Aphor. I 3: XVII B 364,11–15 K. 9 ἐν – ἄρθρων] Hipp. Fract., passim: II 46–110 Kw. = III 412–562 L. ὡς – 15 ἐπήγαγεν] *v.* Hipp. Acut. 28–35 (9): I 122,16–125,19 Kw. = II 280,8–296,1 L. 21 ἰστέον – 24 ἀντίπαλον] *v.* Gal. In Aphor. I 12: XVII B 382,12–15 K.

1 πόσην Z 1sq. ἐπιφέρει θαυμασίως] ὁ αὐτὸς θαυμασίως ἐπιφέρει Z 2 ᾖ *sec. Hipp. scripsi*: ἢ α: *lac. in* Z 4 ἡ δύναμις ἔρρωται Z *post* ὅσον *add.* ἂν A κένωσιν A: *lac. in* Z 5 καὶ τὴν κένωσιν μετρίαν A 6sq. (ἀπο)κενοίημεν – ὑπό(γυιος) *om.* Z, *ut vid.* 7 αὐτῶ α 9 ἀκμῶν ω: *corr.* P²Z² 11 *post* ἅπαξ *add.* δὲ Z 12 μεγάλως Z καὶ[II] *om.* Z δειπνᾶν ω: *correxi* 14 γίνεται A ἐκεῖ γε Z 15 πεποίηκεν] ποιεῖται Z 20 εἰς α 21 ἀθλητικοὺς Z 23 τῇ[I] *om.* α 26 ὑγρῶν] χυμῶν P 28 δέ *om.* Z 29 ἀγῶνα *om.* Z 31 εἰς α 32 δὲ] γὰρ P 34 δηλοῦν *post* εὐεξίας *trsp.* Z

far evacuation should go, he makes admirably clear in the following words: "as far as the constitution of the person to be bled permits", that is to say, as dictated by the patient's strength and the other correlative factors. If resistance is strong, bleed him as much as required; if he is on the weak side, bleeding should be proportionally light, as we can hope to get rid of the residue by the patient's lack of appetite and by massage; if resistance is totally exhausted, we refuse to bleed, for in those cases death is close at hand.

It is further interesting to know that (Hippocrates) here proceeded in the same manner as in Regimen in Acute Diseases and in Fractures and Joints. In Regimen in Acute Diseases, trying to show that a change of habit can cause harm to the body, he said that people accustomed to two meals daily suffer great harm if they have one only, and conversely, and that people accustomed to have lunch, but no dinner, have trouble if they skip lunch and have dinner instead, and conversely – for certain specific symptoms manifest themselves, which he lists in that passage – and then he immediately goes on to describe the cures; this is what he does here, too: after quoting the example of the perfect athletic condition he does not come to the point at once, but discusses the cure, inserting it between the example and the point (it illustrates), the cure being of course evacuation. This is explained by his great eagerness, his impatience to achieve the beneficial results promised by the treatment.

In athletes a top condition is dangerous, when it has reached the extreme limit. By athletes he understands those who make sport their occupation and specialize in wrestling matches. The direct consequence is that those who practice athletics in this sense want to defeat their adversaries, not only by technique or power, but also by sheer bodily weight. We should certainly not think of an "athlete's constitution" in the case of a man who takes occasional exercise in the form of riding, shooting, racing or handling the barbed lance for the purpose of a moderate reduction of fluids and gases accumulating through incomplete digestion due to lack of sleep, over-eating or natural weakness of the innate heat; when the ancients speak of the "athletic constitution", they think of participants in the pentathlon, which consisted of wrestling, boxing, pancratium, foot-race and discus-throwing.

A top condition. The word top has a double meaning: it may denote the highest excellence, as when we say that a man belongs by birth to the top rank of society, but it may also denote a reaching of the farthest limit, beyond which there is nothing else. Hippocrates uses top in the second meaning, that of the farthest limit of a healthy condition, but not of a balanced and perfect condition, as is proved by his advice to break it up as dangerous. To forestall the objection:

μή τις εἴπῃ αὐτῷ· «Τί φῄς, ὦ Ἱπποκρατες; εὐεξίαν λύειν βούλει τοῦ σώματος, ἥτις ἐστὶν ἡ τούτου ἀρίστη κατασκευή;» τὴν ὁμωνυμίαν αὐτοῦ διαστελλόμενος εἶπε τὸ τῆς εὐεξίας ὄνομα μὴ μόνον ἐπὶ τῆς ἀρίστης φαίνεσθαι κατασκευῆς, ἀλλὰ καὶ ἐπὶ τοῦ ἐσχάτου καὶ ἀκροτάτου τῆς ὑγείας ὅρου, ὅπερ δηλοῖ διὰ τοῦ εἰπεῖν ἢν ἐν τῷ ἐσχάτῳ ἔωσι, τουτέστι μεθ' ὃ οὐκ ἐπιδέχεται ἐπίδοσιν ἡ ὑγεία. σφαλερὰ γὰρ πᾶσα ἀμετρία καὶ ἀκρότης, οὐ μόνον ἐν τοῖς παρὰ φύσιν, ἀλλὰ καὶ ἐν τοῖς κατὰ φύσιν.

I 5 [I 3: IV 458,12–13 L.] Οὐ γὰρ δύνανται μένειν ἐν τῷ αὐτῷ οὐδὲ ἀτρεμέειν.

Ἀσαφὲς εἶναι δοκεῖ τὸ παρὸν χωρίον, ὅθεν καὶ διαφόρως αὐτὸ οἱ παλαιότεροι τῶν ἐξηγητῶν ἐξηγήσαντο. οἱ μὲν γάρ φασιν, ὅτι διὰ τοῦτο αἱ ἐς ἄκρον εὐεξίαι σφαλεραὶ ἐπὶ τῶν γυμναστικῶν, διότι τῷ πλήθει τοῦ αἵματος βαρυνόμεναι αἱ δυνάμεις ἠρεμεῖν ἀναγκάζονται, ὅπερ ἄτοπον. ἀπορήσει δέ τις πρὸς τὴν τοιαύτην ἔννοιαν ⟨ὅτι «Τίνος⟩ ἕνεκεν τὴν ἡσυχίαν τῶν δυνάμεων διαβάλλει ὁ Ἱπποκράτης; ὁρῶμεν γάρ, ὅτι πρός τινα καιρὸν ἀναπαυόμεναι αἱ δυνάμεις ἐρρωμενέστεραι πρὸς τὰς ἐφεξῆς ἐνεργείας εὑρίσκονται.» πρὸς ὃ ῥητέον, ὅτιπερ αἱ δυνάμεις διὰ τὴν ἐνέργειαν γεγόνασι καὶ ἐν τῷ κινεῖσθαι καὶ ἐνεργεῖν ἡ ἀρετὴ αὐτῶν διαδείκνυται· οὐδὲν γὰρ ἕτερον αὐτῶν ἡ ἡσυχία καὶ ἀνενεργησία ἐστὶν ἢ εἰκὼν θανάτου. οὕτως γοῦν ἐν ἄλλοις ὁ Ἱπποκράτης «κίνησις μετεξετέρη κρατύνει, ἀργίη δὲ τήκει». ὁπόσον δὲ ἡ ἠρεμία αὐτῶν βλαβερὰ ὑπάρχει, ἐπιφέρει λέγων· [I 3: IV 458,13 L.] ἐπειδὴ οὐκ ἀτρεμέουσι· καὶ μὴ νομίσῃς τὸ οὐκ ἀτρεμέουσι τὸ «οὐκ ἠρεμοῦσι» δηλοῦν, ἀλλ' ὅτιπερ ἠρεμεῖν μὲν οὐ πεφύκασι, νῦν δὲ ἠρεμοῦσι καὶ ἕτερον τρόπον ἡσυχίας παρὰ τὴν ἀνάπαυσιν ἡσυχάζουσιν. ἐπὶ γὰρ τῶν πληθώραν αἱματικὴν ἐχόντων αἱ δυνάμεις κάμνουσι, φησί, καὶ βαρυνόμεναι καὶ ναρκῶσαι, ὅπερ οὐκ ἔστιν ἄνεσις, ἀλλὰ παθητικὴ κίνησις· [I 3: IV 458,13–460,1 L.] οὐκέτι γὰρ ἐπὶ τὸ βέλτιον ἐπιδιδόναι δύνανται, λείπεται οὖν ἐπὶ τὸ χεῖρον μεταπίπτειν αὐτάς. ὁ δὲ Γαληνὸς ἑτέρως ἐξηγεῖται τὸ χωρίον, ὅστις καὶ μᾶλλον ἐπαληθεύει τῷ λόγῳ. φησὶ γάρ, ὅτι περὶ τῶν ἐν ἡμῖν δυνάμεων τοῦθ' Ἱπποκράτης εἴρηκε, καὶ μάλιστα τῶν φυσικῶν· αἱ γὰρ ψυχικαί ποτε καὶ ἠρεμοῦσιν, ὡς ἐν τοῖς ὕπνοις, καὶ τοῦτο ἐν τῷ κατὰ φύσιν, ἐπείπερ ἐν τῇ πληρώσει βαρυνόμεναι ἀνενέργητοι κἂν τῷ ἐγρηγορέναι μένουσι. δεῖ οὖν, ὡς εἴρηται, ἐπὶ τῶν φυσικῶν [ἐπὶ τῶν κατὰ φύσιν] ἐκλαβεῖν τὸ λεγόμενον, αὗται γὰρ ἀεννάως ἐκ διαδοχῆς ἐνεργοῦσιν. ἔργον δὲ αὐτῶν ἡ πέψις τῶν

19 κίνησις – τήκει] Hipp. Off. med. 20: II 42,19 Kw. = III 324,13 L. *cf.* Hipp. Artic. 52: II 192,8–9 Kw. = IV 230,7–8 L. *Stephano similior* Psell., De omnifaria doctrina 182   26sq. ὁ δὲ Γαληνὸς – χωρίον] *v.* Gal. In Aphor. I 3: XVII B 364,2–9 K.

1 βούλει λύειν P   2 διαστελλόμενοι P   3 μὴ] οὐ Z   5 μεθ'] καθ' Z   ὃ] ὧν A   8 δύναται P   αὐτέω Z   9 ἀτρεμέειν] -ν *eras. in* P   10 αὐτῶ A   παλαίτεροι Z   11 εἰς A   12 διότι] δηλαδή· ὅτι Z   13 *post* ὅπερ *add.* ἐστιν Z   ἀπορήσειε δ' ἂν Z   14 ὅτι «Τίνος *addidi*   τῶν δυνάμεων, τὴν ἡσυχίαν Z   διαβάλλει – 16 ῥητέον] διαπροσρητέον Z   15 ἐρρωμενέστερον P   17 δείκνυται A: ἐνδείκνυται Z   18 *post* καὶ *add.* ἡ Z   ἀνεργησία P   19 *ante* ἐν *add.* καὶ Z   *post* Ἱπποκράτης *add.* φησὶ Z   μετ' ἐξωτέρη Z   20 ἠρεμίη Z   αὐτοῖς Z   ἐπειδὴ] ἐπεὶ δὲ *Hipp.* (ἐπειδὴ δὲ C')   21 δηλοῖ Z   22 μὲν *om.* Z   23 παρὰ *scripsi*: περὶ ω   ἐπὶ] ἐπεὶ Z   24 φησί] φύσει Z   25 *ante* κίνησις *add.* ἡ Z   26 οὖν *om.* Z   αὐτοὺς Z   27 *post* τὸ *add.* τοιοῦτον Z   28 ἱπποκράτ(ης) εἴρηκ(ε) Z: ἱπποκράτου εἴρηκα α   μᾶλλον Z   29 ποτε *om.* A   31 ἐπὶ τῶν κατὰ φύσιν *delevi*   *ante* ἐπὶ[II] *add.* καὶ Z   32 αὐτῶν] τούτων Z

"What is this, Hippocrates? Do you want to break up the healthy condition of the body, which is its most desirable state?" he distinguishes between the two meanings, explaining that the term healthy condition is found not only in the sense of the most desirable state, but also in that of the farthest borderline of health; he makes this clear by adding when it has reached the extreme limit, i.e. the point beyond which health admits of no increase. Indeed, any disproportionate and extreme condition is dangerous, not only in the range of the abnormal, but also in that of the normal.

I 5. For they cannot remain at the same point or be in repose.

The present passage seems to be obscure, hence the different interpretations offered by the older commentators. Some say that a top condition is dangerous in athletes because the faculties, weighed down by the excess of blood, are forced to stay in repose, which is unnatural. To this idea one may object: "Why should Hippocrates warn against the faculties being in repose? What we actually see is that by a temporary rest the faculties gain strength for subsequent activities." The answer to this is that the faculties exist for the sake of their functions and their soundness becomes manifest in motion and action; rest and inactivity in them is but an image of death. Thus Hippocrates says elsewhere: "A certain amount of motion strengthens, idleness debilitates." To what degree rest is detrimental to them, he shows by adding: since they cannot stay in repose; and do not think that not stay in repose means "not rest"; it means that though it is against their nature to be in repose, they are in repose now and in a state of rest which is different from relaxation. For in cases of plethora of the blood, he means, the faculties suffer from overloading and numbness, which is not relaxation, but a passive motion: as they can no longer make progress for the better, what remains is changing for the worse. Galen, however, has a different explanation of the passage, and his view comes closer to the truth. He says that Hippocrates is speaking of our faculties, in particular the natural ones; the psychic faculties do rest sometimes, as in sleep, and then this condition is normal – obviously, when they are overloaded by repletion, they can remain inactive even in the waking state –. Therefore, as we said, the words must be understood as referring to the natural faculties, which work continuously in relay. Their task is digestion of food, breaking down of humors, absorption of nutriment,

σιτίων, ἡ κατεργασία τῶν χυμῶν, ἡ πρόσθεσις τῆς τροφῆς, ἡ ἐξομοίωσις καὶ ἡ θρέψις. τούτων ἀεννάως ἐνεργουμένων, καὶ πολλῷ μᾶλλον διὰ τὴν τοῦ αἵματος πληθώραν ἢ πρότερον, τοῦ δὲ σώματος ἐν ἄκρᾳ πληρώσει καὶ ἐσχάτῃ εὐεξίᾳ ὑπάρχοντος σκόπει τὸ ἐντεῦθεν. δῆλον γάρ, ὡς, ἐπείπερ ἐπὶ τὸ βέλτιον χωρεῖν οὐ δεδύνηνται, πάντως ἐπὶ τὸ χεῖρον χωρήσαιεν, ὡς κἀπὶ τῶν ἔξωθεν ἔχει κλιμάκων· ἀνελθὼν γάρ τις ἕως τῆς ἐσχάτης βαθμίδος καὶ πρόσω σπεύδων ἀνελθεῖν, ἐπεὶ μὴ βαθμὶς ἄλλη πρόκειται, κάτω χωρεῖν ἀναγκάζεται. ἐπὶ γὰρ τῆς πληρώσεως τῶν ἀγγείων διὰ μὲν τὸ τὰ νεῦρα πληροῦσθαι σπασμοὶ καὶ ἐπιληψίαι καὶ ἀποπληξίαι ἕπονται, διὰ δὲ τὸ τὰς φλέβας καὶ τὰς ἀρτηρίας, πνιγμοὶ καὶ ῥήξεις καὶ ἀναγωγαὶ ἀμέτρου αἵματος, ἅτινα πάντα ὀξεῖς ἐπάγει θανάτους.

I 6 [I 3: IV 460,1–3 L.] Τουτέων οὖν ἕνεκεν μὴ βραδέως τὴν εὐεξίην λύειν ξυμφέρει, ἵνα πάλιν ἀρχὴν ἀναθρέψεως λαμβάνῃ τὸ σῶμα.

Πεπλήρωται μέχρι τῶν ἐνταῦθα τὸ παράδειγμα, ἄρχεται δὲ ἡ θεραπεία. ὁ δὲ τρόπος τῆς θεραπείας ἐστὶν ἡ κένωσις, ταύτῃ γὰρ λύεται ἡ εὐεξία. σκόπει μέντοι τέχνην Ἱπποκράτους· ἃ γὰρ ὁ Γαληνὸς διὰ πολλῶν λόγων ἐνεδείξατο, ταῦτα ὁ Ἱπποκράτης διὰ βραχέων ἐδήλωσε. φησὶ γὰρ ὁ Γαληνὸς τέσσαρας εἶναι τοὺς κεφαλαιώδεις θεραπευτικοὺς σκοπούς, τὸν ἀπὸ τοῦ ποσοῦ καὶ τοῦ ποιοῦ καὶ τοῦ καιροῦ καὶ τοῦ τρόπου τῆς χρήσεως. ταῦτα γοῦν πάντα σπερματικῶς ἐδήλωσεν ὁ Ἱπποκράτης, ἀφ' ὧν πάντες ὡδηγήθησαν. διὰ μὲν γὰρ τοῦ εἰπεῖν τὴν εὐεξίαν λύειν τὸν τρόπον ἐδήλωσε τῆς χρήσεως, ὅτι δεῖ φλεβοτομῆσαι· διὰ δὲ τοῦ εἰπεῖν μὴ βραδέως τὸν καιρὸν παρέστησε· διὰ δὲ τοῦ εἰπεῖν ἵνα πάλιν ἀρχὴν ἀναθρέψεως τὸ σῶμα λαμβάνῃ, τὸ ποσόν, ἵνα μήτε πολὺ κενώσωμεν μήτε ὀλίγον, ἀλλὰ πρὸς ὃ ὑπαγορεύει ἥ τε τῆς δυνάμεως εὐρωστία καὶ ἡ τοῦ νοσοῦντος φύσις· τὸ δὲ ποιὸν ἀναφαίνεται ἐκ τοῦ πλεονάζοντος χυμοῦ, αἷμα δέ ἐστι τὸ ὑποκείμενον.

Ἐπίστησον δὴ καὶ τοῦτο – ἔμψυχος γὰρ ἡ λέξις –· μὴ βραδέως φησὶ τὴν εὐεξίην λύειν. καταβέβληνται γὰρ αἱ δυνάμεις ἤδη τῷ πλήθει καὶ τῷ βάρει τοῦ αἵματος· εἰ δὲ σὺ ὑπερθῇ τὸν καιρὸν τῆς κενώσεως, πολλῷ μᾶλλον καταβληθήσονται αἱ δυνάμεις, εἶτα ἐν τῇ κενώσει τοῦ χυμοῦ πολλαπλασιασθήσεται ἡ ταλαιπωρία τῶν δυνάμεων. πᾶσα γὰρ κένωσις οἶδε καταβάλλειν τὰς δυνάμεις, κἂν ἄχρηστον ᾖ τὸ κενούμενον, τῷ συνδιαφορεῖσθαι λεληθότως καί τινα τῶν χρηστῶν, καὶ μάλιστα τὸ ζωτικὸν πνεῦμα· κίνδυνος οὖν ἐνταῦθα, μή τι οὐκ ἐξαρκεῖ τὸ ὑπολειφθὲν ἄχρις ἀναθρέψεως, ἀρρώστων τῶν δυνάμεων ὑποκειμένων, ἅπασαι γὰρ τηνικαῦτα βλάπτονται. αὐτὸς μέντοι διὰ τῆς θρεπτικῆς καὶ τὰς ἄλλας συμπεριέλαβεν, ὕλης γὰρ λόγον

16 φησὶ – 18 χρήσεως] *v.* Gal. Ad Glauc. I 1: XI 2,1–4 K. *supra*, p. 46,9–11; *infra*, p. 114,12–13; vol. III, fol. 177r 25–30 κενούμενον] *cf.* Gal. In Aphor. I 3: XVII B 364,11–16 K.

1 πρόθεσις α 2 τούτων θρέψις Z 4 γάρ *om.* Z 5 κλημάτων Z 6 σπεύδειν α 8 ἐπιλήψεις Z *post* ἀποπληξίαι *add.* τῶ ζώω Z 9 τὰςI *om.* P ἀναγωγοὶ P 11 μὴ βραδέως *post* ξυμφέρει *(lin. 12) colloc. Hipp.* εὐεξίαν Z 12 ἀναθρέψηος Z 13 *post* δὲII *add.* γε Z 14 ἡ κένωσις ἐστὶ Z 15sq. ἃ – Ἱπποκράτης *om.* Z 16 *post* βραχέων *add.* ῥημμάτων, πόσην τοῦ λόγου τέχνην Z 17 τὸν] ὁ Z 18 πάντα *om.* Z 18sq. ὁ ἱπποκράτης ἐδήλωσεν Z 19 ἐφ' P 20 τῆς χρήσεως ἐδήλωσεν Z 21 παρέστησε *om.* α εἰπεῖν *om.* α ἀναθρέψηος Z 23 ὃ] ὅπερ Z τῶν νοσούντων Z *post* δὲ *add.* γε Z 25 τούτου α μὴ] καὶ P 26 ε ὐεξίαν Z 27 ὑπέρθη AZ: ὑπάρθη P: *correxi* 28 πολλαπλασθήσεται Z 28sq. ἡ τῶν δυνάμεων ταλαιπωρία Z 29 γὰρ *om.* P 30 τινα] τι Z 31 οὐκ *om.* Z

assimilation and nutrition. As these work unintermittently, and more intensively than before owing to the plethora of the blood, and the body is in a state of utter repletion and extreme vigor, consider what happens next. It is clear that, since they cannot change for the better, they must necessarily change for the worse, just as in daily life it is with a ladder: you have climbed it to the last step and you want to go up farther, but since there are no more steps, you have no choice but to go down. Applied to repletion of the vessels, this results, if the nerves are clogged, in convulsions and epileptic and apoplectic fits, and if the veins and arteries are, in suffocation, bursting veins, bringing up of excess blood, all of which lead to sudden death.

I 6. For this reason it is best to break up the healthy condition without losing time, so that the body can start a new period of growth.

Here the example ends and the treatment begins. The method of treatment is evacuation, which breaks up the condition of health. Meanwhile observe the skill of Hippocrates: what Galen demonstrated in a circumstantial discussion, Hippocrates put in a few words. Galen says that there are four principal points to be considered in therapeutics: the quantity, the quality, the moment and the application. Hippocrates indicated each of these implicitly, and all the others have followed his guidance. When he said break up the healthy condition, he indicated the application, that it must be done by bleeding; by saying without losing time, he betokened the moment; by adding so that the body can start a new period of growth, the quantity, that is to say, we should evacuate neither too much nor too little, but in the measure prescribed by the power of resistance and the patient's constitution; as for the quality, it can be inferred from the redundant humor, which in this case is blood.

Note also the liveliness of the style: Break up the condition, he says, without losing time. The patient's faculties have already been impaired by the quantity and the pressure of the blood; and if you delay the moment of evacuation, the faculties will be impaired even more, after which in the process of evacuating the humor the poor state of the faculties will become many times worse. Any kind of evacuation will impair the faculties, even if the matter evacuated is useless, because imperceptibly some useful matter will be dissipated with it, especially the vital pneuma; so here we have the danger that the remainder will not survive to be restored, the faculties being already weak, for in this situation they all suffer damage. (Hippocrates), however, though he mentioned only the nutritive faculty, included the others with it, because it has the function of basic

πρὸς ἐκείνας αὕτη ἐπέχει· θρέψεως γὰρ μὴ γενομένης κακῶς αἱ ζωτικαὶ καὶ αἱ ψυχικαὶ διατίθενται.

I 7 [I 3: IV 460,3–5 L.] Μηδὲ τὰς ξυμπτώσιας ἐς τὸ ἔσχατον ἄγειν, ἀλλ' ὁκοίη ἂν ἡ φύσις ᾖ τοῦ μέλλοντος ὑπομένειν, ἐς τοῦτο ἄγειν.

Φησίν, ὅτι τὸ ποσὸν τῆς κενώσεως ὁριζέτω σοι ἡ ἐκ τῆς τοῦ κάμνοντος δυνάμεως ἔνδειξις· ἀλλὰ καὶ ἡλικίαν δεῖ θεωρῆσαι καὶ ὥραν καὶ χώραν καὶ τὰ λοιπὰ σύστοιχα, εἰ μέλλοιμεν εὖ διατιθέναι τὴν κένωσιν. ταῦτα πάντα ὁ βραχύλογος διὰ μιᾶς ἐδήλωσε λέξεως, φημὶ δὴ τοῦ τῆς φύσεως ὀνόματος, εἰρηκὼς ἀλλ' ὁκοίη ἂν ἡ φύσις ᾖ τοῦ μέλλοντος ὑπομένειν, εἰς τοῦτο ἄγειν. διὰ δὲ τῆς συμπτώσεως αὐτὸ τὸ ἑπόμενον ἐδήλωσε, λέγω δὴ τὴν κένωσιν· κενουμένων γὰρ τῶν ἐν τοῖς ἀγγείοις περιεχομένων τὸ τῆς συμπτώσεως ἕπεται πάθος. ἐν γοῦν τοῖς δυσὶ τούτοις ἀφορισμοῖς καθάρσεως ἐμνημόνευσεν, εἶτα κενεαγγείης, εἶτα κενώσεως, εἶτα νῦν ξυμπτώσεως. ἔστι δὲ τὰ μὲν ⟨. . .⟩ αἰτιατὰ καὶ ἑπόμενα, ἡ κενεάγγεια δηλαδὴ καὶ ἡ ξύμπτωσις.

I 8 [I 3: IV 460,5 L.] Ὡσαύτως δὲ καὶ αἱ κενώσιες.

Ἐξηγοῦνταί τινες τὸ χωρίον τὸν τρόπον τοῦτον, ὅτι οὐ μόνον ἐπὶ τῶν ἀθλητικῶν σωμάτων ἔστιν εὑρεῖν τὴν γυμναστικὴν εὐεξίαν, ἀλλὰ καὶ ἐπὶ τῶν γεωργικῶν καὶ ἁλιευτικῶν. καὶ διαφέρει αὕτη ἐκείνης τῆς εὐεξίας τῷ μὴ ἀσκεῖν μέγεθος σώματος, ὅπερ ἐκείνοις σπουδάζεται, διὰ δὲ τοῦτο αὐτὸ οὐδὲ σφαλερὰ τυγχάνει ἡ τοιαύτη εὐεξία· ἐπιδέχεται γὰρ τὴν ἐπὶ τὸ ἄκρον ἐπίδοσιν. ἐπειδὴ οὖν ὁμώνυμός ἐστιν ἡ εὐεξία, διελέχθη δὲ περὶ τῆς ἀθλητικῆς, νόμιζε αὐτὸν τὴν ὑπερτέραν τέχνην μιμούμενον, λέγω δὴ τὴν φιλοσοφίαν, ἀπὸ τῶν μερικωτέρων ἐπὶ τὰ καθόλου τὸν λόγον ἀνάγειν καὶ περὶ πάσης εὐεξίας ἀποφαίνεσθαι, ὅτι οὐ μόνον ἐπὶ τῆς ἀθλητικῆς εὐεξίας, ἀλλ' ἐπὶ πάσης χαλεπὸν ἡ ἄμετρος κένωσις, διότι καταλύει τὴν δύναμιν. εἰπὲ δὲ καὶ δευτέραν ἐξήγησιν, ὅτι ὑποθέμενος τὸ παράδειγμα καὶ οὕτως τὴν θεραπείαν ἐπαγαγὼν νῦν ἐπ' αὐτὸ τὸ πρᾶγμα ἐχώρησε. καὶ νόησον οὕτως τὸ λεγόμενον· ὥσπερ ἐπὶ τῆς ἀθλητικῆς εὐεξίας ἡ εἰς ἄκρον ἄφιξις τῆς ὑγείας σφαλερά ἐστιν, ὁμοίως δὲ καὶ ἡ εἰς τὸ ἔσχατον ἀφικνουμένη κένωσις, οὕτως καὶ ἐπὶ παντὸς σώματος ἡ ἄμετρος κένωσις καὶ ἡ εἰς ἄκρον ἀνάθρεψις χαλεπή.

16 Ἐξηγοῦνταί – 24 δύναμιν] *v.* Gal. In Aphor. I 3: XVII B 362,5–363,16; 364,11–16 K.
25 εἰπὲ – 29] *cf.* Gal. In Aphor. I 3: XVII B 364,16–365,6 K.

1 ὑπέχει Z   3 εἰς α   *post* ἄγειν *praeb.* σφαλερὸν γάρ *Hipp.*   4 εἰς α   7 *post* βραχύλογος *add.* οὑτοσὶ Z   8 ᾖ] ἡ α: *corr.* P^2 9 ἄγει A(?)P   10 λέγω] φημὶ Z   *fort.* τῇ κενώσει *scribendum est*   11 τοῖν δυοῖν τούτοιν ἀφορισμοῖν Z   12 εἶτα^{II}] μεθ' ὃ Z   εἶτα^{III}] εἶτ' αὖ Z   νῦν] νὺξ P: *om.* A   13 *lacunam indicavi, supplenda huiusmodi quaedam*: αἴτια καὶ προηγούμενα, τυχὸν ἡ κάθαρσις καὶ ἡ κένωσις, τὰ δὲ   ἡ^{II} *om.* Z   σύμπτωσις P   16 τινες *om.* α   17 σωμάτων – γεωργικῶν *om.* Z   γυμναστικὴν] σωματικὴν A   18 *ante* καὶ^{II} *add.* κἂν Z   διαφέρῃ Z   τῷ] τὸ Z   μέγεθος] τὸ μέγεθος τοῦ Z   19 ἐκείνοις *sscr.* A: ἐκείνης α   21 *post* δὲ *add.* καὶ Z   22 λέγω] φημὶ Z   24 *post* εὐεξίας *add.* ὡς εἴρηται Z   *post* πάσης *add.* δηλαδὴ Z   *post* χαλεπὸν *add.* ἐστιν Z   διότι] ἐπειδὴ Z   25sq. καὶ^{II} – νόησον *om.* Z   26 οὑτωσὶ Z   28 δὲ *om.* A   ἡ^{I} *om.* P   οὕτως – 29 κένωσις *om.* P   καὶ^{II} *om.* A   *ante* ἡ^{II} *add.* καὶ A

matter with respect to the rest: nutrition failing, the vital and psychic faculties are in a bad way.

I 7. Do not carry the collapse to its extreme point, however, but only as far as the constitution of the patient to be bled permits.

He says that you must determine the degree of the evacuation on the evidence of the patient's power of resistance; further, we should consider his age, the season, the region, and the other correlative factors, if we are to handle the evacuation well. Being a man of few words, (Hippocrates) expressed all this in one single term, the noun "constitution", when he said, but only as far as the constitution of the patient to be bled permits. By the word collapse he indicated the direct consequence, i.e., of the evacuation; when the contents of the vessels are cleared out, the phenomenon of collapse follows. Thus in these two aphorisms he spoke, first, of "purging", then of "emptying of the vessels", then of "evacuation", lastly, here, of "collapse". Of these, two are +causes and antecedents, viz. purging and evacuation, the other two+[1] effects and consequences, i.e. emptying of the vessels and collapse.

I 8. Similarly, too, evacuations.

Some explain this passage in the sense that the athletic condition is found, not only in athletes, but also in farmers and fishermen. The healthy condition of the latter is different from the other kind in that there is no deliberate body-building, as practiced by athletes, and therefore this type of healthy condition involves no risk; it can stand an increase to the maximum degree. Therefore, since "healthy condition" has a double meaning, and (Hippocrates) has already discussed the healthy condition of the athlete, you may conclude that, in imitation of the higher art, i.e. philosophy, he now proceeds from the more particular to the universal and gives his opinion on the healthy condition in general, saying that not only in dealing with the healthy condition of the athlete, but in any other case, immoderate evacuation is perilous, because it undermines the power of resistance. You may add a second explanation: having first stated the example and subsequently its treatment, he now comes to the main point. The meaning should then be understood as follows: just as in the case of the athletic condition extreme health is dangerous and extreme evacuation is equally dangerous, so for any other constitution immoderate evacuation and excessive building-up of strength are precarious things.

[1] +causes – two+: these words translate a proposed restoration; see the app. crit.

I 9 [I 4: IV 460,7–8 L.] Αἱ λεπταὶ καὶ ἀκριβέες δίαιται καὶ ἐν τοῖσι μακροῖσιν αἰεὶ πάθεσι καὶ ἐν τοῖσι νοσήμασιν οὗ μὴ ἐπιδέχεται σφαλεραί.

Ἐλευθερώσας ὁ Ἱπποκράτης τὸ σῶμα τῆς τε κατὰ ποιότητα τῶν χυμῶν βλάβης καὶ τῆς κατὰ ποσότητα πλεονεξίας καὶ ἀπέριττον ὡς οἷόν τε ἀπεργασάμενος, ἐπιστάμενος ὅτι «τὰ μὴ καθαρὰ τῶν σωμάτων ὅσον ἂν θρέψῃς, μᾶλλον βλάψεις», καθαρὸν αὐτὸ νῦν τῷ λόγῳ ὑποθέμενος ἐπὶ τὴν δίαιταν ἐχώρησεν ἄμεμπτον αὐτοῦ τὴν ὑγείαν θεμελιῶσαι προθέμενος· δίαιταν δὲ διδάσκει τὴν ἐν τροφῇ παραλαμβανομένην.

Τέτρασι δὲ κεφαλαίοις περιγράφεται ἡ παροῦσα θεωρία. καὶ ἐν μὲν τῷ πρώτῳ κεφαλαίῳ λοιδορεῖ ὁ Ἱπποκράτης τὴν λεπτὴν δίαιταν καὶ σφαλερὰν αὐτὴν ἀποκαλεῖ ἐπὶ τῶν ὑγιαινόντων σωμάτων. ἰστέον δέ, ὅτι τριπλεκές ἐστι τὸ ἡμέτερον σῶμα, ἀπό τε στερεῶν καὶ ὑγρῶν καὶ πνευμάτων συγκείμενον· ἀσιτίας οὖν παραλαμβανομένης ἐπὶ τῶν ὑγιαινόντων ἕκαστον τούτων ἐκδαπανᾶται, τήκεται μὲν γὰρ τὰ στερεά, κενοῦται δὲ τὰ ὑγρά, διαφορεῖται δὲ τὰ πνεύματα· ἐφ' οἷς ταράττονται πᾶσαι αἱ δυνάμεις καταπίπτουσαι, φυσικαί, ψυχικαί. βλάπτει οὖν ἀσιτία τοὺς ὑγιαίνοντας οὐ κατὰ πρῶτον λόγον, κατὰ συμβεβηκὸς δέ, τῷ μὴ ἀναπληροῦσθαι τὸ ἀπορρέον καὶ διαφορούμενον ἐκ τῶν σωμάτων ἐπιδόσει τροφῆς ἑτέρας. οὐ μὴν ἀλλὰ καὶ ἐπὶ τῶν νοσούντων βλαβερά ἐστι. καὶ μὴ ἀπορήσῃς ἐκ τῶν Περὶ διαίτης ὀξέων εἰρημένων, ὅτι «Τὰ ἅπαξ μεταβολὴν ἐσχηκότα σώματα ἐπὶ νόσον τί ἔχει ἀδικῆσαι ἡ λεπτοτάτη δίαιτα; ἐπὶ μὲν γὰρ τῶν ὑγιαινόντων σφαλερὰ καθίσταται, ἐπειδὴ ἀμετάβλητα τέως ἐν ὑγείᾳ τυγχάνοντα μεταβολὴν ἐπὶ νόσον παρασκευάζει, ἐπὶ δὲ τῶν νοσούντων ἤδη ἐν νοσερᾷ μεταβολῇ ὑπαρχόντων οὐδὲν ἀσιτία ἀδικῆσαι δυνήσεται.» πρὸς ὅ φημι, ὅτι δύο τινὰ ἐν ταῖς νόσοις πραγματευόμεθα, τὰ μὲν παρὰ φύσιν τοῦ σώματος ἀνελεῖν, τὴν δὲ δύναμιν φυλάξαι. ἀναιροῦμεν δὲ τὸ νόσημα τῇ τῶν ἐναντίων προσαγωγῇ, φυλάττομεν δὲ τὴν δύναμιν τῇ τῶν ὁμοίων ἐπιδόσει· τί δὲ ὅμοιον ἢ οἰκειότερόν ἐστι τῇ δυνάμει τροφῆς; εἰ τοίνυν τὴν δύναμιν ἡ τροφὴ ὑποστηρίζει καὶ φυλάττει, ἐὰν ἀσιτίαν παραλάβωμεν ἐπὶ τῶν νοσούντων, ἔκ τε τοῦ νοσήματος καὶ ἐκ τῆς ἀσιτίας καταλυομένη ἡ δύναμις εἰς φθορὰν τρέπεται. οὐδὲν δὲ ἧττον καὶ ἐπὶ τῶν χρονίων βλαβερὰ ἡ ἀσιτία καθέστηκε. τῷ γὰρ μήκει τοῦ χρόνου ταλαιπωρουμένη ἡ δύναμις, κάμνουσα δὲ καὶ τῇ ἀσιτίᾳ, καταλύει τὸν τόνον αὐτῆς καὶ οὐχ οἷά τέ ἐστι συμπέψαι τὰ αἴτια· κατὰ σύμπεψιν γὰρ εἴωθε τὰ χρόνια τῶν νοσημάτων ἀποπαύεσθαι. μεμάθηκας οὖν τὴν διαβολὴν τῆς λεπτοτάτης διαίτης, ὡς ἔστι χαλεπὴ καὶ ἐπὶ τῶν ὑγιαινόντων καὶ τῶν νοσούντων.

Δεύτερον δὲ κεφάλαιόν ἐστιν, ἐν ᾧ τὰς διαφορὰς αὐτῆς ἀπαριθμούμεθα. ἐπεὶ γὰρ

4–8 προθέμενος] *cf.* Gal. In Aphor. I 4: XVII B 367,14–16 K. Theoph. In Aphor.: II 261, 12–17 Dietz 6 τὰ – βλάψεις] Hipp. Aphor. II 10: IV 472,6–7 L. 19 καὶ – 23 δυνήσεται] *Stephanus* Hipp. Acut. 36–37 α' (10): I 125,20–127,9 Kw. = II 298,1–302,5 L. *explicans*

2 ἀεὶ α νοσήμασιν] *cf. infra, p. 76,20*: ὀξέσιν *Hipp., Theoph.* U''V'' (ὀξέσι νοσήμασιν C', *Theoph.* S) σφαλεραί *om.* P 5 *post* τῆς *add.* γε Z 6 βλάψης ω: *correxi* καθαρὰν Z 7 αὐτῶ ω (νῦν αὐτῶ A): *correxi* ἐπὶ τὴν *om.* Z 12 δέ *om.* Z 15 κενοῦνται Z ταράττονται *scripsi*: πράττονται ω 16 καταπίπτουσαι] καὶ καταπίπτουσιν Z φυσικαί] αἵ τε φυσικαὶ καὶ αἱ Z *post* ψυχικαί *addiderit* ζωτικαί *Duffy* 22 *fort.* μεταβαλεῖν *scribendum est* 23 δυνήσεται] δύναιτ' ἂν Z 25 τὴν δὲ] τὰ δὲ, τὴν Z 27 *ante* τῇ *add.* τῆς Z τῆς τροφῆς A 31 τόνον] χρόνον Z 32 οἷα ω: *correxi* 34 *post* καὶ[II] *add.* ἐπὶ Z 35 ἀπαριθμοῦμεν Z

I 9. A spare and rigid diet is dangerous, in prolonged affections always, in (acute) diseases, where not admissible.

Hippocrates has first relieved the body of the harm caused by the quality of the humors as well as of excess in quantity, thus making it free from superfluous matter as far as feasible; for he is well aware that "if a body is not clean, the more you feed it, the more you will harm it"; and so, starting from the assumption that it is now clean, he passes on to the subject of diet, with the purpose of providing a flawless foundation for its health; the diet he discusses is that which is to be followed in nutrition.

The present general survey consists of four main points. The first point is Hippocrates' harsh criticism of a spare diet, which he calls dangerous for a healthy body. Let us remember that our body has three kinds of components, solids, fluids and gases; now if abstinence from food is prescribed in the case of healthy persons, all of these are spent: the solids dissolve, the fluids run out, the gases disperse; whereupon all the faculties are disturbed and fail, the natural as well as the psychic. Abstinence from food causes harm to the healthy, not directly, but incidentally, because the matter that runs out and is dispersed from the body is not replenished by the administering of new food. It is also harmful, however, to the sick. Do not object, on the ground of what is said in Regimen in Acute Diseases: "But if the body has already gone through the change to sickness, what harm can even the sparest diet cause? In the case of the healthy it is dangerous because it brings about a change to sickness in bodies which until then were in a stable condition of health, but in the sick, who are already subject to the change to sickness, abstinence from food can cause no harm." My answer is that in illness our purpose is twofold: to eliminate the abnormal, and to preserve the patient's strength. We eliminate the disease by administering what is opposed to it, while we preserve strength by supplying what is similar to it; and what can be more similar or more conducive to strength than food? Food, therefore, supports and preserves the patient's resistance; so, if we prescribe abstinence from it for the sick, resistance is sapped both by the disease and by the lack of food, and goes to ruin. Finally, abstinence from food is no less damaging in chronic diseases. For if the patient's resistance, which is already poor as a result of the long duration, suffers further through lack of food, it loses its tone and is unable to concoct the causes (of the disease); chronic diseases are terminated by a process of concoction. You must have understood from this the warning against an extremely spare diet, that it is dangerous both for the healthy and for the sick.

Our second point is listing the various kinds of diets. Since we have re-

περὶ λεπτοτάτης διαίτης λόγον ἐποιησάμεθα, ἀκόλουθον ἡγούμεθα πᾶν εἶδος διαίτης τοῖς ὀνόμασι διαστεῖλασθαι. ἔστι τοίνυν ἐσχάτως λεπτὴ δίαιτα κατὰ μέν τινας τὸ μελίκρατον, καθ' ἑτέρους δὲ ἡ ἀσιτία· ἡ δὲ μετὰ ταύτην λεπτοτέρα ὁ χυλὸς τῆς πτισάνης· ἡ δὲ ἁπλῶς λεπτὴ πτισάνη σὺν κόκκοις· μέση δὲ πεπλυμένος ἄρτος καὶ ἴτριον· ἁδρὰ δὲ τὰ ᾠά· ἁδροτέρα δὲ ἰχθὺς καὶ λάχανα καὶ ἄρτος· ἁδροτάτη δὲ ὄρνις καὶ κρέατα καὶ τὰ τοιαῦτα.

Τρίτον κεφάλαιόν ἐστιν, ἐν ᾧ πρόκειται ἡμῖν τὴν χρείαν τῆς λεπτοτάτης διαίτης παραθέσθαι· μηδὲ γὰρ πάντῃ ἀπόβλητον αὐτὴν νομίσῃς διὰ τὴν λοιδορίαν καὶ καταδρομὴν τοῦ Ἱπποκράτους. χρησιμεύει τοίνυν ἡ λεπτοτάτη δίαιτα ἐπὶ τῶν κατοξέων νοσημάτων. ἐπειδὴ δὲ τῶν κατοξέων νοσημάτων ἐμνημονεύσαμεν, ἵνα γνῶμεν, τίς ἡ φύσις τῶν τοιούτων νοσημάτων, διαιρέσεώς τινος ἀναμνησθῶμεν περὶ τὸν χρόνον συνισταμένης. τῶν τοίνυν νοσημάτων τὰ μέν ἐστιν ὀξέα, τὰ δὲ χρόνια. καὶ χρόνια μὲν κυρίως λέγονται τὰ τὴν τεσσαρεσκαιδεκάτην ἡμέραν ὑπερβαίνοντα· αὐτὸς γὰρ ὁ Ἱπποκράτης ἐν τῷ Περὶ διαίτης ὀξέων ἔσχατον ὅρον τῶν ὀξέων νοσημάτων τὴν τεσσαρεσκαιδεκάτην ἡμέραν ποιεῖται. ἔστιν οὖν ἐκεῖνα χρόνια εἴτε αὐτόθεν οὕτως ἀρξάμενα εἴτε ἐκ μεταπτώσεως ὀξέων γινόμενα. τῶν δὲ ὀξέων τὰ μὲν ὁμωνύμως ἐστὶν ὀξέα, ὥσπερ τὰ μέχρι τεσσαρεσκαιδεκάτης ἀφικνούμενα· – τὰ γὰρ ἀπεντεῦθεν μέχρι τῆς τεσσαρακοστῆς ἐκτεινόμενα ἐκ μεταπτώσεώς ὀξέα ὡς ἐπὶ πᾶν λέγεται· – τὰ δὲ ἁπλῶς ἐστιν ὀξέα, ὥσπερ τὰ μέχρι τῆς ἑβδόμης προϊόντα ἢ καὶ τῆς ἐνάτης τὸ μήκιστον· τὰ δὲ κατόξεα, τὰ ἐντὸς τῆς τετάρτης περιγραφόμενα. ζητητέον οὖν, ἐπὶ ποίων τῶν μνημονευθέντων νοσημάτων ἡ λεπτοτάτη δίαιτά ἐστι χρήσιμος. καὶ δῆλον, ὅτι ἐπὶ τῶν κατοξέων νοσημάτων χρησιμεύει τὸ εἶδος τοῦτο τῆς διαίτης· ἐνταῦθα γὰρ ἐξαρκεῖ ἡ δύναμις, εἴτε ἐπὶ μελικράτῳ μόνῳ διαιτήσομεν ἢ ἄσιτον τὸν ἄνθρωπον παραφυλάξομεν. κατόξεα δὲ λέγεται νοσήματα, ἵνα μὴ μόνον ἐκ τοῦ τῶν ἡμερῶν ἀριθμοῦ γνωρίζειν ἔχωμεν αὐτῶν τὴν φύσιν, ἀλλὰ καὶ ἐπιστημονικῶς διά τινων ταύτην σημείων ἐπιγινώσκωμεν, τὰ ἔχοντα σφοδροὺς καὶ ὀξυτάτους πυρετοὺς καὶ πόνους ἐσχάτους, «πόνων» δηλονότι ἐνταῦθα τῶν συμπτωμάτων νοουμένων. οὕτω γὰρ αὐτός φησιν· «Ὅκου κάτοξυ νόσημα», διὰ τὸ θερμὸν καὶ δριμὺ καὶ ἐρεθιστικὸν τῆς ὕλης ὀξεῖς πυρετοὺς καὶ μεγάλους ἀναπτούσης «αὐτίκα τοὺς ἐσχάτους πόνους ἔχει καὶ τῇ ἐσχάτως λεπτοτάτῃ διαίτῃ ἀναγκαῖον χρέεσθαι.»

Τέταρτον κεφάλαιόν ἐστιν, ἐν ᾧ κανόνας καὶ προ⟨σ⟩διορισμοὺς θαυμασίους πάσης καθόλου διαίτης τυποῖ ἡμῖν ὁ Ἱπποκράτης. ὡς τινος γὰρ ἀποροῦντος ὅτι «Πῶς οἶδα, ἐπὶ ποίῳ νοσήματι τίνα μεταχειρίσομαι δίαιταν;» τοῦτο, φησί, δύνασαι συνιδεῖν ἔκ τινων τριῶν· ἐκ τοῦ εἴδους τοῦ νοσήματος, ἐκ τοῦ καιροῦ τοῦ

2 ἔστι – 6 τοιαῦτα] *cf.* Gal. In Aphor. I 4: XVII B 368,4–7; 369,12–370,2 K. Theoph. In Aphor.: II 262,9–15 Dietz 13 αὐτὸς – 15 ποιεῖται] *immo* Hipp. Aphor. II 23: IV 476,9–10 L. = Praen. Coac. 143: V 614,5–6 L. *cf.* Gal. In Aphor. I 4: XVII B 369,1–7 K. 16 τῶν – 24 παραφυλάξομεν] *v.* Theoph. In Aphor.: II 261,23–30 Dietz 28 Ὅκου – νόσημα *et* 29sq. αὐτίκα – χρέεσθαι] Hipp. Aphor. I 7: IV 462,12–13 L.

1 περὶ] τῆς Z 2 διαστεῖλλεσθαι Z 3 ἑτέρους *scripsi*: ἑκάτερα P: ἕτερα (κά supra) A: ἑκατρ Z 5 ἰτρίον ω: *correxi* ἁδρο^τρ P 9 ἱπποκράτου A 11 *post* τοιούτων *add.* δηλαδὴ Z 13 κυρίως λέγονται] ἐστι κυρίως Z 14 *post* τῷ *add.* τῆς A ἔσχατον – ὀξέων^II *om.* Z 17 τὰ^I] τῶν Z τεσσαρισκαιδεκάτ(ης) Z: ιδ' α ἀφικνουμένων Z 19 *post* δὲ *add.* γε Z ἐστιν *om.* Z 21 χρήσιμός ἐστι Z 23 *post* ἢ *add.* καὶ Z 24 νοσήματα λέγεται Z 25 ἔχομεν A 26 ταύτη P ἐπιγινώσκομεν α: *corr.* A² 28 *post* θερμὸν *add.* δηλαδὴ Z 30 χρῆσθαι Z 31 προδιορισμοὺς ω: *corr. Duffy* 34 *post* τριῶν *add.* συμβολαίων Z ἐκ^I] ἀπό τε Z ἐκ^II *om.* Z 34sq. τοῦ νοσήματος *om.* Z

ferred to the strictest diet, the next thing to do is, we believe, to distinguish each kind of diet by its own name. The "extremely light" diet, then, is, according to some, honey-and-water, according to others, abstinence; the "lighter" diet, next to this, is barley-water; the "light" diet simply, barley-gruel; the "intermediate" diet is fine bread and cake; the "heavy" diet, eggs; the "heavier", fish, vegetables and bread; the "heaviest", chicken, meat, etc.

As a third point we propose to explain the usefulness of the lightest diet; for you should not think, because of Hippocrates' strong disapproval and criticism, that it is to be rejected entirely. The extremely light diet is useful, then, in the case of very acute diseases. Now that we have mentioned very acute diseases, let us remember a classification according to time, so as to understand the nature of such diseases. Diseases are either acute or chronic. Chronic diseases properly so called are those which exceed the fourteenth day; it is Hippocrates himself, in Regimen in Acute Diseases, who makes the fourteenth day the utmost limit of acute diseases. They either have been chronic from the very beginning or have become so through a change in character of acute diseases. Of acute diseases, some are called acute in a wider sense, namely those that last until the fourteenth day; – those extending beyond this until the fortieth day are usually spoken of as acute diseases which have changed their character; – others are strictly acute, those that continue to the seventh day, or, at the longest, to the ninth; others are very acute, those that do not go beyond the fourth day. We must ask now, for which of the diseases mentioned the lightest diet is beneficial. It is clear, then, that this kind of diet is useful in very acute diseases; in that case there is a sufficient reserve of strength, whether we keep the patient on a diet of honey-and-water, or allow him no food at all. Now very acute diseases – I add this so that we may be able not only to recognize their character from the number of days, but also to discern it scientifically by means of certain signs – are those which involve violent and very sudden fevers and extreme discomforts, "discomforts" of course to be understood here as the symptoms. These are (Hippocrates') own words: "Where there is a very acute disease, (the patient)" – as a result of the hot, sharp and irritating quality of the matter, which causes sudden high fevers – "is immediately in extreme discomfort, and one must use the most rigorously strict diet."

The fourth point are the admirable rules and specifications for all diet generally which Hippocrates outlines for us. As if the question were asked: "How can I tell which diet to employ for which disease?" he says that you can infer this from three things: the kind of disease, the moment of the disease and

νοσήματος καὶ ἐκ τοῦ τόνου τῆς δυνάμεως. εἰς μὲν γὰρ τὸ εἶδος τοῦ νοσήματος ἀποβλέπων διαιτήσεις τὸν τρόπον τοῦτον. πρό⟨σ⟩σχες, εἰ τριταῖός ἐστιν, εἰ καῦσός ἐστιν, εἰ σύνοχός ἐστιν· εἰ γάρ ἐστι, θερμή ἐστιν ἡ ὕλη δηλονότι καὶ ὀξὺ τὸ νόσημα καὶ ὀλιγοχρόνιον, καὶ λεπτῇ διαίτῃ ὅσον ἐπὶ τούτῳ δέον χρήσασθαι. εἰ δὲ ἀμφημερινὸς ὑπόκειται ἢ τεταρταῖος, ψυχρά ἐστιν ἡ ὕλη καὶ χρόνιον τὸ νόσημα, καὶ ἁδροτέρᾳ διαίτῃ προσηκόντως χρησόμεθα. εἰς δὲ τὸν καιρὸν ἀποβλέποντες διαιτήσομεν τὸν τρόπον τοῦτον. εἰ μὲν πλησίον ἐστὶν ἡ ἀκμή, κατὰ τὸν χρόνον ἐκεῖνον καὶ μικρὸν πρὸ ἐκείνου τὴν λεπτοτάτην παραληψόμεθα δίαιταν, εἰ δὲ πόρρω, τὴν ἁδροτέραν. εἰ γὰρ θρέψομεν κατὰ τὸν καιρὸν τῆς ἀκμῆς, δυοῖν ἀτόποιν θάτερον ἕψεται κακόν· ἢ γὰρ περὶ τὴν τροφὴν ἀπασχολουμένη ἡ δύναμις καταφρονεῖ τῆς ἐργασίας τῆς περὶ τὰ αἴτια, κἀντεῦθεν ἐπιτίθεται καὶ σκιρτᾷ τὸ νόσημα τῷ σώματι τυραννίδι τινὶ καὶ αὐτονομίᾳ κατ' αὐτοῦ ἅτε μηδενὸς ἀνθισταμένου χρώμενον· ἢ πρὸς μὲν τὰ αἴτια ἀπασχολεῖται, περιορᾷ δὲ τὴν πέψιν τῆς τροφῆς, ἥτις ἀπεπτουμένη τῇ νοσοποιῷ ὕλῃ προστίθεται καὶ τὸ μέγεθος αὔξει τοῦ νοσήματος. ὥστε οὖν ἐν ταῖς ἀκμαῖς τῶν νοσημάτων ἀσίτους δεῖ τηρεῖν τοὺς ἀρρώστους· χρὴ γὰρ «τοὺς παροξυσμοὺς ὑποστέλλεσθαι, ἐπεὶ τὸ προστιθέναι βλαβερόν». παρούσης οὖν ἢ πλησιαζούσης τῆς ἀκμῆς καὶ δηλούσης ὅσον οὔπω μέλλουσαν ἔσεσθαι κρίσιν, οἷον περὶ τὴν εἰκοστὴν ἡμέραν, ἀπὸ τῆς ἑπτακαιδεκάτης ἀσιτίαν παραλαμβάνειν δέον. καὶ φυλαττέσθω τῶν κατοξέων ὁ λόγος καὶ ἐπὶ τῶν τοιούτων πάντων· ἀπὸ γὰρ τῆς ἑπτακαιδεκάτης μέχρι καὶ τῆς εἰκοστῆς τετάρτης εἰσὶν η' ἡμέραι, ἐν αἷς τὸ μόριον τοῦτο τοῦ νοσήματος περιγράφεται, φημὶ δὴ ἡ ἀκμή. εἰς δὲ τὸν τόνον τῆς δυνάμεως ἀφορῶντες διαιτῶμεν τὸν τρόπον τοῦτον. δεῖ ἅψασθαι τῆς ἀρτηρίας· καὶ εἰ μὲν εὕρωμεν ἐρρωμένην τὴν δύναμιν, ἀσιτίαν παραλαμβάνομεν, εἰ δὲ καταβέβληται, τρέφομεν καὶ ταύτῃ τὸ πᾶν κῦρος παρέχομεν, λέγω δὴ τῇ δυνάμει. αὐτῇ γὰρ δεῖ κατακολουθοῦντας, εἰ καὶ τὰ λοιπὰ ἐναντίως ἔχει, τὸ τῆς διαίτης εἶδος ἁρμόζειν. πολλάκις γὰρ καὶ τὸ νόσημα ὀξὺ ὑπόκειται καὶ ὁ καιρὸς τῆς ἀκμῆς πλησίον ἐστίν, ἀσθενεῖ δὲ ἡ δύναμις, καὶ ἀναγκαζόμεθα θρέψαι βοηθοῦντες τῇ δυνάμει· οὐ γὰρ ἔχομεν ἑτέρῳ τινὶ τὰ νοσοποιὰ αἴτια καταγωνίσασθαι. ὥσπερ οὖν καὶ ἀνάπαλιν χρόνιον ὑπόκειται πολλάκις νόσημα καὶ ἡ ἀκμὴ πόρρω, ἔρρωται δὲ ἡ δύναμις, καὶ ἐπὶ διαίτῃ λεπτοτάτῃ τὸν ἄνθρωπον διεξάγομεν θαρροῦντες εἰς τὴν δύναμιν.

Αἱ λεπταὶ καὶ ἀκριβέες δίαιται. ὁ Ἱπποκράτης κατὰ συγκεχυμένον τρόπον προφέρει τὰ λεγόμενα, καὶ διαλεγόμενος περὶ τῶν διαφορῶν τῆς διαίτης τὴν λοιδορίαν τῆς ἐσχάτως λεπτῆς διαίτης ἐν τῷ μέσῳ τίθησι. διὰ μὲν γὰρ τοῦ εἰπεῖν αἱ λεπταὶ δίαιται τὸ εἶδος τῆς διαίτης ἐδήλωσε, καὶ οὕτως ἐπήγαγε τὴν διαβολήν· ἐπεὶ δὲ ᾔσθετο τὸ τῆς λεπτῆς διαίτης ὄνομα ὁμώνυμον εἶναι, ἵνα μὴ καθ' ἑκατέρου

15sq. τοὺς – βλαβερόν] Hipp. Aphor. I 11: IV 464,11–12 L.

1 ἐκ *om.* Z τόνου] νοῦ P 2 πρόσχες ω: *correxi* 3 ἐστιν[I et II] *om.* Z γάρ ἐστι *om.* Z ἐστι, θερμή *om.* A ἡ *om.* α 4 τοῦτο ω: *correxi* 5 ἡ *om.* Z 6 χρησάμεθα Z 7 τοῦτον τὸν τρόπον Z 9 θρέψοιμεν Z 13 ἀπεπτουμένη] ἀποπεμπομένη A: ἀπασχολουμένη Z 14 μέγεθος] μέγα P 16 ἐπειδὴ Z 18 *post* εἰκοστὴν *add.* δηλαδὴ Z *post* ἀπὸ *add.* γε Z παραλαμβάνειν δέον] παραλαμβάνεσθαι δέον P: δεῖν παραλαμβάνειν Z 20 καὶ *om.* Z η' *scripsi*: αἱ Z: *om.* α 21 ἐπιγράφεται Z 22 εἰ] ἢν Z εὕρομεν α ἐρρῶσθαι A 23 παραλαμβάνωμεν P τρέφωμεν α 24 παρέχωμεν α κατακολουθεῖν Z 25 ἔχοι Z 30 διεξάγωμεν Z 32 διαφόρων Z 33 ἐσχάτως *scripsi*: ἐσχάτ *(ambig.)* Z: ἐσχάτης α 34 *ante* τὴν *add.* ἐδήλωσε α *post* διαβολήν *add.* ἤτοι τὸ ἀκριβέες Z 35 δὲ] γὰρ Z ἵνα μὴ] ἵν' ἀεὶ Z

the force of the patient's resistance. In view of the kind of disease you will determine the diet as follows. Observe whether it is a tertian fever, whether it is a causus, whether it is non-remittent; if so, the matter is obviously hot and the disease is acute and brief, and as far as this is concerned we should prescribe a light diet. If, however, it is a question of a quotidian or quartan fever, the matter is cold and the disease chronic, and we may properly use a heavier diet. From the point of view of the moment of the disease our dieting rules will be these. If the acme is near, we will at that time, and shortly before, use the very lightest diet, if it is far away, the heavier. For if we administer food at the moment of the acme, one out of two unpleasant consequences will follow: either the patient's energy will be absorbed by the food and neglect its task of fighting the causes of the disease, so that the disease can assault the body at will and rule it with the absolute power of a despot, since it meets with no opposition; or else (this energy) is concentrated on the causes and it neglects the digestion of the food, which, when it remains undigested, is added to the matter that causes the disease and thus increases its power. During the acme of a disease we must therefore make the patient abstain from food; for one should "use restraint in the paroxysms, because then any addition is harmful". So when the disease is at, or near, its height and it is clear that the crisis may set in at any moment, e.g. about the twentieth day, abstinence from food should be prescribed from the seventeenth day onward. The rule for very acute diseases must be observed in all those cases: from the seventeenth to the twenty-fourth day there are 8 days within which that part of the disease falls, i.e. the acme. Then, with a view to keeping up the patient's strength, we regulate his diet in the following manner. We feel the pulse; and if we find that his strength holds out, we prescribe abstinence from food, but if it is low, we feed him and give first priority to that consideration, the power of resistance. It is to this, even if the other things point the opposite way, that we must adapt the diet. Often indeed, when we have to do with an acute disease and the moment of the acme is near, but resistance is weak, we are forced to administer food in order to maintain the patient's strength, which is our only means to overcome the causes of the disease. Similarly in the opposite case: often when the disease is chronic and its acme far away, but resistance is strong, we keep the patient on the lightest diet because we have confidence in his strength.

A spare and rigid diet. Hippocrates presents his statements in a jumbled order: while dealing with the different kinds of diets he inserts his criticism of the extremely light diet. When he said A spare diet, he indicated the kind of diet and then followed up with the warning; however, as he was aware that the term "spare diet" is ambiguous and wanted to prevent us from

σημαινομένου τὴν μέμψιν ὑπονοήσωμεν λέγεσθαι, οὐκ ἠρκέσθη μόνον εἰπεῖν αἱ λεπταί, ἀλλ' ἐπήγαγε τὸ ἀκριβέες, ἵνα διὰ τούτου τὴν ἐσχάτως λεπτὴν νοήσωμεν δίαιταν. καὶ μή τις μέμψηται τὸν Ἱπποκράτην ἐπ' ἀσιτίᾳ τὸ τῆς διαίτης ὄνομα θέντα· ἰδιώματι γὰρ παλαιῷ ἐχρήσατο, καθ' ὃ πᾶσαν τὴν περὶ τὸν κάμνοντα γινομένην ἐπιμέλειαν οἱ παλαιοὶ δίαιταν καλεῖν εἰώθησαν, ὥστε οὐκ ἂν ἁμάρτῃς φλεβοτομίαν ἢ κλυστῆρα ἢ ἐπεμβροχὴν ἢ ἕτερόν τι τῶν οὕτω γινομένων δίαιταν ὀνομάζων παρὰ τὸ ἐν αὐτοῖς διαιτᾶσθαι τὸν κάμνοντα. ὡσαύτως καὶ ἡ ἀσιτία ἐπιμέλεια οὖσα εἰκότως ἂν καλοῖτο κατὰ τὸ ἀκόλουθον δίαιτα.

Τί δὲ δηλοῖ τὸ οὗ μὴ ἐπιδέχεται; λέγει ὁ Γαληνός, ὅτι ἡ ἐσχάτως λεπτοτάτη δίαιτα καὶ ἐπὶ τῶν χρονίων καὶ ἐπὶ τῶν ὀξέων νοσημάτων οὐκ ἐνδέχεται δεχθῆναι, καταλύεται γὰρ ὑπ' αὐτῆς ἡ δύναμις. ἔστι δὲ καὶ [ἡ] ἄλλη ἐξήγησις· χαλεπὴν τὴν ἐσχάτως ⟨λεπτοτάτην⟩ δίαιταν ἀπεφήνατο οὐ μόνον ἐπὶ τῶν χρονίων καὶ ὀξέων νοσημάτων, ἀλλὰ καὶ ἐπὶ τῶν κατοξέων, οὐ πάντῃ ἀπόβλητον αὐτὴν ἀποφηνάμενος, ἀλλ' ἐπαγαγὼν οὗ μὴ ἐπιδέχεται, τουτέστιν ἐφ' ὧν ἡ δύναμις ἀσθενεῖ, ἐφ' ὧν τὸ στόμα τῆς γαστρὸς ταχέως ἐκχολοῦται, ἐφ' ὧν ἀραιόπορον φύσει καὶ εὐδιαφόρητον ὑπάρχει τὸ σῶμα. πρὸς δὲ τούτοις δεῖ ἐπιθεωρεῖν καὶ τὴν τῶν συστοίχων φύσιν ἀποβλέποντας εἰς ὥραν καὶ χώραν καὶ ἡλικίαν καὶ τὰ τοιαῦτα. ἐπὶ μὲν οὖν τῶν χρονίων τὸ ἀεὶ τέθηκεν, ἐπὶ δὲ τῶν ὀξέων οὗ μὴ ἐπιδέχεται· καὶ γὰρ ἐπὶ μὲν τῶν χρονίων νοσημάτων ἡ λεπτὴ δίαιτα χαλεπή, ἐπὶ δὲ τῶν ὀξέων οὐκ ἐπὶ πάντων διὰ τὰ κατόξεα. ἐπὶ μέντοι τῶν χρονίων πάθος εἶπεν, ἐπὶ δέ γε τῶν ὀξέων νόσημα.

I 10 [I 4: IV 462,1–2 L.] Αἱ εἰς τὸ ἔσχατον λεπτότητος ἀφιγμέναι δίαιται χαλεπαί· καὶ αἱ πληρώσιες αἱ εἰς ἔσχατον ἥκουσαι χαλεπαί.

Εἰρηκὼς χαλεπὴν εἶναι τὴν ⟨λεπτὴν⟩ δίαιταν, ἵνα μή τις ὁμωνύμῳ φωνῇ σὺν κόκκοις νοήσῃ πτισάνην ἢ ἄρτον πεπλυμένον ἤ τι τοιοῦτον, ἐπήγαγε «καὶ ἀκριβέες», ὡς ἀνωτέρω εἴρηται· εἶτα ἐπειδὴ οἶδεν, ὅτι λεπτὴ καὶ ἀκριβὴς δίαιτά ἐστι καὶ τὸ μελίκρατον, εὐλαβηθείς, μή τις ὑπονοήσῃ αὐτὸν περὶ τούτου λέγειν, ἐπήγαγεν αἱ εἰς ἔσχατον λεπτότητος ἀφιγμέναι δίαιται χαλεπαί, ἀντὶ τοῦ «ἡ ἀσιτία».

Ἀναφαίνεται δὲ ἀπορία[ν] ἐνταῦθα ἐκ τοῦ Τοπικοῦ παραγγέλματος· φησὶ γὰρ Ἀριστοτέλης, ὅτι ὧν τὸ ἐναντίον βλάπτει, τὸ ἐναντίον ὠφελεῖ· ἐὰν οὖν ἡ ἔνδεια βλάπτῃ, ἡ πλεονεξία ὠφελεῖ. λοιπὸν ἵνα μή τις ἐκ τοῦ τοιούτου κανόνος ὁρμώμενος εἴπῃ ὅτι «Ἐὰν ἡ ἐσχάτως λεπτὴ δίαιτα βλάπτῃ, πάντως ἂν ἡ πάνυ ἁδρο-

9 λέγει – 11 δύναμις] *cf.* Gal. In Aphor. I 4: XVII B 367,16–368,4; 370,2–5 (?) K. 25 ὡς ἀνωτέρω εἴρηται] *v. supra*, p. 74,35–76,2 29–30 ὠφελεῖ] *v.* Aristot. Top. VI 9: 147 a 32–35 *infra*, vol. III, fol. 178v

1 λέγεσθαι *om.* Z 2 ἵνα] ὡς ἂν Z 4 γενομένην A 5 ἐπιμέλειαν] δίαιταν A εἰώθεσαν Z 6 ἐπεμβροχῇ P ὀνομάζειν Z 7 *ante* καὶ *add.* δὲ Z ἐπιμέλεια] ἐπὶ μέσα Z 9 οὐ α λέγει] καὶ φησὶν Z 11 [ἡ] ἄλλη ἐξήγησις] ἡ *delevi*: ἄλλως ἐξηγήσασθαι Z 12 *ante* τὴν *add.* γὰρ Z λεπτοτάτην *addidi* 15 ἐκχυλοῦται A: ἐκκεχολοῦται Z ἐνδιαφόρητον Z 17 ἀποβλέπτοντας Z ὥρην Z χώρην Z ἡλικίην Z 20 *post* κατόξεα *add.* δηλαδή· καὶ ὅτι Z μέντοι] μὲν Z γε *om.* Z νοσήματα Z 22 καὶ] *item infra, p. 78,6, Hipp.* C′: καὶ γὰρ *Hipp., Theoph.* πληρώσεις α εἰς ἔσχατον ἥκουσαι] *item infra, p. 78,7*: ἐς τὸ ἔσχατον ἀφιγμέναι *Hipp.* 23 τὴν *om.* P λεπτὴν *addidi* 24 νοῆσαι A τι τοιοῦτον] τοιοῦτον P: τοιοῦτόν τι Z 26 *ante* τὸ *add.* αὐτὸ δὴ Z 27 ἐς P λεπτοτάτ *(ambig.)* P 28 *post* ἀσιτία *add.* δηλαδή Z 29 ἀπορίαν ω: *correxi* 30sq. ἐὰν – ὠφελεῖ *om.* Z 31 λοιπὸν] οὐκοῦν Z 32 Ἐὰν] ἔστ' ἂν Z

understanding his disapproval as extending to both meanings, he did not simply say spare, but added and rigid, to make us think of the extremely light diet. One should not find fault with Hippocrates for applying the word diet to abstention from food; he used an old idiom, by which the ancients called the entire treatment given to the patient "diet", so that you would be perfectly correct in calling a bleeding, an enema, an embrocation or any similar proceeding a "diet", because the patient is treated (*diaitān*) in that way. Thus the withholding of food, being a form of treatment, can rightly be called a "diet" on the analogy of these.

But what is meant by where not admissible? Galen says that neither chronic nor acute diseases admit of the extremely light diet, because it breaks down the power of resistance. There is another possible interpretation: he declared the extremely light diet dangerous, not only in chronic and acute diseases, but also in the very acute ones, not meaning to reject it absolutely, but with the addition where not admissible, i.e. in cases where resistance is weak, or the orifice of the stomach is apt to be flooded with bile, or the body is by nature loosely structured and subject to quick dispersal. In addition to this, we must observe the character of the correlative factors, taking into consideration the season, the region, the age group, etc. So with regard to chronic diseases he says always, with regard to acute ones, where not admissible, because in chronic diseases a light diet is dangerous, in acute diseases not always, on account of the very acute ones. With reference to chronic cases he speaks of affection, with reference to acute ones, of disease.

I 10. A diet that is spare to excess is dangerous; and excessive repletion is also dangerous.

After saying that a spare diet is dangerous, he added "and rigid", as we have said above, to prevent this from being understood as barley-gruel, or fine bread, or something of the kind, owing to the ambiguity of the term; next, as he knows that honey-and-water is also a spare and rigid diet and is afraid of being understood as meaning this, he continued: A diet that is spare to excess is dangerous, that is to say, abstinence from all food.

Here a difficulty presents itself, which arises from the maxim in the Topics, where Aristotle says that, if of a pair of opposites one is harmful, its opposite is beneficial; so if a deficiency is harmful, a surplus is beneficial. Now in case anybody should argue on the ground of this rule: "If an excessively light diet

τάτη ὠφελοίη τοὺς τοιούτους ἀρρώστους», αὐτὸς προϋπέφθασε λέγων, ὅτι ἡ ἄκρως ἁδρὰ δίαιτα χαλεπή ἐστιν ἐπ' αὐτῶν. οὐδὲ γὰρ αὕτη ἀντίκειται τῇ ἐσχάτως λεπτοτάτῃ διαίτῃ, ἀλλ' ἡ μέσως λεπτή. ὥστε ὁμοίως διαβάλλει ἐπὶ τῶν τοιούτων νοσημάτων καὶ τὴν ἄκρως λεπτὴν δίαιταν, φημὶ δὴ τὴν ἀσιτίαν, καὶ τὴν ἁδροτάτην· ἑκατέρα γὰρ ξενισμὸν ἐμποιεῖ τῇ φύσει ἐν ἀμετρίᾳ θεωρουμένη, αἱ μέσαι δὲ δίαιται ὡς σύμμετροι τὸ βλαβερὸν ἀποφεύγουσιν. ὅθεν καλῶς εἶπεν, ὅτι καὶ αἱ πληρώσιες αἱ εἰς ἔσχατον ἥκουσαι χαλεπαί.

I 11 [I 5: IV 462,3 L.] Ἐν τῇσι λεπτῇσι διαίτῃσιν ἁμαρτάνουσιν οἱ νοσέοντες.

Ἔτι καὶ νῦν διαβάλλει τὴν λεπτὴν δίαιταν ὁ Ἱπποκράτης βλαβερὰν αὐτὴν ἀποκαλῶν. ἡ δὲ βλάβη αὐτῆς διχῶς γίνεται ἐπὶ τῶν νοσούντων, ἢ γὰρ ἑκόντες ἢ ἄκοντες βλάπτονται. καὶ ἵνα σαφὲς εἴη τὸ λεγόμενον, ἐξ ὑποθέσεως ὁ λόγος γυμναζέσθω. ὁρῶμέν τινα ἄρρωστον κάτοξυ νόσημα ἔχοντα, λίχνον δὲ πάσης τροφῆς, καὶ τοῦτον ἀσιτῆσαι κελεύομεν. εἶτα ἡμῶν ἀναχωρησάντων βαρείας τῆς ἐπιταγῆς καὶ οἷον ἀδυνάτου αἰσθάνεσθαι δοκεῖ ὁ νοσῶν, καὶ πεισθείς, ὡς ἐντεῦθεν ἄτονος γενήσεται, τροφὴν ἐπιζητεῖ καὶ προδήλως βλάπτεται. καὶ οὕτω μὲν βλάπτονται οἱ νοσοῦντες ἑκουσίως ἁμαρτάνοντες. ἐπὶ οὖν τῶν τοιούτων ἀρρώστων, εἰ καὶ χρεία ἐστὶν ὅσον ἐπὶ τῇ νόσῳ ἀσιτίας, λεπτὴν δεῖ παραλαμβάνειν δίαιταν καὶ προλέγειν αὐτοῖς τὴν φιλοτιμίαν, ὅτι «Ὅσον μὲν ἐπὶ τῷ καλῶς ἔχοντι ἔδει σε ἀσιτῆσαι, ἀλλ' ἐπειδὴ πρό⟨σ⟩κεισαι τῇ τροφῇ, πρὸς τὸ κεχαρισμένον σοι ταύτην ἐπετράπης.» κἀντεῦθεν ἐκεῖνος λογιζόμενος ὅτι «Ἐπὰν ἔδει με ἀσιτῆσαι, κατὰ φιλοτιμίαν δὲ ταύτην ἐπετάγην τὴν τροφήν, πεισθῆναι δεῖ τῇ ἐπιταγῇ τοῦ ἰατροῦ καὶ ταύτῃ μόνῃ τῇ τροφῇ ἀρκεσθῆναι» — οὕτω γὰρ διαιτώμενος οὐκ ἀδικεῖται. καὶ τοῦτο εἰδὼς ὁ Ἱπποκράτης προϊών φησιν ὅτι «Τὸ σμικρὸν χεῖρον καὶ πόμα καὶ σιτίον, ἥδιον δέ, τῶν βελτιόνων μέν, ἀηδεστέρων δέ, μᾶλλον αἱρετέον.»

Ἀκουσίως δὲ βλάπτονται οἱ νοσοῦντες οὕτως. ὑποκείσθωσαν ἄρρωστοι δύο τὸ αὐτὸ ἔχοντες νόσημα· καὶ ὁ μὲν μελίκρατον λαμβανέτω, ὁ δὲ ᾠά, καὶ ἑκάτερος ἐπὶ τὸ βέλτιον προκοπτέτω καὶ πρὸς ἀπαλλαγὴν τοῦ νοσήματος βλεπέτω. ἔνθα λοιπὸν καὶ ἁδρᾶς διαίτης ἐπίδοσις γίνεται, καὶ δὴ παρέχομεν ἀμφοτέροις ὄρνιν. ἐπὶ γοῦν τῇ τροφῇ ταύτῃ ὁ μὲν εἰς ἐβλάβη, ὁ ἐπὶ τῷ μελικράτῳ διαιτώμενος, ὁ δὲ ἐπὶ τοῖς ᾠοῖς διαιτώμενος ὠφελήθη μὴ ἀθρόᾳ χρησάμενος μεταβολῇ. οὐ μόνον δὲ ἐπὶ τῶν νοσούντων, ἀλλὰ καὶ ἐπὶ τῶν ὑγιαινόντων τοῦτο συμβαίνει. πολλάκις γάρ τις εἴθιστο λεπτῶς διαιτᾶσθαι διὰ σώφρονα καὶ σεμνὸν βίον· τούτῳ συνέβη πλεῦσαί ποτε,

10 Ἔτι – 12 βλάπτονται] *cf.* Gal. In Aphor. I 5: XVII B 371,12–15 K. 10sq. Ἔτι – ἀποκαλῶν] *v.* Theoph. In Aphor.: II 263,3–5 Dietz 24sq. Τὸ – αἱρετέον] Hipp. Aphor. II 38: IV 480,17–18 L.

1 προϋπέφθασε λέγων, ὅτι] προλαβὼν εἶπεν Z 2 ἀβρὰ A ἐπ' αὐτῶν] αὐτοῖς Z ἀντίκειται αὕτη Z λεπτοτάτῃ] λεπτῇ Z 5sq. ὡς σύμμετροι] ἅτε ξύμμετροι οὖσαι Z 6 ὅτι] ὡς Z πληρώσεις α 8 τοῖσι Z 11 δὲ] γοῦν Z 13 ἔχοντα νόσημα Z 14 ἀσιτεῖσθαι A 16 γενήσεσθαι Z 17 νοσέοντες Z ἑκοντὶ Z οὖν] γοῦν Z 18 τῇ] τῆς P ἀσιτίας νόσω Z 19 σε *om.* A 20 πρόκεισαι AZ: *corr.* P κεχαρησμένην Z 21 ἀναλογιζόμενος Z Ἐπὰν] ἐπεὶ Z με ἀσιτῆσαι] μοι, ἄσιτος μενεῖν Z 22 δεῖν Z 25 ἀειδέστερον A 26 ἑκουσίως α νοσέοντες Z 27 νόσημα ἔχοντες Z 29 ἁδρῆς α *post* παρέχομεν *add.* αὖ Z γοῦν] μὲν οὖν A 30 βέβλαπται Z 31 διαιτώμενος *om.* Z δὲ] γ' Z 32 *ante* τοῦτο *add.* αὐτὸ Z 33 *post* τούτῳ *add.* γοῦν Z

is harmful, the very heaviest will necessarily be beneficial to such patients", (Hippocrates) forestalled him by saying that an extremely heavy diet is bad for them. Indeed, it is not this diet which is the opposite of the excessively light diet, but the moderately light. Therefore in diseases of this kind he equally disapproves of the excessively light diet, i.e. abstinence, and of the heaviest; for since both are characterized by excess, both cause violent changes in the constitution, while the intermediate diet, which is moderate, avoids such harm. Hence (Hippocrates) said rightly that excessive repletion is also dangerous.

I 11. In a light diet patients will make mistakes.

Once more Hippocrates warns against the light diet, calling it harmful. The harm is of two kinds, as far as the patients are concerned, for either it is due to their own free will, or it is not. To make our meaning clear, let us apply the point to a hypothetical case. We see a man who suffers from a very acute disease, but is fond of any kind of food, and we tell him to fast. Then after our departure the patient feels that the order is hard and practically impossible to obey, and being convinced that it will sap his strength he asks for food and suffers visible harm. This is the kind of damage caused by the patient's own free will. In such cases, even if fasting is required as far as the disease is concerned, you may prescribe a light diet, while making it clear that you are stretching a point: "For your own good you should really fast, but since you are so keen on food, you are allowed this much as a special favor." He will then reason: "Since I should really fast, and this food has been prescribed by way of concession, I had better obey the doctor's orders and be content with it" – if he follows this regimen, it will not injure him. Knowing this, Hippocrates says further down: "Drink and food which are a little less wholesome, but tastier, should be preferred to what is better, but less palatable."

On the other hand, patients may suffer harm without it being their own fault, as follows. Let us take two men suffering from the same disease; and suppose the one takes honey-and-water, the other eggs, and both are making progress and recovery is in sight. It is now time for a heavy diet, and we let them both have a chicken. After this meal one becomes worse – the one who lived on honey-and-water –, while the other, who lived on eggs, improves, because he has not undergone a sudden change. This holds good, not only of sick people, but of the healthy, too. A frequent case is the following: a man was used to a spare diet, because he pursued an abstemious, religious way of life; one day

συνέπλεε δὲ αὐτῷ ἕτερός τις, ἁδροτέρᾳ διαίτῃ συνήθως χρώμενος. εἶτα εἰς πολλὰς ἡμέρας τοῦ πλοῦ ἐκταθέντος συνέβη ἐν ἀπορίᾳ καταστῆναι τὸν λεπτῶς διαιτώμενον κἀντεῦθεν συνδιαιτηθῆναι τῷ ἑτέρῳ καὶ ὀσπριοφαγίαις ἐξ ἀνάγκης χρήσασθαι· ἐφ' αἷς οὗτος μὲν ἐβλάβη τὰ μέγιστα, ὁ δ' ἕτερος ἀβλαβὴς διέμεινε, τῇ συνήθει γὰρ τροφῇ καὶ νῦν ἐχρήσατο.

I 12 [I 6: IV 462,10–11 L.] Εἰς δὲ τὰ ἔσχατα νοσήματα αἱ ἔσχαται θεραπεῖαι ⟨ἐς ἀκριβείην κράτισται⟩.

Ἔσχατα μὲν καλεῖ νοσήματα τὰ κατόξεα, ὧν οὐκ ἔστιν ἐπινοῆσαι ὀξυτέραν ἐν νόσῳ κίνησιν, εἰ μή τι ἄρα τὸν ἐφημερινόν· ἐσχάτην δὲ θεραπείαν τὴν λεπτοτάτην δίαιταν, τουτέστι τὴν ἀσιτίαν. αὐτίκα γὰρ ἡ ἀσιτία κρατίστη ἐστὶν ἐπὶ τῶν κατοξέων, εἰ μὴ ἀσθενὴς ὑπόκειται ἡ δύναμις ἢ στόμα τῆς γαστρὸς ἐκχολούμενον κατὰ τὰ ἀνωτέρω εἰρημένα.

I 13 [I 7: IV 462,12–13 L.] Ὅκου μὲν οὖν κάτοξυ τὸ νόσημα, αὐτίκα ⟨τοὺς ἐσχάτους πόνους ἔχει καὶ τῇ ἐσχάτως λεπτοτάτῃ διαίτῃ ἀναγκαῖον χρέεσθαι⟩.

Ἐκεῖνο τοίνυν ἐστὶ τὸ κάτοξυ νόσημα, τὸ σφοδρὸν ἔχον τὸν πυρετὸν καὶ χαλεποὺς πόνους ἤγουν συμπτώματα, ἀγρυπνίαν φημὶ καὶ ἄλογον δίψος καὶ ῥιπτασμὸν καὶ ὅσα τοιαῦτα.

Τὸ δὲ αὐτίκα δηλοῖ ἐνταῦθα τὸν περιγραφόμενον χρόνον ἐντὸς τῶν τριῶν ἡμερῶν· ἐπὶ γὰρ τῶν κατοξέων νοσημάτων ὅλος οὗτος ὁ χρόνος, φημὶ ὁ τριήμερος, ἀκμή ἐστιν.

I 14 [I 7: IV 462,14–15 L.] Ὅκου δὲ μή, ἀλλ' ἐνδέχεται ἁδροτέρως διαιτᾶν, ⟨τοσοῦτον ὑποκαταβαίνειν, ὁκόσον ἂν ἡ νοῦσος μαλθακωτέρη τῶν ἐσχάτων ᾖ⟩.

Εἰρηκὼς τὴν κατὰ μέρος δίαιταν, ὅτι ἐν τοῖς κατόξεσι νοσήμασιν ἀσιτίαν παραληπτέον, ἐπὶ τὰ καθόλου ἄνεισι· καὶ πολλῆς οὔσης τῆς τῶν νοσημάτων σειρᾶς πᾶσαν περιέλαβεν ἐν τῷ φάναι· ὅκου δὲ μή, ἀλλ' ἐνδέχεται ἁδροτέρως διαιτᾶν.

8–12] *v.* Gal. In Aphor. I 6: XVII B 372,8–12 K. Theoph. In Aphor.: II 264,29–35 Dietz 12 κατὰ – εἰρημένα] *v. supra*, p. 76,14–15 16–18] *v.* Theoph. In Aphor.: II 265,18–20 Dietz 16–17 συμπτώματα] *cf.* Gal. In Aphor. I 7: XVII B 373,4–7 K. 19–21] *v.* Gal. In Aphor. I 7: XVII B 373,11–13 K. Theoph. In Aphor.: II 265,20–21 Dietz

1 *post* αὐτῷ *add.* καὶ Z ἐς Z 2 ἐν] ἐπ' Z ἐπιστῆναι Z 3 κἀντεῦθεν *om.* Z καὶ] ὥστ' ἐντεῦθεν Z χρήσασθαι] χρωμένω Z 4 ὁ δ' ἕτερος] οὗτος δὲ Z συνήθως Z: συνήθ *(ambig.)* A 7 ἐς – κράτισται *in textu hab.* P, *inser.* Z² 8 νοσήματα *om.* Z 9 τι] τοι Z ἐφήμερον Z 10 *post* δίαιταν *add.* ἰστέον Z 11 μὴ] μήπως Z 12 ἀνώτερα P 13 οὖν *om.* A 14 *ante* τοὺς *add.* καὶ *infra, pp. 114,16; 142,30; vol. III, fol. 194ʳ, Hipp. plerique (C'), Theoph.: om. supra, p. 72,29, Hipp. quidam* τοὺς – 15 χρέεσθαι *in textu hab.* A, *inser.* Z² ἐσχάτως] ἐσχάτη A 16 τὸ[I] *om.* Z τὸν *om.* Z 18 ῥυπασμὸν A 19 δηλοῖ ἐνταῦθα *om.* Z *post* χρόνον *add.* δηλοῖ τὸν Z 23 διαιτᾶν *om.* P τοσοῦτον – 24 ᾖ *in textu hab.* A, *inser.* Z²: *om.* P ὅσον A: *corr.* A² 24 ἡ *e corr.* A² 25 ὅτι] ὡς Z *post* κατόξεσι *add.* τουτοισὶ Z 26 μέτεισι Z

he goes on a voyage, in the company of another man, who is accustomed to a heavier diet. As the voyage lasts many days, the one on the light diet finds himself out of provisions, so that he has to share with the other and is compelled to eat pulse, which causes considerable trouble for him, while the other goes scotfree, since he has taken his usual food.

I 12. For extreme diseases cures of extreme rigidity are the best.

By *extreme diseases* he means the very acute, for it is impossible to imagine a faster process in disease, except perhaps in ephemeral fever; by an *extreme cure*, the lightest diet, i.e., abstinence from food. Thus abstinence is best in cases of very acute disease, except in a situation of weak resistance, or when the orifice of the stomach is flooded with bile, as explained above.

I 13. When the disease is very acute, (the patient) is immediately in extreme discomfort, and one must use the most rigorously strict diet.

This, then, is *the very acute disease*, the one attended by violent fever and great discomfort, i.e. symptoms such as sleeplessness, unexplained thirst, tossing about, etc.

Immediately here means within a compass of three days; in very acute diseases this entire period – the three days – is the acme.

I 14. Otherwise, when it is possible to use a heavier diet, you can be more permissive in the same proportion as the disease is slower than the extreme form.

Having first indicated one particular kind of diet – in very acute diseases fasting is to be prescribed –, he now passes on to a general statement; and, the list of diseases being a long one, he included them all in the words: *Otherwise, when it is possible to use a heavier diet.*

Μαλθακὸν δὲ τὸ ἔκλυτον περὶ τὴν κίνησιν καὶ μοχθηρὸν κατὰ χρόνον ὠνόμασε νόσημα.

Πᾶσα οὖν ἡ τοῦ μνημονευθέντος ἀφορισμοῦ ἔννοια τοῦτον ἔχει τὸν τρόπον· ἐπὶ μὲν τῶν κατοξέων ἀσιτίαν παρέλαβεν, ἐφ' ὧν δὲ πάλιν ἐνδέχεται ἁδροτέρως διαιτᾶν, τουτέστιν ἐπὶ τῶν μὴ ἐπιδεχομένων ἀσιτίαν, ἁδροτέρᾳ χρῆσαι τροφῇ· ὅρον δὲ τῆς τοιαύτης ἐπιδόσεως τὸ μῆκος τοῦ χρόνου τὸ μέχρι τῆς οἰκείας ἀκμῆς τοῦ νοσήματος ἔλαβε. τοῦτο γὰρ δηλοῖ τὸ μαλθακωτέρη, τὸ δὲ ἔσχατον τὴν ἀκμήν.

I 15 [I 8: IV 464,1–2 L.] Ὁκόταν ἀκμάζῃ τὸ νόσημα, τότε τῇ λεπτοτάτῃ διαίτῃ ἀναγκαῖον χρέεσθαι.

Ἐπεὶ γὰρ περὶ χρονιωτέρων διείλεκται νοσημάτων καὶ ἁδροτέρᾳ ἐπ' αὐτὰ κεχρῆσθαι τῇ τροφῇ νενομοθέτηκεν, ἵνα μὴ νομίσῃς, ὅτι δι' ὅλου ἐπὶ τῶν τοιούτων τοιαύτῃ δεῖ διαίτῃ κεχρῆσθαι, ἐπήγαγεν ὁκόταν ἀκμάζῃ τὸ νόσημα, τότε τῇ λεπτοτάτῃ διαίτῃ ἀναγκαῖον χρέεσθαι. καὶ ἁρμόζει τὸ λεγόμενον οὐ μόνον ἐπὶ τῶν ὀξέων, ἀλλὰ καὶ ἐπὶ τῶν χρονίων νοσημάτων· πολλὰ γὰρ συμβαίνουσιν ἄτοπα ἐκ τοῦ ἀφυλάκτως ἡμᾶς ἐν ταῖς ἀκμαῖς διαιτᾶν.

I 16 [I 9: IV 464,3–6 L.] Συντεκμαίρεσθαι δὲ δεῖ καὶ τὸν νοσέοντα, εἰ ἐξαρκέσει τῇ διαίτῃ ⟨πρὸς τὴν ἀκμὴν τῆς νούσου, καὶ πότερον ἐκεῖνος ἀπαυδήσει πρότερος καὶ οὐκ ἐξαρκέσει τῇ διαίτῃ ἢ ἡ νοῦσος πρότερον ἀπαυδήσει καὶ ἀμβλυνεῖται⟩.

Διὰ μὲν τοῦ εἰπεῖν συντεκμαίρεσθαι τὸν νοσέοντα χρὴ πρὸς τὴν δύναμιν ἀφορῶντας τὸ εἶδος ὑποτυποῦν τῆς διαίτης παρακελεύεται. πᾶσαν μὲν γὰρ κατὰ γένος δύναμιν ἐπισκοπεῖσθαι δεῖ, ψυχικάς, ζωτικάς, φυσικάς· κατ' ἐξαίρετον δὲ τὸ εἶδος τῆς τροφῆς ἀκριβοῦν βούλεται. περὶ δὲ τοῦ καιροῦ ἐδήλωσεν εἰρηκὼς καὶ πρὸς τὴν ἀκμὴν τῆς νόσου· διὰ δὲ τοῦ εἰπεῖν ἡ νοῦσος πρότερον ἀπαυδήσει καὶ ἀπαμβλυνεῖται τὸ εἶδος τοῦ νοσήματος ἐδήλωσεν, εἴτε ὀξὺ εἴτε χρόνιον. παραμετρεῖν οὖν δεῖ, ὡς αὐτός φησι, τὴν δύναμιν τῷ νοσήματι· καὶ εἰ μὲν ταύτην πρὸς τὸ εἶδος τοῦ νοσήματος εὕροις ἀρκοῦσαν, τὸ νόσημα δὲ ἀπολῆγον, λεπτῶς διαίτησον· εἰ δὲ ἀνάπαλιν εὕροις τὸ μὲν νόσημα ἐπὶ πολὺ ἐξαρκοῦν, τὴν δὲ δύναμιν κατὰ μέρος ὀκλάζουσαν, ἁδροτέρως διαίτησον, ἵνα δυνηθῇ ἡ δύναμις ἀνταγωνίσασθαι πρὸς τὸ νόσημα.

20–21 παρακελεύεται] *v.* Gal. In Aphor. I 9: XVII B 378,1–3 K. 25 παραμετρεῖν – 30] *v.* Theoph. In Aphor.: II 267,5–12 Dietz

3 τουτονὶ Z 4 *fort.* παράλαβε *scribendum est* 5 χρῆσθαι Z 7 νοσήματος] σώματος Z γὰρ] δὲ Z 8 ὅταν P *post* Ὁκόταν *hab.* δὲ *Hipp.* (γὰρ C′) *ante* τῇ *add.* καὶ A, *Theoph.* U″ V″ τῇ *non hab. Hipp. plerique* 9 χρῆσθαι Z 10 ἐπειδὴ Z 11 ὅτι] ὡς Z 12 τῇ *om.* α 14 ἐπὶ[I] – νοσημάτων] τοῖς ὀξέσιν· ἀλλὰ καὶ τοῖς χρονίοις νοσήμασι Z ἐπὶ[I] *om.* P 16 δεῖ] χρὴ *Hipp.* 17 πρὸς – 19 ἀμβλυνεῖται *in textu hab.* A (18sq. ἡ – ἀμβλυνεῖται *inser.* A², *ut vid.*), *inser.* Z² νόσου A 18 πρότερος *Hipp. pauci*: πρότερον *Hipp. cett.* (C′), *Theoph.* ἐξαρκέσῃ A 24 ἡ νοῦσος *om.* A πότερον A *ante* καὶ *add.* τὲ A 26 τῷ νοσήματι] τῶν νοσημάτων Z 28 *post* δὲ[I] *add.* τὸ Z *post* ἀνάπαλιν *add.* ἤγουν εἰ Z μὲν *om.* Z δύναμιν δὲ Z 29 ἀβροτέρως A

Slow describes a disease which is sluggish in its progress and bad from the point of view of duration.

The entire purport of the above aphorism, then, is this: in cases of very acute disease (Hippocrates) forbade all food, while in those cases where a heavier diet is possible, i.e., where all food cannot be refused, you may use more substantial food; as the criterion of this increase he took the length of time till the natural acme of the disease. This is expressed by the word slower, and the extreme form is the acme.

I 15. When the disease is at its height, one must use the lightest diet.

Because he has discussed longer-lasting diseases and has prescribed a heavier diet for them, he does not want you to think that in these cases you should apply such a diet throughout, and therefore he continues: When the disease is at its height, one must use the lightest diet. This statement fits not only acute, but also chronic diseases; indeed, many untoward things happen, if we neglect the diet while a disease is at its height.

I 16. One must also observe the patient and see if he will hold out on this diet until the acme of the disease: whether he will be the first to give up, not being able to survive on the diet, or whether the disease will give in first and weaken.

By saying One must (also) observe the patient (Hippocrates) tells us to prescribe the kind of diet with a view to the patient's resistance. We should pay attention to faculties of all categories: the psychic, the vital, the natural faculties; but in particular he wants us to ascertain his eating habits. The moment is indicated by the words until the acme of the disease; while the phrase the disease will give in first and weaken indicates the character of the disease, whether it is acute or chronic. You must therefore, as (Hippocrates) himself advises, measure the resistance with reference to the disease; and if you find that resistance is strong enough for the type of disease, and that the disease is on its decline, use a light diet; if, on the other hand, you find that the disease is strong enough to continue for a long time, but that the patient's strength is wavering at some point, use a heavier diet, so that he gains power to fight the disease.

I 17 [I 10: IV 464,7–10 L.] Ὁκόσοισι μὲν οὖν αὐτίκα ἡ ἀκμή, αὐτίκα λεπτῶς διαιτᾶν· ⟨ὁκόσοισι δὲ ἐς ὕστερον ἡ ἀκμή, ἐς ἐκεῖνο καὶ πρὸ ἐκείνου σμικρὸν ἀφαιρετέον, ἔμπροσθεν δὲ πιοτέρως διαιτᾶν, ὡς ἂν ἐξαρκέσῃ ὁ νοσέων⟩.

Λέγει, ὅτι δεῖ σκοπεῖν, πότε ἡ ἀκμὴ παραγίνεται, ἄρα τῇ τεσσαρακοστῇ; καὶ δεῖ τότε διαιτῆσαι κατὰ μὲν τὴν ἀρχὴν ἁδροτέρως, ἵνα ἐξαρκέσῃ πρὸς τὴν ἀκμὴν ἡ δύναμις, ἐπὰν δὲ μέλλῃ ἐγγίζειν ἡ ἀκμή, τότε δεῖ σε λεπτῶς διαιτῆσαι, ἀλλὰ μὴ ἀθρόως ἀπὸ ἁδροτέρας διαίτης εἰς τὴν λεπτοτάτην ἐλθεῖν· ἀλλ' εἰ μέλλει τυχὸν ἡ ἀκμὴ τῇ τεσσαρακοστῇ ἡμέρᾳ ἐπιστῆναι, τὴν μὲν ἀρχὴν ἁδροτέρως διαίτησον, ἐπὰν δὲ ὁ νοσῶν τὴν λϛ̅ ἡμέραν φθάσῃ, λεπτοτέρᾳ διαίτῃ χρῆσαι, καὶ τότε δὲ μὴ ἀθρόον, ἀλλ' ἐὰν ἐλάμβανεν εἰ τύχοι ᾠὰ ἢ ἴτριον, μέτελθε ἐπὶ χυλὸν πτισάνης, εἶτα ἐπὶ μελίκρατον· καὶ οὐδὲν ἀδικεῖς τῇ κατὰ λόγον ὑφαιρέσει εἰς ἀσιτίαν τρεπόμενος.

Τὸ δὲ σμικρὸν ἀφαιρετέον οὐ κατὰ τὴν ποσότητα τῆς τροφῆς ληπτέον, ἀλλὰ κατὰ τὸν χρόνον. εἰς ἐκεῖνο, γάρ φησι, τὸ μέρος τοῦ χρόνου, τὸ τῆς ἀκμῆς δηλαδή, καὶ πρὸ ἐκείνου μικρόν, τουτέστι πρὸ δύο ἢ τριῶν ἡμερῶν, ἀφαιρετέον τὰ τῆς τροφῆς.

I 18 [I 11: IV 464,11–12 L.] Ἐν δὲ τοῖσι παροξυσμοῖσιν ὑποστέλλεσθαι χρή, ⟨τὸ προστιθέναι γὰρ βλάβη⟩.

Φησίν, ὅτι τοὺς παροξυσμοὺς ὑποστέλλεσθαι χρή, τουτέστι μὴ τρέφειν. παροξυσμὸς δέ ἐστι τὸ σφοδρότερον μέρος τῆς ὅλης περιόδου· περίοδος δέ ἐστιν ἡ ἀπὸ τοῦ αὐτοῦ εἰς τὸ αὐτὸ ἀποκατάστασις. οἷον εἰσέβαλε σήμερον ὁ παροξυσμός, ὥρᾳ πρώτῃ· ἐθερμάνθη ὁ ἄνθρωπος καὶ ἔμεινε πυρέττων ὥρας ιβ̅· κατέλαβεν ἱδρώς, ἐπαύσατο ὁ πυρετὸς καὶ ἔσχε διάλειμμα ὅλην τὴν νύκτα καὶ τὸ ἐπιὸν ἡμερονύκτιον· καὶ πάλιν τῇ τρίτῃ ἡμέρᾳ εἰσέβαλεν ὁ πυρετὸς ἤγουν ὁ παροξυσμὸς περὶ ὥραν πρώτην. οὗτος ὁ χρόνος ὁ ἀπὸ τῆς πρώτης ὥρας τῆς πρώτης ἡμέρας μέχρι τῆς πρώτης ὥρας τῆς τρίτης ἡμέρας, ἀπὸ τοῦ αὐτοῦ εἰς τὸ αὐτὸ ἀποκατάστασις ὤν, περίοδος λέγεται. ἐκ τούτων τῶν περιόδων τοὺς παροξυσμοὺς γινώσκομεν, ὡς εἴρηται.

Καὶ ἰστέον, ὅτι τῶν πυρετῶν οἱ μέν εἰσι συνεχεῖς, οἱ δὲ διαλείποντες. καὶ τῶν διαλειπόντων οἱ μὲν καθ' ἑκάστην ἡμέραν παροξύνουσιν, οἵτινες ἐπὶ φλέγματι ἀνάπτονται καὶ ἀμφημερινοὶ ὀνομάζονται· οἱ δὲ διὰ μιᾶς παροξύνουσιν ἐπὶ χολῇ ἀναπτόμενοι,

14 εἰς – 16] *v.* Theoph. In Aphor.: II 268,2–4 Dietz 19 Φησίν – τρέφειν] *v.* Theoph. In Aphor.: II 268,28–29 Dietz 20sq. περίοδος – ἀποκατάστασις] *v.* Theoph. In Aphor.: II 269, 10–12 Dietz *cf.* [Gal.] Def. med. 199: XIX 401,15–18 K.; 466: 459,10 K. *infra*, vol. II, fol. 118r

1 ἀκμή] δύναμις Z 2 ὁκόσοισι – 4 νοσέων *in textu hab.* A, *inser.* Z2 δὲ ἐς *inser.* A2 ἡ ἀκμή *om.* A εἰς A 6 ἵνα] ὡς ἂν Z *post* πρὸς *add.* γε Z 7 μέλλει A: μέλλ *(ambig.)* P 8 τήν *om.* Z λεπτὴν Z ἐλθεῖν] δίαιταν ἐλθεῖν A: διελθεῖν Z τυχεῖν Z 9 τὴν μὲν] κατὰ μὲν τὴν Z 10 λϛ̅] τριακοστὴν Z φθάσει Z λεπτοτάτη A χρῆσαι] δεῖ χρήσασθαι Z δὲII] μὲν A 11 ἐὰν] εἴπερ Z εἰ τύχοι *om.* Z ᾠῶν ἢ ἰτρίου Z ἴτριον α: *correxi* *post* ἐπὶII *add.* τὸ Z 12 *post* καὶ *add.* τούτου γιγνομένου Z ἀδικήσ(εις) Z 17 Ἐν – παροξυσμοῖσιν] τοὺς (δὲ) παροξυσμοὺς *supra, p. 74,15; infra, pp. 90,3; 114,17, Hipp.* 18 τὸ – βλάβη *in textu hab.* A, *inser.* Z2 21 εἰσέβαλλ(ε) A ὁ *om.* Z 22 κατέβαλεν PZ: *corr.* A 24 *post* καὶ *add.* αὖ Z τῇ τρίτῃ ἡμέρᾳ] κατὰ τρίτην ἡμέραν Z εἰσέβαλλεν A ἤγουν] εἶτοὖν Z 25 *post* οὗτος *add.* δ' οὖν Z τῆςI *om.* Z *post* μέχρι *add.* καὶ Z 26 *ante* ἀπὸ *add.* ἡ Z ὢν *om.* Z 27 λέγοιτ' ἂν Z *ante* τῶν *add.* γὰρ Z 29 φλέγματος Z 30 διὰ μιᾶς] μετὰ μίαν Z

I 17. In cases where the acme follows immediately, start the light diet immediately; in cases where the acme follows later, reduce it a little before as well as at that time, but in the preceding period you may allow a richer diet, so that the patient's strength will hold out.

(Hippocrates) says that you should observe when the disease will be at its height; let us say on the fortieth day. Then you should permit a more substantial diet at the beginning, so that the patient's strength will suffice for the acme, but when the acme draws near, you must prescribe a light diet, without, however, passing abruptly from the heavier diet to the extremely light. If, for instance, the acme is expected on the fortieth day, begin with a heavier diet, and when the patient reaches the 36th day, set a lighter diet, but even then not suddenly; if for example (the patient) used to get eggs or cake, change to barley-water (first), and then to honey-and-water; in this way you will cause no harm, if by a gradual diminution of the diet you arrive at a total fast.

We should not read reduce it a little as referring to the quantity of the food, but relate it to the time. What (Hippocrates) says is: reduce the food, a little before, i.e. two or three days before, as well as during that period, namely, the acme.

I 18. During paroxysms one should use restraint, for then any addition is harmful.

When he tells us to use restraint in paroxysms, this means not to feed the patient. A "paroxysm" is the most violent part of the entire period; and a "period" is a return from the same point to the same point. For example, the paroxysm set in today, at the first hour; the temperature rose and the patient remained in a fever for 12 hours; then sweating began, the fever ceased and there was an interval lasting that entire night as well as the following twenty-four hours; on the third day the fever or paroxysm began again at the first hour. This time from the first hour of the first day to the first hour of the third day, being a return from the same point to the same point, is called a period. On the basis of these periods we determine paroxysms, as stated.

As regards fevers, some are non-intermittent, some intermittent. Of the intermittent ones, some have a daily paroxysm; they are kindled upon phlegm and are called quotidian fevers; others have a paroxysm every other day; they

οἳ καὶ τριταῖοι καλοῦνται· οἱ δὲ διὰ δύο ἐπὶ μελαγχολικῷ χυμῷ ἀναπτόμενοι, οἳ καὶ τεταρταῖοι λέγονται. αἵματος δὲ οὐκ ἐμνήσθημεν, ἐπειδὴ τὸ αἷμα παρατρεπόμενον σύνοχον πυρετὸν ἀπεργάζεται, ὅστις παροξυσμὸν οὐκ ἔχει εἰ μὴ ἕνα. τοῦτον τοίνυν τὸν τρόπον διηρθρωμένων τῶν διαλειπόντων πυρετῶν οἱ παροξυσμοὶ καὶ περίοδοι γίνονται· αὕτη δὲ ἡ περίοδος ἐκ δύο τινῶν σύγκειται μορίων, ἔκ τε τοῦ παροξυντικοῦ καὶ ἐκ τοῦ ἀνετικοῦ μορίου τοῦ χρόνου περιγραφομένη. τοῦτο τοίνυν τὸ ἀνετικὸν μόριον ἐπὶ μὲν τῶν διαλειπόντων διάλειμμα ὀνομάζεται, ἐπὶ δὲ τῶν συνεχῶν μειοπυρεξία καὶ παρακμὴ ὀνομάζεται. διαφέρει δὲ μειοπυρεξία διαλείμματος, ὅτι ἡ μὲν διάπνοιά ἐστιν ὀλίγη τῆς θερμασίας, τὸ δὲ τῆς ὅλης θερμασίας ἐστὶ διαφόρησις, καὶ ὅτι τῷ μὲν διαλείμματι ἕπεται ἀπυρέκτους γίνεσθαι, τῇ δὲ μειοπυρεξίᾳ λείψανον θερμασίας ἐν τῷ σώματι καταλιμπάνεσθαι.

Καὶ ταῦτα μὲν οὕτως· ἔλθωμεν δὲ λοιπὸν ἐπὶ τὸ σπουδαζόμενον καὶ ζητήσωμεν τὸ τοῦ καιροῦ μέρος, ἐν ᾧ δεόντως τὴν τροφὴν ἐπιδώσωμεν. ὥς τινος γὰρ ἐρωτῶντος· «Ἐν ποίᾳ ὥρᾳ ἔχω θρέψαι, ἆρα ἐν πρώτῃ ἢ ἐν δευτέρᾳ ἢ ἐν τρίτῃ ἢ ἐπέκεινα;» φησίν, ὅτι τοῦτο κατορθοῦται οὐκ ἀπὸ τῆς ποσότητος τῶν ὡρῶν, ἀλλὰ ἀπὸ τῶν περιόδων. ἐν μὲν γὰρ τοῖς διαλείπουσιν οὐ δεῖ ἐν τοῖς παροξυσμοῖς τρέφειν, ἀλλ' ἐν τῷ διαλείμματι· ἐν δὲ τοῖς συνεχέσιν ἄπορος εἶναι δοκεῖ ὁ λόγος. εἰ γὰρ τοὺς παροξυσμοὺς εὐλαβεῖσθαι δεῖ καὶ μὴ ἐπιδιδόναι ἐν αὐτῷ τροφήν, ὁ δὲ πᾶς χρόνος τῆς ὅλης περιόδου τῶν συνεχῶν ἐν παροξυσμῷ θεωρεῖται, πῶς ἕξομεν τὸν καιρόν, καθ' ὃν θρέψαι χρή; πλήν γε δεῖ καὶ ἐπ' αὐτῶν τὴν μειοπυρεξίαν ἤτοι τὴν παρακμὴν ἐπιτηρεῖν· τότε γὰρ ὀλίγην ἄνεσιν ἡ φύσις ἔχουσα ἀπασχολεῖται πρὸς τὴν τροφὴν καὶ ἀβλαβῶς αὐτὴν προσίεται. ὥστε ὃν λόγον ἐπὶ τῶν διαλειπόντων ἔχει τὸ διάλειμμα, τοῦτον ἐπὶ τῶν συνεχῶν ἡ μειοπυρεξία. διὰ τοῦτο δὲ εὐλαβεῖται ὁ Ἱπποκράτης ἐν τοῖς παροξυσμοῖς τροφὴν ἐπιδιδόναι, ἐπειδὴ τότε ἡ φύσις ἐρεθιζομένη ὑπὸ τῶν αἰτίων περὶ αὐτὰ ἀσχολεῖται καὶ τὸν οἰκεῖον κάματον καταβάλλεται, καὶ καλόν ἐστι μὴ ἀντιπερισπάσαι τῇ τῆς τροφῆς ἐπιδόσει. ἓν γὰρ δυοῖν ἀτόποιν τὸ τηνικαῦτα ἀναγκαίως ἐπακολουθήσει· καὶ τοῦτό ἐστι τὸ εἰρημένον, τὸ προστιθέναι γὰρ βλάβη.

Οἱ δὲ παλαιότεροι τῶν ἐξηγητῶν οὐκ ἐπὶ τροφῆς μόνον, ἀλλὰ καὶ ἐπὶ παντὸς ἄλλου ἰατρικοῦ εἴδους τοῖς ἀρρώστοις προσαγομένου τοῦτο τὸ ῥητὸν ἐξελάβοντο, εἴτε κατάπλασμα εἴη τυχὸν εἴτε ἐμβροχὴ εἴτε κλυστὴρ εἴτε ληξιπύρετον εἴτε ἑτέρα τις φαρμακεία· πάντα γὰρ ταῦτά φασιν ἐν τοῖς παροξυσμοῖς δεῖν ὑποστέλλεσθαι ὡς βλάβην ἀπεργαζόμενα. οὐχ οὕτως δὲ ἔχει τἀληθές· ἐν αὐτοῖς γὰρ τοῖς παροξυσμοῖς πολλάκις βοηθήμασί τισι χρώμεθα καταπραῧναι καὶ παρηγορῆσαι τὰ συμπτώματα σπεύδοντες, καὶ ληξιπυρέτοις δὲ τὸ τηνικαῦτα χρώμεθα καὶ κεφαλὴν ἀλείφομεν καὶ

16 ἐν – 23 μειοπυρεξία] *v.* Theoph. In Aphor.: II 269,6–9 Dietz   26sq. ἓν – ἐπακολουθήσει] *cf. supra*, p. 74,9–14

1 διὰ] μετὰ Z   3 τοίνυν] νῦν Z   4 διωρθωμένων Z   διαλειφθέντων A   *post* καὶ *add.* οἱ Z   5 αὐτὴ Z   6 ἐκ *om.* Z   μορίου *om.* Z   περιγραφόμενον ω: *correxi*   7 συνόχων ω: *corr.* A²   9 *post* διάπνοιά *add.* γε Z   10 ἀπυρέκτως Z   15 οὐκ ἀπὸ] οὐ κατὰ Z   ἀπὸ^II] κατὰ τὸ Z   18 *fort.* αὐτοῖς *scribendum est*   19 τῶν συνεχῶν *sscr.* A: τῶν συνόχων ω   22 ἀβλαβῶς] εὐλαβῶς Z   23 συνόχων ω: *correxi*   26 ἓν] ἐν Z   27 ἀναγκαίως *om.* A   *post* εἰρημένον *add.* ὅρα καὶ ἑτέραν ἐξήγησιν τοῦ ἐν δὲ τοῖσι παροξυσμοῖσιν ὑποστέλλεσθαι χρὴ α *(ad lin. 29 sqq. pertinentia)*   γὰρ *om.* Z   29 παλαίτεροι Z   30 ἄλλου *om.* Z   31 εἴτε^III et IV] ἢ Z   ληξιπύρετος Z   εἴτε^V] ἢ Z   33 βλάβην] βλάπτειν P   ἀπεργαζόμενα] ἐμποιεῖ τῷ σώματι Z   35 κεφαλὴν *om.* Z

are kindled upon bile, and are also called tertian fevers; others have intervals of two days, are kindled upon the atrabiliar humor, and are called quartan fevers. We have not mentioned blood because blood when it deteriorates causes non-remittent fever, which has one single paroxysm. To this classification of intermittent fevers paroxysms and periods correspond; such a period consists of two parts: we distinguish a phase of paroxysm and one of relaxation. This phase of relaxation is called an "interval" in the case of intermittent fevers, and "remission of fever" or "abatement" in the case of non-intermittent fevers. A remission of fever differs from an interval in that the former is a slight degree of exhalation of the fever-heat, while the latter is a complete dispersion of the heat; an interval sets us free from fever, a remission of fever leaves a remnant of heat in the body.

Thus much for this; let us now come to the matter that concerns us here and discuss the suitable moment to administer food. As if the question had been asked: "At what time should I administer food: at the first, the second, the third hour, or later?" (Hippocrates) says that the right result is achieved by starting, not from the number of the hours, but from the periods. In intermittent fevers one should provide food, not during the paroxysms, but during the intervals; in non-intermittent fevers, however, the point seems problematic. If, indeed, one should be wary of the paroxysms and not administer food during them, and meanwhile the entire time of a complete period of non-intermittent fevers consists of a condition of paroxysm, how can we find an opportunity to feed (the patient)? However, in these fevers too we should observe the remission of fever, or abatement; at that time the constitution has a slight reprieve, it finds time for food and can take it without harm. The role, then, which is played by the interval in intermittent fevers, is played by the remission of fever in non-intermittent ones. The reason why Hippocrates is afraid to provide food during paroxysms, is that at that time the constitution, irritated by the causes of the disease, is busy with them and hard at work in its own way, so that it is better not to divert it from its task by providing food. If we do, one out of two unpleasant consequences will necessarily follow; this is the sense of the words for then any addition is harmful.

The older commentators understood this text as referring not only to food, but to any other kind of medical treatment given to the sick, whether, for instance, a poultice, or an embrocation, or an enema, or a febrifuge, or another kind of medication; they say that during paroxysms all these should be avoided as harmful. This, however, is not true; precisely in paroxysms we often use certain remedies trying to soothe and alleviate the symptoms: we then use drugs to stop the fever, we anoint the head, we allay the pain by thermal treatment

ὀδύνην διὰ πυρίας ἢ κλυστῆρος παύομεν καὶ πλείστας ἁπλῶς προσεξευρίσκομεν ἐν τοῖς παροξυσμοῖς ϑεραπείας, ἡνίκα μετὰ συμπτωμάτων τινῶν ὑπαντήσωσιν ἢ γενέσϑαι προσδοκηϑῶσιν. ὥστε οὖν περὶ τῆς ἐπιδόσεως τῆς τροφῆς λέγει ὁ Ἱπποκράτης εὐλαβεῖσϑαι τοὺς παροξυσμούς. τοῦτο γὰρ καὶ ἐξ αὐτῆς τῆς λέξεώς ἐστι κυρῶσαι, τὸ προστιϑέναι γὰρ ἔφη· οὐδὲν γὰρ τῷ ἡμετέρῳ προστίϑεται σώματι πλὴν τροφῆς, τὰ δὲ λοιπὰ πάντα ὁμιλεῖ μὲν τῷ σώματι, οὐ προστίϑεται δὲ αὐτῷ.

Δεῖ δὲ καὶ τοῦτο ἐπιστῆσαι ἐνταῦϑα, ὅτι πολλάκις καὶ ἐν τοῖς παροξυσμοῖς τρέφομεν, ἡνίκα ἀσϑενῆ τὴν δύναμιν εὕρωμεν καὶ χαλεπὰ προσδοκᾶται τῷ παροξυσμῷ τὰ συμπτώματα, ὥστε αὐτὴν ῥωσϑεῖσαν ἀπομαχέσασϑαι ταῖς τῶν αἰτίων ἐπιδρομαῖς· ὅϑεν καὶ τηνικαῦτα παρέχομεν τροφήν, εἰ καὶ πυρέττοντες τύχοιεν, ὡς ἐπὶ τῶν συνεχῶν ἢ καὶ ἐπὶ τῶν διαλειπόντων, ἡνίκα μὴ κατὰ τὴν πρώτην εἰσβολὴν τοῦ παροξυσμοῦ εἰσβάλλωσι τὰ συμπτώματα, ἀλλ' ἐν τῇ ἀναβάσει ἢ τῇ ἀκμῇ.

Ἰστέον δέ, ὅτι τὸ τοῦ παροξυσμοῦ ὄνομα καὶ ἐπὶ τῶν διαλειπόντων καὶ ἐπὶ τῶν συνεχῶν ἁρμόζει. ἀλλ' ἐπὶ μὲν τῶν διαλειπόντων παροξυσμὸς ἁπλῶς λέγεται, ἐπὶ δὲ τῶν συνεχῶν ἐπιπαροξυσμός. ἐνταῦϑα οὖν τῷ τοῦ παροξυσμοῦ ὀνόματι καταχρώμενος ἐπὶ τῶν συνεχῶν τέϑηκεν. ἐπιπαροξυσμὸς δὲ λέγεται, ὅτι ἐπὶ τῷ πρώτῳ παροξυσμῷ μένοντι ὁ δεύτερος γίνεται, καὶ τούτου μένοντος ὁ τρίτος, καὶ ἐφεξῆς ὡσαύτως.

I 19 [**I 11: IV 464,12–13 L.**] Καὶ ὁκόσα κατὰ περιόδους παροξύνεται, ἐν τοῖσι παροξυσμοῖσιν ὑποστέλλεσϑαι.

Δῆλον ἐκ τούτου, ὅτι τῷ προτέρῳ τοῦ παροξυσμοῦ ὀνόματι ἐπὶ τῶν συνεχῶς παροξυνομένων ἐχρήσατο· ἰδοὺ γὰρ ἐνταῦϑά φησι· καὶ ὁκόσα κατὰ περιόδους παροξύνονται, ἀντὶ τοῦ διὰ μιᾶς ἡμέρας ἢ διὰ δύο ἢ καϑ' ἑκάστην, καὶ ἐπὶ τούτων εὐλαβεῖσϑαι δεῖ τοὺς παροξυσμούς. ἔστι δὲ τἀληϑέστερον εἰπεῖν, ὅτι, ἔνϑα φησί· [**I 11: IV 464,11 L.**]«παροξυσμοὺς ὑποστέλλεσϑαι δεῖ», περὶ τῶν πυρεκτικῶν πάντων παϑῶν δεῖ τὸν λόγον ἐκδέξασϑαι, εἴτε συνεχεῖς εἶεν οἱ πυρετοὶ εἴτε καὶ διαλείποντες· ἐν οἷς δέ φησι καὶ ὁκόσα κατὰ περιόδους παροξύνεται, περὶ τῶν χωρὶς πυρετοῦ περιοδιζόντων παϑημάτων δεῖ νοῆσαι τὸ λεγόμενον, ὅτι καὶ ἐπ' αὐτῶν δεῖ τοὺς παροξυσμοὺς ὑποστέλλεσϑαι. οὕτω γοῦν κωλικὰς διαϑέσεις καὶ ὠταλγίας καὶ νεφριτικὰς καὶ ἀρϑριτικὰς ὡς ἐπὶ πᾶν ϑεώμεϑα ἄνευ πυρετῶν κατά τινα παροξυνούσας περίοδον. δεῖ οὖν καὶ ἐπ' αὐτῶν εὐλαβεῖσϑαι τοὺς παροξυσμοὺς καὶ μὴ ἐπιδιδόναι ἐν αὐτοῖς τροφήν· εὑρίσκομεν γάρ, ὅτι ὅσον οὔπω καὶ ἐμοῦσι τὰ τῆς τροφῆς χάριν παραλαμβανόμενα.

Γνῶϑι δὲ καὶ τοῦτο, ὅτι συνεχῶς τρέφομεν ἐν τοῖς παροξυσμοῖς, ἡνίκα ἐπὶ κενεαγγείᾳ ἢ ἐκκαύσει γένωνται, ἵνα, εἰ μὲν δυσκρασία ᾖ ἐπὶ ἐκκαύσεως, κατασβεσϑῇ,

13–15 ἐπιπαροξυσμός] *v.* Theoph. In Aphor.: II 268,29–33 Dietz 24 ἔστι – 33] *v.* Theoph. In Aphor.: II 269,1–6 Dietz

1 κλυστῆρος ἢ πυρίας Z 2 ὑπαντήσουσιν α 5 προστιϑέναι] $\overline{\text{προς}}$ Z 9 αἰτίων] ἐναντίων Z 11 $\overset{\text{δια}}{\text{παρα}}$λειπόντων A 12 εἰσβάλωσι P *post* ἀναβάσει *add.* τυχὸν Z 15 ἐπιπαροξυσμός] ἐπεὶ ὁ παροξυσμὸς P χρώμενος Z 16 συνόχων PZ: *corr.* A ἐπιπαροξυσμὸς] ἐπεὶ παροξυσμὸς P τῷ *om.* P 17 ἑξῆς Z 18 ὡσαύτως] ἄλλος Z 20 *post* ὑποστέλλεσϑαι *add.* χρή A²Z, *Hipp. plerique* 21 προτέρῳ τοῦ] τοῦ προτέρου P συνεχῶν Z 23 παροξύνεται Z 24 δὲ *om.* Z 25 *ante* παροξυσμοὺς *add.* τοὺς Z 26 *verbo* λόγον *des.* Z *(cf. supra, p. 15)* ἐκλέξασϑαι α: *correxi* 29 *fort.* ὠταλγικὰς *scribendum est* 33 λαμβανόμενα P

or an enema, in a word, there are a great many additional cures which we contrive during paroxysms, when they are attended by certain symptoms, or are expected to be so. It is therefore in connection with the administration of food that Hippocrates tells us to pay attention to paroxysms. This is borne out by the wording, too, since he spoke of addition; now nothing is added to our body except food, while all the rest, though brought into contact with the body, is not added to it.

Here it must also be observed that we often provide food even during paroxysms, when we find resistance weak and expect serious symptoms attending the paroxysm, so that resistance may become strong enough to fight off the onset of the causes; hence, under those circumstances, we feed (patients) even during fever, as in cases of non-intermittent fever, or even of intermittent fever, when the symptoms start, not at the first onset of the paroxysm, but during the increase or the acme.

It is further to be noted that the word "paroxysm" applies both to intermittent and to non-intermittent fevers. But in intermittent fevers we simply speak of paroxysm, in non-intermittent fevers, however, of "epiparoxysm". Here, (Hippocrates) uses the word "paroxysm" improperly of non-intermittent fevers. We speak of "epiparoxysm" because the second paroxysm supervenes upon (*epi*) the first, while it still continues, and the third during the second, and so forth.

I 19. Also in diseases with periodical paroxysms, restraint should be used during the paroxysms.

This proves that, when he used the word "paroxysm" the first time, it is with reference to paroxysm in non-intermittent fevers, since here he says: Also in diseases with periodical paroxysms – i.e. with intervals of one day, or two days, or occurring daily – there, too, we should be wary of paroxysms. A more correct explanation is that where he says: "During paroxysms one should use restraint", this statement should be understood of all affections attended by fever, whether non-intermittent or intermittent, while the words in diseases with periodical paroxysms should be taken to apply to periodical affections without fever, telling us to use restraint during paroxysms in those as well. Thus, in cases of colic, ear-ache, nephritis and arthritis we generally observe paroxysms of a certain periodicity, but without fever. Here, too, we must be on our guard during the paroxysms and not administer food while they last; otherwise we shall find that very soon patients throw up what was intended as nourishment.

It should also be noted that we continue feeding in paroxysms, when they follow upon emptying of the vessels or sunstroke, with the purpose of quenching any possible distemper after sunstroke, or, in the case of emptying of the vessels,

εἰ δὲ κενεάγγεια ᾖ, ἀντεισαχθῇ μέρος τοῦ κενωθέντος. δεῖ σε οὖν τούτων μεμνῆσθαι τῶν προσδιορισμῶν, ἵνα τέλειος ᾖ καὶ ἀψευδὴς ὁ Ἱπποκράτειος λόγος ὁ λέγων· [I 11: IV 464,11–12 L.] «τοὺς δὲ παροξυσμοὺς ὑποστέλλεσθαι, τὸ προστιθέναι γὰρ βλάβη.»

I 20 [I 12: IV 464,14–17 L.] Τοὺς δὲ παροξυσμοὺς καὶ τὰς καταστάσιας δηλοῦσιν αἱ νοῦσοι καὶ αἱ ὧραι τοῦ ἔτεος καὶ αἱ τῶν περιόδων πρὸς ἀλλήλας ἐπιδόσιες, ⟨ἥν τε καθ' ἡμέρην ἥν τε παρ' ἡμέρην ἥν τε καὶ διὰ πλείονος χρόνου γίγνονται⟩.

Ὡς τινος ἐρωτῶντος· «Καὶ πόθεν ἔχομεν γνῶναι τοὺς μέλλοντας γίνεσθαι παροξυσμούς;» αὐτός φησιν, ὅτι τοὺς παροξυσμοὺς καὶ τὰς καταστάσιας γνωρίσεις πρῶτον μὲν τεχνικῷ στοχασμῷ, δεύτερον δὲ σημειώσει τεχνικῇ καὶ τρίτον ἐπιστημονικῇ διαγνώσει. καὶ τεχνικῷ μὲν στοχασμῷ χρώμενος εὑρήσεις τοὺς παροξυσμοὺς ἀπὸ τοῦ εἴδους τοῦ νοσήματος ἤγουν τῆς ὕλης. εἰ μὲν γὰρ χολῶδές ἐστι τὸ νόσημα, τριταῖος ὑπάρχει ὁ πυρετὸς καὶ διὰ μιᾶς οἱ παροξυσμοὶ γίνονται· εἰ δὲ ἐπὶ μελαγχολικῷ, τεταρταῖος καὶ διὰ δύο ὁ παροξυσμὸς ὑπαντᾷ. ἐκ τούτου οὖν δύνασαι παραλαβεῖν τὸν καιρόν, ἐν ᾧ ὀφείλεις θρέψαι, ἐκφεύγων τοὺς παροξυσμούς. καλῶς εἴρηται «τεχνικῷ στοχασμῷ», ἐπειδὴ τὸ ἀκριβὲς ἡ τοιαύτη σημείωσις οὐκ ἔχει· οὐδὲ γὰρ πάντως, εἰ διὰ μιᾶς ὁ παροξυσμὸς γίνεται, ἤδη καὶ τριταῖός ἐστιν ὁ πυρετός, γίνεται γὰρ ἔστιν ὅτε διπλοῦς πεμπταῖος· οὐδὲ εἰ καθ' ἑκάστην, πάντως ἀμφημερινός ἐστι, δύναται γὰρ διπλοῦς τριταῖος εἶναι· ἀλλ' οὐδὲ ὁ διὰ δύο πάντως ἐστὶ τεταρταῖος, πολλάκις γὰρ διπλοῦς ἑβδομαῖός ἐστι. τεχνικῇ δὲ σημειώσει χρώμενοι γινώσκομεν τοὺς παροξυσμοὺς ἐκ τῶν συστοίχων, οἷον ἀπὸ ὥρας, χώρας, ἡλικίας, κράσεως, βίου καὶ τῶν τοιούτων. ἀπὸ μὲν ὥρας οὕτως· θέρους ὄντος γνῶθι, ὅτι τὸ νόσημα χολῶδες καὶ τριταῖος ὡς ἐπὶ πᾶν ὁ πυρετὸς καὶ διὰ μιᾶς ὁ παροξυσμός· εἰ δὲ χειμών, φλέγμα ὑπόκειται καὶ ἀμφημερινὸς ὁ πυρετὸς καὶ καθ' ἡμέραν οἱ παροξυσμοί. τὰ αὐτά μοι καὶ περὶ χώρας ὑπονόησον· ὡσαύτως δὲ καὶ περὶ ἡλικίας, εἰ ἀκμαστικὴ ὑπόκειται ἡλικία, εἰ παρακμαστική, εἰ γεροντική, εἰ παιδική. δῆλον γὰρ ἐντεῦθεν, ποῖος ἑκάστῃ πρέπει χυμὸς καὶ ποῖος χυμὸς ποῖον εἶδος ἀνάπτει πυρετοῦ καὶ ἕκαστος τῶν πυρετῶν πῶς παροξύνει, ὡς καὶ ἐπὶ τοῖς προλαβοῦσιν εἴρηται. ταῦτα δὲ καὶ περὶ κράσεως νοείσθω καὶ περὶ τοῦ προηγουμένου βίου, ἵνα μὴ καθ' ἕκαστα ἐπεξερχόμενοι μηκύνωμεν τὸν λόγον. εἰ μὲν γὰρ φροντιστικὸς καὶ ταλαίπωρος καὶ ἐπίπονος καὶ ἄγρυπνος ⟨ὁ⟩ προηγησάμενος βίος, χολὴ μᾶλλον ἠθροίσθη καὶ τριταῖος ὁ πυρετὸς καὶ διὰ μιᾶς ὁ παροξυσμός. εἰ δὲ τρυφηλὴ τράπεζα καὶ βίος ἀργὸς καὶ λουτρῶν ἄκαιρος χρῆσις πρὸ πέψεως παραλαμβανομένη, φλέγμα ἠθροίσθη καὶ ἀμφημερινὸς ὁ πυρετὸς καὶ καθ' ἡμέραν ὁ παροξυσμός. ταύτῃ τοίνυν τῇ τεχνικῇ σημειώσει τῇ ἀπὸ τῶν συστοίχων χρώμενος δυνήσῃ προγνῶναι τοὺς καιροὺς τῶν παροξυσμῶν καὶ τούτους παραφυλάττεσθαι, τρέφειν δὲ ἐν ταῖς ἀνέσεσιν.

9–92,5] *cf.* Gal. De crisib. I 4–5. 6: IX 560,1–563,3; 569,6–570,7 K.; III 4: 711,16–712,17 K. 13 εἰ – 15 ὑπαντᾷ] *cf.* Theoph. In Aphor.: II 269,28–270,5 Dietz 23 ἀπὸ – 26 παροξυσμοί] *cf.* Theoph. In Aphor.: II 270,6–10 Dietz

6 δηλοῦσιν *Hipp.* C′, *Theoph.*: δηλώσουσιν *Hipp. plerique* 7 ἐπιδόσιες] *item infra, p. 90,15, Hipp. quidam* (C′), *Theoph.*: ἀνταποδόσιες *Hipp. plerique, cf. infra, p. 94,8* 7sq. ἥν – γίγνονται *in textu add.* A: *om.* P 18 γὰρ *om.* P 19 εἰ] ἡ P 30 *fort.* ταὐτὰ *scribendum est* 32 ὁ *addidi* 34 παραλαμβανομένης P: παραλαμβανόμενος A: *correxi*

replacing a part of what was evacuated. Remember these restrictions, if you want to have a complete and correct understanding of the Hippocratic maxim: "During paroxysms one should use restraint, for then any addition is harmful."

> I 20. Paroxysms and constitutions can be inferred from the disease, the season of the year, and the increase in the periods as compared to each other, whether they come daily, or every other day, or at longer intervals.

As if the question had been asked, "How can we predict future paroxysms?" (Hippocrates) says that you can know paroxysms and constitutions, first by technical conjecture, secondly by technical inference, thirdly by scientific diagnosis. By means of technical conjecture you can infer the paroxysms from the character of the disease, i.e., of the matter. If the disease is bilious, the fever is a tertian and the paroxysms come every other day; if it is atrabilious, the fever is a quartan and the paroxysm sets in after an interval of two days. From this you can deduct the time when you should administer food, avoiding the paroxysms. We called it "technical conjecture" with good reason, because this kind of inference is not exact; for if the paroxysm comes with one day's interval, it does not follow necessarily that the fever is a tertian, since sometimes a double quintan occurs; nor, if there is a daily paroxysm, is the fever always a quotidian, but it may be a double tertian; finally, a fever with a two days' interval is not necessarily a quartan, for often it is a double septiman. By means of technical inference we derive the paroxysms from the correlative factors, such as the season, the region, the age, the temperament, the occupation, etc. From the season as follows: if it is summer you may conclude that the disease is bilious, the fever usually a tertian and paroxysm occurs every other day; if it is winter, the cause is phlegm, the fever a quotidian and paroxysms occur daily. You can make similar conjectures on the ground of the region; and so, too, on the ground of age, according as the patient is in his prime, past his prime, an old man, a child. For from this it is clear what humor belongs to each age, and what humor starts what kind of fever, and how paroxysms occur in each kind, on the same lines as explained above. The same may be held to apply to temperament and past occupation, so that there is no need to lengthen the discussion by going into detail. If, for example, the preceding life was one of worry, hardship, toil and lack of sleep, the probability is that bile collected and that the fever is a tertian and paroxysm comes every other day. If it is a case of a gourmet table, a life of leisure, ill-timed use of baths before digestion, phlegm must have collected, the fever is a quotidian and paroxysm will be daily. By applying this kind of technical inference on the ground of the correlative factors you will be able to prognosticate the times of paroxysms and to take your precautions, administering food during

ὡς οὖν φιλοσύντομος ὁ Ἱπποκράτης τῆς ὥρας καὶ μόνης μνημονεύσας πάντα τὰ λοιπὰ ἡμῖν συνεπινοεῖσθαι κατέλιπε σύστοιχα. ἡ δὲ ἐπιστημονικὴ διάγνωσις [σημείωσις] κατορθοῦται ἡμῖν ἐκ τῶν ἐπιφαινομένων· περὶ ἧς μικρὸν ὕστερον ἐροῦμεν ἐν τῷ χωρίῳ ἐκείνῳ, ἐν ᾧ φησιν· [I 12: IV 464,17 L.] «Ἀτὰρ καὶ τοῖσιν ἐπιφαινομένοισι».

Κατάστασις δέ ἐστιν ἡ τοιάδε σύνθεσις καὶ περιπέτεια τῶν νοσημάτων· ἐκ τούτων γάρ, τῆς τε συνθέσεώς φημι καὶ περιπετείας, δύνασαι διαγνῶναι τοὺς καθόλου καιροὺς καὶ πρὸς τούτους τὸ εἶδος τῆς διαίτης ὑποτυπῶσαι. εἰ μὲν γὰρ ⟨ἐπὶ⟩ χολῇ συνέστη τὸ νόσημα, καὶ τριταῖος τυχόν, γίνωσκε, ὅτι ὀξύ ἐστι καὶ πλησίον ἡ ἀκμή· εἰ δὲ ἐπὶ φλέγματι, καὶ ἀμφημερινός, ὅτι χρόνιον καὶ πόρρω ἡ ἀκμή. χρησιμεύει δὲ τὸ μὲν ἐπίστασθαι τὰς καταστάσεις τοῦ νοσήματος πρὸς τὸ καθόλου τῆς διαίτης εἶδος, ὅπερ ἐξ ἀρχῆς ἁρμόσαι δυνάμεθα πρὸς τὴν τῶν νοσημάτων ἀκμὴν ἀποβλέποντες· τῷ δὲ τοὺς παροξυσμοὺς γινώσκειν πρὸς τὴν κατὰ μέρος δίαιταν ἀεὶ χρώμεθα.

Εἶτά φησι· καὶ αἱ τῶν περιόδων πρὸς ἀλλήλας ἐπιδόσιες· τοῦτο δὲ μικρὸν ἀναμεινάτω, σαφηνιζέσθω δὲ ἤν τε καθ' ἡμέρην ἤν τε παρ' ἡμέρην ἤν τε καὶ διὰ πλείονος χρόνου γίνωνται. λέγει ὅτι σκόπει τὸ εἶδος τοῦ νοσήματος καὶ τὰ σύστοιχα καὶ τὸν τύπον τῶν περιόδων, καὶ ἐκ τούτων εὑρήσεις τὸ εἶδος τοῦ παροξυσμοῦ. ταῦτα γὰρ ἀνασκοποῦντι καὶ σημειουμένῳ καθ' ἑαυτόν, εἴτε καθ' ἡμέραν εἴτε διὰ μιᾶς εἴτε διὰ δύο ἡμερῶν οἱ παροξυσμοὶ ὑπαντῶσι, ῥᾷον ὁποῖός ἐστιν ὁ παροξυσμός σοι διαγνωσθήσεται. δευτέρα τούτου ἐξήγησις· σκόπει τὸ εἶδος τοῦ νοσήματος καὶ τὰ σύστοιχα καὶ τὸν τύπον τῶν περιόδων, κἀντεῦθεν τὸ εἶδος τοῦ παροξυσμοῦ καὶ τὴν κατάστασιν ἐπιγνώσῃ, εἴτε σφοδροτέρως εἴτε ἀμυδροτέρως γένηται, καὶ εἰ πλησίον ἡ ἀκμὴ τοῦ ὅλου νοσήματος ἢ διὰ πλείονος αὕτη χρόνου ἀπαντήσειε· πρὸς ὃ τὸ εἶδος τῆς καθόλου διαίτης ὑποτυπώσειας, ὡς δοκεῖν πρὸς τοὺς καθόλου καιροὺς τοῦ νοσήματος εἰρῆσθαι τὸ λεγόμενον. τρίτη ἐπὶ τούτοις ἐξήγησις αὕτη· τέσσαρσι καιροῖς τρεπομένοις ὁ σύμπας ἐνιαυτὸς περιγράφεται, ἔστι γὰρ ὁ μὲν ἐαρινός, ὁ δὲ θερινός, ὁ δὲ φθινοπωρινός, ὁ δὲ χειμερινός. εἰς τέσσαρας δὲ τροπὰς ἀναλογούσας τοῖς τέσσαρσι καιροῖς τοῦ ἐνιαυτοῦ καὶ τὸ ἡμερονύκτιον διαιρεῖται· τὸ μὲν γὰρ ἑωθινὸν τῆς ἡμέρας ἀναλογεῖ τῷ ἔαρι, εὐκρατότερον ὂν τοῦ οἰκείου ἡμερονυκτίου παντός, τὸ δὲ μεσημβρινὸν ἀναλογεῖ τῷ θέρει, ἐπειδὴ ὁ ἥλιος κατὰ κορυφὴν ὑπάρχων παντὸς τοῦ ἡμερονυκτίου θερμότερον ἐκεῖνο τὸ τοῦ χρόνου μέρος ἐργάζεται, τὸ δὲ δειλινὸν τῷ φθινοπώρῳ ἀναλογεῖ διὰ τὸ ἀνώμαλον, ὅπερ γίνεται τῇ τοῦ ἡλίου ἀναχωρήσει, ἡ δὲ νὺξ τῷ χειμῶνι, ψυχροτέρα γινομένη διὰ τὸ ἀπεῖναι τὸν ἥλιον. τούτων οὕτως ληφθέντων νόμιζε τὸν Ἱπποκράτην ταῦτά σε διὰ τῶν παρόντων γινώσκειν προτρέπεσθαι, ὥστε σκοπεῖν τὸ τοῦ νοσήματος εἶδος καὶ τὰ σύστοιχα καὶ τὸν τύπον τῶν περιόδων. εἰ διὰ μιᾶς ὁ παροξυσμὸς γίνεται, δῆλον γάρ, ὅτι χολῶδες τὸ νόσημα καὶ τριταῖος ὁ πυρετός, καὶ ὡς ἐπὶ τὸ πλεῖστον ἐν μεσημβρινῇ ὥρᾳ παροξύνει, ἐν τῷ θερμοτέρῳ τοῦ ἡμερονύκτου χρόνῳ· εἰ δὲ τεταρταῖος, τῇ δείλῃ τὸν παροξυσμὸν ἔκδεξαι ὡς ἐπὶ τὸ πλεῖστον· εἰ δὲ

6–14] *cf.* Gal. In Aphor. I 12: XVII B 387,3–9 K.

2 κατέλειπε A 3 σημείωσις (-ιν P) *delevi, cf. supra, p. 90,12* 6 περιπέτεια τῶν *scripsi*: περιπετεινῶν A: περιπετειῶν P 8 ἐπὶ *addidi* 9 χολὴ P 17 γίνονται A 19 ἐνασκοποῦντι A: ἐν ἀσκοποῦντι P: *correxi* 33 τοῦ χρόνου] τῆς ἡμέρας A 40 εἰ[I]] *spat. 4 litt. in* P εἰ[II]] *spat. 3 litt. in* P

periods of abatement. Because of his predilection for brevity Hippocrates mentioned only the season, leaving it to us to fill in the remaining correlative factors. As for scientific diagnosis, we arrive at it on the ground of supervening symptoms; we shall deal with it presently in connection with the passage beginning "Moreover, we can go by supervening symptoms".

Constitution means the specific conformation and development of diseases; from these, conformation and development, you can discern the decisive moments in general and prescribe the type of diet accordingly. Thus if the disease results from bile, being for instance a tertian fever, you will know that it is acute and that the acme is near; if from phlegm, with a quotidian fever, this shows that it is chronic and that the acme is still far away. It is useful to know the constitutions of the disease with a view to the general type of diet, so that we can arrange it from the outset according to the acme of the diseases; on the other hand, knowledge of the paroxysms helps us in each case to settle the details of the diet.

The next words, and the increase in the periods as compared to each other, can wait a moment; we will first explain the phrase whether they come daily, or every other day, or at longer intervals. He tells us to watch the kind of disease, the correlative factors and the type of period, then from these we shall be able to infer the character of the paroxysm. If you consider and mark these points, whether paroxysms occur daily or every other day or with an interval of two days, you will find it easier to diagnose the nature of the paroxysm. Another explanation of this: watch the kind of disease, the correlative factors, and the type of period, then from these you will be able to identify the character of the paroxysm and the constitution (of the disease), whether (the paroxysm) will be on the violent or on the weak side, and whether the acme of the entire illness is near or will occur after a considerable time; in view of this you can prescribe the kind of diet generally, so that it would seem that the text applies to the decisive moments of the disease generally. A third explanation, besides these, is the following: the entire year is determined by a succession of four seasons, spring, summer, fall and winter. But the day-and-night period is also divided into four quarters analogous to the four seasons of the year: the morning is analogous to spring, being more temperate than the entire day-and-night period to which it belongs, midday is analogous to summer, because the sun's position in the zenith makes that part of the time hotter than the entire day-and-night period, the evening is comparable to the fall owing to its unevenness, which is th e resut of the declining of the sun, the night to winter, for it becomes colder by the ablsence of the sun. This being understood, you must take it that this is what Hippocrates in the present passage instructs you to learn and for which you have to study the kind of disease, the correlative factors and the type of period. If the paroxysm comes every other day, it is surely obvious that the disease is bilious and the fever a tertian, in which case the paroxysm will usually fall in the noontime, the hottest part of the day-and-night period; if it is a quartan, you can generally expect the paroxysm in the evening; if the paroxysm

καθ' ἑκάστην ἡμέραν ὁ παροξυσμὸς γίνεται, ἐπὶ φλέγματος ἡ κίνησις, καὶ ὡς ἐπὶ τὸ πλεῖστον ἐν νυκτὶ οἱ παροξυσμοὶ ὑπαντῶσι. τούτοις οὖν προσέχων τὸν νοῦν δύνασαι προγινώσκειν τοὺς ἐσομένους παροξυσμούς, ὥστε μὴ τρέφειν ἐν αὐτοῖς. ἐπειδὴ δὲ ὁ σύνοχος πυρετὸς ἀεὶ ἀδιάκοπον ἔχει τὴν θερμασίαν, ἐν τῷ ἑωθινῷ μέρει τῆς ἡμέρας τρέφειν τοὺς ἀσθενοῦντας ἁρμόδιον, οὐκ ἐπὶ συνόχων μόνον, ἀλλὰ καὶ ἐπὶ πάντων τῶν συνεχῶν, ὡς ἀναλογοῦντος τούτου τῷ ἔαρι καὶ εὐκρατοτέρου τυγχάνοντος. τότε γὰρ ἐν ἀνέσει μᾶλλον οὖσα ἡ δύναμις προσίεται καὶ πέττει τὴν τροφήν.

Δεῖ δὲ γινώσκειν, ὅτι «ἀνταπόδοσις» ἐν περιόδῳ λέγεται ἡ τῶν αὐτῶν ὑποστατικῶν ἤτοι χαρακτηριστικῶν τοῦ παρῳχηκότος παροξυσμοῦ ἀνακύκλησις· ἐπίδοσις δὲ ἐν περιόδῳ λέγεται ἡ ἐν τῷ ἐφεξῆς παροξυσμῷ ἐπίτασις ἤγουν αὔξησις τῶν ὑπαρξάντων τῷ προηγησαμένῳ παροξυσμῷ.

I 21 [I 12: IV 464,17–466,1 L.] Ἀτὰρ καὶ τοῖσιν ἐπιφαινομένοισιν· οἷον πλευριτικοῖσι πτύελον ⟨ἢν⟩ αὐτίκα ἐπιφαίνηται ⟨ἀρχομένου μὲν βραχύνει, ἢν δ' ὕστερον ἐπιφαίνηται, μηκύνει⟩.

Λέγει ὅτι, εἰ θέλεις ἐπιστημονικῶς διαγνῶναι τοὺς παροξυσμοὺς καὶ τὰς καταστάσεις τῶν νοσημάτων, ἐξ ὑποθέσεως τῆς πλευρίτιδος λάβε τὴν σαφήνειαν. ὑποκείσθω γὰρ πλευρῖτις καὶ χαρακτηριζέσθω τοῖς παθογνωμονικοῖς αἰτίοις, φημὶ τῷ ὀξεῖ πυρετῷ καὶ δυσπνοίᾳ καὶ τῇ βηχὶ καὶ τῷ νυγματώδει ἀλγήματι. ἀλλὰ ταῦτα μὲν αὐτὴν χαρακτηρίζει εἰς τὸ δεῖξαι, εἴτε ὀξύ ἐστι τὸ ὑποκείμενον νόσημα εἴτε χρόνιον, μείζονα δὲ τὴν τοιαύτην σημείωσιν καὶ βεβαιοτέραν ποιεῖται τὰ ἐπιφαινόμενα. ταῦτα τοίνυν τὰ ἐπιφαινόμενα τριττά ἐστιν· ἢ γὰρ σωτηρίας ἢ ὀλέθρου ποιοῦνται δήλωσιν, ἢ κρίσεως ἢ ἀκρισίας, ἢ πέψεως ἢ ἀπεψίας. τὰ δύο τοίνυν γένη τῶν ἐπιφαινομένων ἐνταῦθα παραλιπὼν ὁ Ἱπποκράτης, φημὶ τὰ κριτικὰ καὶ τὰ σωτηρίας ἢ ὀλέθρου δηλωτικά, περὶ ὧν πολὺν λόγον ἐν τῷ Περὶ κρίσεων καὶ Κρισίμων ἡμερῶν ὁ Γαληνὸς καταβάλλεται, τὰ τῆς πέψεως μόνης καὶ ἀπεψίας νυνὶ σημεῖα μεταχειρίζεται. ταῦτα δὲ ἐν τοῖς ἐκκρινομένοις θεωρεῖται, ἅτινα τριττά ἐστιν, ἐν πτύσμασιν, ἐν διαχωρήμασιν, ἐν οὔροις. καί φησιν ὅτι ἐπὶ τῆς πλευρίτιδος, εἰ μὲν ἐν ἀρχαῖς εὕροις ἀναγόμενον τὸν πτύελον, γνῶθι, ὅτι πλησιέστερον ἡ ἀκμὴ καὶ πρὸς τὸ ἐπιφαινόμενον τὸ διαίτης εἶδος ὑποτύπωσον· εἰ δὲ περὶ τὴν ἑβδόμην ἢ τὴν ἑνδεκάτην εὕροις ἀναγόμενον τὸ πτύελον, γνῶθι, ὅτι πορρωτέρω ἡ ἀκμὴ καὶ ἁδρότερον ἐν ἀρχῇ διαίτησον.

Πρό⟨σ⟩σχες δέ, ὅτι πτύελον εἶπε καὶ οὐχὶ «πτύσμα»· ὁ γὰρ Ἱπποκράτης πτύελον μὲν τὸ πεπεμμένον, πτύσμα δὲ τὸ ἄπεπτον καλεῖ.

Καὶ τοῦτο δὲ γνῶθι, ὅτι ἄλλο ἐστὶ τὸ ἐπιφαινόμενον σύμπτωμα καὶ ἄλλο

9 ἐπίδοσις – 11] *v.* Gal. In Aphor. I 12: XVII B 387,14–16 K. 21 ταῦτα – 31] *v.* Theoph. In Aphor.: II 274,24–275,2 Dietz 21sq. ταῦτα – ἀπεψίας] *cf.* Gal. In Aphor. I 12: XVII B 390,4–8 K. 24sq. περὶ ὧν – καταβάλλεται] *cf.* Gal. In Aphor. I 12: XVII B 383,16–18; 391, 7–14; 399,7–8; 400,10 K. 32sq.] *v.* Gal. De crisib. I 5: IX 564,3–7 K. Theoph. In Aphor.: II 275,2–4 Dietz 34–96,3] *cf.* Gal. In Aphor. I 12: XVII B 390,4–13 K.

1 ἡμέραν *om.* A 5 *ante* τρέφειν *add.* καὶ P 6 ἔαρι *scripsi*: ἀέρι α *(ἀέ eras. est in* A*)* εὐκρατεστέρου α: *correxi* 13 *post* οἷον *hab.* ἐν *Hipp.* ἢν *sec. Hipp. add.* A² 13sq. ἀρχομένου – μηκύνει *in textu add.* A: *om.* P 14 μὲν *hab. Hipp. quidam* (C', V): *om. Hipp. cett., Theoph.* μηκύνη A: *corr.* A² 17 αἰτίοις] *immo* συμπτώμασι *vel* σημείοις, *ut Duffy mihi ostendit; cf. infra, lin. 34sq.* 24 κράσεων α: *correxi* 26sq. ἐν πτύσμασιν *scripsi*: ἐμπτύσματα P: ἐμπτώματα A 28 τὸν] ν *eras. est in* A 32 πρόσχες α: *correxi*

comes daily, the disturbance is due to phlegm, and paroxysms will usually come in the night. By paying attention to this you can foretell future paroxysms, so as to avoid administering food during them. As for non-remittent fever, since its heat is always uninterrupted, it is suitable to feed the patients in the early part of the day – this holds not only for non-remittent fevers, but for all non-intermittent fevers –, because the morning is comparable to the spring, i.e. more moderate. At that time the power of resistance is under less pressure, so that it can take in and digest the food.

Let us further remark that "correspondence" in a period means the recurrence of the same essentials or characteristics as in the preceding paroxysm, while increase in a period means a greater intensity or a growth, in the next paroxysm, of the characteristics present in the preceding one.

I 21. Moreover, we can go by supervening symptoms; for example in cases of pleurisy, if sputum appears immediately at the beginning, this indicates a shorter sickness, but if it appears later, a longer one.

In other words, if you want to diagnose paroxysms and constitutions of diseases scientifically, we may explain it by a hypothetical case of pleurisy. Suppose a case of pleurisy, and suppose it is characterized by the distinctive causes, i.e., acute fever, shortness of breath, coughing and that shooting pain. These characterize the underlying disease as to whether it is acute or chronic, but this kind of inference is made more comprehensive and more reliable by supervening symptoms. There are three classes of these: they may indicate survival or death, a crisis or no crisis, concoction or no concoction. Here, Hippocrates leaves aside the two (other) kinds of supervening symptoms, i.e. those pointing to a crisis and those indicating survival or death – these are discussed extensively by Galen in his works On Crises and On Critical Days –, and now deals only with signs of concoction and no concoction. They are seen in excretions, of which there are three kinds: sputamen, feces, urine. (Hippocrates) says that in a pleurisy, if you find that sputum is brought up at the beginning, you may infer that the acme is close at hand and prescribe the kind of diet on the ground of the supervening symptoms; if, however, you see that sputum is brought up only toward the seventh or eleventh day, you must conclude that the acme is farther off and give a more substantial diet at first.

Note that it says sputum and not "sputamen"; Hippocrates uses sputum for the concocted, and "sputamen" for the crude matter.

Note further that there is a distinction between a supervening and a distinc-

τὸ παθογνωμονικόν. τὰ μὲν γὰρ παθογνωμονικὰ ἐξ ἀρχῆς εὐθὺς συνεισβάλλει τῷ νοσήματι, χαρακτηριστικὰ καὶ ὑποστατικὰ τῆς τούτων ὄντα ὑπάρξεως, τὰ δὲ ἐπιφαινόμενα τελευταῖον αὐτῷ ἐπιγίνεται.

Μὴ ἀπορήσῃς δέ, εἰ ἐπὶ τῆς πλευρίτιδος σημειώσεις ἀπὸ οὔρων καὶ διαχωρημάτων ποιεῖται· εἰκότως γὰρ ἀπὸ οὔρων σημειούμεθα, ἐπειδὴ πυρετὸς ὑπόκειται ἐπὶ χυμοῖς σηπομένοις ἀναπτόμενος, τὸ δὲ οὖρον δηλωτικὸν τῆς διαθέσεως τῶν ἐν ἡμῖν χυμῶν ὑπάρχει. τὰ δὲ διαχωρήματα ὁρῶμεν, ἵνα γνῶμεν ἐντεῦθεν, μή πως ἡ γαστὴρ κεκάκωται καὶ πῶς τὸ ὅλον ἔχει σῶμα.

Τὸ δὲ Ἀτὰρ τὴν πλατικὴν ἀρχὴν σημαίνει, ἥτις ἐν τρισὶ περιγράφεται ἡμέραις· ὡς ἔστι συναγαγεῖν τὸν λόγον καὶ εἰπεῖν ὅτι, ἐὰν ἐπιφαίνηται τὸ πτύελον ἐν τῇ τρίτῃ τῶν ἡμερῶν ἐπὶ τῶν πλευριτικῶν, γνῶθι, ὅτι ὀλιγοχρόνιόν ἐστι τὸ νόσημα καὶ ὅσον οὔπω μέλλουσαν ἔσεσθαι τὴν ἀκμὴν δηλοῖ, εἰ δὲ τελευταῖον ἐπιφανῇ τὸ πτύελον, πολυχρονιώτερον δηλοῦται τὸ νόσημα καὶ πόρρω ἡ ἀκμή. οὐ μόνον δὲ τὰ ἐπιφαινόμενα δηλοῦσιν ἡμῖν τὸ ὀξὺ καὶ χρόνιον, ἀλλὰ καὶ εἰ εὔκριτον μέλλει γενέσθαι τὸ νόσημα ἢ δύσκριτον καὶ φιλυπόστροφον, εἰ σωτήριον ἢ ὀλέθριον. πρὸς ὃ ἀποβλέποντες καὶ τὴν δίαιταν ἁρμόζειν ἐν τούτοις διδασκόμεθα.

I 22 [I 13: IV 466,5 L.] Γέροντες εὐφορώτατα νηστείην φέρουσιν.

Νῦν βούλεται ὁ Ἱπποκράτης περὶ ἡλικιῶν διαλεχθῆναι καὶ διδάξαι ἡμᾶς, πῶς ἐπ' αὐτῶν ἔχει ὁ τόνος τῆς δυνάμεως. φησὶ γάρ· Γέροντες εὐφορώτατα νηστείην φέρουσιν, οἱ δὲ παῖδες οὐ φέρουσιν ἀσιτίαν. καὶ ἰστέον, ὅτι κατὰ τρεῖς αἰτίας εὐφόρως φέρουσι τὴν ἀσιτίαν οἱ γέροντες. ἀλλ' ἵνα τοῦτο σαφῶς ὑποστήσωμεν, εἴπωμεν τὰς χρείας, δι' ἃς ἡ τροφὴ παραλαμβάνεται ἐν τῷ ἡμετέρῳ σώματι. χρειώδης τοίνυν ἡμῖν ἡ τροφὴ κατὰ δύο αἰτίας, κατά τε ἀναπλήρωσιν τοῦ διαφορουμένου λαμβανομένη καὶ κατὰ αὔξησιν τοῦ ἐμφύτου θερμοῦ. ἐπεὶ οὖν ταῦτα οὕτως ἔχει, κατὰ τρεῖς αἰτίας εὐφόρως φέρουσι τὴν ἀσιτίαν οἱ γέροντες· μίαν μέν, ὅτι οὐκ ἔστιν ἐπ' αὐτῶν εὐδιαφόρητον τὸ σῶμα ψυχρότερον τῇ κράσει ὑπάρχον· ἧττον γὰρ τὰ ψυχρὰ διαφορεῖται. δευτέρα αἰτία, ὅτι καὶ ὀλίγον κατ' οὐσίαν ἐστὶ τὸ ἐν αὐτοῖς θερμόν, καὶ οὐ μόνον κατὰ ποσότητα, ἀλλὰ καὶ κατὰ ποιότητα ἀσθενέστερον, ψυχρὸν γὰρ ὑπόκειται τὸ σῶμα φύσει· οὕτως οὖν διακείμενον πλείονος τροφῆς παρεχομένης καταπνίγεται τοῦτο καὶ ἀποσβέννυται. τρίτη αἰτία, ὅτι πολὺς ἐπ' αὐτοῖς ἐστιν ὁ ψυχρὸς καὶ ὠμὸς χυμὸς δυσκρασίαν ἐν ἑαυτῷ περιέχων· ὅστις καὶ κατὰ φύσιν εὑρίσκεται ἐν τῷ στόματι τῆς γαστρός, καὶ μάλιστα ἐπὶ τῶν γερόντων. καὶ πρό⟨σ⟩σχες, ὅτι «ὠμὸν» χυμὸν εἶπον καὶ οὐκ «ὀξώδη» ἢ «ἀλυκόν», οὗτοι γὰρ προσπεφύκασιν. ἐκ τούτου οὖν τοῦ ὠμοῦ χυμοῦ ἐν ταῖς ἐνδείαις τῆς προσαγωγῆς ἡ φύσις ἁρπάζει καὶ ἀλλοιοῖ ἐπιτηδείως πρὸς ταῦτα ἔχοντος καὶ ἐξαιματοῦσα τὴν χρείαν τῆς τροφῆς ἐξ αὐτοῦ ἀποπληροῖ. οὗτος δὲ ὁ χυλός, εἰ μὴ πρότερον τὴν τοῦ φλέγματος ἀνεδέξατο φύσιν, οὐκ ἄν ποτε γένοιτο αἷμα, καὶ δῆλον ἐντεῦθεν· τὰ σιτία πεττόμενα ἐν τῇ γαστρὶ εἰς χυλὸν μεταβάλλεται, καὶ οὗτος ὁ χυλὸς ἀνάγεται εἰς ἧπαρ καὶ ἐξαιματοῦται, ὁ δὲ λευκός ἐστι τῇ χροιᾷ καὶ ὑγρὸς τῇ συστάσει. ἐκ τούτου

9 *cf.* Gal. In Aphor. I 12: XVII B 391,7–11 K. *infra*, p. 128,29–33

6 *ante* τῆς *add.* ἐστι A 7 ὑπάρχει *om.* A 26 ψυχροτέρα P 29 *ante* φύσει *add.* τῇ A 31 ἐστιν ἐπ' αὐτοῖς A 33 πρόσχες α: *correxi* 36 αὐτῆς A χυλὸς *ex* χυμὸς *corr.* A[2] 37 φλέγματος] αἵματος A ἀναδέξεται A

tive symptom. Distinctive symptoms set in at once at the beginning, simultaneously with the disease, being characteristic and constitutive of its respective essence, while supervening symptoms appear at the end.

Do not wonder if, in a case of pleurisy, he draws conclusions from the examination of urine and feces; we examine the urine for the obvious reason that we have to do with a fever, which is caused by the decay of humors; now the urine indicates the state of the humors in the body. As for the feces, we examine them to ascertain whether by any chance the stomach has been affected and what the condition of the entire body is.

The sentence Moreover, (etc.) refers to the beginning in the wider sense, which has a compass of three days; so we can sum up this statement by saying that, if in a pleurisy case the sputum appears on the third day, it is clear that the disease is a short one and will reach its height almost immediately, but if the sputum appears at the end, this proves that the disease will last longer and the acme is still far away. Not only do the supervening symptoms indicate whether the disease is acute or chronic, but also if it will have an easy crisis or a difficult one, with the danger of recurrence, and if the patient will survive or perish. In view of this we are instructed in this passage to prescribe a corresponding diet.

I 22. Old men bear fasting most easily.

From here on Hippocrates' subject is age groups and his purpose is to explain to us the force of resistance in each. He says that old men bear fasting most easily, while children cannot endure going without food. The reasons why old men tolerate lack of food well are threefold. In order to make this clear, let us mention the functions which food fulfills in our body. Food is necessary, then, for two reasons: it serves to supply what is dispersed and to increase the innate heat. This being so, there are three reasons why old men bear fasting well: first, in their case there is less dispersal, their bodies having a colder temperament, and what is cold is less easily dispersed. Secondly, lack of heat is an essential mark of their age, and not only is it limited in quantity, but it is also qualitatively weaker, since their bodies are naturally cold; this being so, if too much food is given, the innate heat is choked and extinguished. Thirdly, they contain a great deal of cold and crude humor, which in itself is of bad temperamental proportion; this humor is also found normally in the orifice of the stomach, especially in old men. Note that I said a "crude" humor, not "acid" or "salty", which are extraneous. Now at times when not enough food is taken, Nature appropriates and changes some of this crude humor, which lends itself to this, and by turning it into blood satisfies the need of food by means of it. If this juice did not first assume the nature of phlegm, it could never become blood, which is proved as follows: food digested in the stomach is converted into chyle, and this chyle is conveyed to the liver and changed into blood; it is white in color and fluid as regards consistency. Of this food which has been converted into chyle, a certain

οὖν τοῦ χυλοποιηθέντος ἀποθησαυρίζεται μοῖρά τις ἐν τῷ στόματι τῆς γαστρὸς καὶ ἀποφλεγματοῦται, ἵνα ἐν ταῖς ἀσιτίαις ταῖς κατά τινα περίστασιν συμπιπτούσαις τῷ ζῴῳ καθάπερ ἀπὸ ταμείου τινὸς ἀρυομένη ἡ φύσις ἐκ τοῦ ἐνταῦθα ἀποθησαυρισθέντος χυλοῦ μέρος τι καὶ τοῦτο ἐξαιματοῦσα θρέψῃ τὸ ζῷον.

Οἱ μέντοι παῖδες, κἂν ἐρρωμένην ἔχωσι τὴν δύναμιν, οὐ φέρουσι τὴν ἀσιτίαν διὰ ταύτας τὰς προειρημένας αἰτίας ὑπεναντίως ἐπ' αὐτῶν ἐχούσας. πρῶτον μέν, ὅτι εὐδιαφόρητον αὐτῶν τὸ σῶμα διὰ τὴν περιουσίαν τοῦ ἐμφύτου θερμοῦ· δεύτερον δέ, ὅτι πλούσιον ἐπ' αὐτῶν τὸ ἔμφυτον θερμὸν κατ' οὐσίαν ὑπάρχει· καὶ τρίτον, ὅτι κατὰ δύο τρόπους ἐστὶν αὐτοῖς ἀναγκαία καὶ χρειώδης ἡ προσφερομένη τροφή· οὐ μόνον γὰρ πρὸς ἀναπλήρωσιν τοῦ διαφορουμένου, ἀλλὰ καὶ πρὸς ἐπίδοσιν τοῦ μεγέθους τοῦ σώματος ἀναγκαία ἐστὶ τοῖς παισὶν ἡ τροφή, τὸ μὲν γὰρ πρῶτον θρέψις, τὸ δὲ δεύτερον αὔξησις προσαγορεύεται. ὥστε οὖν ἐπὶ τῶν παίδων ἀσιτίαν παραλαβεῖν οὐ δυνάμεθα, οὐδὲ ἐν τῷ κατὰ φύσιν οὐδὲ ἐν τῷ παρὰ φύσιν· ἐπὶ δὲ τῶν γερόντων ἀδεῶς τὴν ἀσιτίαν παραλαμβάνομεν καὶ ἐν τῷ κατὰ φύσιν καὶ ἐν τῷ παρὰ φύσιν.

Ἐπεὶ δὲ περὶ ἡλικιῶν ὁ λόγος, δεῖ καὶ περὶ αὐτῶν βραχέα διαλεχθῆναι. ἰστέον οὖν, ὅτι ποικίλως διαιρεῖ τὰς ἡλικίας ὁ Ἱπποκράτης· πῇ μὲν γὰρ εἰς ἑπτὰ διαιρέσεις αὐτάς ἐστι τέμνων, ὡς ἐν τῷ Περὶ ἑβδομάδων εἴρηται, πῇ δὲ εἰς τέσσαρας, ὥσπερ δὴ κἀνταῦθα πεποίηκε, τὴν παιδικήν, τὴν μειρακιώδη, τὴν παρακμαστικὴν καὶ τὴν γεροντικήν. δεῖ δὲ γινώσκειν, ⟨ὅτι⟩ κατὰ τὴν διάφορον ἡλικίαν διάφορόν ἐστι καὶ τὸ ἔμφυτον θερμόν. ἐπὶ μὲν γὰρ τῶν παιδίων πλούσιόν ἐστι τὸ ἔμφυτον θερμὸν κατ' οὐσίαν, ἐπὶ δὲ τῶν μειρακίων αὔξει, ἐπὶ δὲ τῶν ἀκμαζόντων στάσιν ἔχει, ἐπὶ δὲ τῶν παρακμαζόντων ἧττον μειοῦται, ἐπὶ δὲ τῶν γερόντων μᾶλλον. ἡμεῖς μὲν οὖν πέντε ἡλικιῶν ἐμνήσθημεν, ὁ δ' Ἱπποκράτης τεσσάρων, τῆς γὰρ ἀκμαστικῆς αὐτὸς οὐκ ἐμνήσθη, ἐπειδὴ ἐν στάσει ἐστί, καὶ διὰ τοῦτο αὐτῆς οὐκ ἐμνήσθη.

Ἰστέον δὲ καὶ τοῦτο, ὅτι γέροντας ἐνταῦθα οὐ τοὺς ἐσχατογήρους λέγει, οἵ γε δὴ καὶ κυφογέροντες ἐπιλέγονται, ἢ παρὰ τὸ γῆς ἐρᾶν κυρίως οὕτω λεγόμενοι γέροντες πλησίον ὄντος αὐτοῖς τοῦ θανάτου ἢ παρὰ τὸ τὴν γῆν ὁρᾶν, τῷ κεκυφέναι καὶ πρὸς αὐτὴν νενευκότας περιπατεῖν. πᾶσαι γὰρ ἐπ' αὐτῶν καταλέλυνται αἱ δυνάμεις, καὶ οὐδαμῶς τὴν παντελῆ ἀσιτίαν οὗτοι φέρουσιν· οὐ τοίνυν τοὺς τοιούτους δεῖ νοεῖν ὑφ' Ἱπποκράτους εἰρῆσθαι γέροντας, ἀλλά γε τοὺς ὠμογέροντας, τοὺς τὰ ἑξήκοντα ἔτη φθάσαντας καὶ ἢ μικρόν τι ἐκβάντας ἢ βραχύ τι ἐλαττουμένους. οὗτοι γὰρ ἔτ' ὀλίγον ἐρρωμένην τὴν δύναμιν ἔχοντες ἀλύπως φέρειν τὴν ἀσιτίαν ἰσχύουσι.

Νηστείαν δὲ λέγει ἢ τὴν ὀλιγοσιτίαν ἢ τὴν παντελῆ ἀσιτίαν, ἑκάτερον γὰρ οὗτοι εὐχερῶς φέρουσι.

Τὸ δὲ εὐφόρως διχῶς νοητέον, τό τε ἀλύπως καὶ τὸ ἀβλαβῶς· ἀλύπως μὲν καθὸ οὐκ ὀρέγονται, ἀβλαβῶς δὲ καθὸ οὐκ ἀδικοῦνται ὑπὸ τῆς ἀσιτίας μὴ διαφορουμένου αὐτοῖς τοῦ σώματος.

17sq. πῇ – εἴρηται] Hipp. Hebd. 5: VIII 636 = IX 436 L. 23 ἡμεῖς – 25] *cf.* Gal. In Aphor. I 13: XVII B 402,4–11 K. 27 ἢ – 34] *v.* Gal. In Aphor. I 13: XVII B 402,17–403,6 K. 30 οὐ – 32 ἐλαττουμένους] *v.* Theoph. In Aphor.: II 276,8–10 Dietz 35sq.] *cf.* Gal. In Aphor. I 13: XVII B 403,6–11 K. 37–39] *v.* Gal. In Aphor. I 13: XVII B 401,3–4 K.

3 ἀπὸ] ἐπὶ P 4 τούτου α: *correxi* 6 εἰρημένας P αὐτῶν] αὐ A 8 ὑπάρχει *ex* ὑπάρχον *corr.* A² 9 αὐτοῖς *om.* A 13 δεόμεθα P 20 ὅτι *addidi* κατὰ *scripsi*: καὶ α 21 παίδων A *(cf. infra, p. 100,13. 18)* 28 τῷ *scripsi*: τὸ α 32 τι ἐκβάντας] ὑπερβάντας P 33 ἐρρωμένην *om.* A

part is stored in the orifice of the stomach and changed into phlegm, so that, if in any particular situation the organism has to do without food, Nature can draw from this store-room, as it were, part of the chyle accumulated there, turn it into blood and thus feed the organism.

Children, on the other hand, even if their resistance is strong, cannot endure abstinence from food for the reasons mentioned above, which in their case work in the opposite way. First, their bodies have a high degree of dispersal because of the abundance of innate heat; secondly, a wealth of innate heat is an essential characteristic of their age; thirdly, the food they take is necessary and useful to them in two ways: the food is needed not only to replace what is dispersed, but children need it also to increase the size of the body, the former being known as nutrition, the latter as growth. Consequently, where children are concerned, we cannot resort to abstinence from food, neither in normal nor in abnormal circumstances; but in the case of old men we do not scruple to do so in either situation.

Since the subject of age groups has been broached, let us go into it a little farther. Hippocrates has several classifications according to age: sometimes he distinguishes seven groups, as in the treatise On Hebdomads, sometimes four, as he does here: childhood, youth, middle age, old age. Note that the innate heat differs according to the difference in age. In children abundant innate heat is characteristic of their age, in young men it increases, in men in their prime it is at a standstill, in the middle-aged it decreases to a lesser extent, in old men the decrease goes farther. We have mentioned five ages, as against the four in Hippocrates, who does not include the prime of life, because it is static, for which reason he leaves it out.

It should be noted further that old men here does not mean those in extreme old age, sometimes described as "old men bent with age", to whom the word *gerontes* ("old men") strictly applies, either as "longing for the earth" (*gēs erōntes*), because death is near to them, or as "looking at the earth" (*gēn horōntes*), because their backs are bent and they stoop to the ground as they walk. In these people all the faculties are weakened and they are certainly unable to stand complete fasting; we should not understand these by the old men mentioned by Hippocrates, but rather elderly men, those who are sixty years of age, or a little over or a trifle under that. They have still retained a certain amount of vigor, so that they can bear fasting without trouble.

By fasting he means eating either little or nothing at all; old men can easily endure either of these.

Easily has the double sense of without trouble and without harm; without trouble, insofar as they have no appetite, without harm insofar as the lack of food causes no damage to them because there is no dispersal of their bodies.

123 [I 13: IV 466,5–7 L.] Γέροντες εὐφορώτατα νηστείαν φέρουσι, δεύτερον οἱ καθεστηκότες, ἥκιστα τὰ μειράκια, πάντων δὲ μάλιστα τὰ παιδία· τουτέων δὲ αὐτέων ἃ ἂν τύχῃ αὐτὰ ἑωυτέων προθυμότερα ἐόντα.

Καθεστηκότας φησὶ τοὺς ἐν παρακμῇ τυγχάνοντας ἐκ τοῦ ἑπομένου καὶ γινομένου τὸ ἡγούμενον αἰνιττόμενος. ἡ μὲν γὰρ ἀκμαστικὴ ἡλικία πλούσιον ἔχουσα τὸ ἔμφυτον θερμὸν καὶ κατὰ ποιότητα ἐπιτεταμένον εὐκίνητός τέ ἐστι περὶ τὰς πράξεις καὶ θυμώδης καὶ ἐν δόξαις καὶ λογισμοῖς εὐμετάβλητος· οἱ δὲ παρακμάζοντες ἅτε λοιπὸν μειουμένου τοῦ ἐμφύτου θερμοῦ οὔτε περὶ τὰς πράξεις οὔτε περὶ τὸν θυμὸν εὐκίνητοί εἰσιν, ἀλλὰ καὶ τὸν λογισμὸν σώφρονες καὶ βεβηκότες ὑπάρχουσιν, ὅπερ αὐτὸς ἔφη καθεστηκότες, διὰ τὸ τὸ ζέον τοῦ θυμοῦ λωφηθῆναι καὶ κατασταλῆναι. φέρουσιν οὖν καὶ αὐτοὶ τὴν ἀσιτίαν ἀλύπως καὶ ἀβλαβῶς, ἧττον μὲν ἤπερ οἱ ὠμογέροντες, μᾶλλον δὲ ἢ τὰ μειράκια καὶ οἱ παῖδες. καὶ ἐπ' αὐτοῖς δὲ τοῦτο συμβέβηκε διὰ τὴν ὀλιγότητα τοῦ ἐμφύτου θερμοῦ. τὰ γὰρ μειράκια ἐπ' ὀλίγον φέρουσιν ἀσιτίαν, ὃ δηλοῖ παρ' Ἱπποκράτει τὸ ἥκιστα· τοῦτο γὰρ παρὰ μὲν τοῖς ῥήτορσι τὸ οὐδαμῶς σημαίνει, παρὰ δὲ τῷ Ἱπποκράτει τὸ ἐπ' ὀλίγον, ὡς δηλοῖ τὸ ἐπίτασιν αὐτὸν λαμβάνειν ἐπὶ τῶν παίδων ἐν τῷ λέγειν πάντων δὲ μάλιστα τὰ παιδία. τοῦ γὰρ οὐδαμῶς οὐκ ἔστιν εἰπεῖν οὐδαμώτερον, ὥσπερ ἐπὶ τοῦ ὀλίγον ἔστιν εἰπεῖν ὀλιγώτερον. ἐπ' ὀλίγον οὖν αὐτὴν καὶ τὰ μειράκια φέρουσι διὰ τὸ αὔξειν ἐπ' αὐτοῖς τὸ ἔμφυτον θερμόν. καὶ ὅσον μὲν κατὰ τοῦτον τὸν τρόπον ἀσιτεῖν οὐδὲ ταῦτα δύνανται· ἐπειδὴ δὲ οὐδαμῶς φέρουσι τὴν ἀσιτίαν οἱ παῖδες, λείπεται τὰ μειράκια πρὸς μὲν τοὺς παῖδας μᾶλλον φέρειν αὐτήν, ἧττον δὲ πρὸς καθεστηκότας καὶ γέροντας.

Ὥστε οὖν μεμάθηκας, ποῖαι τῶν ἡλικιῶν φέρουσιν ἀσιτίαν, καὶ ποῖαι μὲν μᾶλλον, ποῖαι δὲ ἧττον, ποῖαι δὲ οὐδαμῶς. λοιπὸν δεῖ σε ἐν τοῖς νοσήμασι τῷ κανόνι τούτῳ παρακολουθοῦντα τοῖς μὲν ἁδροτέραν παρέχειν τροφήν, τοῖς παισὶ λέγω, τοῖς δὲ ἧττον ἁδράν, τοῖς μειρακίοις φημὶ καὶ ἀκμάζουσιν, ἐπὶ δὲ τῶν παρακμαζόντων καὶ ὠμογερόντων τὴν ἐσχάτως λεπτοτάτην [περὶ τὸ μᾶλλον καὶ ἧττον] παραλαμβάνειν δίαιταν· οὗτοι γὰρ φέροντες ἀσιτίαν οὐκ ἀδικοῦνται.

Οὐκ ὤκνησε δὲ ἐνταῦθα ὁ Ἱπποκράτης καὶ προσδιορισμῷ ἀναγκαίῳ χρήσασθαι ἐν τῷ φάναι τουτέων δὲ αὐτέων ἃ ἂν τυγχάνῃ αὐτὰ ἑωυτέων προθυμότερα ἐόντα, τουτέστιν ἐπὶ πάσης ἡλικίας τῶν ἤδη ὑποτεθεισῶν κατὰ τὸ μᾶλλον καὶ ἧττον τὴν ἀσιτίαν οἱ ἄνθρωποι φέρουσιν· ἐπὶ μὲν τῆς γεροντικῆς τοὺς γέροντας, ἐπὶ δὲ τῆς ἀκμαίας τοὺς ἀκμάζοντας καὶ ἐφ' ἑκάστης ἁπαξαπλῶς τοὺς ἐπὶ ταύτης θεωρουμένους μᾶλλον καὶ ἧττον ἰδεῖν ἔστι τὴν ἀσιτίαν, ὡς εἴρηται, φέροντας, καὶ γὰρ μᾶλλον καὶ ἧττόν ἐστιν ἐπ' αὐτοῖς τὸ ἔμφυτον θερμόν. δῆλον οὖν, ὡς ἐπὶ πάσης ἡλικίας οἱ προθυμότεροι τῇ περιουσίᾳ τοῦ ἐμφύτου θερμοῦ ἧττον φέρουσι τὴν ἀσιτίαν. δεῖ οὖν ἐπὶ τῶν νοσούντων, ἔνθα θερμοτέρα ἡ φύσις ἐστίν,

5 Καθεστηκότας – 19 ὀλιγώτερον] *v.* Theoph. In Aphor.: II 276,10–19 Dietz Καθεστηκότας – τυγχάνοντας] *v.* Gal. In Aphor. I 13: XVII B 401,17–402,3 K. 14 τὰ – 18 παιδία] *cf. infra,* vol. II, fol. 15ʳ 15sq. τοῦτο – σημαίνει] *v.* Phot., Suda s. v. ἥκιστα

2 τὰ^{I} *hab. Hipp.* C′: *non hab. Hipp. plerique, Theoph.* τὰ^{II} *non hab. Hipp.* 11 τὸ^{II} *om.* P θυμοῦ *scripsi*: θερμοῦ α λωβηθῆναι P 17 αὐτῶν A: *fort.* αὐτὸ *scribendum est* 21 δύναται P 22 προκαθεστηκότας P 28 περὶ – ἧττον *delevi (cf. lin. 32–36)*

I 23. Old men bear fasting most easily, then those of settled age, young men to a very slight extent, children worst of all; and of these again, those who measured by their own standard are the most active.

By those of settled age (Hippocrates) means the middle-aged, leaving it to us to infer the preceding state from the following, present one. People in their prime, indeed, in whom innate heat is abundant as well as intense in its quality, are easily stirred to action, quick-tempered, and prone to change their opinions and their reasonings; while the middle-aged, whose innate heat is now on the decline, are not easily stirred to action or to anger and are also sober and sedate in their thought; this is what (Hippocrates) called of settled age, because the hotness of the temper has cooled down and abated. These, too, can bear lack of food without trouble or harm, less well, it is true, than people in incipient old age, but better than young men and children. With them, it is again the result of the dearth of innate heat. As for young men, they can bear to forgo food for a short time, which is what Hippocrates means by *hēkista*, a word which in the orators means "not at all", but in Hippocrates "slightly", as appears from the fact that he attributes a higher degree to children when he says children worst of all. In relation to "not at all" there can be no "not-at-aller", as in relation to "slight" there is a "slighter". Even young men, then, can bear it only to a slight extent, because in them the innate heat is on the increase. As far as this goes, they are also unable to endure lack of food; but since children cannot bear it at all, the upshot is that young men endure it better if compared to children, less well if compared to the middle-aged and the old.

So you have learned which of the age groups can endure lack of food, which of them better, which less well, which not at all. What you have to do now in cases of illness is, in accordance with this standard, allow children a more substantial diet, young men and those in their prime a less heavy one, while for the middle-aged and elderly you may prescribe the extremely light diet, because they can endure abstinence from food without suffering harm.

Here, Hippocrates did not hesitate to add the necessary restriction and of these again, those who measured by their own standard are the most active, i.e., within each of the age groups already distinguished, people have different degrees of tolerance for abstinence from food: we see that old men in their own group, men in their prime in theirs, and in a general way, all in their own group, have, as we said, different degrees of tolerance for fasting, because they have innate heat in different degrees. Obviously, then, it is the most active individuals in each age group who, being rich in innate heat, are less capable of fasting. It follows that in cases of sickness we must be cautious in prescribing

εὐλαβεῖσθαι παραλαμβάνειν τὴν ἀσιτίαν. τὸ γοῦν πάντων μάλιστα τὰ παιδία· τουτέων δὲ αὐτέων ἃ ἂν τύχῃ αὐτὰ ἑωυτέων προθυμότερα ἐόντα οὑτωσὶ νοητέον, ὅτι τῶν παίδων οἱ μὲν θερμότεροι ὑπάρχουσι καὶ διὰ τοῦτο προθυμότεροι, οἱ δὲ οὐχ οὕτως ἔχουσι φύσεως· ὅσοι οὖν τῶν παίδων εἰσὶ θερμότεροι καὶ διὰ τοῦτο προθυμότεροι, ἀδυνάτως φέρουσι τὴν ἀσιτίαν.

Καὶ ἰδοὺ τῇ πρὸς ἕτερον παραβολῇ τὸ αὐτὰ ἑωυτέων ἐξηγησάμεθα· ἁρμόζει δὲ καὶ πρὸς ἕνα καὶ τὸν αὐτὸν τουτὶ νοηθῆναι, καί φαμεν οὕτως. αὐτὸς καθ' ἑαυτὸν ὁ εἷς καὶ ὁ αὐτὸς παῖς ποτὲ μὲν θερμοτέρως διατίθεται καὶ προθυμότερός ἐστι, ποτὲ δὲ ψυχροτέρως, ἢ διὰ τοιαύτην κατάστασιν ἀέρος ἢ διὰ τροφῆς ψυχροτέρας ἐπίδοσιν· καὶ ποτὲ μὲν ποσῶς φέρει τὴν ἀσιτίαν, ποτὲ δὲ οὐδαμῶς, ἡνίκα δηλονότι προθυμότερος ἑαυτοῦ ἐστιν. ἐκ γὰρ τῆς προθυμίας τὸ ποιοῦν ἐδήλωσε, τὴν περιουσίαν φημὶ τοῦ θερμοῦ· πᾶσα γὰρ πρᾶξις καὶ πᾶσα κίνησις διὰ τοῦ ἐν ἡμῖν θερμοῦ γίνεται.

I 24 [I 14: IV 466,8 L.] Τὰ αὐξανόμενα πλεῖστον ἔχει τὸ ἔμφυτον θερμόν.

Ἐνταῦθα γενόμενος ὁ Γαληνός φησιν, ὅτι ὁ «γὰρ» σύνδεσμος λείπει, ὡς εἶναι τὸ λεγόμενον τοιοῦτον· «πάντων δὲ μάλιστα τὰ παιδία χαλεπῶς φέρουσι τὴν ἀσιτίαν· τὰ γὰρ αὐξανόμενα πλεῖστον ἔχει τὸ ἔμφυτον θερμόν.» διὰ μὲν τοῦ εἰπεῖν τὰ αὐξανόμενα [I 14: IV 466,8–9 L.] πλείστης δεῖται τροφῆς ἐδήλωσε τὸ διττὸν τῆς χρείας, λέγω δὴ τήν τε ἀναπλήρωσιν τοῦ διαφορηθέντος καὶ τὴν αὔξησιν τῶν μορίων· διὰ δὲ τοῦ εἰπεῖν πλεῖστον ἔχει τὸ ἔμφυτον θερμὸν τὴν περιουσίαν εἰσήγαγε τῆς ἐν αὐτοῖς ἐμφύτου θερμασίας· διὰ δὲ τοῦ εἰπεῖν [I 14: IV 466,9 L.] εἰ δὲ μή, τὸ σῶμα ἀναλίσκεται τὸ εὐδιαφόρητον τῆς τῶν παίδων ἕξεως παρεγύμνωσεν, ὅπερ κατὰ δύο τρόπους ἐπὶ τῶν παίδων ὑπαντᾷ, καθ' ἕνα μὲν τῷ ὑγρῷ καὶ διακεχυμένῳ τῆς τῶν μορίων αὐτῶν φύσεως, καθ' ἕτερον δὲ τῷ δραστηρίῳ τῆς ἐμφύτου θερμασίας, αὕτη γὰρ μὴ ὑποκειμένης τροφῆς αὐτὴν τὴν οὐσίαν ἐξαναλίσκει τοῦ σώματος.

Ἀπορεῖ δὲ ἐνταῦθα γενόμενός τις λέγων· «Εἰ τῷ κατὰ φύσιν θερμῷ πέττονται τὰ σιτία, τί δήποτε τοῖς μὲν παισὶ πολλὴν δίδοσθαι τὴν τροφὴν ὁ Ἱπποκράτης νομοθετεῖ, τοῖς δὲ ἀκμάζουσιν ἀπαγορεύει; καίτοι πολλῷ πλέον ἔχουσι τὸ ἔμφυτον θερμὸν ἤπερ οἱ παῖδες.» ἀλλὰ δεῖ εἰδέναι, ὅτι ἐν ἑκατέρᾳ τῶν ἡλικιῶν περιουσία ἐστὶ τοῦ ἐμφύτου θερμοῦ, οὐ μέντοι γε ἴσως ἑκάστῃ, ἀλλὰ τῇ μὲν κατ' οὐσίαν ἡ πλεονεξία, ὥσπερ ἐπὶ τῶν παίδων, τῇ δὲ κατὰ ποιότητα, ὥσπερ ἐπὶ τῶν ἀκμαζόντων. καὶ ὅτι ἀληθὲς τὸ λεγόμενον, δῆλον ἐκ τοῦ τοὺς μὲν ἀκμάζοντας πολλὰ πέττειν μὴ δύνασθαι, πέττειν δὲ ὅμως τὰ δυσκατέργαστα καὶ δυσαλλοίωτα, βόεια κρέα φημὶ καὶ χοίρεια καὶ τυρὸν καὶ τὰ τοιαῦτα – γίνεται γὰρ ἡ τούτων πέψις τῇ δριμύτητι

1 τὸ – 5] *cf.* Gal. In Aphor. I 13: XVII B 402,11–16 K. Theoph. In Aphor.: II 276,19–277,5 Dietz 16–18 θερμόν] *v.* Gal. In Aphor. I 13: XVII B 401,10–17 K. Theoph. In Aphor.: II 278,1–4 Dietz 22 διὰ – 27] *cf.* Gal. In Aphor. I 14: XVII B 411,16–412,5 K. Theoph. In Aphor.: II 278,4–8 Dietz 28–33 ἀκμαζόντων] *cf.* Gal. In Aphor. I 14: XVII B 407,4–10; 409,9–410,14 K.

1 τὸ] τῶν P 3 *post* τῶν *add.* μὲν P 18sq. πλεῖστον – αὐξανόμενα *om.* P 20 δὴ] δὲ P 22 τῆς ἐν αὐτῆς P: *om.* A: *correxi* 23 παρεδήλωσεν A γύμνωσεν 34 τοῦ τοὺς] τούτους P

abstinence, where the constitution is relatively hot. Hence the words children worst of all; and of these again, those who measured by their own standard are the most active, should be understood to mean that among children, some are hotter and therefore more active, while others are of a different constitution; those children, then, who are hotter and therefore more active, are unable to endure fasting.

Thus we explain the phrase measured by their own standard in terms of comparison with another individual; but it can be understood also with reference to one and the same individual, as follows. Viewed by itself, the identical child is sometimes of a hotter disposition and is then more active, and at other times it is colder, either owing to a similar condition of the air, or because food of a colder type has been given; and sometimes (the child) can bear a certain measure of fasting, at other times none at all, namely, when it is at its most active. (Hippocrates) used the activity as evidence of its cause, i.e. the abundance of heat; indeed, all action and all motion is due to our intrinsic heat.

I 24. Growing bodies have the most innate heat.

Dealing with this passage, Galen says that the conjunction "for" is missing, the sense being "children endure fasting worst of all, for growing bodies have the most innate heat." When he said, Growing bodies need the most food, (Hippocrates) indicated its double purpose, i.e. the replacement of what has been dispersed and the growth of the parts of the body; when he said, They have the most innate heat, he introduced the point of the abundance of the innate heat in them; and when he said, Otherwise the body wastes away, he made it clear that the healthy condition of children is easily dispersed; this happens to them in two ways: on the one hand, by the fluid and diffuse nature of the parts of their bodies, on the other hand, by the force of the innate heat, which, when no food is available, consumes the substance of the body itself.

At this point somebody raises the objection: "If food is digested by natural heat, why does Hippocrates prescribe plenty of food for children, while refusing it to those in their prime, despite the fact that they have far more innate heat than children do?" However, it should be remarked that, though in each of the two age groups there is an abundance of innate heat, it does not have the same character in both: while in the case of children the abundance is essential, it is qualitative in the prime of life. Proof of the truth of this statement is that men in their prime, while they cannot digest much, can nevertheless digest food that is difficult to break down and to convert, such as beef, pork, cheese, etc., the di-

τοῦ ἐν ἐκείνοις θερμοῦ –, τοὺς δέ γε παῖδας τὰ μὲν δυσκατέργαστα οὐ πέττειν διὰ τὸ μὴ εἶναι ἐπ' αὐτῶν τὸ θερμὸν καυστικόν, πολλὴν δὲ τροφὴν δύνασθαι κατεργάζεσθαι τῇ περιουσίᾳ τῆς κατ' οὐσίαν ἐμφύτου θερμασίας. πλεῖστον ἔχει τὸ ἔμφυτον θερμόν· τὸ γὰρ πλεῖστον ποσότητα δηλοῖ καὶ οὐ ποιότητα.

I 25 [I 14: IV 466,9–10 L.] Γέρουσι δὲ ὀλίγον τὸ θερμόν· διὰ τοῦτο ἄρα καὶ ὀλίγων ὑπεκκαυμάτων δέονται.

Φησίν, ὅτι ὀλίγον ἐστὶν ἐπὶ τῶν γερόντων τὸ ἔμφυτον θερμόν, καὶ διὰ τοῦτο ὀλίγων ὑπεκκαυμάτων δέονται, τουτέστι τροφῆς, εἰ μὴ μέλλοιεν τὸ τῆς λυχνιαίας φλογὸς πείσεσθαι σύμπτωμα ἀθρόου αὐτῆς καὶ πολλοῦ τοῦ ἐλαίου καταχεθέντος. «ὑπεκκαύματα» δὲ καλοῦσιν οἱ παλαιοὶ τοῦ πυρὸς τὰ λεπτὰ τῶν ξύλων καὶ αὐτὰ τὰ ξύλα, καὶ διὰ τοῦτο ὁ Ἱπποκράτης ὑπέκκαυμα τὰς τροφὰς ἐκάλεσεν ὡς ὕλην οὔσας τοῦ ἐν ἡμῖν ἐμφύτου θερμοῦ.

I 26 [I 14: IV 466,11–12 L.] Διὰ τοῦτο καὶ οἱ πυρετοὶ τοῖσι γέρουσιν οὐχ ὁμοίως ὀξέες· ψυχρὸν γὰρ τὸ σῶμα.

Ἐνταῦθα βούλεται ὁ Ἱπποκράτης καὶ ἀπὸ τῶν νοσημάτων, ὧν μάλιστα πάσχουσιν οἱ γέροντες, δεῖξαι, ὅτι ὀλίγον ἐστὶ τὸ ἐν αὐτοῖς θερμὸν καὶ εὐφόρως φέρουσι τὴν ἀσιτίαν. καὶ νῦν μὲν πυρετοῦ μόνου μέμνηται βληχροτέρου καὶ ἧττον ἔχοντος τὸ θερμὸν καὶ τὸ ζέον· προϊὼν δὲ πολλὰ πάθη οἰκεῖα καταλέγει τοῖς γέρουσιν, ἅτινα δεῖ ἐπὶ τοῦ παρόντος εἰπεῖν πρὸς πίστωσιν τῶν λεγομένων. πάσχουσιν οὖν ὡς ἐπὶ πᾶν οἱ γέροντες κάρους, ἀποπληξίας, βῆχας, κορύζας, κατάρρους, πταρμοὺς καὶ τὰ τοιαῦτα. συγγενῆ γὰρ τῇ κράσει αὐτῶν ὑπάρχει τὰ τοιαῦτα πάθη, ψυχρὰ ὄντα καὶ ὑγρά, οἷστισι καὶ ἀναλίσκονται. ταύτης ἕνεκεν τῆς αἰτίας οὐκ εὐχερῶς πυρετῷ περιπίπτουσιν· εἰ δὲ καὶ γένωνται αὐτοῖς πυρετοί, διὰ τὴν φυσικὴν ψῦξιν τοῦ σώματος αὐτῶν οὐχ εὑρίσκονται θερμοὶ καὶ διακαεῖς, κολάζεται δὲ ἐν αὐτοῖς τὸ ζέον· εἰ δέ γε συμβῇ ποτε σφοδροὺς ἐπ' αὐτῶν ὑποστῆναι πυρετούς, εἰδέναι δεῖ, ὅτι ὅσον οὔπω τεθνήξονται.

I 27 [I 15: IV 466,13–14 L.] Αἱ κοιλίαι χειμῶνος καὶ ἦρος θερμόταται φύσει, καὶ ὕπνοι μακρότεροι.

Δεῖ σκοπεῖν ἐπὶ τῶν ὑγιαινόντων τὰς ὥρας καὶ τὴν ποιότητα αὐτῶν καὶ τὸ εἶδος τῆς διαίτης ὑποτυποῦν· ἀλλὰ καὶ ἐπὶ τῶν νοσούντων εἰδέναι, ποῖαι μέν εἰσι θερμότεραι, ποῖαι δὲ ψυχρότεραι, ἵν' ἐντεῦθεν εἰδῇς, ὅτι αἱ μὲν θερμαὶ ὧραι εὐδιαφόρητα ποιοῦσι τὰ σώματα καὶ τὸ στόμα τῆς γαστρὸς ἑτοίμως ἐκπικροῦσιν, αἱ δὲ ψυχραὶ τὸ ἀνάπαλιν, ὥστε καὶ τὴν δίαιταν πρόσφορον ἁρμόζειν. φησὶ γάρ· Αἱ

5–12] *v.* Gal. In Aphor. I 14: XVII B 413,6–17 K. Theoph. In Aphor.: II 278,8–12 Dietz 18 προϊὼν – 21 τοιαῦτα[I]] *cf.* Hipp. Aphor. III 31: IV 500,15–502,2 L. 22 ταύτης – 26] *v.* Gal. In Aphor. I 14: XVII B 414,8–12 K. ταύτης – 25 ζέον] *v.* Theoph. In Aphor.: II 278,12–17 Dietz

1 οὐ] μὴ P 3 *fort.* ⟨ἐπεὶ⟩ πλεῖστον *scribendum est* 6 καὶ *non hab. Hipp.* 7 τοῦτο *ex* τὸ *corr.* P[2] 8 ὀλίγων *ex* -ον *corr.* P[2] 10 δὲ *om.* P 21 τὰ[I] *om.* A 23 γένονται α: *correxi* 25 αὐτοὺς A 27 θερμόταται *ex* θερμότεραι *corr.* A[2] 28 μακρότεροι *ex* -αι *corr.* A[2]: μακρότατοι *infra, pp. 106,1; 110,32, Hipp.* 32 καὶ – ἐκπικροῦσιν *om.* A στόμα *scripsi*: σῶμα P

gestion being due to the sharpness of the internal heat at this age; children, on the other hand, cannot digest food that is difficult to break down because in them the heat is not caustic, but they can deal with a great quantity of food thanks to the abundance of essential natural heat. They have the most innate heat: the word most indicates quantity, not quality.

I 25. Old men have little heat; therefore they also need little kindling.

He says that there is little innate heat in old men, and therefore they need little "kindling", i.e. food, else they might suffer the fate of the flame of the lamp, when too much oil at a time is poured upon it. "Kindling" is a word used by the ancients for thin pieces of firewood and for firewood generally, and this is why Hippocrates called food kindling, as fuel for our innate heat.

I 26. This is also why fevers in old men are less acute, their bodies being cold.

Here Hippocrates tries to derive further proof from the diseases that are commonest in old men, to show that there is little heat in them, so that they can easily endure abstinence from food. For the present he mentions only that fever is lower, and less hot and scalding; later on he lists many affections that are proper to old men; we will mention them now in support of the argument. Old men, then, as a general rule are subject to torpors, apoplectic fits, coughs, colds, catarrhs, sneezing, etc. Affections of this kind are akin to their temperament, being cold and wet; they are also consumed by them. This is the reason why they do not easily contract a fever; and if fevers do occur, the natural coldness of their bodies will prevent the fever from being hot and burning, and reduce its scalding heat; but if they ever happen to incur a violent fever, you may be sure that death will follow soon.

I 27. The cavities are naturally hottest in winter and spring, and sleep is (then) longer.

We must examine the seasons and their qualities with respect to the healthy and outline the kind of diet accordingly; but with respect to the sick, too, you must know which (seasons) are hotter, which are colder, so that you will realize that the hot seasons make the body subject to dispersal and the orifice of the stomach to acidity, while the cold (seasons) have the contrary effect; thus you can vary the diet accordingly. What (Hippocrates) says is: The cavities are

κοιλίαι χειμῶνος καὶ ἦρος θερμόταται φύσει, καὶ ὕπνοι μακρότατοι – καὶ δεῖ πλείονα τροφὴν παρέχειν.

Ἰστέον δέ, ὅτι κατὰ δύο αἰτίας θερμόταται γίνονται αἱ κοιλίαι χειμῶνος, μίαν μὲν φυσικήν, ἑτέραν δὲ Ἀριστοτελικήν. φησὶ γὰρ ἐκεῖνος, ὅτι ἀντιπεπονθότως ἔχουσι πρὸς ἑαυτὰ τὰ στοιχεῖα, καὶ ἀνθυποχωροῦσιν ἀλλήλαις καὶ ἀντιπεριίστανται αἱ ποιότητες. ὅτε μὲν γὰρ ἐν βάθει ἐστὶν ἡ θερμασία, καταλαμβάνει τὴν ἐπιφάνειαν ἡ ψῦξις· καὶ ἔμπαλιν εἰς τὸ βάθος ὑποχωρούσης τῆς ψύξεως εἰς τὴν ἐπιφάνειαν ἐφαπλοῦται ἡ θερμασία. ἐν τῷ χειμῶνι τοίνυν τῆς ψύξεως περὶ τὴν ἐπιφάνειαν σχολαζούσης εἰς τὸ βάθος ὑποστέλλεται ἡ θερμασία· ἐν δὲ τῷ θέρει τῆς θερμασίας τὴν ἐπιφάνειαν καταλαβούσης ἐπὶ τοῦ βάθους ἡ ψῦξις ἐνδομυχεῖ. δευτέρα δὲ αἰτία ἐστὶ κατὰ τοὺς ἰατροὺς αὕτη. θερμαί εἰσιν ἐν ταῖς ὥραις ταύταις αἱ κοιλίαι τρόπῳ τοιούτῳ· πεπύκνωται ἡ ἐπιφάνεια τοῦ σώματος, ἐπείγεται τὸ ἔμφυτον θερμὸν ὡς ἀεικίνητον ἐπὶ τὸ ἐκτὸς ἀχθῆναι, οὐχ εὑρίσκει διέξοδον, εἶτα ἀντανακλᾶται καὶ ἀνθυπονοστεῖ ἐπὶ τὰ ἐντός· καὶ τούτου πολλάκις γινομένου τοῦ διαύλου πολλαπλασιάζεται καὶ δριμύτερον ἑαυτοῦ γίνεται κἀντεῦθεν ποιεῖ τὰς κοιλίας θερμάς.

Κοιλίας δὲ καλεῖ ἐνταῦθα οὐ μόνον τὴν σιτοδόχον γαστέρα, ἀλλὰ πᾶσαν κοιλότητα ἐν τῷ βάθει κειμένην πλὴν τοῦ θώρακος. ἐπειδὴ γὰρ ἡ τοῦ θώρακος κοιλότης διὰ τῆς εἰσπνοῆς εἰσάγει ἀέρα τῇ καρδίᾳ, καὶ ὡς ἂν διατεθῇ τὸ κατάστημα, οὕτως εἰσπνέομεν, ἐν δὲ τῷ χειμῶνι ψυχρόν ἐστι τὸ περιέχον, ἀνάγκη καὶ τὸν θώρακα οὕτως διατεθῆναι. ἐνταῦθα οὖν θερμὰς ἐν χειμῶνι κοιλίας ἀκουστέον τὴν τοῦ ἐγκεφάλου, τῆς καρδίας, τοῦ στομάχου, τῆς γαστρός, τοῦ ἥπατος, τῶν ἐντέρων, τῶν νεφρῶν, τῆς κύστεως.

Καὶ ἀποροῦσί τινες λέγοντες· «Πῶς ὁ Ἱπποκράτης ἐν χειμῶνι θερμὰς τὰς κοιλίας εἶναι λέγει; καὶ μὴν ὁρῶμεν ἐν τῷ θέρει αὐχμὸν πολὺν ἐν τοῖς σώμασιν καὶ δίψος ἀφόρητον καὶ καῦμα καὶ ζέσιν κατὰ τὴν γαστέρα καὶ τὸ βάθος συνισταμένην, ὧν οὐδὲν ἐν χειμῶνι ὡς ἔτυχε γίνεται.» πρὸς ὃ ῥητέον, ὅτι τῇ ποιότητι τῆς λέξεως προσεχόντων ἡμῶν οὐχ ἕξει ἀπορίαν τὸ λεγόμενον· Αἱ γὰρ κοιλίαι χειμῶνος καὶ ἦρος θερμόταται φύσει, τουτέστι τὸ κατὰ φύσιν θερμὸν ἔχουσαι, τὸ οἰκεῖον, τὸ πεπτικὸν τῶν χυμῶν, οὐ μὴν τὸ παρὰ φύσιν ὥσπερ ἐπὶ τῶν πυρεσσόντων, οὔτε μὴν τὸ οὐ φύσει, ἀλλ' ἐπίκτητον ὥσπερ τὸ ἐν τῷ θέρει συμβαῖνον. τηνικαῦτα γὰρ ὑπὸ τοῦ παρὰ φύσιν καὶ ἐπικτήτου θερμοῦ ὡς ἀλλοτρίου ὑπάρχοντος διαφορεῖται μὲν τὸ κατὰ φύσιν καὶ οἰκεῖον καὶ ἀσθενέστερον ἑαυτοῦ καθίσταται τῇ δυσκρασίᾳ καταβαλλόμενον, ἀντεισάγεται δὲ τὸ ἀλλότριον καὶ πρὸς ἑαυτὸ διατίθησι τὸ σῶμα.

Ἔστι δὲ πάλιν ἀπορῆσαι· «Εἰ διὰ τὸ πεπυκνῶσθαί πως τὴν ἐπιφάνειαν ἐν τῷ χειμῶνι καὶ ἐν τῷ ἔαρι τὸ βάθος ἐστὶ θερμόν, τί δήποτε μὴ διαφορουμένου τοῦ σώματος λέγει, ὅτι δεῖ τρέφειν ἐν χειμῶνι; οὐδὲν γὰρ ἕτερόν ἐστι τροφὴ εἰ μὴ τοῦ διαφορηθέντος καὶ λείποντος ἀναπλήρωσις.» καὶ ἐπιλυόμεθα οὕτως, ὅτι οὐ μόνον ἔνθα μὴ γίνεται διαφόρησις οὐ δεῖ τρέφειν, ἀλλὰ καὶ ἔνθα ὀλίγον ὑπάρχει τὸ ἔμφυτον θερμὸν καὶ στόμα γαστρὸς μὴ ἐκχολούμενον. ἐνταῦθα οὖν, εἰ καὶ διαφόρησις οὐ γί-

4 φησὶ – 10 ἐνδομυχεῖ] *v.* Gal. In Aphor. I 15: XVII B 416,9–15 K. φησὶ – 6 ποιότητες] *cf.* Aristot. Meteora I 12: 348 b 2–8. 15–17 10 δευτέρα – 15] *v.* Theoph. In Aphor.: II 279,12–281,6 Dietz 16–22] *v.* Theoph. In Aphor.: II 279,10–12 Dietz

1 θερμότ$^{\rho}$ A μακρότεροι A 3 θερμότεραι A 3sq. μίαν – Ἀριστοτελικήν] *immo* μίαν μὲν φυσικὴν καὶ Ἀριστοτελικήν, ἑτέραν δὲ ἰατρικήν 4 ἀντιπεπονθότος A 11 αἱ *om.* A 13 ἀνθυποστροφεῖ A 14 τοῦτο P 28 θερμότεραι A 29 μὴν^{II}] οὖν A 35 ἔαρι] ἀέρι P 39 *fort.* μὴ *delendum est*

naturally hottest in winter and spring, and sleep is (then) longest – so you must allow more food.

Two reasons can be stated why the cavities become hottest in winter, one of them physiological, the other Aristotelian. (Aristotle) says that there is mutual antipathy between the elements, and that the qualities make way for each other and change places with each other. When the heat is deep inside, the cold takes hold of the surface; and conversely, when the cold withdraws to the depth, the warmth spreads over the surface. In winter, therefore, when the cold is made free of the surface, the warmth retires to the inside; but in summer, when the warmth has taken possession of the surface, the cold hides inside. The second, medical, reason is this. In these seasons the cavities become hot in the following way: the surface of the body has contracted; the innate heat, being in perpetual motion, strives to make its way outside, but, as it finds no passage, it then rebounds and returns to the inside; and by the frequent repetition of this motion to and fro it multiplies, becomes keener than it was, and thus it makes the cavities hot.

Cavities in this case means not only the stomach, the receptacle of food, but any deep-lying cavity with the exception of the chest. For since the thoracic cavity through inhalation supplies air to the heart, since the air we inhale varies according to weather conditions, and since in winter the surrounding air is cold, such will necessarily be the condition of the chest, too. In this passage, therefore, the cavities that are hot in winter must be understood as those of the brain, the heart, the stomach, the belly, the liver, the intestines, the kidneys and the bladder.

Some raise the objection: "How can Hippocrates say that the cavities are hot in winter? What we actually observe is that in summer there is much desiccation of the body, intolerable thirst, a burning, scalding heat which settles in the region of the stomach and in the depth of the body, none of which occurs in winter unless for a special reason." The answer is that if we pay attention to the exact wording, there is no problem: The cavities are naturally hottest in winter and spring means that they have their normal, own heat, which concocts the humors, not the abnormal heat of fever patients, nor the non-natural, adventitious heat that occurs in summer. In those cases the abnormal and adventitious heat, which is alien (to the body), disperses its normal, own heat, so that it loses strength and is overcome by distemper; and the alien heat takes its place and lends its own disposition to the body.

Another possible objection is: "If a sort of contraction of the surface in winter and spring is the cause of the heat inside, why does (Hippocrates) tell us to administer food in winter, though there is no dispersal of the body? Surely food is nothing but a replacement of matter dispersed and wanting." Our solution is that food should be withheld where not only there is no dispersal, but innate heat is also scarce and the orifice of the stomach is not flooded with bile. In the present instance now, though there is no dispersal to speak of, yet innate heat is strong,

νεται ἀξιόλογος, ἀλλ' οὖν ἐρρωμένον ἐστὶ τὸ ἔμφυτον θερμόν, καὶ δεῖ πολλὴν τροφὴν παρασχεῖν τῷ σώματι, ἵνα μὴ τῇ ἀπορίᾳ τῆς ὕλης ἀπομαρανθῇ ἢ κατὰ τῶν στερεῶν χωρήσῃ μορίων καὶ ἐκτήξῃ αὐτά. ἐπιλυόμεθα δὲ καὶ οὕτως, ὅτι ἐν χειμῶνι πολλὴ γίνεται διαφόρησις, εἰ καὶ ἀνεπαίσθητός ἐστι. τοῦ γὰρ ἐμφύτου θερμοῦ ἐν τῷ βάθει πλεονάζοντος πάντα τὰ ἔργα τῆς φύσεως, πέψις φημί, ἀνάδοσις, πρόσθεσις, πρόσφυσις, ἐξομοίωσις, λέπτυνσις, ὅσα τοιαῦτα, ὑγιῶς ἐπιτελεῖται. λεπτυνόμενοι οὖν οἱ χυμοὶ εἰς ἀτμοὺς ἀναλύονται καὶ διὰ τῆς ἀδήλου διαπνοῆς ἀνεπαισθήτως διαφοροῦνται. καὶ τοῦτο ἔξεστί σοι μαθεῖν ἐκ τῆς τοῦ στόματος ἀποφορᾶς· τότε γὰρ μέγα ἀποφυσῶμεν καπνοῦ δίκην παχυμεροῦς τῆς ἀναπνοῆς ἐν χειμῶνι ἐξαγομένης· κατὰ γὰρ τὸν αὐτὸν τρόπον καὶ διὰ παντὸς τοῦ σώματος ἀδήλου διαπνοῆς διαφόρησις γίνεται, ἀνεπαισθήτως μέντοι διὰ τὴν λεπτότητα τοῦ διαπνεομένου. ἐν μέντοι τῷ θέρει ἀσθενοῦς ὄντος τοῦ ἐν ἡμῖν θερμοῦ καὶ μὴ δυναμένου λεπτοποιῆσαι τοὺς χυμοὺς εἰς ἀτμούς, οὗτοι παχυμερεῖς ἀναδίδονται κἀντεῦθεν ἱδρῶσι τὰ σώματα περιρρέονται. ἔστι δὲ καὶ ἄλλως εἰπεῖν, ὅτι οὐ μόνον ἀτμοειδῶς καὶ ἀνεπαισθήτως διαφορεῖται ἐν χειμῶνι τὸ ἡμέτερον σῶμα, ἀλλὰ καὶ αἰσθητῶς κατὰ τοὺς φυσικοὺς ὑπονόμους. πολλὴ γὰρ ἡ τῶν ὑγρῶν ἔκκρισις γίνεται· πεπυκνωμένης γὰρ τῆς ἐπιφανείας καὶ τῶν ἀτμῶν ἐπὶ τὰ ἐκτὸς μὴ εὑρισκόντων διέξοδον ὑπονόστησις γίνεται ἐπὶ τὸ βάθος καὶ φέρεται ἐπὶ κύστιν καὶ ἔντερα καὶ μυκτῆρα τὰ περιττά, ὅθεν καὶ οὔρων πολλὴ ἐν χειμῶνι ἔκκρισις γίνεται καὶ διαχωρημάτων καὶ μύξης πολλὴ διαφόρησις καὶ πτυέλων καὶ τῶν τοιούτων. εἰ οὖν πολλὴ διαφόρησις ἐν χειμῶνι, πῇ μὲν διὰ τῶν φυσικῶν ὑπονόμων, πῇ δὲ διὰ τῆς ἀδήλου διαπνοῆς, πῇ δὲ καὶ διὰ τῆς ἀκριβοῦς κατεργασίας τῶν χυμῶν, δῆλον, ὅτι καὶ πολλὴ χρεία τῆς ἀντεισαγωγῆς.

Πάλιν δέ τινες ἀποροῦσιν ὅτι «Πῶς ὁ Ἱπποκράτης ἐν χειμῶνι θερμὰς εἶναι τὰς κοιλίας λέγει; καὶ μὴν ὁρῶμεν τὰ ἕρποντα τῶν ζῴων νεκρούμενα ἐν τῷ χειμῶνι, ὥστε καὶ ταῖς χερσὶν ἀναλαμβάνεσθαι μηδὲν ὅλως ἀδικοῦντα.» πρὸς οὕς φαμεν, ὅτι ἐκεῖνα τῶν ζῴων θερμὰς ἔχει τὰς κοιλίας ἐν χειμῶνι, ὅσα μεταξὺ τῆς κοιλότητος καὶ τῆς ἐπιφανείας πολὺ φέρουσι τὸ ἐν μέσῳ διάστημα καὶ ὅσα εὔσαρκά εἰσι· τὰ δὲ μήτε πολὺ τὸ μεταξὺ διάστημα ἔχοντα μήτε εὔσαρκα, ἀλλ' οἷον ἀβαθῆ καὶ ὀλιγόσαρκα, ψυχρὰ δι' ὅλου ἐν χειμῶνι εὑρίσκονται. τὰ οὖν ἕρποντα καὶ ἰοβόλα τῶν θηρίων ἅτε ὀλιγόσαρκα καὶ ἀβαθῆ μὴ πολλοῦ τοῦ μεταξὺ τῆς κοιλότητος καὶ τῆς ἐπιφανείας ὄντος αὐτοῖς διαστήματος ψύχεται καὶ ναρκοῦται χειμῶνος. φθάνει γὰρ περὶ τὸ βάθος ἀφικέσθαι ψῦξις, ὥστε καὶ αὐτοῦ τοῦ ἐμφύτου θερμοῦ αὐτῶν ἅπτεσθαι, οὕτινος καταψυχομένου νεκροῦνται τὰ τοιαῦτα ζῷα. διχῶς οὖν ἐδείχθη ψυχόμενα, τῷ τε ἀβαθῆ εἶναι τρόπον τινὰ καὶ τῷ μὴ ἔχειν προβόλους σάρκας ἀπομάχεσθαι τῇ ψύξει δυναμένας. καὶ ὅτι τοῦτ' ἀληθές, αὐτὸς ὁ Ἱπποκράτης παρακατιὼν πιστοῦται λέγων· «Ἔστι δὲ ὅκου ἐπὶ τετάνῳ νέῳ εὐσάρκῳ θέρεος μέσου ἄνευ ἕλκεος ψυχροῦ πολλοῦ κατάχυσις θέρμης ὑπανάκλησιν ποιέεται· θέρμη[ν] δὲ ταῦτα ῥύεται», ὡς ἂν τῆς τῶν σαρκῶν περιουσίας καὶ πολυαιμίας τὰ μεγάλα τῷ τρόπῳ τούτῳ τῆς θάλψεως συμβάλλεσθαι δυναμένης, τῆς δὲ ἐνδείας τοὐναντίον. φοβούμενος γὰρ τὴν

3 ἐπιλυόμεθα – 13 περιρρέονται] *cf.* Gal. In Aphor. I 15: XVII B 419,18–422,2 K. 14 ἔστι – 22] *cf.* Gal. In Aphor. I 15: XVII B 422,6–11 K. 23–35 δυναμένας] *cf.* Gal. In Aphor. I 15: XVII B 417,10–418,9 K. 36sq. Ἔστι – ῥύεται] Hipp. Aphor. V 21: IV 538,10–12 L.

3 χωρήσει A ἐκτήξει A 4 εἰ *om.* P 5 πρόθεσις A 18sq. οὖρον πολὺ P 27 μήτε] μήπω A 28 ἀλλοῖον A 29 εὑρίσκεται A 36 τετάνων α: *sec. Hipp. (v. l.) correxi* 37 ἐπανάκλησιν *Hipp.* θέρμην α: *corr.* A² 39 θλίψεως A

so we must provide much food for the body, otherwise (the heat) might be smothered for want of fuel, or it might invade the solid parts of the body and dissolve them. Another solution is that in winter there *is* a great deal of dispersal, though it remains unnoticed. Owing to the abundance of innate heat within, all the functions of nature, i.e. digestion, distribution, absorption, adhesion, assimilation, comminution, etc., are performed in a healthy way. In the process of comminution the humors dissolve into vapors and are dispersed imperceptibly by invisible exhalation. You can see this from the air that is breathed out; for then, in winter, we blow out a big cloud and breath comes thick like smoke; in the same way there is dispersal by invisible exhalation from the entire body, which, however, remains unnoticed because of the thinness of the matter exhaled. In summer, on the other hand, the heat in us being too weak to dissolve the humors into vapors, they come to the surface in a dense form, so that sweat drips from the body. You can also explain it in another way, namely, that in winter the body is subject to dispersal, not only imperceptibly by evaporation, but also visibly through the natural channels. There is much excretion of fluids then; since the surface is contracted and the vapors find no way out, a reflux toward the depth takes place, and the waste matter is conveyed to the bladder, the intestines and the nose; hence much urine is passed in winter, and there is also a great deal of dispersal in the form of stools, mucus, sputum, etc. If, therefore, we have all this dispersal in winter, partly through the natural channels, partly through invisible exhalation, and partly through the complete breaking down of the humors, there is obviously also a great need for replacement.

Again, some raise the question: "How can Hippocrates maintain that in winter the cavities are hot? Yet we see that in winter reptiles become torpid, so that they can even be handled without doing harm." We answer that only those animals have hot cavities in winter, in which there is a considerable distance between the cavity and the surface, and those which are fleshy; but those which lack that distance and that fleshiness and have, in a manner of speaking, no depth and little flesh, are found to be cold throughout in winter. Therefore reptiles and venomous animals, having little flesh and little depth, because the cavity and the surface are not far apart, become cold and numb in winter. The reason is that the cold reaches the depth, so that it invades even the innate heat, and when this cools off, such creatures become torpid. As we have shown, they lose warmth for two reasons, first, because they are, so to speak, without depth, and secondly because they have no protective layer of flesh to keep the cold at a distance. That this is true, Hippocrates himself confirms when he says farther down: "Sometimes in cases of tetanus during midsummer, when the patient is a sturdy young man and there is no wound, a shower-bath with plenty of cold water brings back the heat; and heat is the cure for this disease"; this implies that abundant flesh and rich blood can contribute greatly to this way of warming (the body), while

ἐκ τοῦ ψυχροῦ πλῆξιν ἐπὶ εὐσάρκου τετανικοῦ τὸν τρόπον τοῦτον τῆς θεραπείας παραλαμβάνει.

Ἀποροῦσι δέ τινες πάλιν λέγοντες ὅτι «Εἰ θερμαί εἰσιν ἐν χειμῶνι αἱ κοιλίαι, τί δήποτε τότε φλέγμα πολὺ γεννᾶται ἐν τῇ γαστρὶ καὶ ἐν τοῖς ἐντέροις καὶ πολλὰ ἐν χειμῶνι πτύομεν μᾶλλον καὶ διὰ μυκτήρων φέρομεν καὶ πολλὰ νοσήματα γίνονται, κατάρροιαι τυχὸν καὶ βῆχες καὶ κοιλιακαὶ διαθέσεις καὶ ἰσχιάδες καὶ ἕτερα πλεῖστα νοσήματα, ἅτινα πάντα περιουσίας ψυχρῶν εἰσι γνωρίσματα;» πρὸς οὓς ἔστιν εἰπεῖν· εἰ τοσαύτης μετελαμβάνομεν ἐν χειμῶνι τροφῆς, ὅσην δυνατὸν τὸ ἐν ἡμῖν θερμὸν κατεργάζεσθαι, ὥστε ἀναλογεῖν τὰ αἰρόμενα τῷ πέττοντι, οὐδὲν ἂν τούτων ἐγίνετο. ἀλλ' εἰδότες, ὅτι πολύ ἐστι τὸ ἐν ἡμῖν θερμὸν κατὰ τὴν ὥραν ταύτην, τούτῳ τε πεποιθότες πολλὰς καὶ ὑπὲρ τὴν ἀναλογίαν τροφὰς προσφερόμεθα, ἅστινας πέψαι διὰ τὴν ὑπερβολὴν μὴ δυνάμενοι τῶν τοιούτων αἴτιοι χυμῶν ἡμεῖς ἑαυτοῖς καθιστάμεθα. εἰ δὲ εἴποι τις ὅτι «Εἰ ἀπεπτουμένης τῆς τροφῆς φλέγμα γεννᾶται, τὸ δὲ βάθος θερμὸν ὑπάρχει, ἔδει ὅσον ἐπὶ τούτῳ χολὴν γεννηθῆναι», πρὸς τοῦτό φαμεν, ὅτι οἱ ἐν ἡμῖν στοιχειώδεις χυμοὶ κατὰ φύσιν γεννῶνται. πᾶσα γὰρ ἀνάγκη ἀναλογίαν πρὸς τὸ περιέχον σῴζειν καὶ τὸ περιεχόμενον, ὥσπερ εἴρηται ἐν τῷ θέρει ὅτι τὸ δίψος καὶ τὸ ἀφόρητον καῦσος καὶ ἡ γένεσις τῆς χολῆς τῷ ἐπικτήτῳ θερμῷ συνίσταται· οὕτως δὲ καὶ ἐν ἑκάστῃ ὥρᾳ, ὡς ἔχει τὸ περιέχον, οὕτως ἔχει καὶ τὸ περιεχόμενον. καὶ ἄλλως δέ, εἰ καὶ θερμόν ἐστιν ἐν χειμῶνι τὸ βάθος καὶ τούτῳ θαρροῦντες ὑπὲρ τὴν ἀναλογίαν ἐφιέμεθα τροφῆς, ἀλλὰ ταύτης ἀπεπτηθείσης ἧττον ἑαυτοῦ γίνεται τὸ θερμόν, ὑποστέλλεται γάρ, καὶ ἀνάγκη πᾶσα συνδιατεθῆναι τὸ ἀπεπτηθὲν τῷ περιέχοντι, καὶ διὰ τοῦτο ἐν χειμῶνι συμβαίνει γεννᾶσθαι ἐν ἡμῖν τὸν φλεγματικὸν χυμόν.

Δεῖ δὲ καὶ τοῦτο εἰδέναι, ὅτι περὶ τὰς ἀρχὰς καὶ τὰ μέσα τοῦ ἦρός εἰσι θερμόταται αἱ κοιλίαι, ἐπεί τοί γε ἐν τῷ πέρατι ἅτε πλησιάζοντι τῇ ἀρχῇ τοῦ θέρους οὐχ εὑρίσκομεν θερμὰς οὔσας τὰς κοιλίας. ἄλλως τε δὲ εἰ καὶ ἐν τῷ ἔαρι καὶ τῷ χειμῶνι θερμαί εἰσιν αἱ κοιλίαι, ἀλλ' οὖν ἐν μὲν τῷ ἔαρι καθ' αὑτό τε καὶ κατὰ πρῶτον λόγον εὐκράτου ὄντος τοῦ περιέχοντος καὶ τῷ λόγῳ τῆς εὐκρασίας ἀφθόνου καὶ πλουσίου τικτομένου τοῦ ἐν ἡμῖν θερμοῦ· ἐν δὲ τῷ χειμῶνι κατὰ συμβεβηκός, τῷ ἐκ τῆς πυκνώσεως τῆς ἐπιφανείας τοῦ σώματος ἐν τῷ βάθει συνάγεσθαι τὸ θερμὸν τῇ πολυειδεῖ κινήσει καὶ παλιρροίᾳ.

Καὶ ὕπνοι μακρότατοι. ἐπειδὴ οἶδεν ὁ Ἱπποκράτης ἐν χειμῶνι μεγάλας τὰς νύκτας ἐκεῖνο τὸ μέρος τοῦ ζῳδιακοῦ κύκλου διανύοντος τοῦ ἡλίου, ἐν ᾧ ἐστήρικται τοξότης καὶ αἰγόκερως καὶ ὑδροχόος, μείζονος περιφερείας κατὰ τὸ ὑπὸ γῆν ἡμικύκλιον ἐνταῦθα περιγραφομένης, ὡς ἐντεῦθεν πλείονας ὥρας τοῦ ἡλίου ὑπὸ γῆν διατρίβοντος τῇ χρονίᾳ τούτου ἀπουσίᾳ τὸν ὑπὲρ γῆν ψύχεσθαι τόπον, ὡμολόγηται δὲ καὶ ἐν Προγνωστικῷ καὶ ἐν ἑτέροις τὸν κατὰ φύσιν ὕπνον ἐν νυκτὶ μάλιστα γίνεσθαι, νόμιζε ταῦτά σοι λέγειν αὐτόν, ὅτι ἐν χειμῶνι μεγάλαι εἰσὶν αἱ νύκτες πλεῖστον χρόνον τοῦ ἡλίου ὑπὸ γῆν διατρίβοντος· πλείοσιν οὖν δεῖ κεχρῆσθαι τροφαῖς· εἰ δὲ μή γε, συννεύοντος ἐν τῷ βάθει τοῦ ἐμφύτου θερμοῦ καὶ πολλῷ πλείονος

16 εἴρηται] *cf. supra*, p. 106,23–33 24–26 κοιλίας] *v.* Gal. In Aphor. I 15: XVII B 424,13–16 K. 36 ὡμολόγηται – 38 γίνεσθαι] *v.* Hipp. Progn. 10: p. 205,9–10 Alexanderson = II 134,5–6 L. Praen. Coac. 487: V 694,17–18 L.

4 πολὺ φλέγμα A 13 ἀποπεπτουμένης A 19 τοῦτο α: *correxi* 21 ὑποσυστέλλεται A 24 θερμότρ A 26 *et* 27 ἔαρι] ἀέρι P 29 τῷ[II]] τὸ P 32 μακρότεροι A 33 νύκται α (-αι *eras. in* P): *correxi*

lack of these has the opposite effect. It is out of fear of the impact of the cold that he applies this cure only to the fleshy tetanus patient.

Others again object: "If the cavities are hot in winter, how is it that just then much phlegm is formed in the stomach and in the intestines? Why is there more expectoration in winter, more running at the nose, and why do we have numerous diseases such as catarrh, coughing, intestinal trouble, sciatica and many others, all of which are indicative of a surplus of cold matter?" The answer can be: if in winter we partook of only so much food as our internal heat can digest, so that the intake was in the right proportion to the digestive capacity, none of these things would happen. As it is, knowing that the internal heat in this season is plentiful, and trusting in this, we take too much food in proportion; and since, as a result of such excess, we are unable to digest it, it is our own fault that we are troubled by such humors. Someone may remark: "If defective digestion of food causes the production of the phlegm, and the inside is hot, the humor produced, on the strength of this explanation, should be bile." We reply that the elementary humors in us are produced by a natural process. For inevitably the surrounded will be in keeping with its surroundings, just as we said already that in summer the thirst and the intolerable hotness and the production of bile are due to the adventitious heat; and this holds true of every season: the condition of the surrounded corresponds to that of the surrounding. Moreover, even though in winter the inside is hot and this encourages us to indulge in over-eating, yet when the food remains undigested, the heat diminishes, because it is forced to retreat, and the undigested part of the food necessarily assumes the disposition of its surroundings; this explains why in winter it is the phlegmatic humor that develops in us.

We should add that at the beginning and the middle of spring cavities are hottest; at the end, which comes close to the beginning of summer, we do not find them hot. Besides, while it is true that cavities are hot both in spring and in winter, yet in spring this is so absolutely and primarily, because the surrounding air is temperate and owing to the temperate quality (of the air) internal heat is generated plentifully and abundantly; in winter, however, it is so accidentally, because owing to the contraction of the surface of the body the heat collects in the inside by its multiple motion and reflux.

And sleep is (then) longest. Hippocrates knows that nights are long in winter, when the sun traverses that part of the zodiac in which Sagittarius, Capricorn and Aquarius stand, because a greater part of the circumference is then taken up by the hemicycle underneath the earth, so that the sun spends a greater number of hours under the earth and as a result of its long absence the region above the earth grows cold; further, in Prognostic and elsewhere it has been acknowledged that natural sleep usually occurs at night; consequently, you may conclude that what he means is: In winter nights are long because the sun is the longest time underneath the earth; therefore one should take more food; otherwise, because

διὰ τὸ μέγεθος τῶν νυκτῶν γινομένου, ἐὰν μὴ ὑποστῇ τροφή, ἀδικεῖται τὸ σῶμα συντηκόμενον ὑπ' αὐτοῦ.

Καὶ ἀποροῦσί τινες· «Εἰ παρὰ τὸ εἶναι μεγάλας τὰς νύκτας, παρὰ τοῦτο ἤδη καὶ ὕπνοι μακρότατοι, πῶς ὁρῶμέν τινας ἐν τρισὶν ἢ τέτρασιν ὥραις ἀρκουμένους τῷ ὕπνῳ, οὐ μόνον ἐν ταῖς μεγάλαις νυξίν, ἀλλὰ καὶ ἐν θέρει, ὅτε σμικρόταταί εἰσιν αἱ νύκτες; ἄλλως τε δὲ πολλῆς οὔσης ἐν τῷ βάθει τῆς θερμασίας χειμῶνος πῶς γίνεται ὕπνος μακρός, εἴ γε ἡ θερμασία τῷ ἀεικινήτῳ καὶ ζέοντι ἀγρυπνητικοὺς ἡμᾶς ποιεῖ διανύττουσα τούτῳ καὶ διεγείρουσα, ὁ δὲ ὕπνος ἐν ἀνεργείᾳ θεωρεῖται;» πρὸς οὓς λέγομεν, ὅτι ἐκ τῆς πολλῆς τροφῆς τῆς διδομένης ἀτμοὶ χρηστοὶ τίκτονται τῷ κατ' ὀλίγον γίνεσθαι τὰς πέψεις διὰ τὴν ῥώμην τοῦ ἐμφύτου θερμοῦ· οἵτινες περὶ τὸν ἐγκέφαλον ἀνιόντες καθυγραίνουσιν αὐτόν, καὶ ἐμφράττοντες αὐτοῦ τὰς κοιλίας τὸν ὕπνον ἐπιφέρουσιν. ἢ καὶ ἄλλως· ἰστέον, ὅτι ἐν χειμῶνι πάντα τὰ μόρια τρέφονται ἐκ τοῦ πλήθους τῆς προσαγομένης τροφῆς καὶ ἐκ τῆς περιουσίας τοῦ ἐμφύτου θερμοῦ. ὧν εἷς ἐστι καὶ ὁ ἐγκέφαλος, ὅστις τρεφόμενος καὶ ὑγραινόμενος ἐπιτέγγεται καὶ τοὺς ὕπνους ἐπάγει. ῥητέον καὶ τρίτην λύσιν· ἐν χειμῶνι τὸ περιττεῦον ἐν ἡμῖν θερμὸν τὸ κατ' οὐσίαν ἐστί, τὸ ἀτμωδέστερον καὶ ὡς ἂν εἴποι τις ὑγρότερον καὶ προσηνέστερον τοῦ κατὰ ποιότητα, ὅπερ δριμύτερον καὶ δακνωδέστερον ὑπάρχει. ὡς προσηνὲς οὖν καὶ ἐπὶ τὸν ἐγκέφαλον παραγινόμενον ὑγραίνει αὐτὸν καὶ τοὺς ὕπνους ἐργάζεται. τὸ γὰρ κατὰ ποιότητα τοὐναντίον διανίστησι καὶ διεγείρει καὶ ἀγρυπνίας ἐστὶ ποιητικόν· καὶ τοῦτο δῆλον ἐκ τῶν ἀκμαζόντων, ἄγρυπνοι γάρ εἰσι τὸ ὅλον καὶ πρακτικώτατοι, καὶ ἠρεμεῖν οὐ δύνανται τοῦ κατὰ ποιότητα θερμοῦ ἐνοχλοῦντος αὐτοῖς. οἱ μέντοι παῖδες πλεῖστα καθεύδουσι διὰ τὸ καὶ ἐπ' αὐτῶν τὸ κατ' οὐσίαν πλεονάζειν θερμὸν ἀτμωδέστερον ὄν.

I 28 [I 15: IV 466,14–15 L.] Ἐν ταύτῃσιν οὖν τῇσιν ὥρῃσιν καὶ τὰ προσάρματα πλεῖον δοτέον.

Προσάρματα τὰς τροφὰς ἐκάλεσε. νόμιζε οὖν ταῦτα λέγειν σοι τὸν Ἱπποκράτην· ἐπειδὴ ἐν χειμῶνι πολὺ τὸ ἔμφυτον θερμόν, πλείονος χρεία καὶ τῆς τροφῆς· εἰ δὲ μή γε, χωρεῖ τοῦτο κατὰ τῆς τριμερείας τοῦ σώματος, πνευμάτων φημὶ καὶ ὑγρῶν καὶ στερεῶν, καὶ τὰ μὲν στερεὰ τήκει, τὰ δὲ ὑγρὰ καὶ τὰ πνεύματα διαφορεῖ, κἀντεῦθεν ἀναλίσκεται.

I 29 [I 15: IV 466,16 L.] Σημεῖον αἱ ἡλικίαι καὶ οἱ ἀθληταί.

Λέγει· ὥσπερ ἐπὶ τῆς παιδικῆς ἡλικίας καὶ τῆς ἀθλητικῆς διὰ τὸ πλούσιον τοῦ ἐμφύτου θερμοῦ πλείονος χρεία καὶ τῆς τροφῆς, οὕτω καὶ ἐν τῷ χειμῶνι. ἐν δὲ τῷ παραδείγματι τοῦτο πρώτως καὶ καθ' αὑτὸ ἔλαβε, φημὶ δὴ τὸ ἔμφυτον θερμόν, ἐπὶ [δὲ] τῶν παίδων· τὸ δὲ κατὰ συμβεβηκός, τὸ εἶναι πολὺ τὸ ἐπίκτητον, ἐπὶ τῶν

8 πρὸς – 12 ἐπιφέρουσιν] *v.* Theoph. In Aphor.: II 281,9–13 Dietz 24–27 τροφῆς] *v.* Theoph. In Aphor.: II 281,13–15 Dietz 31–33 χειμῶνι] *v.* Theoph. In Aphor.: II 281,16–17 Dietz

1 ὑποστῇ τροφή] ὑποτῆ τροφῆ P 4 μακρότεροι A 5 ὅτε *ex* ὅτι *corr.* P[2] 6 τε *om.* A 8 ἐνεργεία A 9 τῷ] τὸ P 11 αὐτόν *om.* A 14 ἐπιτέγγεται *scripsi (cf. infra, p. 140,15)*: ἐπιτάγγεται A: ἐπιτάττεται P 15 τριτὴν A: τριττὴν P: *correxi* 16 ὑγρότ[τ] P 20 πρακτικώτ[ρ] A 25 πλεῖον *et infra, vol. II, fol. 9[v]*: πλείω *Hipp.* 26 σοι *om.* P 34 τούτῳ α: *correxi* πρῶτον A 35 δὲ[I] *delevi* δὲ[II] *om.* A

the innate heat converges in the depth and is greatly increased by the length of the nights, the body is consumed by it and suffers harm, unless food is supplied.

Some object: "If the length of the sleep is the immediate result of the length of the nights, why do we see that for some people three or four hours' sleep is sufficient, not only during the long nights, but also in summer, when nights are shortest? Besides, if during winter there is a great deal of heat inside, where does the long sleep come from? Surely heat keeps us wakeful by its restless and scalding quality, by means of which it stimulates and rouses us, whereas sleep consists in inactivity." Our answer is that from the abundant food that is given benignant vapors are produced, because digestion takes place gradually thanks to the strength of the innate heat; these vapors, mounting to the brain, moisten it, and by clogging its cavities bring about the sleep. Another explanation: in winter all the parts of the body are fed from the plentiful food that is taken and from the abundance of innate heat. One of these is the brain, which, with food and fluid supplied to it, becomes moist and brings on sleep. Let us add a third solution: in winter the surplus heat in us is the essential heat, which is more vaporous and, one might say, moister and milder than the qualitative heat, which is more acrid and stinging. When this mild kind of heat reaches the brain, it moistens it and causes sleep. As for the qualitative kind of heat, it has the reverse effect: it activates and rouses, and brings about wakefulness; this is clear from the fact that men in their prime are on the whole wakeful and eminently active; they cannot sit still, because the qualitative heat leaves them no peace. Children, on the other hand, sleep a great deal, because in their case there is a surplus of essential heat, which is more vaporous.

I 28. So in these seasons one should allow more sustenance.

By sustenance he means food. What Hippocrates wants to tell you is this: since in winter the innate heat is plentiful, more food is needed; otherwise the heat will attack the threefold substance of the body, i.e. gases, fluids and solids, dissolving the solids, dispersing the fluids and the gases, and thus (the body) will be consumed.

I 29. Proof of this are the young and the athletes.

That is: just as in the age group of children and in that of athletes the wealth of innate heat demands more food, so it is also in winter. In his example he took this – i.e. the innate heat – in its primary and absolute form when referring to children; in its accidental form, as a surplus of adventitious heat, when he men-

ἀθλητικῶν σωμάτων, καὶ ἐκ τῆς κινήσεως γὰρ τοῦ γυμνασίου θερμότεροι ἑαυτῶν οἱ ἀθληταὶ γίνονται. ἔστιν οὖν τὸν πάντα λόγον οὑτωσὶ συνελεῖν· ἐν χειμῶνι καὶ ἔαρι αἱ κοιλίαι θερμαί εἰσι, καὶ πλεονάζει τότε ἐν ἡμῖν τὸ ἔμφυτον θερμόν· διὸ δεῖται πολλῆς ἐπιλαβέσθαι τροφῆς, ἵνα μὴ τὸ σῶμα ἐκτήκηται. τοῦτο δὲ πιστούμεθα οὐ μόνον ἐκ τῆς παιδικῆς ἡλικίας – τὰ γὰρ αὐξανόμενα τῶν σωμάτων πλεῖστον ἔχει τὸ ἔμφυτον θερμόν –, ἀλλὰ καὶ ἐκ τῶν ἀθλούντων σωμάτων· πολλοῦ γὰρ ἐν τούτοις ὄντος τοῦ θερμοῦ, ἐὰν μὴ πλείων ἡ τροφὴ εἰσαχθῇ, ἐκτήκεται καὶ καταναλίσκεται τούτων τὰ σώματα.

I 30 [I 16: IV 466,17–19 L.] Ὑγραὶ δίαιται πᾶσι τοῖσι πυρεταίνουσι ξυμφέρουσι, μάλιστα δὲ παιδίοις καὶ τοῖσιν ἄλλοισι τοῖσιν οὕτως εἰθισμένοισι διαιτᾶσθαι.

Ἰστέον, ὅτι ἀδύνατόν ἐστι κατορθῶσαι τὴν θεραπείαν μὴ τῶν τεσσάρων τούτων συνερχομένων· τοῦ τε ποσοῦ καὶ τοῦ ποιοῦ καὶ τοῦ καιροῦ καὶ τοῦ τρόπου τῆς χρήσεως. ἐπεὶ τοίνυν καὶ ἡ δίαιτα θεραπεία τίς ἐστι, δεῖ καὶ ἐν αὐτῇ τὰ τέσσαρα ταῦτα θεωρεῖσθαι. καὶ περὶ μὲν τοῦ ποσοῦ ὁ Ἱπποκράτης διελέχθη ἐν οἷς ἔφη· «Ὅκου μὲν κάτοξυ τὸ νόσημα, αὐτίκα καὶ τοὺς ἐσχάτους πόνους ἔχει καὶ τῇ ἐσχάτως λεπτοτάτῃ διαίτῃ ἀναγκαῖον χρέεσθαι.» περὶ δὲ τοῦ καιροῦ, ἔνθα ἔλεγε· «Τοὺς δὲ παροξυσμοὺς ὑποστέλλεσθαι χρή, τὸ προστιθέναι γὰρ βλάβη.» νυνὶ δὲ περὶ τοῦ ἀπὸ τῆς ποιότητος διαιτητικοῦ σκοποῦ τὸν λόγον ποιεῖται φάσκων· Αἱ ὑγραὶ δίαιται πᾶσι τοῖς πυρέττουσι ξυμφέρουσι.

Καὶ ἰστέον, ὅτι τὸ ἐν ἡμῖν θερμὸν ὑγρόν τι χρῆμα καὶ θερμόν ἐστι· καὶ ὅταν μὲν ἔχῃ κατὰ φύσιν, ὑγιαίνει τὸ ζῷον, ἡνίκα δὲ τοῦ συμμέτρου παρατραπῇ καὶ εἰς τὸ ἐναντίον μεταπέσῃ, νόσον πυρεκτικὴν ἀπεργάζεται. ἐπεὶ οὖν ὁ πυρετὸς ξηρόν τι νόσημα καὶ θερμὸν ὑπάρχει, διὰ τῶν ἐναντίων δεῖ θεραπεύειν αὐτό, φημὶ δὴ ὑγρῶν. εἰ δέ τις ἀπορῶν εἴποι μὴ μόνον ξηρόν τι χρῆμα εἶναι τὸν πυρετόν, ἀλλὰ καὶ θερμόν, καὶ χρῆναι πάντως, εἰ μέλλοι γίνεσθαι διὰ τῶν ἐναντίων ἡ θεραπεία, μὴ μόνον ὑγροῖς, ἀλλὰ καὶ ψυχροῖς ἐνταυθοῖ χρήσασθαι, μηδὲ γὰρ ἐνδέχεσθαι τὴν μίαν ποιότητα ταῖς δυσὶν ἀμετρίαις ἀπομαχέσασθαι, φαίημεν ἂν πρὸς τόδε, ὅτιπερ βραχυλογίᾳ προσκείμενος ὁ Ἱπποκράτης τῆς μιᾶς μνησθεὶς ἀντιθέσεως καὶ τὴν λοιπὴν συνεπινοουμένην ἐδήλωσεν. ἔστι μέντοι καὶ ἄλλως εἰπεῖν, ὅτι πρὸς τὸ κατεπεῖγον ὁ Ἱπποκράτης ἱστάμενος – μᾶλλον γὰρ ἡ ξηρότης τὸν νοσοῦντα λυμαίνεται ἤπερ ἡ θερμότης – μόνου διὰ τοῦτο τοῦ ὑγροῦ ἐμνημόνευσε. δέχου καὶ τρίτην λύσιν, ὅτι κἂν τῷ κατὰ φύσιν διακεῖσθαι θερμὸς ὑπάρχει ὁ ἄνθρωπος κἂν τῷ πυρέττειν ὁμοίως διάκειται· οὐ δήπου γὰρ τὴν εἰς τὸ ἐναντίον ἔσχε μεταβολήν, φημὶ δὴ τὴν εἰς τὸ ψυχρόν, ἀλλ' ἢ μόνον ἐπίτασιν θερμασίας ἐδέξατο. ἐπὶ δὲ τῆς ὑγρότητος οὐχ ὡσαύτως ἔχων ἐστίν,

12–13 χρήσεως] *cf.* Gal. Ad Glauc. I 1: XI 2,1–4 K. *supra*, p. 66,16–18 *infra*, vol. III, fol. 177ʳ 15 Ὅκου – 17 χρέεσθαι] Hipp. Aphor. I 7: IV 462,12–13 L. 17 Τοὺς – 18 βλάβη] Hipp. Aphor. I 11: IV 464,11–12 L. 23 ἐπεὶ – 30 ἐδήλωσεν] *v.* Theoph. In Aphor.: II 283,3–12 Dietz

2 γίνονται οἱ ἀθληταί A 7 πλείων ἡ *scripsi*: πλείονι P: πλεῖον A 9 Ὑγραὶ] *item infra, p. 118,19, Hipp.* MV *et al., Theoph.* SV'': Αἱ ὑγραὶ *infra, lin. 19, Hipp.* C', *Theoph.* U'' 13 συνεχομένων P 16 τόνους P 18 βλάβους P περὶ *om.* A 19 διαιτικοῦ P 25 εἴπη A 26 μέλλ *(ambig.)* A ἡ θεραπεία διὰ τῶν ἐναντίων A 28 ἀντιμαχέσασθαι A, *sed cf. infra, p. 118,19* 32 κἂν τὸ P: κάντο A: *correxi* 33 ὑπάρχει *ex* -ων *(?) corr.* A²

tioned the athletic body, because athletes, as a result of the exercise taken in training, become warmer than they normally are. We can sum up the entire argument as follows: in winter and spring the cavities are hot, and at that time the innate heat is abundant in us; therefore it is necessary to take plenty of nourishment, to prevent the body from wasting away. We infer this not only from the age group of the very young – since growing bodies have the most innate heat –, but also from the constitution of athletes: there is so much heat in them that, if no extra food is supplied, their bodies will be consumed and waste away.

I 30. Liquid diets are beneficial to all fever patients, but especially to children and to others who are accustomed to such a diet.

It is impossible for treatment to be successful unless these four go together: the quantity, the quality, the moment and the application. Since diet, too, is a form of treatment, these four should be considered here also. With quantity, Hippocrates has already dealt in the passage: "When the disease is very acute, (the patient) is immediately in extreme discomfort, and one must use the most rigorously strict diet." With the moment he dealt when he said: "During paroxysms one should use restraint, for then any addition is harmful." Now he discusses diet from the point of view of quality, saying: Liquid diets are beneficial to all fever patients.

It should be clear that our internal heat is something moist and hot; when it is in its normal state, the organism is healthy, but when it deviates from the right proportion and changes to the contrary, it causes a disease characterized by fever. Now since fever is a dry and hot disease, it should be cured by the opposite qualities, i.e. by moisture. If someone should object that fever is not only something dry, but also something hot, so that obviously, if a cure is to be attained through opposites, we must use not only moisture but also cold in this case, because one quality cannot fight two disproportionate ones, we could reply that Hippocrates, fond as he is of brevity, mentioned merely the one contrast while implying the other one. However, one can also give a different explanation, namely that Hippocrates, dealing with the most urgent aspect, since dryness hurts the patient more than heat does, on this account referred to heat only. Here is a third solution: man is warm when in his normal disposition, and when he has a fever, his condition is a similar one; he has not undergone a change into the contrary, i.e. cold, but only an increase of heat. Where moisture is concerned, however, the

ἀλλ' ἐν μὲν τῷ κατὰ φύσιν τηρούμενος ὑγρόν πως κέκτηται τὸ σῶμα, πυρετῷ δὲ περιπεπτωκὼς ξηρόν, δῆλον οὖν, ὡς ἐντεῦθεν τὴν εἰς τὸ ἐναντίον ἐδέξατο μεταβολήν. ἐπεὶ οὖν ἡ πρὸς τὸ ἐναντίον μεταβολὴ χεῖρον τῆς τοῦ ὁμοίου ἐστὶν ἐπιτάσεως, διὰ τοῦτο μόνου δοκεῖ μεμνῆσθαι τοῦ ὑγροῦ ὁ τεχνικός.

Πρὸς τούτοις ἔτι ῥητέον· οὐκ ἠδύνατο εἰπεῖν ὁ Ἱπποκράτης, ὅτι αἱ ὑγραὶ καὶ ψυχραὶ δίαιται συμφέρουσι τοῖς πυρέττουσιν. εἰ μὲν γὰρ τοῦτο τέθηκεν, ἀνάγκην ἂν ἔσχε πολλοῖς προσδιορισμοῖς ἐν τῷ λόγῳ χρήσασθαι καὶ εὑρίσκετο ποιῶν τι παρὰ τὸ σύνηθες ἑαυτῷ μηκύνων τὰ λεγόμενα. εἰ δ' ἀπροσδιορίστως αὐτὸ ἐδήλωσε, πολλῶν ἂν κακῶν αἴτιος ἐγεγόνει τοῖς κάμνουσιν ἡμῶν ὡς ἔτυχε χρωμένων ἐπὶ τῶν πυρεττόντων τοῖς ψύχουσιν. ἴσμεν γάρ, ὡς, ὅτε παρασχεῖν ὕδωρ βουληθῶμεν πυρέττοντι, ἀνάγκην ἔχομεν ἀφορᾶν πρὸς τὴν ἡλικίαν καὶ τὸ ἔθος καὶ τὸν καιρὸν τοῦ νοσήματος καὶ τὸν τῆς δυνάμεως τόνον καὶ τὴν θέσιν τῶν σπλάγχνων, ὥστε τὴν μὲν ὥραν θερινὴν εἶναι, τὴν δὲ ἡλικίαν ἀκμαστικήν, τὴν δὲ χώραν θερμήν, πέψιν τῆς ὕλης, ἀκμὴν τοῦ νοσήματος, ἐκ συνηθείας τε ἀβλαβῶς μεταλαμβάνειν τὸν ἀκμάζοντα, καὶ μηδεμίαν φλεγμονὴν ἢ εὐπάθειαν κατά τε τὸ ἧπαρ ἢ τὸν στόμαχον ἢ τὴν γαστέρα ἤ τι τῶν ὑποχονδρίων ὅλως θεωρεῖσθαι, ἔτι γε μὴν καὶ τὴν δύναμιν ἐρρῶσθαι. καὶ ἡνίκα ταῦτα καθάπερ χορὸς συμφωνεῖ, τότε ὕδωρ παρέχομεν· ἑνὸς δὲ τῶν ῥηθέντων ἐναντιουμένου οὐκ ἄν ποτε εἰς ἀγαθὸν τελευτήσῃ ἡ τοῦ ὕδατος ἐπίδοσις. ἐκεῖνο δέ μοι νόει, ὅτι καὶ μετρίαν ψῦξιν ἐργάζεται ἡ τῆς ὑγρότητος προσαγωγή, καὶ οὕτως πρὸς ἑκατέραν ἀντίθεσιν τὰ τῆς δεούσης θεραπείας ἐξισάζεται.

Πάλιν ἀποροῦσί τινες ὅτι «Πῶς φησιν ὁ Ἱπποκράτης τὴν ὑγρὰν δίαιταν ἁρμόζειν τοῖς πυρέττουσι; καὶ ἐπὶ τῶν ὑδεριώντων γάρ, ἐπειδὴ σύνεστι τούτοις πυρετός, δεῖ τοῖς ὑγραίνουσι χρήσασθαι, καίτοι τοῦ ὑδέρου τῶν ξηραινόντων δεομένου ὡς ψυχροῦ καὶ ὑγροῦ πάθους ὑπάρχοντος, ἀλλ' αὐξήσωμεν τὸ πάθος τῇ τῶν ὁμοίων εἰσαγωγῇ;» ἔστιν οὖν εἰπεῖν, ὅτι ἁπλῶν πυρετῶν θεραπείαν ὁ Ἱπποκράτης παραδίδωσιν, οὐ μὴν συνθέτων, τὴν ὑγρὰν δίαιταν, ἡνίκα συμβῇ γενέσθαι τὸν πυρετὸν μετά τινος τῶν ψυχρῶν ἢ ὑγρῶν παθῶν, ὡς ἐπὶ τοῦ λεχθέντος παραδείγματος. ἐπὶ τῶν παθημάτων οὖν, ἐφ' ὧν ἀντένδειξις θεωρεῖται, πρὸς τὸ κατεπεῖγον δεῖ ἐνίστασθαι μηδετέρου παντάπασιν ἀμελοῦντας. οὕτω δὴ κἀνταῦθα, εἰ μὲν τὰ τῆς θερμασίας ἐπὶ τῶν ὑδεριώντων κρατεῖ, ἧττον δὲ τὰ τοῦ ὑδέρου ἐνοχλεῖ, τοῖς ὑγραίνουσι καλῶς χρησόμεθα· εἰ δὲ τοὔμπαλιν, πρὸς τὸν ὕδερον δεῖ μάχεσθαι μηδετέρου ἀμελοῦντας. οὐδὲν δὲ ἧττον μένει ἡ ἀπορία· καὶ γάρ φησιν· «Εἰ καὶ περὶ ἁπλῶν πυρετῶν φαίημεν τὸν λόγον εἰρηκέναι τὸν Ἱπποκράτην καὶ τὸν πυρετὸν καθὰ πυρετὸν διὰ τῆς ὑγρᾶς διαίτης βούλεσθαι θεραπεύειν αὐτὸν καὶ ἐπὶ τῶν ἁπλῶν πυρετῶν ἀληθής ἐστιν οὗτος ὁ λόγος, τὸν ἀμφημερινὸν ἄρα οὑτωσὶ θεραπεύσομεν, ἐπὶ ψυχρᾷ καὶ ὑγρᾷ ὕλῃ καὶ φλεγματικῇ γινόμενον, τοῖς ψύχουσι καὶ ὑγραίνουσι χρώμενοι; αὐξήσομεν γὰρ τὴν ὕλην, ἀφ' ἧς ἀνάπτεται· καίτοι ὁ Γαληνὸς ὀξυμέλιτι κεχρῆσθαι κελεύει ἐπὶ τῶν ἀμφημερινῶν καὶ ζέματι ἀψινθίου καὶ τῷ Διοσπολιτικῷ φαρμάκῳ καὶ ἁπλῶς

10 ἴσμεν — 18 ἐπίδοσις] *cf. infra*, p. 218,9–18 16sq. καὶ^{II} — συμφωνεῖ] *cf.* Gal. Ad Glauc. I 2: XI 9,7–8 K. 21–32 ἀμελοῦντας] *v.* Gal. In Aphor. I 16: XVII B 426,10–427,12 K. 25 ἔστιν — 32 ἀμελοῦντας] *v.* Theoph. In Aphor.: II 284,9–12 Dietz 35sq. τὸν — γινόμενον] *cf.* Gal. De crisib. II 6: IX 663,16–17 K. 37 καίτοι — 118,1 ἐκφράττουσι] *cf.* Gal. Ad Glauc. I 13. 15 : XI 40,16–18; 56,11–12 K.

4 μόνον α: *correxi (cf. p. 114,32)* 7 ἀνάγκη P εὑρίσκεται α: *correxi* 8 αὐτὸ] αὐτῷ A 18 τελευτήσ *(ambig.)* P 22 τούτοις] τεοῖς A 25 θεραπείας A 26 συνθέντων P 30 ὑγιαίνουσι A 35 θεραπεύσωμεν A

case is not the same, but as long as he stays in a normal condition, his body is moist to a certain degree, while when he contracts a fever, it is dry, from which it is clear that he has undergone that change to the contrary. Now the change to the contrary is worse than the increase of the similar, and this, in my opinion, is why the writer of the manual mentions a liquid diet only.

We must add to this that Hippocrates could not say that liquid and cold diets are beneficial to fever patients. If he had put it that way, he would have been forced to qualify his statement by many restrictions, and he would be found to act against his custom by a prolix explanation. If, on the other hand, he had said it without any qualification, he would have caused a great deal of harm to sick people, because we would use cooling drinks in cases of fever at random. As we all know, if we want to give a fever patient water, we must consider age, habit, the moment of the disease, the strength of his resistance, and the condition of the inner organs, in the sense that the season has to be summerlike, the age the prime of life, the region warm, the matter well concocted, the disease at its height, the patient accustomed to drinking water without any bad effects; no inflammation or sensitivity should be noticeable in the liver, the stomach, the belly, or any part of the abdomen, and finally resistance should be strong. When all these are in tune like a chorus, we allow a drink of water; but if only one of the factors mentioned works the other way, giving water can never turn out well. Bear in mind, however, that the administering of fluids already brings about a certain amount of cooling, and thus the correct treatment is adequate to deal with both opposites.

Again, some raise the question: "How can Hippocrates say that a liquid diet is suitable for fever patients? Does this mean that in cases of dropsy, since they are attended by fever, we should apply moisture, in spite of the fact that dropsy, being a cold and moist condition, requires a desiccating treatment? Should we aggravate the disease by introducing matter of a similar nature?" We can answer to this that it is for the treatment of simple fevers that Hippocrates prescribes the liquid diet, not for complex ones, when the fever appears in combination with cold or moist affections, as in the example cited. In those diseases, then, where a counter-indication appears, we should deal with the more urgent need without completely neglecting either one. So here, too: if in cases of dropsy the heat prevails, while the dropsical condition is less troublesome, treatment by moisture will be preferable; in the opposite case, we must fight the dropsy, without neglecting the other side. Yet the problem remains unsolved; (our questioner) will say: "Suppose we admit that Hippocrates refers to simple fevers and wants to treat fever as such by means of a liquid diet, and that this statement holds true for simple fevers; does it follow that we should treat a quotidian fever in this way, by applying a cooling and moistening cure, notwithstanding the fact that it supervenes upon cold and moist, i.e. phlegmatic, matter? We should only increase the matter by which it is kindled; Galen, however, tells us to use oxymel for quotidian fevers, and a decoction of absinthe and the Diospol-

εἰπεῖν τοῖς θερμαίνουσι καὶ λεπτύνουσι καὶ τέμνουσι καὶ ἐκφράττουσι.» λέγομεν δὲ πρὸς τοῦτο, ὅτι οὐδέποτε τὸ φλέγμα πυρετὸν ἀνάψαι δύναται μὴ σηπόμενον, πάντα δὲ τὰ σηπόμενα θερμότερα καὶ δριμύτερα γίνονται, τὰ δὲ δριμύτερα ἐπὶ τὸ ξηρότερον ῥέπει· ὥστε οὖν κἂν τῇ φαντασίᾳ ἐπὶ τῶν ἀμφημερινῶν πυρετῶν ὑγρὸν εἶναι δοκεῖ τὸ φλέγμα, ἀλλὰ τῇ δυνάμει ὡς σεσηπὸς καὶ δριμὺ θερμόν ἐστι καὶ ξηρὸν καὶ εἰκότως τῶν ὑγραινόντων δεηθήσεται κατὰ δίαιταν. ἔστι δὲ καὶ ἄλλως εἰπεῖν, ὅτι διττή ἐστιν ἡ θεραπεία· ἡ μὲν καθ' αὑτό, ἥτις διὰ τῶν ἐναντίων πάντως γίνεται, καθ' ἣν τὰ θερμὰ ψύχομεν καὶ τὰ ψυχρὰ θερμαίνομεν, ἡ δὲ κατὰ συμβεβηκός, ἥτις διὰ τῶν ὁμοίων δοκεῖ γίνεσθαι, κατ' ἀλήθειαν δὲ καὶ αὕτη διὰ τῶν ἐναντίων ἀπαρτίζεται. τούτῳ τῷ κατὰ συμβεβηκὸς εἴδει τῆς θεραπείας χρώμενος ὁ Γαληνὸς θεραπεύει τὸν ἀμφημερινόν· ἀψινθίῳ γὰρ καὶ σελίνῳ καὶ ἀνήθῳ καὶ τοῖς τοιούτοις ἐπὶ τῶν πυρεττόντων ποτὲ χρώμεθα θερμοῖς οὖσιν, οὐχ ἵνα τὸν πυρετὸν αὐξήσωμεν κατὰ πρῶτον λόγον — τοῦτο γὰρ ἴσως γενήσεται —, ἀλλ' ἵνα τὴν ψυχρὰν καὶ παχεῖαν ὕλην τέμωμεν καὶ ἐκφράξωμεν καὶ κενώσωμεν, ὑφ' ἧς σηπομένης ὁ πυρετὸς ἀνάπτεται· ταύτῃ γὰρ κενουμένῃ ὁ πυρετὸς συναποκαθίσταται. ἀλλὰ καὶ χυλὸν πτισάνης παρέχομεν διὰ τὸ ἀπαμβλῦναι τὴν δριμύτητα καὶ ὑγρᾶναι τὴν ξηρότητα.

Ἰστέον δὲ καὶ τοῦτο, ὅτι κατὰ δύο τρόπους τὴν δίαιταν νῦν παραλαμβάνει ὁ Ἱπποκράτης· καθ' ἕνα μέν, ἵνα τὰ ὅμοια φυλάξῃ, καθ' ἕτερον δέ, ἵνα τοῖς ἐναντίοις ἀπομαχήσηται, φησὶ γὰρ οὕτως· Ὑγραὶ δίαιται πᾶσι τοῖς πυρεταίνουσι ξυμφέρουσι. καὶ ὅτι τὸ νόσημα ὁ πυρετὸς ἐναντιώσεως δεῖται, ὡς μὲν ξηρὸν ὑγρότητος, ὡς δὲ θερμὸν ψυχρότητος, καὶ μάλιστα ἐπὶ τῆς παιδικῆς· δεῖται γὰρ αὕτη τῆς ὑγρότητος διά τε τὴν αὔξησιν καὶ τὴν θρέψιν. ἐπειδὴ δὲ καὶ τὸ ἔθος τῶν ὁμοίων δεῖται φύσιν μιμούμενον κατὰ τὸ εἰρημένον «Ἔθος δευτέρα φύσις», ἄκουε τοῦ Ἱπποκράτους λέγοντος καὶ τοῖσιν ἄλλοισι τοῖσιν εἰθισμένοισι διαιτᾶσθαι.

I 31 [I 17: IV 466,20–468,2 L.] Καὶ τοῖσιν ἅπαξ ἢ δὶς ἢ πλεῖον ἢ καὶ κατὰ μέρος· δοτέον δέ τι καὶ τῇ ὥρῃ καὶ τῇ χώρῃ καὶ τῷ ἔθει καὶ τῇ ἡλικίῃ.

Εἴρηται, ὅτι πᾶσα θεραπεία τετραχῶς κατορθοῦται· ἀπὸ ποσότητος, ἀπὸ ποιότητος, ἀπὸ καιροῦ καὶ ἀπὸ τρόπου τῆς χρήσεως· ἐφ' ὧν καὶ ἡ δίαιτα, τῆς θεραπείας μέρος ὑπάρχουσα. καὶ ἡ μὲν κατὰ ποσότητα ὑποτύπωσις τῆς διαίτης καὶ ὁ καιρὸς καὶ τὸ ποιὸν παραδέδοται ἐν τῇ θεωρίᾳ· ὑπόλοιπον οὖν ἐστιν ἐν τῷ λόγῳ τὸν τῆς χρήσεως τρόπον εἰπεῖν, οὕτινος τὴν παράδοσιν νῦν πραγματεύεται ὁ Ἱπποκράτης. κατορθοῦται γὰρ διά τε τοῦ τόνου τῆς δυνάμεως καὶ †τῆς χρήσεως†

4sq. ὥστε – ξηρὸν] *cf.* Gal. Ars med. 28: I 381,14–17 K. 10 τούτῳ – 12 οὖσιν] *v. supra*, p. 116,37–38 17–22 θρέψιν] *v.* Gal. In Aphor. I 16: XVII B 426,1–10 K. 18sq. καθ'I – ἀπομαχήσηται] *cf.* Theoph. In Aphor.: II 283,14–16 Dietz 22 ἐπειδὴ – 24] *v.* Theoph. In Aphor.: II 283,16–18 Dietz 23 Ἔθος – φύσις] *cf.* Iulian. Misopogon 353 A (Julien, Discours II 2, ed. Lacombrade, Paris 1964) 28–30 ὑπάρχουσα] *v. supra*, p. 114,12–15 30sq. καὶ – θεωρίᾳ] *v. supra*, p. 114,15–20 31 ὑπόλοιπον – 120,10 ὀλιγάκις] *v.* Theoph. In Aphor.: II 283,22–30 Dietz 33 κατορθοῦται – 120,1 δεομένου] *v.* Gal. In Aphor. I 17: XVII B 429,12–14 K.

θερμαίνομεν

1 φράττουσι A 7 ἐστιν *om.* P 8 ξηραίνομεν A 10 τῷ] τὸ P 14 τέμνομεν A κυνώσωμεν α: *corr.* P2 19 οὗτος A 23 δευτ(έ)ρ(α) φύ(σις) A: δευτέρας φύσεως P 25 πλείω *Hipp.*, πλείονα *Theoph.* *post* ἢIII *hab.* ἐλάσσω *Hipp.* 26 τι] τε A 31 ἐνII *fort. delendum est* 33 τῆς χρήσεως] *lege vel* τῆς χρείας *vel* τοῦ σώματος *(cf. Theoph.)*

itan drug, in short, remedies which heat, comminute, fragmentize and dislodge." We reply that phlegm can never cause fever unless it is corrupted, and whatever is corrupted becomes hotter and more acrid, and what is more acrid tends to be drier; consequently, though in quotidian fevers we imagine the phlegm as moist, yet in its effect, being corrupted and acrid, it is hot and dry and will obviously call for a moistening diet. Another explanation is that there are two kinds of treatment: one direct, which uses only opposite remedies and consists in cooling the hot and heating the cold; the other indirect, which appears to use similar remedies, but in reality achieves its end also by means of opposites. It is by this indirect kind of therapy that Galen treats quotidian fever; for we sometimes prescribe absinthe, celery, dill and similar kinds of hot medicine for fever patients, not with the primary intention of increasing the fever – as may well happen –, but to fragmentize, dislodge and evacuate the cold thick matter by the corruption of which the fever is kindled, because simultaneously with this evacuation the fever subsides. But we also give barley-water to dull the sharpness and to moisten the dryness.

It is to be observed further that Hippocrates here applies this diet for two purposes: first, to preserve the similar, secondly, to fight off the contrary, his words being Liquid diets are beneficial to all fever patients. Also, that this disease, fever, demands treatment by opposites: insofar as it is dry, by moisture, insofar as it is hot, by cold, and this especially in children, because this age needs the moisture for growth and nutrition. But since custom, imitating nature – according to the saying "Custom is a second nature" – also demands what is similar, hear what Hippocrates says: and to others who are accustomed to such a diet.

I 31. Some need it once, or twice, or more often, or little by little; allowance should also be made for season, region, custom and age.

As we said, the success of all treatment depends on four factors: the quantity, the quality, the moment and the application; this is also true of the diet, which is part of the treatment. Directions for the quantity of the diet, as well as for the moment and the quality, have been given in our general survey; to complete the discussion, the application must be dealt with, and it is to this that Hippocrates turns now. It depends on the strength of the resistance and the need (?) of the

τοῦ ταύτης δεομένου. ἵνα σαφὲς τὸ λεγόμενον γένηται, ὑποκείσθω δύναμις ἐρρωμένη καὶ σῶμα δεόμενον· ἐνταῦθα πολλῇ δεῖ χρήσασθαι τροφῇ καὶ πολλάκις· πολλῇ μὲν διὰ τὴν ἰσχὺν τῆς δυνάμεως· ἐφ' ὅσον γὰρ ὁ ἐργάτης ὀχεῖν δύναται, ἐπὶ τοσοῦτον καὶ τὸ φορτίον βαρύνομεν· πολλάκις δὲ διὰ τὸ δεῖσθαι τὸ σῶμα εὐδιαφόρητον ὄν. ὑποκείσθω πάλιν δύναμις ἐρρωμένη, σῶμα δὲ μὴ δεόμενον· ἐνταῦθα δεῖ πολλὰς μὲν τροφὰς διδόναι, ὀλιγάκις δέ. ὑποκείσθω πάλιν ἀσθενὴς μὲν ἡ δύναμις, τὸ δὲ σῶμα δεόμενον· ἐνταῦθα πολλὰς μὲν οὐ δεῖ τὰς τροφὰς χορηγεῖν, τρέφειν δὲ πολλάκις ὀλίγα καὶ πάλιν ὀλίγα προσφέροντα. λοιπὸν καὶ τέταρτον δύναμις ὑποκείσθω αὐτή τε ἀσθενὴς οὖσα καὶ σῶμα παριστῶσα μὴ δεόμενον· ὀλίγην δεῖ παρέχειν τροφὴν καὶ ὀλιγάκις. ταῦτα διὰ τῶν παρόντων παραδίδωσιν ὁ Ἱπποκράτης, ἐν οἷς φησι· Καὶ τοῖσιν ἅπαξ ἢ δὶς καὶ τὰ ἑξῆς.

Οὗτός ἐστιν ὁ τρόπος τῆς χρήσεως· πρὸς τούτοις δὲ δεῖ καὶ τὰ σύστοιχα γινώσκειν. ἐὰν γὰρ θερμὴ ὑπάρχει ἡ χώρα, πρὸς δὲ καὶ ἡ ὥρα, καὶ ἡ ἡλικία ἀκμαστική, εὑρήσεις δὲ ἐπὶ τούτοις καὶ φύσει τὸ σῶμα εὐδιαφόρητον, δεῖ σε πολλάκις τρέφειν καὶ πολλὰς ἐπιδιδόναι τροφάς· εἰ δὲ πάντα τοὐναντίον, ὀλίγας καὶ ὀλιγάκις.

I 32 [I 18: IV 468,3–4 L.] Θέρεος καὶ φθινοπώροιο σιτία δυσφορώτατα φέρουσι, χειμῶνος δὲ ῥήϊστα, ἦρος δεύτερον.

Ἐπειδὴ ἐν θέρει ἐπὶ τὰ ἐκτὸς νεύει τὸ θερμὸν ὑπὸ τοῦ περιέχοντος πρὸς τὸ ὁμογενὲς ἐξελκόμενον, καὶ τῷ τρόπῳ τούτῳ διαφορούμενον ἀσθενέστερον γίνεται, ὀλίγης χρεία καὶ τῆς τροφῆς. ἐν μέντοι τῷ φθινοπώρῳ ἔξω μὲν τὸ θερμὸν οὐκ ἔστιν, ἀλλ' ἀποκλείεται ἤδη τῆς ψύξεως ἀρχομένης· ὑπὸ δὲ τῆς ἀνωμαλίας τῆς ὥρας πάσχει καὶ καταλύεται ποτὲ μὲν θαλπομένου, ποτὲ δὲ ψυχομένου τοῦ σώματος. καὶ διὰ τοῦτο ὀλίγην παρέχομεν τροφήν, ὅπερ ἐδήλωσε διὰ τοῦ δυσφορώτατα φέρουσι, διὰ τὸ ἄχθεσθαι τὴν δύναμιν, πῇ μὲν τῇ διαφορήσει τῆς ἐν ἡμῖν θερμότητος, ὥσπερ ἐν θέρει, πῇ δὲ τῇ καταλύσει τῆς δυνάμεως τῷ λόγῳ τῆς ἀνωμαλίας, ὥσπερ ἐν φθινοπώρῳ. ἐν δὲ χειμῶνι διὰ τὸ ἐναποκλείεσθαι τὸ ἐν ἡμῖν θερμὸν καὶ πλεονάζειν εὐχερῶς αἱ πέψεις γίνονται, ὅπερ ἐδήλωσε διὰ τοῦ ῥήϊστα. δεύτερον δὲ ἐν τῷ ἔαρί φησιν, ἐπειδὴ τότε μεμερισμένον ἐστὶ τὸ ἐν ἡμῖν θερμόν, καὶ ἔσω καὶ ἔξω, ὑπὸ τῆς θάλψεως τοῦ περιέχοντος ἐπὶ τὰ ἐκτὸς προτρεπόμενον. λοιπὸν κἂν τῷ ἔαρι καλῶς γίνεται ἡ τῶν σιτίων πέψις, ἀλλὰ καὶ δεύτερον ὡς πρὸς χειμῶνα.

I 33 [I 19: IV 468,5–7 L.] Τοῖσιν ἐν τῇσι περιόδοισι παροξυνομένοισι μηδὲν διδόναι μηδ' ἀναγκάζειν, ἀλλ' ἀφαιρέειν τῶν προσθέσεων πρὸ τῶν κρίσεων.

Φησὶν ὅτι 'Σκόπει τὰς ἐμπροθέσμους περιόδους καὶ τοὺς ἐν αὐταῖς γινομένους παροξυσμούς, καὶ μὴ ἐπιδώσῃς ἐν αὐτοῖς τροφὴν μηδ' ἀναγκάσῃς ὅλως', ἐπειδὴ τὰ

1 ἵνα – 4 ὄν] *v.* Gal. In Aphor. I 17: XVII B 430,9–13 K. 6 ὑποκείσθω – 8 προσφέροντα] *v.* Gal. In Aphor. I 17: XVII B 429,15–430,3 K. 8 λοιπὸν – 10 ὀλιγάκις] *v.* Gal. In Aphor. I 17: XVII B 430,5–9 K. 12–15] *cf.* Gal. In Aphor. I 17: XVII B 431,1–432,14 K. 20 ἐν – 27 ῥήϊστα] *v.* Theoph. In Aphor.: II 286,14–18 Dietz 34–122,3 νόσημα] *v.* Theoph. In Aphor.: II 287,6–13 Dietz

6 ὑποκεῖσθαι P 8 τετάρτη α: *correxi* αὐτῇ P 17 δὲ α, *Theoph.* U'': *non hab. Hipp., Theoph.* SV'' 19 ἀσθενεστέρα P 21 ἐρχομένης A 30 δευτέρως P χειμῶν *(ambig.)* A: χειμῶνι P 35 ἐπιδώσεις P

person who requires it. To illustrate what we mean, let us take the case of a strong resistance and a body needing food: then we should give much food and often; much, because of the strong resistance – we make the burden as heavy as the carrier can bear –; often, because the body is quickly dispersed and therefore needs it. Again, let us take a strong resistance and a body that needs no food; then we should allow much food, but rarely. Or take a weak resistance and a body needing food: in that case we should not supply much food, but keep the patient fed by administering a little and again a little at frequent intervals. Fourth and last, suppose the resistance is weak itself and also causes the body to demand no food: then we should prescribe little food and at long intervals. This is what Hippocrates teaches us in the present passage, when he says: Some need it once, or twice, etc.

So much for the application; in addition to this, we must be aware also of the correlative factors. If the region is hot and so is the season, and if the age is the prime of life, and if besides you find that the body has a natural tendency to quick dispersal, you should feed often and supply great quantities of food; if all the contrary circumstances prevail, then little and rarely.

I 32. In summer and autumn food is most difficult to digest, in winter easiest, in spring next easiest.

Because in summer the heat tends outward, being drawn out toward its own kind by the surrounding air, and is weakened by this form of dispersal, little food is needed. In the fall, on the other hand, though the heat is not outside, but is locked in by the beginning cold, yet it suffers from the unevenness of the season and is weakened by it, as the body is now heated, then cooled. For this reason we allow little food, which (Hippocrates) expressed by the words is most difficult to digest, because our strength is taxed, in the one case, in summer, by the dispersal of our internal heat, and in the other, in fall, by loss of resistance as a result of the uneven weather. But in winter, when the internal heat is locked in and is abundant, digestion goes smoothly, as expressed by the word easiest. In the spring, he says, it is next easiest, because then our internal heat is divided between the inside and the outside, being lured outside by the warming air. Consequently food is digested well in the spring too, but it is a second best as compared to winter.

I 33. If paroxysms come in periods, give the patients nothing and force nothing upon them, but diminish addition before crises.

That is, 'Observe the regular periods and the paroxysms that occur in them, and do not give food during them, or force anything upon the patient at all',

μέγιστα βλάψει τὸ τηνικαῦτα τρέφον, ἢ πρὸς ἔμετον παρασκευάζον τὸν κάμνοντα διὰ τοῦ βάρους τῆς τροφῆς καὶ κάματον αὐτῷ ἐμποιοῦν, ἢ τῶν νοσοποιῶν αἰτίων προσθήκη γενήσεται καὶ αὐξήσει τὸ νόσημα. πρόσθεσιν μὲν οὖν τὴν τροφὴν ὀνομάζει, περίοδον δὲ τὴν ὡρισμένως τεταγμένην, τουτέστι τὴν ἀπὸ τοῦ αὐτοῦ εἰς τὸ αὐτὸ ἀποκατάστασιν. εἰ μέντοι ἀδοκήτως εἰσβολή τις γένηται καὶ ἄτακτος εὑρεθῇ ἡ περίοδος, οὐδὲν παρὰ τοῦτο ἁμαρτάνει ὁ ἰατρός, εἰ καὶ πρὸ ὀλίγου τοῦ παροξυσμοῦ ἔθρεψε· θεοῦ γὰρ μόνου ἐστὶ τὸ πάντα γινώσκειν, ὁ μέντοι τεχνίτης τῇ ἐμμεθόδῳ χρῆται προγνώσει, οὐ μὴν καὶ τοὺς ἀτάκτως παρεμπεσόντας παροξυσμοὺς διά τινας οὔσας τῶν οὐρανίων περιόδους συμβαίνοντας οἷός τέ ἐστιν ἐκμελετᾶν καὶ προγινώσκειν. [εἰ] οἷόν τί ἐστι τὸ λεγόμενον, ὁρῶ τινα ἄρρωστον κατὰ περίοδον παροξυνόμενον, ἐν ᾧ προσδοκᾶται ἡ τοῦ προηγουμένου παροξυσμοῦ ἀνταπόδοσις ὥρᾳ δεκάτῃ τῆς ἡμέρας. ἐπὶ τούτου ἔρρωται ἡ δύναμις, κατεπείγει καὶ ἡ χρεία τοῦ σώματος καὶ δεῖ θρέψαι αὐτὸν καὶ πολλὰ καὶ πολλάκις. εἰσερχόμενος οὖν εἰς αὐτὸν ὥραν πρώτην κελεύω δοθῆναι αὐτῷ ποτήριον χυλοῦ μεστόν· εἶτα πάλιν περὶ ὥραν τετάρτην σημειοῦμαι αὐτὸν καὶ εὑρίσκω πέψαντα, καὶ λέγω παρασχεθῆναι αὐτῷ ποτήριον πάλιν μεστόν· εἶτα περὶ ὥραν ὀγδόην εἰσερχόμενος σημειοῦμαι αὖθις αὐτὸν καὶ εὑρίσκω πέψαντα πάλιν αὐτόν· καὶ ἕτερον ὁμοίως ποτήριον δοθῆναι τούτῳ κελεύσαντός μου διὰ τὸ δεῖσθαι τὸ σῶμα τροφῆς καὶ μήν γε καὶ τοῦ ποτηρίου δοθέντος ὁ εἰς ῑᾱ ὥραν ἐπεισβάλλων παροξυσμὸς ἀτάκτῳ τρόπῳ χρησάμενος κατὰ τὴν ὀγδόην ὥραν προσέβαλεν. ἐνταῦθα οὖν οὐ δεῖ τὸν ἰατρὸν μέμψασθαι.

Κρίσιν δὲ καλεῖ τὸν παροξυσμὸν καταχρώμενος, τῷ καὶ αὐτὸν ὡς πρὸς τὴν τοῦ διαλείμματος σύγκρισιν ταραχὴν καὶ θόρυβον καὶ ἀγῶνα ἐμποιεῖν τῇ φύσει τε καὶ τῷ σώματι.

I 34 [I 20: IV 468,8–10 L.] Τὰ κρινόμενα καὶ τὰ κεκριμένα ἀρτίως μὴ κινέειν ⟨μήτε νεωτεροποιέειν⟩ μήτε φαρμακείῃσι μήτε ἄλλοισιν ἐρεθισμοῖσι χρέεσθαι.

Νῦν διδάσκει ἡμᾶς, ὅτι δέον ἐστὶν ἐν ταῖς κρίσεσι τῶν νοσημάτων τὸ πᾶν καταλιμπάνειν τῇ φύσει, μηδὲν δὲ νεωτεροποιεῖν τεχνικὸν ἢ ἐρεθίζειν, εἰ καί ποτε χρὴ καὶ ἡμᾶς αὐτοὺς ἐπικουρεῖν αὐτῇ ἐν ταῖς κρίσεσι καὶ πρὸς λυσιτέλειαν τοῦ κρινομένου τεχνικόν τι συνεισάγειν. καὶ ἵνα σαφὲς γένηται τὸ λεγόμενον, ὑποκείσθω ἄρρωστος, ἐν ᾧ πέψεως σημείων σαφῶν γενομένων δηλοῦται ἡ ἀρχὴ καὶ ἡ ἀνάβασις τοῦ ὅλου νοσήματος παρελθοῦσα, ἡ δὲ ἀκμὴ ἐνισταμένη καὶ πρὸς κρίσιν ἐπειγομένη, ὡς ἡ τῶν προλαβόντων ἐδήλου κίνησις. τὰ δὲ τῆς πέψεως σημεῖα ἔν τε οὔροις καὶ σφυγμοῖς καὶ ποιότητι τῆς θερμασίας γνωρίζεται, τοῦ μὲν σφυγμοῦ ὁμαλοῦ ὄντος, τοῦ δὲ πυρετοῦ μὴ πάνυ δριμεῖαν ποιουμένου τὴν ἐπιφοράν, τοῦ δὲ οὔρου ὑποξάνθου καὶ ὑποπύρρου ὄντος καὶ ὑπόστασιν λευκὴν καὶ λεπτὴν καὶ ὁμαλὴν κεκτημένου. ἅτινα πάντα ἑωρακὼς ὁ τεχνίτης τὴν πρέπουσαν προαγορεύσας δίαιταν ἀνεχώρησε· καὶ συνελθὼν καθ' ἑτέραν περίοδον πάντας εὑρίσκει τοὺς ἐν τῷ οἴκῳ ὀδυρομένους διὰ τὸ ἐν πολλῇ αὐτὸν δυσφορίᾳ καθεστάναι. τούτων ἀκούων ὁ τεχνίτης μειδιάσας εὐφραίνεται καθ'

21–23] *v.* Theoph. In Aphor.: II 287,3–6 Dietz

10 εἰ *delevi* 13 αὐτὸν^{II} *scripsi*: ἑαυτὸν α 18 καὶ^{II} *om.* P 21 τῷ] τὸ P 25 μήτε νεωτεροποιέειν *addidi; cf. infra, p. 126,3. 18*: μηδὲ νεωτεροποιέειν *Hipp.* 26 χρέεσθαι] *item infra, p. 126,5. 18*: ἀλλ' ἐᾶν *Hipp.* 30 εἰσάγοντος A 31 πέψεων α: *correxi* 32 ὡς] καὶ A 34 ποιότητ *(ambig.)* P: ποιότητος A 39 καθιστάναι α: *correxi*

because food taken at that time will cause the greatest harm: either it will dispose the patient to vomiting by the heaviness of the food and it will exhaust him, or it will be added to the causes of the disease and will worsen the illness. By addition he means food, by period only one that has a definite regularity, i.e., a return from the same point to the same point. If, however, an attack sets in unexpectedly and the period is found to be irregular, it is not the doctor's fault, even if he has given food shortly before the paroxysm; for only God knows everything, whereas the skilled physician applies methodical prognosis, without being able, however, to study and foretell irregular paroxysms due to certain existing celestial periods. As an example of what I mean: I visit a patient with periodical paroxysms, in whose case recurrence of the preceding paroxysm is expected at the tenth hour of the day. His resistance is strong, his body urgently needs food, and it should be provided in great quantity and frequently. So when I visit him at the first hour, I prescribe a cupful of barley-water; about the fourth hour I examine him again, and finding that he has digested (the food) I say that he should be given another cupful; next I come in at the eighth hour, I examine him once more and I find that he has again digested (his food); then, when I have prescribed yet another cupful for him, because his body needs food, and the cup has actually been given, the paroxysm that was due at the 11th hour irregularly sets in at the eighth. In such cases the doctor should not be held responsible.

The word crisis is used loosely here of the paroxysm, because, as compared to the interval, it also brings about disturbance, tumult and distress in the constitution and the body.

I 34. During a crisis and after a sound crisis do not disturb anything, do not interfere and do not apply purges or any other irritants.

Here (Hippocrates) teaches us that during the crisis of a disease one should leave everything to nature, without artificial interference or use of irritants, though there are occasions when we have to come to her aid in a crisis and, for the patient's good, use some artificial means as well. To clarify this, let us take the example of a patient who shows manifest signs of concoction, so that it is clear that the beginning and the increasing period of the entire disease are over and that the acme has set in and the crisis is at hand, as indicated by the development in the earlier stages. The signs of concoction appear in the urine, in the pulse and in the quality of the heat: the pulse is even, the impact of the fever not too violent, the urine is yellowish and reddish and has a white, thin and uniform sediment. Having seen all this, the expert physician prescribes the proper diet and goes away; and when he comes for his visit during the next period, he finds everybody in the house in tears because the patient is in great discomfort. Upon hearing them, the

ἑαυτὸν τῇ προγνώσει τῶν τῆς πέψεως σημείων πεποιθὼς καὶ πρὸς κρίσιν ἀγαθὴν ὁρμᾶν τὴν φύσιν λογιζόμενος, ἥστινος χάριν καὶ τὰ τῆς δυσφορίας προηγήσαντο. εἶτα καὶ ποίῳ τρόπῳ μέλλει τὰ τῆς νόσου κριθῆναι, ἐξετάσαι βουλόμενος ἀνακρίνει, εἰ κεφαλαλγία συνέπεσεν, εἰ βάρους συναίσθησις περὶ τὸν τράχηλον γίνεται, εἰ μαρμαρυγαί τινες περὶ τοὺς ὀφθαλμοὺς ἐφάνησαν· ὧντινων ὁμολογουμένων δι' αἱμορραγίας ἐλπίζει τὴν κρίσιν γενέσθαι. εἰ δὲ καρδιωγμοῦ αἴσθησις τῷ πάσχοντι γένηται καὶ τὸ κάτω χεῖλος κραδαίνεται καὶ τὰ ὑποχόνδρια ἀνασπᾶσθαι δοκεῖ, δι' ἐμέτου αὐτῷ ἡ κρίσις προσδοκηθήσεται. εἰ δὲ μηδὲν τούτων πάρεστι, σφυγμὸς δὲ μέγας ἐστὶ καὶ ὑψηλὸς καὶ θερμὸν τὸ ὅλον σῶμα, δι' ἱδρώτων τὴν κρίσιν ἐκδέξεται. εἰ δὲ μηδὲν τούτων περιῇ, ἀνώμαλος δὲ κατὰ τὸ μέγεθος ὑποπέσοι ὁ σφυγμός, ποτὲ μὲν μέγας, ποτὲ δὲ μικρὸς γινόμενος, πλήθους σημεῖον τὸ τοιοῦτον μέλλοντος ἐκκρίνεσθαι, διά τινος τῶν φυσικῶν ὑπονόμων τῶν ἐπὶ τὰ κάτω τὴν πάροδον τῶν περιττωμάτων ποιουμένων· διὰ τοῦτο γὰρ ποτὲ μὲν μέγας ὁ σφυγμός, ποτὲ δὲ καὶ μικρὸς γενήσεται τῆς φύσεως ἐν τῷ βάθει συστελλομένης εἰς ἀποδίωξιν καὶ ἔκκρισιν τοῦ λυποῦντος αὐτὴν πλήθους. ταύτην τοίνυν τὴν κίνησιν εὑρίσκων ὁ τεχνίτης ἐν τοῖς σφυγμοῖς προγινώσκει, ὅτι ὅσον οὔπω ἐκτάραξις τῆς γαστρὸς γενήσεται, ἐφ' ᾗ κριθήσεται τὸ νόσημα. ἐπὶ τούτοις μικρὸν ὑποχωρήσας καὶ πάλιν ἐπανελθὼν εὑρίσκει πάντως ὁποτερονοῦν τούτων γινόμενον. ἡνίκα τοίνυν ταῦτα οὕτως ἔχει, οὐ δεῖ τὸν τεχνίτην καινισμόν τινα ἐν τοῖς γινομένοις ἐπινοεῖν καὶ ταράσσειν τὴν φύσιν, ἀλλὰ μένειν τὴν τελείαν ἔκβασιν τῆς κρίσεως· φύσεως γὰρ ὑπηρέτης ὑπάρχει ὁ ἰατρός. τῆς οὖν φυσικῆς κινήσεως γινομένης παρεῖναί σε δεῖ· καὶ εἰ μὲν πάντα κατὰ λόγον ἐπιτελεῖται, ἀγαθὴ καὶ τελεία δηλονότι ἡ κρίσις ἀπαντήσει τοῦ νοσήματος, ἡνίκα μηδὲν ὅλως τὸν ἰατρὸν ἐπιτηδεύειν χρεών· εἰ μέντοι ὀκλάσει καὶ καταπέσῃ ἐν τούτῳ ἡ φύσις, τότε δεῖ καὶ τὸν τεχνίτην χεῖρα ὀρέξαι καὶ ἐπικουρῆσαι αὐτῇ. καὶ εἰ μὲν διὰ γαστρὸς ἡ κένωσις γίνεται, ταύτης ἐπισχημένης ἀτελοῦς οὔσης τῆς ἐκκρίσεως χρησόμεθα κλυστῆρι· εἰ δὲ δι' ἱδρώτων, τοῖς ἠρέμα ἀραιοῦσι τὸ δέρμα, ὁποῖά εἰσι τὰ χλιαρὰν ἔχοντα τὴν θερμασίαν, ὥσπερ τὸ χαμαιμηλέλαιον. τί γάρ; ὅτι ὥρμησεν ἡ φύσις πρὸς κένωσιν· καὶ αὕτη μὲν καλῶς ὥρμησεν, ἔμφραξις δὲ γέγονεν ἢ περὶ τὰ ἔντερα ἢ περὶ τοὺς ἀδήλους πόρους κἀκεῖθεν οὐ γίνεται κατὰ λόγον ἡ κένωσις. γινομένης μέντοι φυσικῶς κατὰ λόγον τῆς ἐκκρίσεως μηδὲν ὅλως νεωτεροποιήσῃς, ἀλλ' ἐνταῦθα ἡσύχαζε καὶ μηδὲν καινὸν ἐπιτήδευε, γινώσκει γὰρ ἡ φύσις κριτικῶς ἐπεγειρομένη, πῶς δεῖ ποιεῖν τὴν κένωσιν τοῦ λυποῦντος αἰτίου καὶ μέχρι πόσου.

Τὰ κρινόμενα καὶ τὰ κεκριμένα ἀρτίως μὴ κινέειν. ἰστέον, ὅτι τὸ ἀρτίως ἀντὶ τοῦ ὑγιῶς καὶ ὁλοκλήρως καὶ ἀνελλιπῶς εἴρηται. σκόπει οὖν, φησίν, γενομένην ἢ [μὴ] γινομένην κρίσιν, καὶ εἰ εὕροις αὐτὴν ἀνελλιπῶς καὶ ἀπηρτισμένην ἀπαντήσασαν, μηδὲν νεωτεροποιήσῃς, μηδεμίαν κίνησιν ἐπιτηδεύσῃς, οὐδὲ γὰρ δεῖται τὸ τηνικαῦτα ἡ φύσις βοηθείας.

Τὸ δὲ μὴ κινέειν διττόν ἐστι, τὸ μὲν τοπικῶς καὶ σωματικῶς γινόμενον, τὸ δὲ ψυχικῶς, ὁπότε τις ἀκοὴ λόγων λυπηρῶν ἔστιν ὅτε τῷ νοσοῦντι καὶ φοβερῶν

3 εἶτα – 15 πλήθους] *cf.* Gal. De crisib. III 11: IX 752,10–768,18 K. *infra*, vol. III, fol. 236v εἶτα – 8 προσδοκηθήσεται] *cf.* Gal. Ad Glauc. I 16: XI 66,8–67,11 K. 33 ἰστέον – 37] *v.* Theoph. In Aphor.: II 288,4–9 Dietz 33sq. ἰστέον – εἴρηται] *cf.* Gal. In Aphor. I 20: XVII B 437,7–438,9 K.

3 κριθῆναι *om.* A 4 βάρους] κάρου A 10 δὲ *om.* A ὑποπέσ *(ambig.)* P 13 μὲν *om.* A 14 στελλομένης P 18 ὁποτεονοῦν τοῦτου *(sic)* P 23 *immo* ὀκλάσῃ καταπέσ *(ambig.)* P: καταπέσει A 34 φησίν] φύσιν P 35 μὴ *delevi (cf. Theoph.)* 39 ἀκοὴν A

expert smiles and feels satisfied, for he has confidence in his prognosis of the signs of concoction and he considers that nature is on her way to a favorable crisis, to which the preceding signs of discomfort were also due. Next, as he wants to ascertain also what form the crisis of the disease will take, he asks if there has been a headache, if there is a feeling of heaviness around the neck, if flashes of light have appeared before the eyes; if the answer is affirmative, he expects a crisis by hemorrhage. If the patient has a feeling of heartburn, if his lower lip quivers and the hypochondrium seems to retract, a crisis by vomiting is to be foreseen. If none of these symptoms appears, but there is a large and high pulse and the whole body is hot, he will expect a crisis by sweating. Again, if nothing of the kind happens, but the pulse is found to be irregular in magnitude, being now large, now small, this indicates an abundance of matter on the point of being excreted, the waste matter making its way through one of the natural channels below; this explains why the pulse is alternately large and small: the natural force withdraws deep within in order to expel and excrete the surplus that troubles it. So when the expert observes this kind of motion in the pulse, he prognosticates that immediately afterwards there will be a disturbance of the bowels, which will be the crisis of the disease. Upon this he goes away for a short time and when he comes again he necessarily finds that one of these possibilities is coming true. When this is so, the physician must not contrive any interference with the process and thus upset its natural course, but wait for the full completion of the crisis; for the physician is a servant of nature. Hence, when the natural process takes place, you have to be there; and if everything happens according to plan, the crisis of the disease will of course be beneficial and complete, in which case the physician should take no action whatsoever; but if in this process nature falters and breaks down, then the doctor must lend a hand and come to her aid. If the evacuation takes place by way of the bowels and excretion is incomplete owing to constipation, we will use an enema; if through sweating, we use medicines which gently open up the pores of the skin, as do those which possess a tepid warmth, for example camomile oil. Why? Because nature has made an attempt at evacuation; and the attempt was right, only an obstruction has formed either in the intestines or in the invisible pores and hence the evacuation does not proceed according to plan. When, on the other hand, excretion takes place naturally and normally, you should not interfere in any way whatever, but refrain from action and from any initiative, for when nature is roused to a crisis, she knows how to handle the evacuation of the cause of the trouble, and to what extent.

During a crisis and after a sound crisis do not disturb anything. Note that sound means "healthy", i.e. "whole" or "complete". So what he says is: Take heed when a crisis has taken place or is taking place, and if you find that it has been complete and total, do not interfere and do not initiate any disturbance, because in that case nature needs no help.

Do not disturb has a twofold meaning, one spatial and corporeal, the other psychical, when, as sometimes happens, the patient chances to hear a conversation

παρεμπέσοι ἢ ἁπλῶς ἀκαταθυμίων· πολλάκις γὰρ οὗτοι παρεμπεσόντες γινομένην κρίσιν ἀνέκοψαν.

Τὸ δὲ μήτε νεωτεροποιέειν ἀντὶ τοῦ ξενοπρεπῶς τι ἐπιτηδεύειν διὰ τὸ τοῖς παρεστῶσι δεῖξαι ἑαυτὸν ἐπὶ τῆς τέχνης.

Εἶτά φησι· μήτε φαρμακείῃσι μήτε ἄλλοισιν ἐρεθισμοῖσι χρέεσθαι, τουτέστι μήτε ὑπήλατον δοῦναι μήτε κλυστῆρι διερεθίσαι τὴν γαστέρα μήτε μὴν ἐμετικῷ χρήσασθαι φαρμάκῳ μήτε μὴν ἐλαίῳ τινὶ ἀλεῖψαι τὸ σῶμα ἢ ὅλως τι τοιοῦτον ἐργάσασθαι· ἕκαστον γὰρ τῶν τοιούτων φαρμακεία τίς ἐστιν.

Εἶτα ὥς τινος ἀποροῦντος ὅτι «Καὶ πόθεν ἔχομεν γνῶναι, εἰ τελεία γέγονεν ἡ φυσικὴ κρίσις, ἵνα παραφυλαξώμεθα τὴν οἱανδήποτε ἐπιτηδεῦσαι κίνησιν;» λέγει ὁ Ἱπποκράτης· «Εἰ ἐπηκολούθησεν εὐφορία τῷ κάμνοντι ἐκκρίσεως κριτικῶς γενομένης ἢ ὅσον οὔπω μέλλει γενέσθαι.» μεμαθήκαμεν γάρ, ὅτι ἢ παρευθὺς ἢ μετ' οὐ πολὺ τῆς κρίσεως αὕτη γίνεται· τί γάρ; ὅτι πολλάκις εὐαισθήτου ὑποκειμένου τοῦ στομάχου ἢ δριμέων τινῶν κενωθέντων δῆξις κατὰ τὰ ἔντερα ἐναπέμεινεν ἢ ἔκλυσις καὶ λιποθυμία ἐνοχλεῖν ποιεῖ τῷ κάμνοντι, δι' ἃ μέλλει ἡ εὐφορία. οὐ δεῖ οὖν ἐπὶ τούτοις ταράττεσθαι, ὅσον γὰρ οὔπω καθίσταται καὶ σαφῆ τὴν εὐφορίαν ἐπάγει.

Ἔστι δὲ τὸ ὅλον τοῦ ἀφορισμοῦ οὕτως· Τὰ κρινόμενα καὶ τὰ κεκριμένα ἀρτίως μὴ κινέειν μήτε νεωτεροποιέειν μήτε ἄλλοισιν ἐρεθισμοῖσι χρέεσθαι· [I 21: IV 468,11–12 L.] ἃ δεῖ ἄγειν, ταύτῃ ἄγειν, ὅκου ἂν ⟨μάλιστα⟩ ῥέπῃ ἡ φύσις, διὰ τῶν ξυμφερόντων χωρίων. διὰ μὲν τοῦ εἰπεῖν ἃ δεῖ ἄγειν δύο τινὰ ἐδήλωσε, τήν τε ποιότητα τοῦ δεομένου χυμοῦ καθάρσεως πρὸς τελείαν καὶ ἀνελλιπῆ κρίσιν· τὸν γὰρ ὀφείλοντα χυμὸν κενωθῆναι καὶ ὃν ἡ φύσις κενοῦν ἤρξατο, τοῦτον δεῖ καὶ σὲ τὸν τεχνίτην ἐν ταῖς ἀτελέσι κρίσεσιν ἐρεθίζειν, εἴτε ξανθόχολος εἴη εἴτε φλεγματικὸς εἴτε μελαγχολικός, καὶ μὴ ἄλλον ἀντ' ἄλλου κινεῖν. τὸ δὲ ὅκου ἂν μάλιστα ῥέπῃ ἡ φύσις ἀντὶ τοῦ 'δεῖ θεωρῆσαι, ποῦ ἡ φύσις ἐξέρριψε τὸν χυμὸν καὶ πόθεν ὥρμησε ποιεῖν τὴν ἔκκρισιν, κἀκεῖθεν παρασκευάζειν τὴν τῶν καταλειφθέντων κένωσιν'. εἰ μὲν γὰρ μελαγχολικός ἐστιν ἢ φλεγματικὸς ὁ χυμὸς καὶ κάτω βρίθων, δι' ἐντέρων καὶ ἡ φύσις πάντως ὥρμησε τοῦτον ἀποκενοῦν καὶ σὲ δεῖ τὸν ἐρεθισμὸν ποιήσασθαι κλυστῆρι χρώμενον ἢ ὑποθέτῳ τινὶ τῶν ἐπὶ τὰ κάτω ἐρεθιζόντων· εἰ δὲ χολὴ ἤρξατο κενοῦσθαι, ἐπειδὴ ὡς κούφη ἐπιπολάζει, τὰ δὲ ἐπιπολάζοντα μάλιστα διὰ στομάχου ἐκκρίνεται φυσικῶς, δεῖ καὶ σὲ ἐπὶ τῶν ἐγκαταλιμπανομένων ἐμετικὸν πάντως διδόναι βοήθημα. καὶ τουτέστιν ὅκου ἂν μάλιστα ῥέπῃ, ταύτῃ ἄγειν, τουτέστι πρὸς τὴν ῥοπὴν τῆς ὕλης καὶ πρὸς τὴν ὁρμὴν τῆς φύσεως καὶ τὸν τεχνίτην συνεπαμῦναι.

Εἶτά φησι· διὰ τῶν ξυμφερόντων χωρίων, τουτέστιν ἀπὸ κυρίων μορίων ἐπὶ ἄκυρα δεῖ ἕλκειν τὴν ὕλην καὶ διὰ τῶν φυσικῶν ὑπονόμων αὐτὴν ἐρεθίζειν. πρὸς ταῦτά τινές φασι· «Τί φῄς, ὦ Ἱππόκρατες; ἐὰν ἐπὶ στόμαχον εὐπαθῆ ὄντα ῥέψῃ ἡ ὕλη, ἐμετικοῖς χρήσομαι βοηθήμασιν, ὥστε ἐκεῖθεν ἐρεθίσαι τὴν κένωσιν, μὴ εὐλα-

5–8] *cf.* Theoph. In Aphor.: II 288,10–14 Dietz 12sq. μεμαθήκαμεν – γίνεται] *v. supra,* p. 56,3–17 25 τὸ – 33 ἄγειν] *cf.* Theoph. In Aphor.: II 289,3–12 Dietz

3 μὴ P 11 κριτικῆς A 14 ἔκκλυσις P 15 *fort.* ἐνόχλησιν *scribendum est* 19 ταύτῃ ἄγειν] *item infra, p. 128,13, Hipp. pauci: ante* διὰ *colloc. infra, lin. 33; vol. II, fol. 67ʳ; 69ʳ, Hipp. cett., Theoph.* μάλιστα *sec. Hipp. addidi; cf. infra, lin. 25. 33; p. 128,13; vol. II, fol. 67ʳ; 69ʳ* 20 ἡ φύσις] *item infra, lin. 25; p. 128,13, Hipp. pauci* (C'), *Theoph.* V'': *om. infra, lin. 33; vol. II, fol. 67ʳ; 69ʳ, non hab. Hipp. plerique, Theoph. SU''* 24 ξανθίχολος P εἴη *om.* A 25 ῥέπει A 29 δεῖ σε P

that is painful or terrifying to him, or simply distasteful; often such incidental words have checked a crisis already in process.

The words do not interfere refer to out-of-the-way intervention in order to demonstrate one's own skill to those present.

He goes on: and do not apply purges or any other irritants, i.e. one should not give a suppository, irritate the bowels by an enema, use an emetic, rub the body with a particular oil or do anything whatever of the kind, all of these being purges of some sort.

Then, as if somebody had asked the question "How can we tell that the natural crisis has been complete and that consequently we should refrain from contriving any kind of disturbance?" Hippocrates says that (this is the case) if the patient experiences a feeling of euphoria immediately upon critical excretion or shortly afterwards. As we have seen, this state occurs either at once or not long after the crisis. Why? Because frequently, when we have to do with a sensitive stomach or when pungent matter has been evacuated, there is some lingering irritation of the bowels, or prostration and fainting trouble the patient, and this delays the euphoria. Hence one should not worry about these things, for they redress themselves soon and are followed by a manifest feeling of well-being.

The entire aphorism runs as follows: During a crisis and after a sound crisis do not disturb anything, do not interfere and do not apply any other irritants; what has to be removed, you should remove by the way to which nature mainly tends, through the appropriate parts of the body. By saying what has to be removed, (Hippocrates) made two things clear: first, the quality of the humor that has to be purged out for a complete and total crisis: the humor which needs evacuating and which nature has already begun to evacuate, is the humor that you, the professional, should draw forth by irritation in cases of an incomplete crisis, whether it is bilious, phlegmatic, or atrabilious, and you should not stir up the one instead of the other. As for the words to which nature mainly tends, they mean that one should examine where nature has discharged the humor and from where it has attempted the excretion, and then contrive the evacuation of the remainder by that way. Thus, if the humor is atrabilious or phlegmatic and apt to sink downwards, it is certain that nature, too, has attempted to evacuate it through the bowels, and you should draw it forth by means of an enema or some kind of suppository which stimulates evacuation below; but if the humor that has begun to be evacuated is bile, it will rise to the surface because of its lightness, and whatever rises to the surface is most naturally excreted through the stomach, and therefore the only course for you, too, is to administer an emetic as medication for the remainder. This is the meaning of removing by the way to which it mainly tends, in other words, the physician should adapt his share in the rescue action to the trend of the matter and to the impulse of nature.

(Hippocrates) continues: through the appropriate parts of the body, meaning that we should draw the matter from the vital to the unimportant parts and provoke evacuation through the natural channels. Some object: "What do you mean, Hippocrates? If the matter tends to move toward a sensitive stomach, should I use emetics, in order to provoke evacuation by that way,

βούμενος συγκοπὴν ἢ λιποθυμίαν ἢ ἔκλυσιν, ἅτινα πάντα κινδυνώδη τοῖς κάμνουσι καθίσταται;» πρὸς οὓς λέγομεν, ὅτι τὸ διὰ τῶν ξυμφερόντων χωρίων εἰπεῖν ἐδήλωσεν, ὅτι, ἐὰν ἐπὶ τὸν στόμαχον ῥέψῃ ἡ ὕλη φύσει εὐπαθῆ ὄντα καὶ ἐκλυόμενον, διὰ τῶν ξυμφερόντων χωρίων τὴν κένωσιν δεῖ παρασκευάσασθαι ἀπὸ τοῦ κυρίου μορίου ἐπὶ ἀκυρότερα μεταγαγόντα τὴν ὕλην, ἀπὸ στομάχου φημὶ ἐπὶ ἔντερα· δεῖ γὰρ ἀπὸ τῶν κυρίων ὡς εἴρηται μορίων παντὶ τρόπῳ ἐπὶ τὰ ἀκυρότερα ποιεῖσθαι τὴν τῆς ὕλης μετάστασιν. καὶ ἐν αὐτοῖς δὲ τοῖς κυρίοις τὰ μὲν μᾶλλόν ἐστι κύρια, τὰ δὲ ἧττον· ἀπὸ καρδίας γοῦν πολλάκις ἀγαθὸν ἐπὶ στόμαχον μεταστῆσαι τὴν ὕλην, ἀπὸ δὲ ἥπατος ἐπὶ γαστέρα. οὕτω μὲν οὖν πρὸς τὸ προσεχὲς ἐξηγούμεθα τὸν παρόντα ἀφορισμόν.

I 35 [I 22: IV 468,13 L.] Πέπονα φαρμακεύειν καὶ κινέειν, μὴ ὠμά.

Τὴν ἐλλιπῆ ἔκκρισιν προσεχῶς εἰς τὸ τελειότατον ἐπανάγων ὁ Ἱπποκράτης ἔλεγεν· «Ἃ δεῖ ἄγειν, ταύτῃ ἄγειν, ὅκου ἂν μάλιστα ῥέπῃ ἡ φύσις.» εἶτα ἐπειδὴ αἰτία πολλάκις ἀτελοῦς κρίσεως γίνεται ἡ τῶν χυμῶν ἀπεψία, τοῦτο αἰνιττόμενός φησι· Πέπονα φαρμακεύειν καὶ κινεῖν, ἀντὶ τοῦ 'Δεῖ προσέχειν τῇ πέψει τῶν χυμῶν καὶ οὕτω διδόναι τὸ κενωτικὸν φάρμακον'. ἄπεπτοι γὰρ ὄντες οἱ χυμοὶ οὐχ ὑπείκουσι τοῖς ἐρεθίζουσι φαρμάκοις. ἀλλ' ἡ μὲν φύσις πρὸς κίνησιν παρασκευαζομένη ταῖς οἰκείαις δυνάμεσι χρῆται πρὸς πέψιν· ἐκκρίνουσα δὲ ἡ τέχνη φαρμάκοις τισὶ λεπτυντικοῖς, οἷά εἰσι τὰ ἀποζέματα καὶ τὰ δι' ὀξυμέλιτος πινόμενα, συμπέττει τοὺς ὠμοὺς χυμούς, καὶ πάλιν ὑπηλάτῳ χρωμένη τούτους ἐκκαθαίρει τοῦ σώματος. μιμητὰς οὖν τῆς φύσεως ἡμᾶς γινομένους πέπονα δεῖ φαρμακεύειν καὶ κινεῖν· πάντα γὰρ ὑπείκει τῇ κενώσει καὶ ἐκκρίνεται δι' ὧν μορίων τὰς παρόδους ποιεῖται. εἴτε οὖν ἀτελοῦς τῆς φύσεως κρινάσης διά τινα ἔμφραξιν ἢ ἕτερον περιστατικὸν αἴτιον κωλῦσαν ἢ καὶ διὰ τὴν ἐπὶ μέρους ἀπεψίαν τῶν ἐκκρινομένων, εἴτε καὶ αὐτόθεν τῆς τέχνης ἄνευ φυσικῆς ἐκκρίσεως ἐπὶ τὴν κένωσιν ὁρμώσης κάθαρσις παραλαμβάνεται, ἀνάγκη πᾶσα τῷ Ἱπποκρατείῳ λόγῳ ἀκολουθεῖν καὶ τοὺς πεπεμμένους τῶν χυμῶν ἐν προπαρασκευῇ πολλῇ τίθεσθαι. τί δὲ φάρμακον ἐνταῦθα καλεῖ τὸ ὑπήλατον; διὰ τὸ δραστήριον τῆς δυνάμεως αὐτῶν.

[I 22: IV 468,13–14 L.] Μηδὲ ἐν ἀρχῇσι, φησί. ζητητέον, τίνα καλεῖ ἀρχήν. ἀρχὴ γὰρ λέγεται ἥ τε πρώτη καὶ ἀκαριαία εἰσβολὴ τοῦ παροξυσμοῦ καὶ ἡ ἐν πλάτει χρόνου θεωρουμένη, ἥτις διχῶς λαμβάνεται, καθ' ἕνα μὲν τρόπον ἐντὸς τῆς τρίτης ἡμέρας περιγραφομένη, καθ' ἕτερον δὲ τοῖς λοιποῖς τοῦ ὅλου νοσήματος ἀντιδιαστελλομένη καιροῖς, ἥτις καὶ τεχνικὴ προσαγορεύεται· περὶ ἧς καὶ νῦν διαλέγεται ὁ Ἱπποκράτης. ταύτην δὲ τὴν ἀρχὴν ἀδύνατόν ἐστί ποτε πέψεως ἀγαγεῖν σημεῖα· ἀμυδρῶν γὰρ σημείων φανέντων πέψεως πέπαυται μὲν ἡ τοῦ ὅλου νοσήματος ἀρχή, ἄρχεται δὲ ἡ ἀνάβασις· ὥσπερ καὶ σαφῶν καὶ τελείων φανέντων τῶν σημείων πέ-

13 Ἃ – φύσις] Hipp. Aphor. I 21: IV 468,11 L. 17 ἀλλ' – 21 κινεῖν] *cf.* Theoph. In Aphor.: II 290,1–5 Dietz 17sq. ἀλλ' – πέψιν] *cf.* Gal. In Aphor. I 22: XVII B 442,6–9 K. 30 ἀρχὴ – 33 προσαγορεύεται] *cf.* Gal. De crisib. I 6. 8: IX 570,14–17; 580,7–11 K.

1 ἔκκλυσιν A 2 *fort.* εἰπὼν *scribendum est* 3 ἀπαθῆ α: *correxi* 5 ἀκυρώτερον A ἀπὸ] ἐπὶ P 8 οὖν A 12 ὁ ἱπποκράτης ἐπανάγων εἰς τὸ τελειότατον A 19 ὀξυμέλιτι α: *correxi* συμπέπτει A 20 ὑπηλάτων P 22 ὑπείκη A 23 *fort.* ἀτελῶς *scribendum est* παραστατικὸν A 28 *fort.* αὐτοῦ *scribendum est* 31 *post* μὲν *add.* οὖν A

without worrying about a possible collapse, fainting or prostration, all of which are dangerous to the sick?" We answer that by saying through the appropriate parts of the body, he made it clear that, if the matter tends toward a naturally sensitive and weak stomach, the right way to bring about evacuation through the appropriate parts of the body is by conveying the matter from the vital part to less important parts, i.e. from the stomach to the bowels; for, as we said already, one should under all circumstances transfer the matter from the vital parts to the less vital ones. Within the class of the vital parts, some are more vital, others less so; thus it is often beneficial to transfer the matter from the heart to the stomach, from the liver to the bowels. This is our interpretation of the present aphorism in its immediate context.

I 35. Purge and disturb (humors), when ripe, not while crude.

Immediately before this, Hippocrates brought incomplete excretion to completion, when he said: "What has to be removed, you should remove by the way to which nature mainly tends." Next, since an incomplete crisis is often caused by unconcocted humors, he hints at this, when he says Purge and disturb (humors), when ripe, in other words, 'Pay attention to the concoction of the humors, and only then administer the evacuant'. For when humors are unconcocted, they do not yield to the purgatives that should draw them forth. Now, when nature prepares to stir (humors), it uses its own faculties to concoct them; the art, however, when it evacuates, concocts the crude humors by means of certain comminuting medicines, such as decoctions and potions on the basis of oxymel, then by means of a suppository purges them out of the body. It is in imitation of nature, then, that we should purge and disturb (humors), when ripe, because then they all yield to the evacuation and are excreted by way of the parts of the body through which they pass. Therefore, no matter whether there has been an incomplete natural crisis owing to some obstruction, to another accidental obstacle or to the fact that the matter excreted is partially unconcocted, or whether the art on its own initiative, without any natural excretion, makes for evacuation and resorts to a purge, it is absolutely necessary to follow Hippocrates' rule and take every precaution that the humors should be concocted. Why, however, does he call the suppository a purge here? This is because of the efficacy of its power.

He says: nor in the beginning. The question is what he means by "beginning". The word is used both of the first, instantaneous onset of the paroxysm and of this onset considered as having a certain duration, in which case there are two acceptations: one is to limit it to a space of three days, the other to contradistinguish it from the other stages of the entire illness, and this is the technical usage; it is to this sense that Hippocrates refers here. The beginning, taken in this way, can never bring with it signs of concoction; for as soon as weak signs of concoction appear, the beginning of the sickness as a whole is over and the increase begins; similarly, when the signs show themselves clear and complete, the

παυται μὲν ἡ ἀνάβασις, ἄρχεται δὲ ἡ ἀκμή. καὶ εἰ ταῦτα οὕτως ἔχει ἐν ταῖς ἀκμαῖς, δῆλον, ὅτι αἱ κρίσεις ὑπαντῶσι κατὰ λόγον, ἔνθεν καὶ πεπεμμέναι εἰσὶν αἱ ὗλαι.

Μὴ ὠμὰ οὖν φησι κινήσῃς, μηδὲ ἐν ἀρχῇσιν, [I 22: IV 468,14 L.] ἢν μὴ ὀργᾷ, ὡς ἀντιστρέφοντος τοῦ λόγου καθ' ἑκάτερον τῶν σημαινομένων· ἔνθα γὰρ ἀρχή, πάντως ὠμοὶ καὶ ἄπεπτοι οἱ χυμοί· καὶ ὅπου ὠμοὶ οἱ χυμοί, πάντως ἀρχή. κατὰ δὲ τὸ ἕτερον οὐ δοκεῖ ἀντιστρέφειν, λέγω δὴ κατὰ τὸ ὀργᾶν· οὐ γὰρ ταὐτόν ἐστιν ὀργᾶν τὴν ὕλην καὶ πεπέφθαι τοῦ ὀργᾶν τὴν κίνησιν αὐτῶν σημαίνοντος. ἔστιν οὖν συνελόντα εἰπεῖν οὕτως· πεπεμμένους δεῖ κινεῖν τοὺς χυμοὺς καὶ πρὸς ἔκκρισιν ἐκκαλεῖσθαι, ἀλλὰ μὴ ὠμούς. ἐκ δὲ τούτου δῆλον, ὅτι οὐδὲ ἐν ἀρχῇ οὐδὲ ἐν ἀναβάσει νοσήματος ἐρεθίσομεν τὴν ὕλην, εἰ μή τι ἄρα ὀργᾷ, τουτέστιν ἐπιτεταμένως κινεῖται, ὥσπερ ἐπὶ τῶν λεπτῶν καὶ θερμῶν συμβαίνει χυμῶν καὶ τῶν κατοξέων νοσημάτων. τὸ τηνικαῦτα γάρ, εἰ καὶ ἀπεψία ὑπόκειται, ἀλλ' ὅμως διὰ τὸ πολλὴν ἀνίαν ἐγκεῖσθαι τοῖς σώμασιν ἀναγκαῖον ἡγούμεθα πρὸς κένωσιν ὁρμῆσαι καὶ τῆς τοιαύτης ὀχλήσεως ἐλευθερῶσαι τὸ σῶμα. ἔστι γὰρ ἀκοῦσαι τῶν οὕτως πασχόντων ποτὲ μὲν τοὺς ὠμοπλάτας ὀδυνωμένων, ἄλλοτε δὲ τὴν κεφαλήν, νῦν δὲ τὰς πλευράς, εἶτα πάλιν τὰ ἔντερα καὶ τοὺς λαγόνας, ὅπερ σημεῖόν ἐστι τῆς πολυκινήτου φορᾶς τοῦ νοσοποιοῦ αἰτίου. οὐκοῦν εἰ ὀργᾷ, οὐδὲν ἄτοπον καὶ ἐν ἀρχῇ τοῦ νοσήματος παραλαβεῖν τὴν κάθαρσιν, τῷ γὰρ εὐκινήτῳ τῆς ὕλης ἑτοίμως ἡ ἔκκρισις ἀπαντήσει.

[I 22: IV 468,14 L.] Τὰ δὲ πολλὰ οὐκ ὀργᾷ, φησίν, ὅτι ἐνδέχεταί ποτε καὶ ἐν ἀρχῇ ὀργῶσαν εὑρεθῆναι τὴν ὕλην, σπανιάκις δέ. νόμιζε γὰρ αὐτὸν ὀξέα καὶ χρόνια νοσήματα ἐν τούτῳ τῷ λόγῳ θεωρεῖν φυσικῶς καὶ τὰ μὲν ἐν ἀρχῇ ὀργῶντα τῶν κατοξέων νοσημάτων λέγειν εἶναι αἴτια καὶ ἐν τούτοις θερμὴν εἶναι τὴν ὕλην καὶ χολώδη, οὐ πάντως δὲ καὶ λεπτὴν καὶ δριμεῖαν. τούτου γὰρ χάριν ἐπήγαγε· τὰ δὲ πολλὰ οὐκ ὀργᾷ, οὐ μόνον τὴν τῶν χρονίων νοσημάτων ἐντεῦθεν φύσιν παραδηλῶν, ἐφ' ὧν τὴν τελείαν πέψιν, ἥτις ἐν ἀκμῇ γίνεται, ἀναμένει ἡ ὕλη, ἐν ἄλλῳ χρόνῳ κινηθῆναι πρὸς κρίσιν ἐπιτηδείως οὐκ ἔχουσα, ἀλλὰ καὶ τῶν ὀξέων συμπεριλαμβάνων ἐκεῖνα, ἐν οἷς εἰ καὶ θερμὴ ὑπόκειται ὕλη, ἀλλά γε τῷ πάχει τοῦ ὀργᾶν καὶ κινεῖσθαι ἐστέρηται.

I 36 [I 23: IV 470,1–3 L.] [Πέπονα φαρμακεύειν καὶ κινέειν, μὴ ὠμὰ μηδὲ ἐν ἀρχῇσιν, ἢν μὴ ὀργᾷ· τὰ δὲ πολλὰ οὐκ ὀργᾷ.] Τὰ χωρέοντα μὴ τῷ πλήθει τεκμαίρεσθαι, ἀλλ' ὡς ἂν χωρέῃ οἷα δεῖ καὶ φέρει εὐφόρως· καὶ ὅκου δεῖ, ἄχρι λιποθυμίης ἄγειν.

Ἐνταῦθα τὸ μέτρον τῆς ἐκκρίσεως κανονίσαι βουλόμενός φησιν, ὅτι οὐ δεῖ τῇ ποσότητι τῶν κενουμένων προσέχοντας τεχνικῶς σημειοῦσθαι, εἴτε καλῶς γέγονεν ἡ κένωσις εἴτε μή. τί φῄς, ὦ Ἱππόκρατες; ὑπηλάτου δοθέντος φαρμάκου οὐ δεῖ τὸν ἰατρὸν τὸ ποσὸν τῶν ἐκκρινομένων σκοπῆσαι, εἴτε πολλά ἐστι ταῦτα εἴτε ὀλίγα, καὶ εἰ συμφωνεῖ τῷ προθεωρηθέντι σκοπῷ τῆς τέχνης ἡ ἔκκρισις; ἵνα οὖν ταύτην ἐπιλυσώμεθα τὴν ἀπορίαν, ἐκ παραδείγματος εἴπωμεν οὕτως. ὑπο-

6sq. οὐ[II] – σημαίνοντος] *cf.* Gal. In Aphor. I 22: XVII B 441,5–13 K. 21sq. καὶ[II] – αἴτια] *cf.* Theoph. In Aphor.: II 290,9–11 Dietz

12 τὸ[II] *om.* P 21 καὶ[II] *om.* A 24 πολλὰ] *item infra, lin. 30, Hipp.* MV: λοιπὰ A *(cf. Theoph. In aphor.: II 290,11 Dietz)*: πλεῖστα *Hipp.* C', *Theoph.* U'' 29sq. Πέπονα – ὀργᾷ *uncis inclusa in* P: *delevi* 32 ἄχρι] *item infra, p. 132,16. 22; vol. III, fol. 169ᵛ, Theoph.*: μέχρι *infra, p. 132,18, Hipp.* 38 εἴπομεν α: *correxi*

increase is over and the acme begins. And if this is the case in the acme, it is evident that the crisis develops normally, which means that the matter is concocted.

He says, then, that you should not disturb (humors), *while crude, nor in the beginning, unless there is commotion*, the statement being convertible as regards both of these concepts: when a disease is in its beginning, the humors are necessarily crude and unconcocted; and when the humors are crude, the disease is necessarily in its beginning. As far as the remaining one, "commotion", is concerned, it does not seem to be convertible with the others; for commotion of the matter is not the same as concoction, since commotion means that it is disturbed. We can sum up as follows: one should disturb humors and stir them to excretion only when they are concocted, not while they are crude. From this it is clear that we will stir up the matter neither in the beginning nor during the increase of a disease, unless it is in commotion, i.e. in violent disturbance, which happens with thin and hot humors and in cases of very acute diseases. Under those circumstances, even if we have to do with unconcocted matter, yet on account of the extreme physical discomfort we deem it necessary to resort to evacuation and deliver the body from this distress. We hear from patients in this plight that now their shoulder blades ache, now their head, now their sides, now their intestines and flanks, which is evidence of the restless motion of the cause of the disease. Therefore, if there is commotion, it is perfectly reasonable to resort to a purge even at the beginning of the disease, since the excretion will respond readily to the mobility of the matter.

But usually there is no commotion, (*Hippocrates*) continues, (meaning) that sometimes the matter may be found in commotion even at the beginning, but this is rare. You may think that in this statement he gives a physiological account of acute and chronic diseases, saying that whatever is in commotion at the beginning causes very acute diseases and that in these cases the matter is hot and bilious, though not necessarily thin and sharp. This explains the addition *but usually there is no commotion*, by which he intimates not only the character of chronic diseases, in which the matter waits for complete concoction during the acme — the only time when it is fit to be stirred to a crisis —, but also includes those cases of acute diseases when the matter, though hot, shows no commotion and upheaval owing to its thickness.

> **I 36.** *[Purge and disturb (humors), when ripe, not while crude, nor in the beginning, unless there is commotion; but usually there is no commotion.] Do not judge the matter evacuated by bulk, but consider whether it is of the right kind and the patient bears up well; where necessary, go on until he faints.*

Here, wanting to set a rule for the quantity of the excretion, (*Hippocrates*) says that one cannot diagnose expertly whether evacuation has proceeded well or not by observing the quantity of matter evacuated. What do you mean, *Hippocrates*? When a suppository has been administered, should the physician not examine the quantity of the excrement, whether there is much or little, and whether the excretion corresponds to the purpose envisaged beforehand by the art? To answer this objection, let us use the following example. Suppose two

κείσθωσαν δύο τινὲς καθαιρόμενοι, εἴτε φυσική ἐστιν ἡ κάθαρσις εἴτε δι' ὑπηλάτου· τούτων ὁ μὲν εἷς ποιείτω πεντήκοντα ἐπαναστάσεις, ὁ δὲ ἕτερος ποιείτω κένωσιν εἴκοσι λιτρῶν. ἑκάτερος οὖν αὐτῶν πολλὰ λέγεται κενωθῆναι τοῦ πλήθους πῇ μὲν κατὰ τῶν ἐπαναστάσεων φερομένου, πῇ δὲ κατὰ [τὴν] τῆς ποσότητος τῶν ἐκκρινομένων, καὶ οὐδέτερον τούτων ἐπιστημονικὴν ἢ τεχνικὴν ἔχει τὴν σημείωσιν. ἐνδέχεται γὰρ καὶ τὸν πολλὰς ἐπαναστάσεις ποιησάμενον κατ' ὀλίγον κενωθῆναι παχέος καὶ δριμέος ὄντος τοῦ κενουμένου καὶ συνεχῶς αὐτὸν ἐρεθίζοντος καὶ τὸν πολλὰ κενώσαντα μὴ τὸν δέοντα κενῶσαι χυμόν, ἀλλ' ἕτερον ἀντ' αὐτοῦ. τοῦτο οὖν ἐπιστάμενός φησιν, ὅτι τὰ ἐκκρινόμενα οὐ δεῖ τῷ πλήθει τῶν ἐπαναστάσεων σημειοῦσθαι, εἰ καλῶς ἔχει εἴτε μή, ἀλλ' ἐὰν ἐκκρίνηται, οἷα δεῖ καθαίρεσθαι, καὶ πῶς ἂν ταῦτα καθαίρηται σκοπεῖν. τοῦ γὰρ βλαπτικοῦ χυμοῦ ἐκκρινομένου εὐφορία τὸν κάμνοντα διαδέχεται, ὥσπερ καὶ τὸ ἀνάπαλιν δυσφορίαν ἐπάγει ὅσα μή ἐστιν αἴτια τοῦ νοσήματος κενούμενα. τῷ ἰδιώματι δὲ τῷ ἀνωτέρω καὶ νῦν ἐχρήσατο· εἰρηκὼς γὰρ τὸ «οἷα δεῖ» τὸ εἶδος τοῦ χυμοῦ ὑπηνίξατο πρὸς τὴν κατὰ ποιότητα βλάβην ἐνιστάμενος.

Εἶτα ἐπήγαγε· καὶ ὅκου δεῖ, ἄχρι λιποθυμίης ἄγειν. ἰστέον, ὅτι κοινὸν γένος ἡ κένωσις κατά τε τῆς φλεβοτομίας φερομένη καὶ κατὰ τῆς καθάρσεως. καὶ πόθεν τοῦτο δῆλον; ἐκ τοῦ φάναι μέχρι λιποθυμίας ἄγειν. οὐδεὶς ἐπὶ τῶν τεχνικῶς καθαιρομένων ὁρίσαι δύναται τὸ παρεχόμενον βοήθημα, ὥστε μέχρι λιποθυμίας τὴν κάθαρσιν ποιῆσαι, ἀλλὰ τούτου ἐξουσίαν ἐν ταῖς φλεβοτομίαις ὁ τεχνίτης ἔχει. φησὶν οὖν ὁ Ἱπποκράτης· Τὰ χωρέοντα μὴ τῷ πλήθει τεκμαίρεσθαι, ἀλλ' ὡς ἂν χωρέῃ οἷα δεῖ καὶ φέρει εὐφόρως· καὶ ὅκου δεῖ, ἄχρι λιποθυμίας ἄγειν ὡς δῆθεν τῆς μέχρι λιποθυμίας λαμβανομένης κενώσεως ὠφέλιμόν τι πρὸς θεραπείαν τοῖς κάμνουσιν εἰσαγούσης. ζητητέον οὖν, ποίαν λιποθυμίαν δεῖ παραλαβεῖν. ἐπὶ τῶν διὰ φλεβοτομίας κενουμένων πολύτροπος γίνεται ἡ λιποθυμία, τῶν μὲν δι' ἄκραν δειλίαν ἀκοῇ καὶ μόνον τοῦ φλεβοτόμου ταρασσομένων, τινῶν δὲ αὖ ἐκ τοῦ ὁρᾶν τὸ σιδήριον λιποθυμούντων, ἕτεροι δὲ φλεβοτομηθέντες ἐν ἀρχῇ τῆς κενώσεως ἢ περὶ τὰ μέσα χυμοῦ τινος περὶ τὸν στόμαχον συρρεύσαντος τὰς λιποθυμίας ὑφίστανται· ἕτερος δὲ τρόπος λιποθυμίας ὁ παρατεινόμενος πρὸς τὴν τοῦ κάμνοντος δύναμιν τῆς κενώσεως ἐπιγενομένης. περὶ ταύτης τῆς λιποθυμίας νῦν διαλέγεται ὁ Ἱπποκράτης καὶ μέχρι ταύτης ἐφ' ὧν δεῖ παρακελεύεται ἡμῖν τὰς τῆς φλεβοτομίας κενώσεις.

Ἐφ' οἷς ἀκόλουθον ζητῆσαι, τί βούλεται τὸ ὅκου δεῖ· οὐδὲ γὰρ ἐπὶ πάντων τῷ τρόπῳ τούτῳ τῆς κενώσεως βούλεται ἡμᾶς κεχρῆσθαι διὰ τοῦ εἰπεῖν ὅκου δεῖ, τουτέστιν ἐφ' ὧν δεῖ νοσημάτων. καὶ ποῖα νοσήματα τῆς διὰ φλεβοτόμου δέονται κενώσεως μέχρι λιποθυμίας; ἡνίκα ἢ πυρετὸς ὑπόκειται διακαὴς καὶ φλογώδης ἢ φλεγμονὴ μεγίστη ἔν τινι τῶν ὑποχονδρίων ἢ ὀδύνη μεγάλη καὶ σφακελίζουσα. καὶ

8 τοῦτο – 13 ἐχρήσατο] *v.* Theoph. In Aphor.: II 291,1–7 Dietz 14 οἷα δεῖ] Hipp. Aphor. I 2: IV 458,6 L. 16–17 καθάρσεως] *v.* Theoph. In Aphor.: II 291,7–9 Dietz 24 ζητητέον – 32] *v.* Gal. In Aphor. I 23: XVII B 444,15–445,11 K. 35 καὶ – 37 σφακελίζουσα] *v.* Gal. In Aphor. I 23: XVII B 445,11–15 K. 35sq. καὶ – διακαὴς] *v.* Theoph. In Aphor.: II 291,9–11 Dietz 37 καὶ[II] – 134,5 σῶμα] *v.* Theoph. In Aphor.: II 291,13–20 Dietz

3 πολλὰ *scripsi*: πολλάκις α 4 τὴν *delevi* 6 τὸν *scripsi*: τῶν P: τὰς A 16 λυποθυμίας A 18 τεχνικῶν A 20 ὁ τεχνίτης ἐν ταῖς φλεβοτομίαις A 26 μόνου A 29sq. παρατεινόμενος ... ἐπιγενομένης] *fort.* παρατεινομένης ... ἐπιγινόμενος *scribendum est* 31 τῆς *om.* A

patients are purged, no matter whether naturally or by means of a suppository; let one of them have fifty bowel movements and the other excrete twenty pounds. Of each of them it can be said that there has been much evacuation, the quantity referring in the one case to the number of bowel movements, in the other to the bulk of the matter excreted, and neither indication warrants a scientific or technical diagnosis. The man who has had many bowel movements may have evacuated only little each time, because the matter is thick and pungent and continually irritates him, whereas the one who evacuated a great quantity may not have excreted the right kind of humor, but a different one instead. Being aware of this, he says that one should not judge the excrements by the number of bowel movements to decide whether they are right or not, but one should consider whether the right kind of matter is evacuated and how the evacuation takes place. If the harmful humor is excreted, the patient's subsequent feeling will be one of euphoria; on the other hand, evacuation of matter that is not the cause of the disease will result in a feeling of discomfort. (Hippocrates) here used the same idiom as above: when he said "the right kind", he indicated the type of humor, trying to prevent the damage caused by its quality.

He continued: Where necessary, go on until he faints. It should be understood that evacuation is a generic term covering both bloodletting and purgation. This appears from the expression Go on until he faints. For in the case of artificial purging nobody can determine the dose of the medication in such a way as to purge to the point where the patient faints, but in bleeding the skilled physician can control this. So when Hippocrates says, Do not judge the matter evacuated by bulk, but consider whether it is of the right kind and the patient bears up well; where necessary, go on until he faints, he implies that evacuation to the point of fainting can have a beneficial effect for the curing of the sick. Hence the question arises to what kind of fainting one should be willing to go. When evacuation by phlebotomy is applied, many kinds of fainting occur: some are so extremely fearful as to panic at the mere word "lancet", others faint upon seeing the implement, others again have their fainting fits at the beginning of the evacuation or in the middle of it, because a particular humor flows to the region of the stomach; another kind of fainting is that which occurs when evacuation is extended to the limit of the patient's resistance. This is the fainting to which Hippocrates refers here, and it is to this point that he encourages us to carry evacuation by bloodletting in cases where necessary.

The next question to ask is the meaning of where necessary; he does not want us to use this kind of evacuation in every case, as he shows by adding where necessary, i.e. in those diseases which require it. What diseases, then, require evacuation by bloodletting to the point of fainting? When we have to do, either with a burning, fiery fever, or with a severe inflammation in one of the viscera, or with an intense, gangrene-like pain. We shall explain the reason for

τὴν αἰτίαν ἑκάστου τούτων προσφόρως ἀποδώσομεν. οἱ καυσώδεις τῶν πυρετῶν ἐπὶ χυμοῖς ἀνάπτονται σηπομένοις· δύο δ' αἴτια ἡ σηπεδὼν ἔχει, ὕλην τε σεσηπυῖαν καὶ ποιότητα μοχθηρὰν καὶ κακόχυμον. ἡ οὖν μέχρι λιποθυμίας ἐπὶ τῶν τοιούτων πυρετῶν ληφθεῖσα φλεβοτομία καὶ τοῦ ποσοῦ τῆς ὕλης ἀφαιρεῖται καὶ τὴν δριμεῖαν καὶ φλογώδη ποιότητα κατασβέννυσι τῆς λιποθυμίας ψυχούσης ἱκανῶς τὸ σῶμα τῇ διαφορήσει τοῦ ἐμφύτου θερμοῦ καὶ τῷ σκεδασμῷ τοῦ ζωτικοῦ τόνου· οὐδὲν γὰρ ἕτερόν ἐστι λιποθυμία ἢ λεῖψις τοῦ θυμοῦ, εἰκὼν ὑπάρχουσα θανάτου. ἀλλὰ καὶ φλεγμονῆς περὶ τὰ σπλάγχνα ὑφισταμένης, ἐπειδὴ καὶ αὕτη ὕλην τε ἔχει, ἐφ' ἧς γέγονεν, ἔτι μέντοι καὶ δυσκρασίαν, κατὰ τὸν αὐτὸν δεῖ λόγον μέχρι λιποθυμίας φλεβοτομεῖν. ἀλλὰ μὴν καὶ ὀδύνην ἄμετρον καὶ σφακελώδη ἡ τοιαύτη κένωσις παύει, τῇ τε ἀφαιρέσει τῆς ὕλης καὶ τῷ δυσαίσθητον τῇ καταψύξει τῆς λιποθυμίας γίνεσθαι τὸ ὀδυνώμενον μόριον κατὰ τὸ εἰρημένον· «Νάρκη γὰρ μετρίη ὀδύνης ληκτική.»

Ἐπιφέρει δέ· [I 23: IV 470,3 L.] τοῦτο ποιέειν, ἢν ἐξαρκέσῃ ὁ νοσέων, τουτέστιν ἐφ' ὧν ἔρρωται ἡ δύναμις. εἰ γὰρ τοῦτο ὡς μηδενὸς ἄξιον παραδράμωμεν, ἅμα τῇ λιποθυμίᾳ ὁ θάνατος ἐπακολουθήσει· ἔνθα οὖν ἀσθενὴς ὑπόκειται ἡ δύναμις, μηδὲ μέχρις ἐννοίας τοῦτο τολμήσειας διαπράξασθαι.

I 37 [I 24: IV 470,4–5 L.] Ἐν τοῖσιν ὀξέσι νοσήμασιν ὀλιγάκις καὶ ἐν ἀρχῇσι τῇσι φαρμακείῃσι χρέεσθαι, καὶ τοῦτο προεξευκρινήσαντας ποιέειν.

Ἀκολούθως τοῖς προσεχῶς εἰρημένοις καὶ ἡ τοῦ παρόντος ἔννοια δέδοται, καὶ μάλιστα τῷ εἰρημένῳ· «Πέπονα φαρμακεύειν καὶ κινέειν, μὴ ὠμὰ μηδὲ ἐν ἀρχῇσιν, ἢν μὴ ὀργᾷ.» ταῦτα γάρ ἐστιν ἐφ' ὧν ὀργᾷ ἡ ὕλη καὶ δεῖ ἐν ἀρχῇ τὰς κενώσεις ποιεῖσθαι, ὡς ὁ παρὼν ἀφορισμὸς διεξέρχεται, ταῦτα φάσκων εἶναι τὰ ὀξέα νοσήματα. – ὀξέα οὖν ἀκουστέον τὰ μέχρι τῆς ζ̄ ἢ τῆς θ̄ ἢ τῆς ια̅ ἢ τῆς ιδ̅ ἀφικνούμενα. – ἐπειδὴ οὖν ἐκεῖσε ἐπήγαγε· «τὰ δὲ πολλὰ οὐκ ὀργᾷ», ἐνταῦθα ἐκ τοῦ ἐναντίου τῷ ὀλιγάκις ἐχρήσατο. ἐπὶ οὖν τῶν ὀξέων νοσημάτων ὀλιγάκις καὶ ἐν ἀρχῇσι τῇ φαρμακείᾳ δεῖ χρέεσθαι· ὀλιγάκις μὲν διὰ τὸ σπανίως ὀργῶσαν ἐν ἀρχῇ εὑρίσκεσθαι τὴν ὕλην, ἐν ἀρχῇ δὲ διὰ τὸ μὴ πάνυ τὸ τηνικαῦτα κατεπείγειν τὴν θερμασίαν μήτε τὰ συμπτώματα ὥσπερ ἐν ἀκμῇ. ἐπεὶ γὰρ θερμή ἐστιν ἐπ' αὐτῶν ἡ ὕλη καὶ ξηρὰ καὶ διακαῆ πυρετὸν ἀνάπτει, μάλιστα ἐν ἀκμῇ, καὶ τὸ διδόμενον κενωτικὸν φάρμακον θερμὸν καὶ ξηρόν, κίνδυνος μὴ πολλαπλασιασθήσεται ἡ ζέσις καὶ διαφθαρήσεται τὸ ζῷον. διὰ τοῦτο οὖν ὀλιγάκις ἐπὶ τῶν ὀξέων νοσημάτων παραλαμβανόντων ἡμῶν

6sq. οὐδὲν – θανάτου] *cf. infra*, p. 224,25–26; vol. III, fol. 169v 12sq. Νάρκη – ληκτική] Hipp. Aphor. V 25: IV 540,17 L. 14–15 δύναμις] *v.* Theoph. In Aphor.: II 291,11–13 Dietz 21–24 νοσήματα] *v.* Gal. In Aphor. I 24: XVII B 446,14–447,6 K. 22sq. Πέπονα – ὀργᾷ[I]] Hipp. Aphor. I 22: IV 468,13–14 L. 26 τὰ – ὀργᾷ] Hipp. Aphor. I 22: IV 468,14 L.

1 ἀποδώσωμεν A 2 δ' αἴτια] δέ τινα *Theoph.* τε *om.* P 3 ἡ] εἰ A 7 θυμοῦ *scripsi (cf. infra, p. 224,26)* : θερμοῦ α 8 ἐφ'] ὑφ' P ἧς] οἷς A 9 αὐτ˜ P 11 τῷ *scripsi*: τὸ α 14 ποιέεις A ἢν *sec. Hipp. scripsi*: ἵν' P: εἰ A ἐξαρκέσῃ *Hipp. C', Theoph.*: ἐξαρκῇ *Hipp. plerique* 16 παρακολουθήσει A ἡ *om.* A 18 Ἐν] *item infra, vol. II, fol. 52r, Hipp.*: *om. infra, vol. II, fol. 70v, Theoph. V''* νοσήμασιν] πάθεσιν *infra, p. 136,5; vol. II, fol. 52r; 70v, Hipp.* 19 προεξευκρινήσαντας] *item infra, pp. 136,6; 216,31, Theoph.*: -ντα *Hipp. quidam* 22 κινεῖν P 26 τῷ *scripsi*: τὸ α

each of these in due order. Burning fevers break out when humors are corrupted; and their corruption has two causes, corrupted matter and a malignant, unwholesome quality. Hence, in the case of such fevers, bloodletting to the point of fainting both diminishes the bulk of the matter and quenches its pungent, fiery quality, since the fainting cools the body considerably by dispersing the innate heat and dissipating the vital strength; for fainting is nothing but a failure of life, and thus an image of death. Secondly, when an inflammation occurs in the viscera, we must bleed to the point of fainting for the same reason, because here, too, there is matter which causes it, and there is also a distemper. Finally, this kind of evacuation puts an end to excessive, gangrene-like pain by diminishing the matter and by lessening the perception in the affected part owing to the chilling that the fainting-fit brings about, in accordance with the saying: "For a light numbness relieves pain."

He adds: You may do this, if the patient's resistance is sufficient, i.e. if his strength is unimpaired. If we neglect this as of no consequence, the fainting will be followed immediately by death; so when resistance is weak, you must not even consider taking this risk.

I 37. In acute diseases use purges rarely and only at the beginning, and then after thorough preparation.

The idea of the present aphorism is a sequel to the preceding ones, especially to the one that says: "Purge and disturb (humors), when ripe, not while crude, nor in the beginning, unless there is commotion." For those are the cases when the matter is in commotion and when one should evacuate in the beginning, as the present aphorism explains, stating that these are acute diseases. – By acute diseases we must understand those which last until the 7th, the 9th, the 11th or the 14th day. – Now because in the other aphorism he added: "But usually there is no commotion", he used rarely as its counterpart in this one. Thus, in acute diseases one should use purges rarely and only at the beginning: rarely, because the matter is seldom found to be in commotion at the beginning; at the beginning, because at that stage the heat and the symptoms are not urgent, as they are during the acme. For since in these diseases the matter is hot and dry and causes a burning fever, especially during the acme, and since further the evacuant we administer is also hot and dry, there is a danger of the scalding heat multiplying and the organism being destroyed. Therefore, while we rarely resort

κάθαρσιν ἐν ἀρχῇ δεῖ ταύτην παραλαμβάνειν, ὅτε τὰ δυνάμει αἴτια τὸ δραστήριον ἔχει καὶ μόνα, ἅτινα καὶ κενῶσαι δεόμεθα ἔτι τὴν ἑαυτῆς ἰσχὺν τῆς δυνάμεως κεκτημένης.

Πάθος δέ ἐστι τὸ ἐν τῷ γίνεσθαι ἔχον τὸ εἶναι, νόσημα δὲ τὸ ἐν τῷ γεγονέναι τὴν ὕπαρξιν κεκτημένον· νῦν δὲ τὸ πάθος ἀντὶ τοῦ νοσήματος εἴρηκε.

Καὶ τοῦτο, φησί, προεξευκρινήσαντας ποιέειν, τουτέστι προγνόντας τὸν δεόμενον χυμὸν κενώσεως, ἵνα πρὸς αὐτὸν ἁρμόσωμεν τὸ φάρμακον· ἢ καὶ προπαρασκευάσαντας τὴν ὕλην καὶ προλεπτύναντας διὰ τῶν τοῦτο ποιῆσαι δυναμένων ἀποζεμάτων, ὥς φησιν αὐτὸς παρακατιών· «Τὰ σώματα χρή, ὅκου τις βούλεται καθαίρειν, εὔροα ποιέειν.» συνελὼν οὖν εἰπεῖν οὑτωσὶ τὸ πᾶν τοῦ λόγου ῥητέον· «Ἐν τοῖς ὀξέσι πάθεσιν ὀλιγάκις κεχρῆσθαι δεῖ τῇ φαρμακείᾳ, καὶ ἐν ἀρχῇ καὶ προεξευκρινήσαντας.»

Ὁ μέντοι Γαληνὸς ἐνταῦθα γενόμενος ἐπέστησεν, ὡς οὐδέποτε ἐν τοῖς ὀξέσι νοσήμασιν αὐτὸς ἐχρήσατο καθάρσει, ὅπερ οὐδὲ τὸν Ἱπποκράτην διέλαθεν εἰρηκότα, ὅτι δεῖ ἐπ' αὐτῶν ὀλιγάκις κεχρῆσθαι τῇ καθάρσει. «Ἀλλ' ἐφλεβοτόμησα» φησὶν «ἐπὶ τῶν τοιούτων» ὁ Γαληνός, «εἰ καὶ καθάρσεως ἐδεῖτο τὸ σῶμα, τὰ δύο ἐντεῦθεν πραγματευσάμενος, τό τε τὴν ὕλην κενῶσαι καὶ τὴν δυσκρασίαν σβέσαι τῷ μέχρι λιποθυμίας τὴν φλεβοτομίαν παραλαβεῖν· ἐνταῦθα γάρ ἐστιν ἐν ἐμοὶ καὶ στῆσαι, ὅτε βούλομαι, τὴν κένωσιν καὶ μὴ στῆσαι, ὅπερ ἐπὶ τῶν καθαιρόντων οὐκ ἔστι διαπράξασθαι· οὔτε γὰρ ποιῆσαι λιποθυμίαν ἐν ἐμοί ἐστιν οὔτε ἐπιτεταμένην κένωσιν εὐχερῶς ἐπισχεῖν.»

Κύκλον δὲ μιμούμενος ὁ Ἱπποκράτης ὅθεν ἤρξατο ἐκεῖ καὶ παύεται. τὸν κολοφῶνα γὰρ τοῦ λόγου καθαρὸν ἀπεργάζεται σφραγῖδά τινα βεβαίαν καὶ ἀσφαλῆ ἐπιθέμενος τῷ τῆς καθάρσεως λόγῳ, τὴν εὐφορίαν φημί. λέγει γὰρ ἐν ἀρχῇ· [I 2: IV 458,6–7 L. = I 25: IV 470,6–7 L.] Ἢν οἷα δεῖ καθαίρεσθαι καθαίρονται, ξυμφέρει τε καὶ εὐφόρως φέρουσι. τί οὖν; ταὐτολογεῖ πάλιν ταῦτα φάσκων; οὐχί, ἀλλ' ἐκεῖ μὲν φυσικὴν καθαίρων κάθαρσιν καὶ αὐτόματον τῷ ἐπιλόγῳ τούτῳ ἐκέχρητο, νῦν δὲ τεχνικὴν καὶ ἐξ ἐπιτηδεύσεως παρεισάγει γεγενημένην. ἐν οἷς σὺν θεῷ ἡ πρᾶξις καὶ τὸ πρῶτον τμῆμα πεπλήρωται.

4sq.] *v.* Theoph. In Aphor.: II 292,30–31 Dietz 6–9 ἀποζεμάτων] *cf.* Gal. In Aphor. I 24: XVII B 447,6–12 K. Theoph. In Aphor.: II 292,35–36 Dietz 9sq. Τὰ – ποιέειν] Hipp. Aphor. II 9: IV 472,4–5 L. *v.* Gal. In Aphor. I 24: XVII B 449,3–5 K. *cf.* Theoph. In Aphor.: II 293,1 Dietz 13–21] *hae enuntiationes in commentario Galeni in Aphor. I 24 non inveniuntur; cf.* Gal. In Aphor. I 23: XVII B 445,11–446,10 K. 22 Κύκλον – παύεται] *cf.* Eliae In isag.: CAG XVIII 1, p. 23,26–27 David. In isag.: CAG XVIII 2, p. 45,27–46,1 [Elias] 17,1 Westerink (Amstelodami 1967) 24 λέγει – 28 γεγενημένην] *v.* Theoph. In Aphor.: II 293,18–294,2 Dietz λέγει – 26 φάσκων] *v.* Gal. In Aphor. I 25: XVII B 450,4–8 K. 27sq. οὐχί – γεγενημένην] *v.* Gal. In Aphor. I 25: XVII B 450,8–15 K.

1sq. ὅτε – μόνα] *immo* ὅτε τὰ αἴτια τὸ δραστήριον ἔχει δυνάμει καὶ μόνον 4 τὸ ἐν[I] *om.* A 5 τοῦ *om.* P 10 ποιέων α: *corr.* A², ποιέειν *Hipp.* 17 τῷ *scripsi*: τὸ α 25 Ἢν *sec. Hipp. scripsi*: ἵν' α

to purging in acute diseases, we should do so in the beginning, when only the potential causes are effective; we have to evacuate them so long as resistance is still strong.

An affection is that which is in process of becoming, a disease, that which is already in existence; here, however, (Hippocrates) uses affection instead of disease.

And then, he continues, only after thorough preparation, i.e. after determining which humor has to be evacuated, so that we can adapt the purgative to it; or he may mean: after having first conditioned the matter and comminuted it by means of decoctions that have this power, as he says later on: "Bodies, when one wants to purge them, should be made to flow readily." The whole statement can be summed up as follows: "In acute affections purging should be used rarely, and then in the beginning and after due preparation."

Galen, however, commenting on the passage, noted that he himself never resorted to purging at all in acute diseases; but then Hippocrates, too, felt this way, since he says that purging ought to be used rarely in these cases. "Instead", Galen says, "I have applied bloodletting in such diseases, even when the body needed purging, with a twofold purpose: to evacuate the matter, and to quench the temperamental disorder by carrying the bleeding to the point of fainting; for then it is in my power to stop the evacuation when I choose, or to continue, which is not feasible when one uses purgatives; with those, it is not in my power to bring about a fainting-fit nor is it easy to check excessive evacuation."

Following the pattern of a circle, Hippocrates ends where he began. He neatly winds up his argument by attaching to the discussion of purgation a sure and infallible seal, namely, the state of euphoria. At the outset he said: If the matter discharged is of the right kind, this is beneficial and easily tolerated. Is he simply repetitious, then, saying the same over again? No, for in the first instance he arrived at this conclusion dealing with natural, spontaneous evacuation, while here he describes the outcome of an artificial and deliberate procedure. This, with God's help, is the end of the lecture and of the first section.

ΑΡΧΗ ΤΟΥ ΔΕΥΤΕΡΟΥ ΤΜΗΜΑΤΟΣ

II 1 [II 1: IV 470,9–10 L.] Ἐν ᾧ νοσήματι ὕπνος πόνον ποιέει, θανάσιμον· ἢν δὲ ὕπνος ὠφελέῃ, οὐ θανάσιμον.

Ἐνταῦθα τοῦ δευτέρου τμήματος ἀρχόμενος ὁ Ἱπποκράτης σημείωσιν ἀπὸ τῶν ὕπνων διδάσκει, ἀφ' ὧν δυνάμεθα γνῶναι, εἴτε σωτήριον εἴτε ὀλέθριόν ἐστι τὸ ὑποκείμενον νόσημα. ζητήσωμεν δὲ ἡμεῖς τινα κεφάλαια· καὶ πρῶτον μὲν τί ἐστιν ὅλως ὕπνος εἴπωμεν· δεύτερον δὲ τίς ἡ μερικὴ χρεία τοῦ ὕπνου, ⟨καθ' ἣν⟩ τῇ πρώτῃ τῶν ἀρχῶν συμβάλλεται, φημὶ δὴ τῷ ἐγκεφάλῳ· τρίτον τίς ὁ τρόπος τῆς γενέσεως τῶν ὕπνων· ἐν τῷ τετάρτῳ δὲ κεφαλαίῳ τί ⟨τὸ⟩ χρήσιμον τοῦ ὕπνου εἰρήσεται καὶ πῶς τῷ παντὶ χρησιμεύει σώματι.

Καὶ ἀρκτέον ἀπὸ τοῦ πρώτου. ὕπνος τοίνυν ἐστὶν ἡσυχία καὶ ἀνάπαυλα τῶν ψυχικῶν δυνάμεων μετ' ἐπιθέσεως τῶν φυσικῶν ἐνεργειῶν. ἠρεμούσης γὰρ τῆς ψυχῆς καὶ μὴ ἀναγκαζομένης ὑπουργεῖν †τῇ φύσει† λείπεται τοῖς οἰκείοις ἔργοις ἀδιασπάστως ταύτην σχολάζειν.

Δεύτερόν ἐστι κεφάλαιον, ἐν ᾧ δεῖ τὴν μερικὴν χρείαν τοῦ ὕπνου διηγήσασθαι, καθ' ἣν συμβάλλεται τῷ ἐγκεφάλῳ. καὶ ἰστέον, ὡς αἱ κρείττονος ἀξιώματος μεταλαβοῦσαι ἀρχαί, ἐγκέφαλός φημι καὶ καρδία καὶ ἧπαρ, ἡσυχίᾳ τινὶ καὶ ἀναπαύσει τὰς οἰκείας ἀνακτῶνται δυνάμεις. οὕτω γοῦν ἡ καρδία ἐν τῷ συστέλλεσθαι ⟨καὶ τῷ διαστέλλεσθαι⟩ ἠρεμοῦσα ἐνεργεῖ ἑκατέρας τῶν κινήσεων δυσὶν ἡσυχίαις μεσολαβουμένης, μιᾷ ἐντὸς καὶ μιᾷ ἐκτός· οὕτως οὖν ἠρεμεῖ ἡ καρδία, ὡς ἐντεῦθεν ἀναπαυομένην αὐτὴν ἀνακτᾶσθαι τὰς οἰκείας δυνάμεις. οὐ μὴν ἀλλὰ καὶ τὸ ἧπαρ τὴν ἡμέραν πᾶσαν ἐν ἀναπαύσει τινί ἐστιν ἧττον ἐνεργοῦν κατὰ τὰς φυσικὰς δηλονότι δυνάμεις ἐν τῇ ἐγρηγόρσει. ὅτι μὲν οὖν ἠρεμοῦσιν αἱ φυσικαὶ δυνάμεις ἅτε προαιρέσει μὴ δουλεύουσαι, τῶν ὁμολογουμένων καθέστηκεν· ἅμα πάλιν ἐνεργοῦσιν αὗται, δῆλον γάρ, ὅτι τὸ ἧπαρ νῦν μὲν ἕλκει, νῦν δὲ κατέχει, ἐφεξῆς δὲ ἀλλοιοῖ καὶ τέλος ἀποκρίνει. ἀλλὰ γὰρ εἰ καὶ πᾶσαι ἐν κινήσει αἱ τοιαῦται θεωροῦνται ἐνέργειαι, ὥστε κίνησιν ὑπὸ κινήσεως διαδέχεσθαι, ἀλλ' οὐ κατὰ πᾶν μέρος καὶ μόριον ἑαυτοῦ τὸ ἧπαρ ἐν πάσαις ταύταις ἐνεργεῖ ταῖς δυνάμεσιν, ἀλλὰ κατ' ἄλλο μὲν ἕλκει, κατ' ἄλλο δὲ κατέχει. πῶς οὖν οὐκ ἄτοπον τὴν τιμιωτέραν πασῶν ἀρχήν, ἐν ᾗ τὸ ἡγεμονικὸν τῆς ψυχῆς ἐγκαθίδρυται, τὸν ἐγκέφαλον λέγω, μηδεμιᾶς ἀναπαύσεως μετέχειν, καὶ ταῦτα πολυειδῶς κινούμενον ἐν τῷ φαντασιοῦσθαι καὶ λογίζεσθαι καὶ τῆς ἀπαν-

11sq. ὕπνος – ἐνεργειῶν] *cf.* [Gal.] Def. med. 127: XIX 381,17–18 K.

6 *fort.* ⟨δ'⟩ τινα *scribendum est* 7 εἴπομεν α: *correxi* καθ' ἣν *addidi (cf. lin. 16)* 9 τὸ *addidi* 12 φυσικῶν] ψυχικῶν A 13 τῇ φύσει] *requiritur* αὐτῇ τῆς φύσεως 18sq. καὶ τῷ διαστέλλεσθαι *addidi* 20 ἠρεμεῖν α: *correxi* 22 ἐν *om.* P 25 γάρ *om.* A

SECOND SECTION

II 1. A disease in which sleep causes distress, is deadly; but if sleep brings relief, it is not deadly.

Here, at the beginning of the second section, Hippocrates instructs us in inference from kinds of sleep, so that from them we can discern whether the disease with which we deal is curable or fatal. We will examine a number of points: first, we will explain what sleep, in general terms, is; secondly, what the particular function of sleep is, by which it is useful to the first of the principles, i.e. the brain; thirdly, in what manner sleep originates; as a fourth point we shall discuss the usefulness of sleep, and how it extends to the entire body.

Let us begin with the first. Sleep, then, is a rest and relaxation of the psychic faculties with increased activity of the natural functions. For when the soul is quiet and nature[1] is not forced to minister to its needs, it is left free to perform its own activities undisturbed.

The second point is the particular function of sleep, by which it is useful to the brain. It should be known that the higher-ranking principles, i.e. the brain, the heart and the liver, recuperate their faculties by a certain rest and relaxation. Thus the heart in the process of contraction and dilatation works while taking rest, each of the two movements being separated by two moments of rest, one inside and one outside; in this way the heart rests, so that it can relax and recuperate its powers. As for the liver, it rests, in a sense, the whole day, since it is less active – that is, as far as the natural faculties are concerned – in the waking state. It is a matter of general agreement, that the natural faculties rest, since they are independent of the will; on the other hand, they are active at the same time, for it is evident that the liver now attracts, now retains, then transforms, and finally secretes. Nevertheless, though all these functions are seen to consist in motions, so that one motion succeeds another, yet the liver in exercising all these faculties does not work with each of its parts or parts of parts simultaneously, but there is one with which it attracts, another with which it retains. It would be absurd, therefore, if the most precious of all the principles, in which the governing part of the soul is seated, I mean the brain, should be denied all repose, in spite of the fact that it goes through a variety of motions in the processes of imagining, reasoning and governing voluntary motion in any

[1] See the app. crit.

ταχοῦ τῶν μορίων κατὰ προαίρεσιν γινομένης ἐξηγεῖσθαι κινήσεως; οὔτε γὰρ τὸν ἄκρον δάκτυλον ἢ τελευταίαν δακτυλίδα κινῆσαι δυνατὸν ἄνευ τοῦ τὸν ἐγκέφαλον κινηθῆναι, εἴ γε πάσης προαιρετικῆς κινήσεως ἐν ἡμῖν ἐπιτελουμένης φαντασία προηγεῖται, αὕτη δὲ τοῦ ἐγκεφάλου ἔργον. οὕτως οὖν πολυτρόπως κινούμενος ὁ ἐγκέφαλος εἰ οὐδεμίαν ἕξει ἀνακωχὴν καὶ ἀνάπαυλαν, πάντως ἐξασθενεῖ καὶ πολλῶν κακῶν αἴτιος τῷ ζῴῳ γενήσεται, ἀναίσθητον αὐτὸ καὶ ἀκίνητον τῷ καμάτῳ τῆς ἀεννάου κινήσεως ἐργασάμενος. εἰκὸς οὖν ἦν καὶ τὸν ἐγκέφαλον ἀναπαύσεως δεῖσθαι καὶ τὸ ἐφεξῆς ἀμέμπτως ἐνεργεῖν· καὶ δὴ φιλοτιμεῖται αὐτῷ ἡ φύσις διὰ τοῦ ὕπνου τὴν ἄνεσιν.

Ἐν δὲ τῷ τρίτῳ κεφαλαίῳ τὸν τρόπον τῆς γενέσεως τοῦ ὕπνου διεξερχόμεθα. ἰστέον οὖν, ὅτι γίνεται ὁ ὕπνος τρόπῳ τοιῷδε· ἐπειδὴ μάλιστα μετὰ τὴν τροφὴν εἰς ὕπνον ἑαυτοὺς τρέπειν εἰώθαμεν φυσικῶς, συνωθουμένης καὶ συννευούσης ἐν τῷ βάθει τῆς φύσεως περὶ τὴν τῆς τροφῆς ἐργασίαν καὶ τοῦ ἐμφύτου θερμοῦ ἐκεῖσε συντρέχοντος ἀτμοί τινες χρηστοὶ ἐν τῇ ζυμώσει τῶν σιτίων πεττομένων γινόμενοι ἐπὶ τὸν ἐγκέφαλον ἀναδίδονται, οἵτινες ἐπιτέγγουσιν αὐτὸν καὶ ὑγρότερον ἀπεργάζονται, ἔτι γε μὴν καὶ τὰς κοιλίας ἐμφράττουσι καὶ τὸ ψυχικὸν πνεῦμα ἀπολαμβάνουσιν, ᾧτινι ὡς ὀργάνῳ χρωμένη ἡ ψυχὴ πᾶσαν ἑαυτῆς ἐπιτελεῖ τὴν ἐνέργειαν. τοῦτο γὰρ χορηγούμενον ἐπὶ τὰ αἰσθητήρια καὶ πανταχοῦ τοῦ σώματος διηκόντων τῶν νεύρων ἐπεγείρει αὐτὰ εἰς ἐνέργειαν. τούτου οὖν στερούμενον τὸ σῶμα ἀνενέργητον ἀποτελεῖται· αὐτός τε ὁ ἐγκέφαλος ἐμφραττόμενος τῇ περιουσίᾳ τῆς ὑγρότητος ἀπείργεται τῆς ψυχικῆς ὡς εἰπεῖν ἀποφοιτώσης. ταύτης τοιγαροῦν ὡς οἷόν τε ἠρεμούσης καὶ τῶν φυσικῶν δυνάμεων δραστικώτερον ἐνεργουσῶν ἡ καταλαμβάνουσα τὸ σῶμα διάθεσις ὕπνος ὀνομάζεται. ἀδύνατον δὲ ἦν παντελῶς ἀκαταύγαστον γενέσθαι τὸ σῶμα ἔτι ὑπνοῦντος τοῦ ζῴου· διὰ τοῦτο οὖν ἀμυδρῶς πως καὶ ἐν τοῖς ὕπνοις ἐλλάμπεται, ὡς δηλοῖ ἡ τοῦ θώρακος κίνησις καὶ οἱ ὄνειροι, ἀκτινοειδῶς διαδιδράσκοντος διὰ τῆς ἀτμώδους φύσεως τοῦ ψυχικοῦ πνεύματος καὶ τὰς εἰρημένας ἀμυδρῶς ἐπιτελοῦντος ἐνεργείας, ὅπερ καὶ ἐπὶ τοῦ ἡλίου καὶ τοῦ νέφους γίνεται.

Ἀκόλουθον οὖν εἰπεῖν τὸ ἐκ τοῦ ὕπνου γινόμενον τῷ παντὶ σώματι χρήσιμον. συννεύοντος τοῦ ἐν ἡμῖν θερμοῦ κατὰ τοὺς ὕπνους ἐν τῷ βάθει ἐνταῦθά τε ἀπὸ τῆς ἐπιφανείας γινομένου ψύχεσθαι μὲν ἀνάγκη τὰ ἐκτός, ὡς δηλοῖ τὸ περιβλημάτων ἡμᾶς καὶ σκεπασμάτων δεῖσθαι ἐν τοῖς ὕπνοις, ἐπιτεταμένως δὲ καὶ δραστηρίως θάλπεσθαι τὸ βάθος. ἐν γὰρ τῇ ἡμέρᾳ καὶ ἐπὶ τὰ ἐντὸς μερίζεται τὸ ἐν ἡμῖν θερμὸν καὶ ἐπὶ τὰ ἐκτός. ταύτης οὖν τῆς θερμότητος πολλαπλασιαζομένης ἐν τοῖς ὕπνοις κατὰ τὸ βάθος κατὰ λόγον αἱ πέψεις γίνονται· χυλοποίησις, ἐξαιμάτωσις, πρόσφυσις, θρέψις, διάκρισις τοῦ χυμοῦ. καὶ ὅτι ταῦτα πάντα ἀληθῆ, ἡ ἐγρήγορσις πιστοῦται· ἐξ ὕπνου γὰρ ἀναστάντες ἐπὶ τὴν ἔκκρισιν τῶν περιττωμάτων τρεπόμεθα· οὖρον ἀποθέσθαι ἐπειγόμεθα καὶ ἀποπατῆσαι κατὰ τὸ στερεὸν περίττωμα συνωθούμεθα. δυσὶ γὰρ τούτοις ἐτίμησε τὸ ζῷον ἡ φύσις, ὕπνῳ καὶ ἐγρηγόρσει, τὸ μὲν διὰ τὴν τοῦ σώματος ἀνάπαυσιν καὶ τὴν τῆς πέψεως ἀκρίβειαν, τὸ δὲ διὰ τὴν τῆς ψυχῆς πρᾶξιν καὶ τὴν τῶν περιττωμάτων ἀπόθεσιν. ἐδεδοίκει γάρ, μή τι μετὰ τὴν ἐντελῆ πέψιν τὰ περιττὰ τῷ σώματι ἐμβραδύνοντα παχυνθῇ καὶ πλημυρήσῃ καὶ βαρήσῃ τὴν δύ-

28–34 γίνονται] *cf.* Steph. Ad Glauc.: I 252,25–28 Dietz *infra*, vol. II, fol. 125v

8 καὶ[I]] *fort.* πρὸς *scribendum est* 15 ἐπιτάττουσιν P 18 διηκούντων A 22 φυσικῶν] ψυχικῶν A 23 ἦν *scripsi*: ἡ A: εἶ P 25 δηλ˜ A 38 τούτων A 38 *et* 39 τὸ] *fort.* τῷ *scribendum est* 40 ἐδεδείκει A: ἐδεδόκει P: *correxi* γάρ *om.* A 41 ἐμβραδύναντα P

part whatsoever of the body. Indeed, we cannot even move a fingertip or a little finger without the brain being moved, since any voluntary motion that takes place in us is preceded by imagination, and imagination is a function of the brain. So if the brain with all this manifold motion is to have neither reprieve nor repose, it will inevitably weaken and cause great damage to the organism by depriving it of sense and motion as a result of the exhaustion due to everlasting action. It was obvious, then, that the brain, too, needed rest, after which it could go on to function faultlessly; and thus nature bestowed upon it such relaxation through sleep.

The third point we will discuss is the manner in which sleep originates. Sleep is brought about in the following way: since the most natural time to go to sleep is after meals, it happens while the natural forces concentrate and converge in the depth for the purpose of digesting the food, and while the innate heat accumulates there, that certain benign vapors, produced by fermentation in the process of concoction of the food, mount to the brain; they flood it and increase its moisture, and furthermore they block up its cavities and intercept the psychic pneuma, which the soul uses as an instrument for the exercise of all its activities. For it is this pneuma which, distributed among the organs of sense, since the nerves extend through every part of the body, stimulates them to action. The body, deprived of it, becomes inert, while the brain itself, blocked by the excess of moisture, is debarred from the psychic faculty, which in a manner of speaking has departed from it. When, therefore, this faculty is at rest as far as is possible and the natural faculties increase their activity, the resulting condition of the body is called sleep. It was impossible, however, that the body should remain entirely devoid of irradiation while the organism is asleep; therefore it is illuminated dimly even during sleep, as is proved by the movement of the chest and by dreams; the psychic pneuma escapes diffusely through the vaporous substance and by its dim glimmer effects the said activities, just as it happens in the case of sunlight and a cloud.

Our next point is to explain the gain that accrues to the entire body through sleep. When in sleep our internal heat converges in the inner depths and thus recedes from the surface, the outside will inevitably cool off, as our need of blankets and cover during sleep proves, while the inmost part is warmed intensely and efficaciously. The reason is that in the daytime our inner heat is divided between the inside and the outside. When in sleep that heat is multiplied within, the process of digestion takes place normally: conversion into chyle, into blood, adhesion, nutrition, segregation of the humor. The truth of all this is borne out by the waking up: as soon as we get up from sleep, we go to discharge the remainders; we are in a hurry to pass water and we feel the urge to excrete solid feces. These are the two gifts of nature to the organism, sleep and waking, the one for the sake of rest for the body and total digestion, the other for the sake of conscious activity and the discharge of waste matter. Otherwise there would be the danger that after complete digestion the waste matter, remaining in the body, should thicken and overflow, overtax our strength and choke and extinguish

ναμιν καὶ καταπνίξῃ καὶ ἀποσβέσῃ τὸ ἔμφυτον θερμόν. οὐ μόνον δὲ τῆς εἰρημένης πέψεως κατὰ λόγον γινομένης αἴτιος ἡμῖν ὁ ὕπνος γίνεσθαι δείκνυται, ἀλλὰ καὶ τῆς τῶν ὑλῶν πέψεως οὐδὲν ἧττον ἀφορμὴ καὶ πρόφασις τῇ φύσει τυγχάνει· ἐν τούτῳ γὰρ τὰ μὲν παχέα λεπτύνεται, τὰ δὲ λεπτὰ καὶ δριμέα συμμέτρως παχύνεται. ἢ οὐ πολλάκις ὀδύνας ὀφθαλμῶν ἐπὶ λεπτῷ καὶ δριμεῖ ῥεύματι παροξυνομένας καὶ ῥευματικὰς ἄρθρων διαθέσεις γινομένας ἔπαυσε, πῇ μὲν ἀνακοπέντος τοῦ ῥεύματος, πῇ δὲ τῆς δυσκρασίας ἐπικερασθείσης;

Ἔστι δ' ὅτε οὐ μόνον πολλάκις οὐκ ἔπαυσε ῥευματισμὸν ἢ καὶ ὀδύνην ὁ ὕπνος, ἀλλὰ καὶ ἐπέτεινεν, ἡνίκα τις ἀσθενεστέρα ὑπέκειτο δύναμις καὶ πολλὰ ἐν τῷ σώματι τὰ περιττώματα. τί γάρ; ὅτι κινεῖται μὲν ταῦτα ἐν τοῖς ὕπνοις τῇ εἰς βάθος συννεύσει τοῦ θερμοῦ, μὴ δυνηθέντα δὲ πεφθῆναι ἢ διαφορηθῆναι διὰ τὴν τῆς δυνάμεως ἀσθένειαν κατὰ τῶν ἀσθενεστέρων ἐχώρησε τόπων, ὅπερ ἐν ταῖς εἰσβολαῖς μάλιστα τῶν παροξυσμῶν συμβαίνει, ἡνίκα διεγείρομεν τοὺς κάμνοντας μὴ συγχωροῦντες αὐτοὺς καθευδῆσαι τὸ σύνολον δεδιότες, μὴ τῇ εἰς βάθος ὑποστολῇ τῆς φύσεως ἐπαναστῇ τὰ περιττώματα καὶ καταπνίξῃ τὸ ἔμφυτον θερμόν. εἰκὼν δὲ τοῦ λόγου τὸ ἐπὶ τῆς ἐκτὸς πυρᾶς συμβαῖνον, ἡνίκα ἀσθενεστέρᾳ φλογὶ πολλὰ καὶ ὑγρὰ ἐπιβληθῇ ξύλα ἢ τοὔμπαλιν δαψιλεῖ φλογὶ τροφὴ ὀλίγη καὶ ξηρά. καὶ εἰ μὲν ἐν ἀρχῇ παροξυσμοῦ, ὥς φησιν ὁ Γαληνός, τὸ τοιοῦτον συμβαίη, εἰ καὶ ἐπισφαλές, ἀλλ' οὐκ ὀλέθριον· ὅσον γὰρ οὔπω ἐξαφθήσεται τὰ τῆς θερμασίας καὶ τῶν περιττωμάτων τὸ φρύαγμα καταστραφήσεται. ⟨. . .⟩ καὶ μάλιστα ἐν παρακμῇ, πῇ μὲν διὰ τὸν ἀγῶνα καὶ πάλην τῆς φύσεως, πῇ δὲ διὰ τὸ μετὰ τὸν κάματον ἐνέδρας τινὸς χάριν ἀπροόπτως καταδυναστεῦσαι τὰ περιττώματα.

Τοῦτο δηλῶν ἐνταῦθα ὁ Ἱπποκράτης φησίν· Ἐν ᾧ νοσήματι ὕπνος πόνον ποιέει, θανάσιμον. καὶ ζητητέον, ἐπὶ ποίου νοσήματος ἢ σημαινομένου συντέθηται τὸ ὕπνος πόνον ποιέει. ἔθος γὰρ τῷ Ἱπποκράτει πόνους καλεῖν καὶ τὰ γυμνάσια· οὕτω γοῦν φησι· «Πόνοι σιτίων ἡγείσθωσαν», ἀντὶ τοῦ «Γυμνάζειν δεῖ πρὸ τῆς τροφῆς τὰ σώματα». πόνον καλεῖ καὶ τὴν ὀδύνην ἐν οἷς φησι· «Δύο πόνων ἅμα γιγνομένων μὴ κατὰ τὸν αὐτὸν τόπον ὁ σφοδρότερος ἀμαυροῖ τὸν ἕτερον.» ὡσαύτως δὲ καὶ κατὰ τῶν συμπτωμάτων τὸ τοῦ πόνου ἐπιφέρειν εἴωθεν ὄνομα, ὡς ὅταν λέγῃ· «Ὅκου μὲν οὖν κάτοξυ τὸ νόσημα, αὐτίκα καὶ τοὺς ἐσχάτους πόνους ἔχει». καθ' ὃ σημαινόμενον καὶ ἐν τῷ παρόντι λόγῳ τὸ τοῦ πόνου τέθηκεν ὄνομα. καὶ νόμιζε τὸν Ἱπποκράτην ταῦτά σοι λέγειν· σκόπει τοὺς ὕπνους ἐπὶ τῶν νοσούντων· καὶ εἰ μὲν τούτοις πέττονται αἱ ὗλαι, σωτήριον δηλοῦται τὸ νόσημα· εἰ δ' αὖ οὐ μόνον αὗται οὐ πεφθῶσιν, ἀλλὰ καὶ κακόν τινα μετεωρισμὸν δέξονται, ἢ μὴ ὄντα ἐφελκύσουσι, κεφαλαλγίαν ἢ λιποθυμίαν ἢ φλεγμονὴν ἤ τι τοιοῦτον, ἢ ὄντα καὶ προκείμενα αὐξήσουσι, κακὸν τὸ σημεῖον καὶ θανατωδέστατον.

10–16 θερμόν] *v.* Gal. In Aphor. II 1: XVII B 452,13–453,2 K. 16 εἰκὼν – 18 ξηρά] *cf.* Gal. De crisib. III 9: IX 744,11–13 K. Steph. Ad Glauc.: I 277,30–278,5 Dietz 18 καὶ – 22] *v.* Theoph. In Aphor.: II 295,6–296,4 Dietz καὶ – 20 καταστραφήσεται] *cf.* Gal. In Aphor. II 1: XVII B 452,4–6 K. 20 ⟨. . .⟩ – 22] *cf.* Gal. In Aphor. II 1: XVII B 453,11–454,5; 454,14–19 K. 23–32 ὄνομα] *v.* Theoph. In Aphor.: II 295,2–6 Dietz 25 ἔθος – 27] *cf.* Gal. In Aphor. II 16: XVII B 474,8–11 K. 26 Πόνοι – ἡγείσθωσαν] Hipp. Epid. VI 4,23: V 314,3 L. 27sq. Δύο – ἕτερον] Hipp. Aphor. II 46: IV 482,15–16 L. 30sq. Ὅκου – ἔχει] Hipp. Aphor. I 7: IV 462,12–13 L.

4 παχεῖα A 19 ὅσω *ex* ὅσου *mut.* A ἐξαναφθήσεται *Theoph.* 20 καστασταλήσεται *Theoph.* *lac. indicavi, cf. Theoph. In Aphor.: II 295,12–296,4 Dietz* 21 πάλιν α: *correxi* 34 κακοῦ τινος A 35 ἐφελήνσουσι P

the innate heat. But sleep proves to be not only the cause of the normal course of digestion as described, but it is also, for nature, an incentive to, and an opportunity for, the concoction of redundant matter, since in sleep thick substances are comminuted, while thin and sharp ones are thickened to the right degree. Does not sleep often put an end to pain in the eyes resulting from irritation by a thin, pungent flux, as well as to arthritic conditions of the joints, the flux being checked in the first case, and the temperamental disorder corrected by admixture in the second?

There are other, frequent instances when sleep, so far from curing rheumatism or pain, increases them; this happens when for some reason strength was already deficient and a great deal of waste matter is present in the body. Why? Because this matter is disturbed in sleep owing to the inward convergence of the heat, but when it cannot be concocted or dispersed through lack of strength, it finds its way to the weaker places; this occurs especially during the onset of paroxysms; we then rouse the patients, not allowing them to go to sleep at all, lest as a result of the inward retreat of the natural strength the waste matter should rise in revolt and overwhelm the innate heat. An illustration of this point is what happens to a fire in the outside world, when a great quantity of wet wood is thrown upon a weak flame, or, conversely, a small quantity of dry fuel into a blazing fire. If, Galen says, this kind of thing happens at the beginning of a paroxysm, it is dangerous, but not pernicious: the heat will soon be rekindled and the uproar of the waste matter will be quelled. +During the increase, the acme and the abatement, sleep is as a rule manifestly beneficial, and most of all so during the abatement; but it is a deadly sign if sleep causes harm at those times,+ [1] especially during the abatement, partly owing to the battle which nature has fought, partly because after this exhausting fight the waste matter, by a sort of surprise attack, may suddenly get the upper hand.

This is what Hippocrates means here, when he says: A disease in which sleep causes distress, is deadly. And we must pose the question, to what disease the phrase sleep causes distress (*ponos*) relates, and what it signifies. Hippocrates frequently uses the word *ponos* in the sense of exercise; thus he says, "Exertion should precede food", i.e. "One should take exercise before meals". He uses *ponos* also to denote pain, where he says: "When two pains occur simultaneously, but not in the same place, the more violent one obscures the other." Similarly, he often applies the word *ponos* to symptoms, as when he says: "When the disease is very acute, (the patient) is immediately in extreme discomfort"; and it is in this sense that he uses the word *ponos* in the present passage. You may conclude that what Hippocrates tells you is this: Pay attention to the patient's sleep; if during it the matter is concocted, it proves that the disease is curable; if, on the other hand, instead of being concocted, it shows a fatal rise, or evokes symptoms that were not there, such as headache, swooning or inflammation, or if it enhances these symptoms when they were already present, this is a bad and a most deadly sign.

[1] +During – times+: see the app. crit.

Καὶ ὁ μὲν Ἱπποκράτης μερικὸν ἐποιήσατο τὸν λόγον, ἐπὶ ὕπνου καὶ μόνου θεωρήσας τὰ συμπτώματα τῇ ἰσχύι τῶν συμβαινόντων τὸ κῦρος ἀποδιδούς. ὁ γὰρ ὕπνος οὐ κατὰ πρῶτον λόγον κινεῖ τὰς ὕλας, ἀλλὰ κατὰ συμβεβηκὸς τοῦτο ποιεῖ τῆς δυνάμεως ἡττωμένης ὥστε μὴ ἰσχύειν αὐτὰς ἐκπέψαι. πολλάκις μὲν οὖν ὁ ὕπνος οὐ μόνον οὐδὲν ἐπιφέρει κακόν, ἀλλὰ καὶ ὠφέλησεν· ἣν δὲ φαύλως ἔχῃ τὰ περὶ τὴν κατάκλισιν τοῦ νοσοῦντος καὶ τὴν ἀναπνοήν, ἐπικίνδυνον δηλοῖ τὴν ἔκβασιν. ὥστε οὖν μετὰ ὕπνου δεῖ καὶ τἄλλα πάντα θεωρεῖν καὶ συμφωνίαν μὲν ἀγαθὴν ποιούμενα βεβαίαν πρόγνωσιν σωτηρίας εἰσηγεῖσθαι νομίζειν· κακῶς δὲ συμφωνοῦντα τὸ ἐναντίον προλέγειν· εἰ δὲ ἀσύμφωνα εἶεν, ἢ τοῖς πλείοσιν ἢ τοῖς ἰσχυροτέροις δίδου τὴν πίστιν.

Καὶ τοῦτο δὲ δεῖ γινώσκειν, ὅτι, ὥσπερ ἀνωτέρω τὰ ὁμοειδῆ συγκρίνων ἡλικίαν ἡλικίᾳ παρέβαλλε καὶ ὥραν ὥρᾳ ἀντεξήταζεν, οὕτω καὶ νῦν ὁμοειδῶν ποιεῖται τὴν σύγκρισιν· ὕπνον γὰρ ὕπνῳ συγκρίνει καὶ οὐχ ὕπνον ἐγρηγόρσει. φησὶ γὰρ οὕτως· Ἐν ᾧ νοσήματι ὕπνος πόνον ποιέει, θανάσιμον· ἢν δὲ ὕπνος ὠφελέῃ, οὐ θανάσιμον. εἶτα καὶ παραδείγματα τοῦ λόγου σαφηνείας ἕνεκεν τίθησιν· [II 2: IV 470,11 L.] Ὅκου παραφροσύνην ὕπνος παύει, ἀγαθόν. καί φησιν ὁ Γαληνός, ὅτι δεῖ καινοτομῆσαι τὴν λέξιν καὶ τὸν «γὰρ» καταθεῖναι σύνδεσμον, ὥστε μίαν ἀπαρτίζεσθαι συνέχειαν τὸν πάντα σκοπὸν περιλαμβάνουσαν, ὡς εἰ ἔλεγεν οὕτως· Ἐν ᾧ νοσήματι ὕπνος πόνον ποιέει, θανάσιμον· ἢν δὲ ὕπνος ὠφελέῃ, οὐ θανάσιμον· ὅκου γὰρ παραφροσύνην ὕπνος παύει, ἀγαθόν, ὅπερ παράδειγμά ἐστι τοῦ ἀγαθὸν εἶναι τὸν τὰ συμπτώματα παύοντα ὕπνον. καὶ αὐτὸς μὲν ἐκ τοῦ κατ' ἐξαίρετον τὴν τοῦ λογισμοῦ βλάβην ἔλαβε, παυομένην ἐπὶ τοῦ ὕπνου, ὡς ἀγαθὸν σύμβολον σωτηρίας· σὺ δὲ εἰπέ, ὅτι καὶ ὀδύνην ἐὰν παύσῃ, ἀγαθόν, καὶ φλεγμονὴν ἐὰν συμπέψῃ, ἀγαθόν, καὶ ῥεῦμα ἐὰν ἀνακόψῃ καὶ ἀποκρούσηται, οὐδὲν ἧττον ἀγαθόν, καθολικὸν τὸν λόγον ποιούμενος.

II 2 [II 3: IV 470,12–13 L.] Ὕπνος, ἀγρυπνίη, ἀμφότερα μᾶλλον τοῦ μετρίου γινόμενα κακόν.

Ὡς τινος ἀπορεῖν μέλλοντος· «Εἰ ὁ ὕπνος ἐπὶ τῶν τοιούτων νοσημάτων μεγίστης βλάβης αἴτιος γίνεται, ἡ ἐγρήγορσις δηλονότι ἀνακόπτει τὴν βλάβην· μήποτε οὖν χρὴ τοὺς οὕτω πάσχοντας, κἂν ποτε εἰς ὕπνον τραπῶσι, διεγείρειν καὶ ἐγρήγορσιν ἐμποιεῖν· εἰ γὰρ τῷ ὕπνῳ ἡ βλάβη ἕπεται, τῇ ἐγρηγόρσει πάντως ὡς ἐναντίῳ ἡ ὠφέλεια ἕποιτ' ἄν» – ταῦτα οὖν διορθούμενος ὁ Ἱπποκράτης λέγει· οὐχ ὁ ὕπνος ὀλέθριον, ἀλλ' ἡ κακοήθεια τοῦ νοσήματος ⟨ . . . ⟩ σημεῖον γίνεται. τοῖς μὲν γὰρ ἄλλοις σώμασι παντὸς ἀγαθοῦ παραίτιός ἐστιν, ἐπὶ δὲ τοῦ χαλεπῷ κατεχομένου νοσήματι οὐδ' αὐτὸς ὁ εὐεργετῆσαι δυνάμενος τὸν κάμνοντα ὤνησεν. οὐ μὴν ἀλλὰ καὶ ἡ ἄμετρος ἀγρυπνία κακή ἐστι καὶ ἐπιβλαβής. κακὸς τοίνυν καὶ ὁ ὕπνος καὶ ἡ ἀγρυπνία, ὅταν πλέον γένωνται τοῦ μετρίου, τῇ γὰρ συμμετρίᾳ χαίρει ἡ φύσις.

Ἰστέον δέ, ὅτι καὶ ὁ ὕπνος καὶ ἡ ἀγρυπνία τῶν πρός τί ἐστι· πρὸς γὰρ τὴν

11 ἀνωτέρω] *v.* Hipp. Aphor. I 13–18: IV 466,5–468,4 L. 16 καί – 21 ὕπνον] *v.* Gal. In Aphor. II 2: XVII B 456,2–6 K. 21 καὶ – 25] *v.* Gal. In Aphor. II 2: XVII B 456,6–11 K.

4 ἐκπέμψαι P 5 φαῦλος P ἔχει A 12 παρέβαλε P 13 ὕπνον[I]] ὕπνω A 14 ὠφελέει *in* ὠφελέῃ *corr.* A[2] 15 *fort.* παράδειγμα *scribendum est* 26 Ὕπνον α: *corr.* A[2] 28 ἀπορεῖν μέλλοντος] ἀποροῦντος A 32 ἕποιτ'] ἕπειτ' P 33 *lac. indicavi, supple fere* ἧς ὁ ὕπνος 37 γένονται α: *correxi*

Hippocrates deals with one particular aspect, by studying the symptoms with reference to sleep only; the decisive point to him is the strength of the actual events. The fact is that sleep does not stir up the diseased matter directly, but it does so incidentally, when resistance is too weak to concoct it. Often, therefore, sleep, so far from causing any harm, is beneficial; but if the patient's posture and his breathing are wrong, this indicates that the issue may be fatal. It follows that, in conjunction with sleep, one should consider all the other circumstances, and if they are uniformly favorable, one may feel free to make a confident prediction of recovery; or, if they are uniformly bad, one may prognosticate the contrary; but if they disagree, you may trust either the majority or the stronger indications.

It should further be noted that, just as above he compared things of the same kind, setting age group against age group and contrasting season with season, so here, too, he compares like with like, that is, sleep with sleep, not sleep with the waking state. He says: *A disease in which sleep causes distress, is deadly; but if sleep brings relief, it is not deadly.* Then he adds examples to illustrate his point: *Where sleep puts an end to delirium, this is a good sign.* *Galen* proposes to alter the text by inserting the conjunction "for", so that one continuous sentence is formed comprising the entire purport of the argument, as if he had written: *A disease in which sleep causes distress, is deadly; but if sleep brings relief, it is not deadly; for where sleep puts an end to delirium, this is a good sign*, as an example of the beneficial effect of a sleep which cures the symptoms. Now (*Hippocrates*) himself has selected the most striking case, that of damage to the reasoning faculty redressed by sleep, as an encouraging token of recovery; but you yourself can add that it is also a good sign, if it puts an end to pain, and that it is a good sign, if it concocts an inflammation, and that it is no less good, if it checks and suppresses a rheumatic condition, thus giving the statement universal validity.

II 2. *Sleep and sleeplessness are both bad signs, if in excess of the normal.*

As if someone is going to object: "If, in diseases of this kind, sleep becomes a cause of the greatest harm, obviously being awake will control the harm; so perhaps we should wake up patients in this condition, even when they fall asleep, and we should induce a state of remaining awake; for if the harm results from sleep, improvement will necessarily come from waking, as its opposite"; – *Hippocrates*, to correct this idea, says: It is not the sleep that is deadly, but the malignancy of the disease, +of which the sleep+[1] is a sign. To other bodies it is beneficial in every way, but in the case of a grave disease, even this potential benefactor is of no use to the patient. On the other hand, excessive sleeplessness is also bad and harmful. Thus both sleep and sleeplessness in excess of the normal are bad, since nature likes right proportion.

Note, however, that sleep and sleeplessness are relative, in that they happen

[1] +of – sleep+: see the app. crit.

διάφορον ἡλικίαν καὶ τὴν διάφορον ὥραν ἐπιγίνεται, καὶ τινὶ μὲν κατὰ φύσιν, ἑτέρῳ δὲ παρὰ φύσιν ἐστίν. οἱ μὲν γὰρ παῖδες πλείους τῶν ὀκτὼ ὡρῶν καθεύδειν πεφύκασιν· ἐπὶ τοσοῦτον δὲ ἢν ὁ ἀκμάζων καθευδήσῃ, ἀμέτρως ὑπνοῖ, οἱ γὰρ ἀκμάζοντες ἓξ ὥρας τὸ μήκιστον καθεύδειν δύνανται τῷ λόγῳ τῆς ξηρότητος. ὁμοίως ἐν χειμῶνι πλείους ὥρας καθεύδειν πεφύκαμεν διὰ τὸ τῶν νυκτῶν μέγεθος, ἐν δὲ τῷ θέρει ἧττον καθεύδομεν διά τε τὴν βραχύτητα τῶν νυκτῶν καὶ τὸ ἐρεθιστικὸν τοῦ ἔτους, καυσώδους ἡμῖν περικειμένου ἀέρος. τούτων οὖν οὕτως ἐχόντων ἐὰν ἐν θέρει πολλὰ καθευδήσωμεν, ἐν χειμῶνι δὲ ὀλίγον, ἀσύμμετρος ὁ ὕπνος γίνεται.

Ἔστι δὲ καὶ ἕτερος διορισμός, ὅστις ἀπὸ καιροῦ λαμβάνεται, οἷον ἐάν τις ἐν νυκτὶ μὲν ἀγρυπνῇ, ἐν ἡμέρᾳ δὲ εἰς ὕπνον ἕλκηται· ἢ ἐάν τις πυρετοῦ πολλοῦ καὶ διακαοῦς ἐπὶ σηπεδόνι ἀναπτομένου καὶ ζέσεως ἐπικειμένης ὕπνῳ βέβληται καὶ ῥέγχειν δοκεῖ, ἀσύμμετροι οἱ τοιοῦτοι ὕπνοι διὰ τὸ μὴ ἐν καιρῷ δέοντι γίνεσθαι. ὁ μὲν γὰρ ὀφείλων ἐκ τῆς ζέσεως τοῦ πυρετοῦ διεγηγερμένως καὶ ἐν ἀγρυπνίᾳ διατελεῖν κωματωδῶς δηλονότι καθεύδει καὶ ἀποπληξίαν μηνύει· ὁ δὲ δυσφημίας τινὸς ὑποπιπτούσης καὶ δυσδιαφόρητον ἔχων τὴν καρδίαν, τῆς φύσεως τὴν ἀπόσβεσιν καὶ πνιγμονὴν τοῦ ἐμφύτου θερμοῦ δεδοικυίας εἰς νύκτα μὲν οὐ καθεύδει διὰ τὴν στεγάνωσιν, ἐν ἡμέρᾳ δὲ μᾶλλον ὑπνοῖ τῇ τοῦ περιέχοντος διαφορήσει φυσικῶς θαρρῶν.

Δεῖ δέ σε εἰδέναι, ὅτι ὁ ἀσύμμετρος ὕπνος καὶ ἡ ἐγρήγορσις καὶ ὡς σημεῖα καὶ ὡς αἴτια κακά ἐστιν· ὁ μὲν ὕπνος ὡς σημεῖον, ἐπειδὴ δηλοῖ πλῆθος ὕλης καὶ ἀσθένειαν δυνάμεως, ὡς αἴτιον δέ, ἐπειδὴ ἐπιτείνει τὸ πλῆθος μὴ συγχωρῶν αὐτὸ διαφορηθῆναι, αἱ γὰρ διαφορήσεις ἐν τῇ ἐγρηγόρσει γίνονται. ἡ δὲ ἐγρήγορσις ὡς μὲν σημεῖον πολλὴν ἐνδείκνυται ξηρότητα, ὡς δὲ αἴτιον, ἐπειδὴ ταύτην ἐπιτείνει τῇ διαφορήσει. ἐνταῦθα δὲ τὴν ἀγρυπνίαν ἀντὶ τῆς ἐγρηγόρσεως εἴρηκεν ὁ Ἱπποκράτης.

Ἀποροῦσι δέ τινες λέγοντες ὅτι «Οὐδέποτε ὁ ὕπνος πέφυκε κακόν τι ἐργάζεσθαι ἀεὶ ἐν συμμετρίᾳ θεωρούμενος· ὁ δὲ ἄμετρος οὐχ ὕπνος, ἀλλὰ κῶμα λέγεται.» φαμὲν οὖν, ὅτι ἄλλο κῶμα καὶ ἄλλο μακρὸς ὕπνος, καὶ ταῦτα διορίζει ἡ δυσχερὴς καὶ εὐχερὴς ἐξανάστασις. οἱ γὰρ ὑπνοῦντες διεγειρόμενοι μετά τινος κραυγῆς ἢ δονήσεως ἑτοίμως εἰς ἐγρήγορσιν ἄγονται, ὁ δὲ κωματωδῶς καθεύδων οὐδὲ μετ' ἐπιτάσεως τῶν διατάσεων ἐγρηγορέναι δύναται· βεβλαμμένας γὰρ ἔχει τὰς αἰσθητικὰς ἐνεργείας διὰ τὸ τὸν ἐγκέφαλον πάσχειν καὶ νοσώδη εἶναι. ἄλλως τε τὸ μὲν κῶμα καὶ ποσότητι τῆς ψυχρᾶς ὕλης καὶ ποιότητι τῇ ὑγραινούσῃ τὸν ἐγκέφαλον γίνεται, ὁ δὲ μακρὸς ὕπνος ὑγρότητι μόνῃ. οὐκ ἠγνόησεν οὖν ὁ Ἱπποκράτης, ὡς διαφέρει μακρὸς ὕπνος κώματος, ἀλλ' ἐπιστάμενος, ὅτι χωρὶς κώματος ἔστι μακρὸς ὕπνος καὶ ἀγρυπνία μακρὰ ἄνευ ἐγρηγόρσεως, ἑκατέρου τὸ ἄμετρον ἐκώλυσεν.

II 3 [II 4: IV 470,14 L.] Οὐ πλησμονή, οὐ λιμός, οὐδ' ἄλλο οὐδὲν ἀγαθόν.

18–22 διαφορήσει] *cf.* Gal. In Aphor. II 3: XVII B 457,1–2 K. Theoph. In Aphor.: II 297, 9–16 Dietz 24–30 εἶναι] *cf.* Gal. In Aphor. II 3: XVII B 457,1–14 K. 24–29 δύναται] *v.* Theoph. In Aphor.: II 297,16–20 Dietz

7 ἔτους] *fort.* θέρους *scribendum est* 10 ἀγρυπνῇ *ex* ἀγρυπνεῖ *corr.* A[2] ἕλκεται A 18 ἄμετρος A 25 ἐν *om.* P 32 ὑγρότητι *scripsi*: ὑγρότητ *(ambig.)* A: ὑγρότητα P 34 ἐκάλεσεν P

proportionally to the different ages and seasons, and while normal for the one, they are abnormal for the other. For children it is natural to sleep over eight hours; but if a man in his prime sleeps as long as that, he sleeps too much, for those in their prime can sleep six hours at most because of their dry constitution. Similarly, in winter it is natural for us to sleep for more hours owing to the length of the nights, but in summer we sleep less because of the shortness of the nights and the restlessness caused by the summer weather, when we are surrounded by scorching hot air. This being so, much sleep in summer, and little sleep in winter, become disproportionate.

There is still another specification, derived from time, namely when a man is sleepless at night, but drops off to sleep in the daytime; or if, in a case of a strong, burning fever kindled upon putrefaction, while the patient is in a state of seething heat, sleep overcomes him and he seems to snore; then such sleep is disproportionate, because it does not come at the right moment. The man who, because of his seething fever, ought to be awake and sleepless all the time, lies in an obviously comatose sleep, which points to apoplexy; the other, owing to some bad news that has reached him, suffers from lack of dispersal in the heart, and thus, since nature fears the extinction and the smothering of the innate heat, he does not sleep at night because of the tightening of the pores, but he prefers to go to sleep in the daytime, when the dispersing action of the surrounding air restores his natural confidence.

One should be aware that disproportionate sleep and waking are bad both as symptoms and as causes; sleep is bad as a symptom, because it indicates a surplus of matter and weakness of the power of resistance, and as a cause, inasmuch as it increases the surplus by preventing its dispersal, for processes of dispersal take place in the waking state. As for waking, as a symptom it points to excessive dryness, and as a cause it aggravates this dryness by dispersal. Hippocrates here uses the word sleeplessness instead of "waking".

Some object that sleep by its very nature can never cause any harm, because it always appears in right proportion; the disproportionate kind is not called sleep, but coma. We answer that a coma and a long sleep are different; they are distinguished by the difficulty or ease with which the patient can be roused. Those who are asleep, when they have to be waked, can be readily brought back to the waking state by shouting or noise, while the patient in a comatose condition cannot be waked even by increased efforts; for his sensory activities are impaired by the fact that the brain is affected and diseased. Furthermore, coma is brought about both by the quantity of cold matter and by the quality that moistens the brain, whereas long sleep is due to moisture only. Hippocrates, then, was perfectly aware that a long sleep differs from a coma, but while knowing that a long sleep is possible without a coma and long waking without insomnia, he warned against excess in both.

II 3. Neither repletion nor hunger, nor anything else is good.

Φησίν, ὅτι οὐ μόνον ὁ ὕπνος καὶ ἡ ἐγρήγορσις ἀσυμμέτρως ἐπιγινόμενα κακόν ἐστιν, ἀλλὰ καὶ πλησμονὴ καὶ κόρος ὑπερβάλλων καὶ λιμὸς ἐπιτεταμένος ἐπιβλαβὴς τυγχάνει τοῖς σώμασι, καὶ σκληρότης καὶ μαλακότης, καὶ πυκνότης καὶ ἀραιότης, θερμασία καὶ ψῦξις, ἴσχναν σις καὶ πάχυνσις, καὶ πάντα τὰ πλεῖστον ἀλλήλων διεστῶτα. οὕτως ἀπὸ τῶν μερικῶν ἐπὶ τὰ καθόλου τὴν μέθοδον ἀνήγαγε. πλησμονὴ μέντοι καὶ λιμὸς ἐναντίον, ὧν μετὰ τὸν ὕπνον καὶ τὴν ἐγρήγορσιν ἐμνημόνευσεν ὡς αἰτίων ἐκείνων· ὁ μὲν γὰρ πολὺς ὕπνος τῇ πλησμονῇ τῶν βρωμάτων γίνεται, ἡ δὲ ἐπιτεταμένη ἀγρυπνία τῷ ὑπερβάλλοντι λιμῷ ξηρότητα τοῖς σώμασι καὶ αὐτῷ τῷ ἐγκεφάλῳ ἐμποιοῦντι.

II 4 [II 5: IV 470,16 L.] Κόποι αὐτόματοι φράζουσι νούσους.

Ἰστέον, ὅτι ὁ κόπος διττὸς ἐν τῷ καθόλου· ὁ μὲν γὰρ ἐπὶ προκαταρκτικῇ γίνεται αἰτίᾳ ἀσυμμέτρου προληφθέντος τοῦ γυμνασίου, ὁ δὲ ἐπὶ προηγουμένῃ. νῦν οὖν οὐ περὶ τοῦ ἐπὶ προκαταρκτικῇ αἰτίᾳ γινομένου κόπου ὁ λόγος τῷ Ἱπποκράτει, ἀλλὰ [καὶ] περὶ ⟨τοῦ⟩ ἐπὶ προηγουμένῃ αἰτίᾳ, ὡς δηλοῖ διὰ τοῦ εἰπεῖν αὐτόματοι, τοῦ αὐτομάτου ἀφ' ἑαυτοῦ γινομένου καὶ ἀφανῶς καὶ οὐ κατ' αἴσθησιν ἔχοντος τὴν αἰτίαν. μεμάθηκας οὖν, ὅτι τῆς αἰτίας τὰ μὲν δῆλα, τὰ δὲ ἄδηλα. οὗτος ὁ κόπος τριχῶς γίνεται· καὶ ὁ μὲν λέγεται ἑλκώδης, ὅστις ὅταν ὥσπερ ἢ ἀπὸ βελόνης ἢ ἀκανθῶν τινων νύττεσθαι δοκῶμεν γίνεται· ὁ δὲ λέγεται τονώδης, οἵτινες τείνεσθαι καὶ διασπᾶσθαι δοκοῦσι καὶ ῥήγνυσθαι· ὁ δὲ λέγεται ὀστοκοπώδης, ὅστις ἀμφότερα τὸ σῶμα πάσχειν ποιεῖ, δοκεῖ γὰρ ἐκτείνεσθαι ἅμα καὶ νύττεσθαι. καὶ ὁ μὲν ἑλκώδης ἐπὶ δριμέσι χυμοῖς γίνεται, ὁ δὲ τονώδης ἐπὶ πλήθει καὶ παχείᾳ ὕλῃ, ὁ δὲ ὀστοκοπώδης ἐπὶ πολλοῖς ἅμα καὶ δριμέσι χυμοῖς. ὥστε ἐντεῦθεν καὶ τὴν θεραπείαν ὑποτυποῦσθαι συμβαίνει ἐκ τοῦ τὸν πόνον ποιοῦντος χυμοῦ τὴν ἔνδειξιν τῆς ἰάσεως ποιουμένους. διὸ ἐπὶ μὲν τοῦ ἑλκώδους καθάρσει χρηστέον, ἐπὶ δὲ τοῦ τονώδους φλεβοτομίᾳ, ἐπὶ δὲ τοῦ ὀστοκοπώδους τῷ συναμφοτέρῳ.

Σκόπει δὲ ἀκρίβειαν τοῦ παλαιοῦ εἰρηκότος· Κόποι αὐτόματοι φράζουσι νούσους, τουτέστι μηνύουσιν, οὐ πάντως δὲ ποιοῦσιν, ἐὰν φθάσας ὁ τεχνίτης προεκκόψῃ τὴν μελετωμένην ἔφοδον.

II 5 [II 6: IV 470,17–18 L.] Ὁκόσοι πονέοντές τι τοῦ σώματος τὰ πολλὰ τῶν πόνων μὴ αἰσθάνονται, τουτέοισιν ἡ γνώμη νοσεῖ.

Προειρηκὼς «Κόποι αὐτόματοι φράζουσι νούσους» καὶ πᾶσαν κακίαν καὶ βλάβην ἢ οὖσαν ἢ μελετωμένην διά τινος ἑτέρου πολυτρόπως διαλαβὼν καθολικῶς νῦν

1–5 διεστῶτα] *cf.* Gal. In Aphor. II 4: XVII B 458,12–459,2 K. 4sq. τὰ – διεστῶτα] *cf.* Aristot. Categ. 6: 6 a 17–18 5 οὕτως – ἀνήγαγε] *v.* Theoph. In Aphor.: II 298,9–11 Dietz πλησμονὴ – 9] *v.* Theoph. In Aphor.: II 298,5–9 Dietz 11–16 αἰτίαν] *cf.* Gal. In Aphor. II 5: XVII B 459,5–10 K. 16 οὗτος – 22 χυμοῖς] *v.* Gal. In Aphor. II 5: XVII B 459,10–15 K. De sanit. tuenda IV 2: CMG V 4,2, p. 104,5–106,15 De sympt. caus. II 5: VII 178,6–179,9 K. Theoph. In Aphor.: II 298,20–27 Dietz 26sq. Κόποι – μηνύουσιν] *v.* Theoph. In Aphor.: II 298,27–28 Dietz 31–150,2 ὀδύνης] *cf.* Theoph. In Aphor.: II 299,14–16 Dietz Κόποι – νούσους] Hipp. Aphor. II 5: IV 470,16 L.

2 κόρον A 10 νόσους P 12 προσληφθέντος A προηγουμένου A 13 τῶν ἱπποκράτου P: τοῦ ἱπποκράτ *(ambig.)* A: *correxi* 14 καὶ *delevi* τοῦ *addidi* 16 οὗτος α: οὗτος *ex* οὕτως *corr.* A 17 ὥσπερ *om.* A 32 διαλαβεῖν A: *fort.* διαβαλὼν *scribendum est*

He says that not only sleep and waking are bad when they come in undue measure, but that excessive repletion and satiety and intense hunger are also harmful to the body, and so are hardness and softness, deneness and rarity, heating and cooling, emaciation and fattening, and all things that are most distant from one another. Thus he has methodically progressed from the particular to the universal. As for repletion and hunger, they are opposites which he mentioned after sleep and waking because they are their causes: long sleep is brought about by repletion with food, and prolonged sleeplessness by excessive hunger, which causes dryness in the body and in the brain itself.

II 4. Spontaneous fatigue points to disease.

Generally speaking, there are two kinds of fatigue: the one results from an immediate cause, after immoderate exercise, the other from an antecedent cause. Here, Hippocrates does not refer to the fatigue resulting from an immediate cause, but to the kind that comes from an antecedent cause, as he makes clear by the word spontaneous: the spontaneous happens all by itself and it has a cause which is hidden and beyond the range of the senses. You have learnt that of causes, some are manifest, some are obscure. Such fatigue appears in three forms: the one is described as "smarting", when we seem to feel something like the pricking of a needle or thorns; the second is called "straining", when patients feel as if they were stretched and drawn and torn apart; the third is called "racking", which causes the body to suffer both: it seems to be stretched and stabbed at the same time. The "smarting" kind is caused by pungent humors, the "straining" kind by an excess of thick matter, and "racking" fatigue by humors which are both excessive in quantity and pungent. This also contains the guidelines for treatment; the cure can be inferred from the humor that causes the pain. So for smarting fatigue we must apply purging, for straining fatigue bleeding, for racking fatigue both.

Observe the ancient author's accuracy, when he says: Spontaneous fatigue points to disease, i.e. indicates it, but not necessarily causes it, if the expert takes timely action to suppress the impending attack.

II 5. Those who, while suffering some affection of the body, remain on the whole unaware of their suffering, are affected in their minds.

In the preceding he has said, "Spontaneous fatigue points to disease" and has dealt with all kinds of damage and harm, either present or impending, which in a variety of ways are brought about through something else; now he states

ἀποφαίνεται, ὅτι πᾶσα ὀδύνη ἀναισθήτως γινομένη μεῖζον κακόν ἐστι τῆς αἰσθητῆς ὀδύνης, πλείω γὰρ τὴν βλάβην καὶ κυριωτέρων μορίων δηλοῖ. αὕτη μὲν ἡ τάξις τοῦ ἀφορισμοῦ, ἡ δὲ ἔννοια ἀκολούθως εἴρηται· ἐάν τις, φησίν, ὀδυνηρὰν ἔχων διάθεσιν ἐν οἱῳδήποτε μέρει τοῦ σώματος, αἰσθητικῷ δηλονότι, μὴ αἰσθάνηται τῆς ὀδύνης, χαλεπὸν τὸ τοιοῦτον, δηλοῖ γάρ, ὅτι ὁ ἐγκέφαλος πέπονθε. καὶ ἵνα σαφὴς γένηται ὁ λόγος, ἐφ' ὑποθέσει τινὶ τὸ λεγόμενον διευκρινήσωμεν. ὑποκείσθω τοίνυν ἄρρωστος ἔχων φλεγμονὴν περὶ τὸν μηρὸν μετὰ τῶν συνεδρευόντων δηλονότι συμπτωμάτων, ἐρεύθους, ζέσεως καὶ τάσεως καὶ τῶν τοιούτων. τοῦτον ὁρῶν εὑρίσκω ὀδυνώμενον κατὰ λόγον καὶ τῆς δεούσης ἀξιώσας παραμυθίας ἀπηλλάγην· εἶτα τῇ ἑξῆς ἐλθὼν ἤκουσα παρὰ τῶν συνόντων αὐτῷ, ὅτι ὅλως οὐκ ᾔσθετο ὀδύνης ἐν τῇ νυκτὶ ταύτῃ καίτοι πρὸ τούτου μὴ φέρων αὐτήν. ἐνταῦθα οὖν καθ' ἑαυτὸν λογίζομαι· «Μή τι ὅτι διεφορήθη ὁ τοιοῦτος ὄγκος ἢ μετωχετεύθη ἢ ἐρράγη καὶ τοῦ περιεχομένου κενωθέντος ἀνώδυνος γέγονεν;» εἶτα ἀκριβῶς ἐρευνήσας οὐδὲν τούτων εὗρον, τὸν δὲ αὐτὸν ὄγκον ἐν τῷ μηρῷ ἐθεασάμην ὑποκείμενον· κἀντεῦθεν ἐτεκμηράμην ἢ παραφρονῆσαι τὸν ἄνθρωπον ἢ ὅσον οὔπω μέλλειν παραφρονεῖν, ἐβλάβη γὰρ τὸ κρῖνον, ὡς μὴ συναισθάνεσθαι αὐτὸν τῆς ὀδυνηρᾶς διαθέσεως.

Δεῖ δὲ ζητῆσαι, τί σημαίνει τὰ π ο λ λ ὰ ἐν τῷ παρόντι ἀφορισμῷ. καί φαμεν ὅτι τὸ ὡς ἐπὶ πᾶν καὶ ὡς ἐπὶ πολύ, τοῦ λόγου ἀληθεύοντος ἐπὶ τῶν πλείστων παθῶν. δεῖ γὰρ εἰδέναι, ὅτι διὰ καθαρότητα ψυχῆς ἧττον περὶ τὸ σῶμα ἀναστρεφομένης ἐνδέχεται μὴ συναισθάνεσθαι τοῦ πάθους ἤτοι τῆς ὀδύνης τὸν κάμνοντα διὰ τὸ περί τινα θεωρίαν ὑψηλὴν ἀσχολεῖσθαι τὸν νοῦν.

'Απορουσι δέ τινες εἰς ἀντίφασιν τὰ λεγόμενα περιάγοντες· φασὶ γάρ· «Εἰ ἐπὶ τῆς ὀδύνης τὸ τοῦ π ό ν ο υ ὄνομα παρείληπται, ἡ δὲ ⟨ὀδύνη⟩ ὀδυνηρά ἐστι συναίσθησις, πῶς ἐνδέχεται τὸν αὐτὸν καὶ πονεῖν» — λέγω δὴ ὀδυνηρὰν ἔχειν συναίσθησιν — «καὶ μὴ αἰσθάνεσθαι; εἰ γὰρ πονεῖ, δῆλον, ὅτι καὶ αἰσθάνεται, εἰ δὲ μὴ αἰσθάνεται, οὐδὲ πονεῖ.» λύομεν δὲ αὐτὴν οὕτως· ὁ Ἱ π π ο κ ρ ά τ η ς ἀντὶ τοῦ ποιοῦντος τὸ γινόμενον εἶπεν· ἀντὶ γὰρ τῆς ὀδυνηρᾶς διαθέσεως τὸν π ό ν ο ν ἤτοι τὴν ὀδύνην τέθηκε. νόμιζε οὖν ταῦτά σοι λέγειν τὸν Ἱ π π ο κ ρ ά τ η ν· «'Οκόσοι ὀδυνηρὰν διάθεσιν ἔν τινι μέρει τοῦ σώματος ἔχοντες, φημὶ δὴ φλεγμονὴν ζέουσαν καὶ διατείνουσαν, μὴ αἰσθάνονται τῆς ὀδύνης, τούτων τὸ κρῖνον βέβλαπται.» γ ν ώ μ η ν μὲν γὰρ εἶπε τὴν διάνοιαν· εἰ δὲ καὶ τὸν λογισμὸν ἀκούοις, οὐδὲν ἁμάρτοις. ὅτι δὲ ἄλλο ὀδύνη καὶ ἄλλο ὀδυνηρὰ διάθεσις, δῆλον· ὀδύνη μὲν γάρ ἐστιν ἡ ἀνιαρὰ τοῦ πάσχοντος μορίου συναίσθησις, ἡνίκα αἰσθητικὸν ὑπάρχει, ὀδυνηρὰ δὲ διάθεσις αὐτὸ τὸ νόσημα, ἀφ' οὗ ἡ ὀδύνη γίνεται, τάσις φημί, ἢ δυσκρασία, ταὐτὸν δὲ εἰπεῖν φλεγμονὴν ἐρυσιπελατώδη καὶ τὰ τοιαῦτα.

II 6 [II 7: IV 470,19–20 L.] Τ ὰ ἐ ν π ο λ λ ῷ χ ρ ό ν ῳ λ ε π τ υ ν ό μ ε ν α σ ώ μ α τ α ν ω θ ρ ῶ ς ἐ π α ν α σ τ ρ έ φ ε ι ν, τ ὰ δ ὲ ἐ ν ὀ λ ί γ ῳ ὀ λ ί γ ω ς.

3 ἐάν – 16] *v.* Theoph. In Aphor.: II 299,16–30 Dietz 17–18 πᾶν] *v.* Theoph. In Aphor.: II 299,30–31 Dietz 22–27 τέθηκε] *v.* Gal. In Aphor. II 6: XVII B 460,4–8 K. 30 γνώμην – διάνοιαν] *v.* Gal. In Aphor. II 6: XVII B 460,13–14 K. 31 ὅτι – 35] *v.* Gal. In Aphor. II 6: XVII B 460,8–12 K.

13 τούτω P 16 αἰσθάνεσθαι A 22 φησὶ P 23 περιείληπται α: *correxi* ὀδύνη *addidi* ἐστι συναίσθησις *scripsi*: ἐστιν ἡ θέσις α *(spat. 6 litt. rel. ante* ἡ *in* P*)* 24 λέγει P 32 ἀνιαρὰ *scripsi*: ἀμαυρὰ α 37 ἐπαναστρέφειν] *item infra, p. 152,9, Theoph.* SV'': ἐπανατρέφειν A², *Hipp., Theoph.* U'' *(cf. infra, p. 152,8. 10)*

in general terms that any hurt that remains unnoticed is a greater evil than a perceptible hurt, since it indicates a greater harm, by which more vital parts are affected. So much for the place of this aphorism; the thought is expressed in conformity with this: If someone, he says, who has a painful condition no matter in which part of his body – a sensitive part, of course – is unaware of the pain, this is serious, for it shows that the brain has suffered. To make this statement clear, let us elucidate its purport by means of a hypothetical case. Suppose there is a patient who has an inflammation in the thigh, of course with the usual accompanying symptoms, redness, seething heat, tension, etc. On my visit I find him in pain as expected, and having done what is necessary to give him relief I go away; then, when I come the following day, I hear from those around him that during that night he has felt no pain at all, though until then it was unbearable. So then I ask myself: "Can it be that this swelling has been dispersed or diverted or has broken through and become painless by the effusion of the content?" Upon careful examination I find that none of these is the case, but I see the same swelling still there in the thigh; and from this I conclude that the man either is delirious or will be so pretty soon, for his faculty of judgment has been affected, so that he is not conscious of his painful condition.

The point arises what on the whole means in the present aphorism. The answer is, "generally" or "mostly", since the statement applies to most affections. For it should be observed that the purity of a soul which is not much preoccupied with the body may be the reason why the patient is not aware of his ailment or of the pain, because his mind is engrossed by some sublime subject of contemplation.

Some raise a problem by arguing that the text is self-contradictory; if, they say, the word suffering is used here in the sense of pain, and pain is a painful sensation, how is it possible for the same man to suffer – meaning to have a sensation of pain – and not to be aware of it? If he suffers, he is obviously aware of it, and if he is not, he does not suffer either. We solve this problem as follows: Hippocrates mentioned the process instead of the cause, i.e. instead of the painful condition he spoke of suffering or pain. So what Hippocrates says can be considered equivalent to this: "Those who, while having a painful condition in some part of the body, let us say an inflammation with seething heat and swelling, remain unaware of the pain, have suffered impairment of their faculty of judgment." By mind he means reasoning; however, if you understand it as reason itself, you will not be wrong. That pain is different from a painful condition is evident: pain is the unpleasant sensation of the affected part, if it is a sensitive one, but a painful condition is the disease itself to which the pain is due, I mean tension or distemper, in other words, an inflammation of the erysipelas type or something like it.

II 6. Bodies that lose weight over a long period of time should be restored slowly, those that have lost weight quickly, fast.

Φησὶν ὁ Ἱπποκράτης ὅτι «Σκόπει τὸ νόσημα, εἴτε χρόνιόν ἐστιν εἴτε ὀξύ.» ἐπειδὴ γὰρ τὸ ἡμέτερον σῶμα τριπλεκές ἐστιν ἔκ τε πνευμάτων καὶ ὑγρῶν καὶ στερεῶν συγκείμενον καὶ ἐπὶ μὲν τῶν χρονίων νοσημάτων ἕκαστον τούτων †γίνεται†, διαπνεῖται μὲν τὰ πνεύματα, ἀπορ⟨ρ⟩εῖ δὲ τὰ ὑγρὰ καὶ διαφορεῖται, καὶ συντήκεται τὰ στερεὰ μέχρι καὶ αὐτῶν τῷ χρόνῳ τῆς λύμης προϊούσης, κἀντεῦθεν ἰσχναίνεται παντοίως καὶ συμπίπτει ὁ τοῦ σώματος ὄγκος καὶ δηλονότι καὶ αἱ δυνάμεις ἑκάστου τῶν μορίων στρεβλοῦνται, ἐπὶ τῶν τοιούτων νοσημάτων ἐν τῇ ἀνακομιδῇ ὀλίγας δεῖ καὶ εὐπέπτους διδόναι τὰς τροφάς, ὅπερ δηλοῖ τὸ τὰ ἐν πολλῷ χρόνῳ λεπτυνόμενα σώματα νωθρῶς ἐπαναστρέφειν, τουτέστι λεπτῶς καὶ κατ' ὀλίγον ἀμυδράν τινα δύναμιν τῆς τροφῆς παρεχομένης. εἰ δὲ ὀξὺ ὑπόκειται νόσημα, ἐπειδὴ οὐ πάντα πέπονθε τὴν τῆς [ση]μειώσεως βλάβην τὰ μέρη – τὰ μὲν γὰρ πνεύματα πάντως ὡς εὐπαθέστερα διεσκέδασται, οὐ μὴν ἀλλὰ καὶ τῶν ὑγρῶν ἀπέρρευσέ τι, τὰ δὲ στερεὰ οὐ συνετάκη, οὐδὲ τῶν δυνάμεων ἡ βλάβη ἐπὶ πολὺ γέγονε –, δεῖ ἐπὶ τῶν τοιούτων πλείονα διδόναι τροφὴν καὶ σύντομον ποιεῖσθαι τὴν ἀνακομιδήν, εἰ καὶ ἥττονος δεῖται προσαγωγῆς· καὶ τοῦτό ἐστι τὸ τὰ δὲ ἐν ὀλίγῳ ὀλίγως, ἢ τὸ ἁδροτέρως πρὸς τὸ νωθρῶς ἢ τὸ ἐν ὀλίγῳ χρόνῳ.

II 7 [II 8: IV 472,1–3 L.] Ἢν ἐκ νόσου τροφὴν λαμβάνων τις μὴ ἰσχύῃ, σημαίνει, ὅτι τὸ σῶμα πλείονι τροφῇ χρέεται· ἢν δὲ τροφὴν μὴ λαμβάνοντος τοῦτο γίνεται, σημαίνει, ὅτι κενώσεως τοῦτο δεῖται.

Φησίν, ὅτι προσῆλθέ σοί τις λέγων ὅτι «Ἄρτι ἀπενόσησα καὶ πολλῶν τροφῶν ὀρέγομαι καὶ πολλὴν τροφὴν λαμβάνω· ἀδύνατος δέ εἰμι καὶ σῶμα ἰσχνὸν ἔχω.» καὶ ζητῶν σὺ τὴν αἰτίαν εὑρίσκεις, ὅτι αἱ φυσικαὶ δυνάμεις αὐτοῦ ἀσθενοῦσι καὶ οὔτε χυλοποίησις κατὰ λόγον οὔτε ἐξαιμάτωσις οὔτε πρόσθεσις οὔτε ἐξομοίωσις γίνεται καὶ δηλονότι οὐδὲ θρέψις, κἀκεῖθεν ἰσχνὸν μένει τὸ σῶμα. ἡ γὰρ τροφὴ οὐχ ὡς τροφὴ παραλαμβάνεται, ἀλλ' ἐπὶ καταλύσει τῶν δυνάμεων· οὐδὲ γὰρ ἀφ' ἑαυτῆς πέττεται, ἀλλὰ πολλοῦ δεῖται καμάτου ἡ φύσις ὥστε κατεργάσασθαι τὴν προσαγομένην τροφήν. ταῦτ' οὖν ἐννοήσας λέγοις ἂν τῷ κάμνοντι ὡς «Ὑπὲρ τὴν δύναμίν σού ἐστιν ἡ τροφή, ἣν λαμβάνεις, καὶ δεῖ ὀλιγώτερα ὧν ὀρέγῃ προσφέρεσθαι, ἵνα κατακρατῇ αὐτῶν ἡ δύναμις, ἀλλὰ μὴ κρατεῖται ὑπ' αὐτῶν.» εἶθ' ἕτερος προσέρχεται ἄρρωστος ἐκ νόσου ἀνακομιζόμενος λέγων ὅτι «Οὐκ ὀρέγομαι ὅλως τροφῆς»· ἔστι δὲ καὶ αὐτῷ ἰσχνὸν τὸ σῶμα καὶ ἀδύναμον. συλλόγισαι οὖν κἀπὶ τούτου, τίς ἡ αἰτία, ὅτι παυσαμένου τοῦ νοσήματος οὐκ ὀρέγεται τροφῆς ὁ ἄνθρωπος· καὶ λέγε, ὅτι ἀτελὴς γέγονεν

1 Φησὶν – ὀξύ] *v.* Theoph. In Aphor.: II 300,4–6 Dietz 2 ἐπειδὴ – 10 παρεχομένης] *v.* Gal. In Aphor. II 7: XVII B 461,4–12 K. 10 εἰ – 15 προσαγωγῆς] *cf.* Gal. In Aphor. II 7: XVII B 461,12–15 K. 20–29 αὐτῶν] *cf.* Gal. In Aphor. II 8: XVII B 462,13–463,1 K. 21 καὶ[III] – 24 θρέψις] *v.* Theoph. In Aphor.: II 301,4–6 Dietz 29 εἶθ' – 154,5] *cf.* Gal. In Aphor. II 8: XVII B 463,1–4 K.

3 γίνεται] *aut* ⟨μεῖον⟩ γίνεται *aut* μειοῦται *scribendum est* 4 ἀπορεῖ α: *corr.* A² 7 ὀλίγους P 8 ἀπέπτους α: *correxi* τὸ] τῷ P 9 ἐπαναστρέφειν] *cf. ad p. 150,37* 11 σημειώσεως α: *correxi* 14 εἰ *om.* P 17 *post* νόσου *add. et del.* τροφὴν λαμβάνοντός τινος μὴ ἰσχύῃ τὸ σῶμα A: *non hab. Hipp. (cf. infra, pp. 158,23; 206,20)* 18 ὅτι – τροφῇ] *Hipp. quidam*: τὸ σῶμα ὅτι πλείονι τροφῇ *infra, p. 206,20–21, Hipp.* C' (τῷ σώματι), *Theoph.*: ὅτι πλείονι τροφῇ *infra, p. 158,23, Hipp.* V: ὅτι πλείονι τροφῇ τὸ σῶμα *Hipp.* M *et multi* 19 τοῦτο] *item infra, p. 156,10*: *om. infra, p. 158,24, non hab. Hipp.* 22 σοι α: *correxi* 25 περιλαμβάνεται P 28 ὀλιγώτερα *scripsi*: ὀλιγώτ^ρ A: ὀλιγωτέραν P κατακρατ῀ A 29 προσφέρεται A

Hippocrates tells us to observe the disease, whether it is chronic or acute. Our body, indeed, is threefold, being composed of gases, fluids and solids; in cases of chronic illness each of these is diminished[1]: the gases are blown away, the fluids flow away and are dispersed, and the solids dissolve, because at last the injury extends even to them; hence the volume of the body is emaciated and shrinks in every way, while of course the power of each of the parts is also maimed; therefore, in diseases of this kind, one should allow only small quantities of easily digestible food during convalescence; this is expressed in the words Bodies that lose weight over a long period of time should be restored slowly, i.e. by light food and gradually, the food providing a certain minimal resistance. On the other hand, if we have to do with an acute disease, not all the parts have suffered diminution; for while the gases, as less resistant, have inevitably been dispersed, and a part of the fluids also has flowed away, yet the solids have not been dissolved, nor has the harm done to the powers advanced far; therefore in these cases one should allow more food and work toward a quick recovery, even though (the patient) needs less nutriment; this is the sense of those that have lost weight quickly, fast, i.e., either by a heavier diet as opposed to slowly, or in a short time.

II 7. If after sickness a person, while taking food, does not gain strength, this is a sign that his body receives too much food; if it happens without his taking food, that is a sign that it needs evacuation.

Somebody comes to you, (Hippocrates) says, and tells you: "I have just recovered from an illness, I have an appetite for plenty of food and I do eat a great deal; yet I am weak and my body remains thin." When you inquire into the cause, you find that his natural faculties are weak, and neither conversion into chyle takes place as it should, nor conversion into blood nor absorption nor assimilation, and thus there is naturally no nutrition, and as a result the body remains thin. This is because the food does not serve as food, but for the demolition of the faculties, since it is not digested of itself, but the constitution has to do a great deal of hard work to convert the food that is taken. Considering this, you might say to the patient: "The food you are taking is in excess of your strength, you must eat less than you want to, so that your strength can master it and will not be mastered by it." Then another convalescent comes to you and tells you, "I have no appetite at all", and his body too is thin and weak. In this case also, you must find the reason why, though the disease is over, the man has no appetite for food; and the answer will be that the crisis has appar-

[1] See the app. crit.

ἡ κρίσις, ὡς ἔοικε, καὶ τὸ ἐγκατάλειμμα τοῦ μοχθηροῦ χυμοῦ κακοῖ τὸν στόμαχον αὐτοῦ καὶ καταλύει τὴν ὄρεξιν, καὶ διὰ τοῦτο τροφῆς οὐκ ἐφίεται. σκόπει λοιπόν, τί βούλεται ἡ τέχνη· καὶ εὑρήσεις, ὅτι κενώσεως δεῖται τὸ ἐναποκείμενον ἐγκατάλειμμα τοῦ χυμοῦ ἐν τῷ σώματι, ἵνα τούτου ἀπαλλαττομένου ὁ στόμαχος τὴν οἰκείαν ἀνακτήσηται ὄρεξιν.

Δεῖ δὲ τοῦτο εἰδέναι, ὅτι ἄλλο ἐστὶν ὄρεξις καὶ ἄλλο θρέψις ἤγουν πέψις. τὸ μὲν γὰρ ὀρέγεσθαι ἔργον ἐστὶ φυσικὸν τοῦ στομάχου μετὰ ψυχικῆς γινόμενον συναισθήσεως, ἡ δὲ πέψις τῆς ἐν ἑκάστῳ μορίῳ ἀλλοιωτικῆς δυνάμεως ἐνέργεια· καὶ οὐδὲν ἄτοπον ἐρρῶσθαι μὲν τὴν ὀρεκτικὴν δύναμιν, διὰ δὲ ψυχρὰν ὡς εἰκὸς δυσκρασίαν καταλαβοῦσαν τὸ στόμιον τῆς γαστρὸς τὰς ἄλλας βαρεῖσθαι δυνάμεις τῷ πλήθει τῆς προσφερομένης τροφῆς.

Ἀποροῦσι δέ τινες ὅτι «Πῶς δέον ὂν ἐπὶ τῶν ἀκαθάρτων σωμάτων μὴ προσάγειν τροφὴν πρὸ καθάρσεως, ἵνα μὴ ἐκ τῆς τοιαύτης τροφῆς ὕλη τῇ κακοχυμίᾳ προστίθηται, ἐπὶ τῶν πυρεττόντων τροφαῖς χρώμεθα, καὶ μάλιστα ἡνίκα ἐπὶ χυμοῖς ὦσιν οἱ πυρετοί;» φαμὲν οὖν, ὅτι οὐ κυρίως τροφῇ χρώμεθα ἐπ' αὐτῶν, ἀλλὰ φαρμακώδει τροφῇ· ἡ γὰρ πτισάνη καὶ αἱ θριδακῖναι καὶ τὸ ὀξύμελι καὶ τὰ τοιαῦτα φαρμάκου τάξιν ἐπέχει. ἄλλως τε ἐπὶ τῶν πυρετῶν διὰ τὴν δύναμιν τρέφομεν, ἵνα ταύτην ὑποστηρίζωμεν, ὥστε διαμαχήσασθαι καὶ διανικῆσαι τὰ νοσοποιὰ αἴτια.

II 8 [II 9: IV 472,4–5 L.] Τὰ σώματα χρή, ὅκου ἄν τις βούληται καθαίρειν, εὔροα ποιέει⟨ν⟩.

Λέγει, ὅτι τὸν βουλόμενον καθαίρειν τὸ σῶμα χρὴ εὔροιαν ἐπιτηδεύειν, τουτέστι σκοπεῖν, ποίοις μάλιστα μορίοις τοῦ σώματος ἐπιτήδειος ὁ χυμὸς καὶ ποῦ τὴν ῥοπὴν ποιεῖται, ἵνα, εἰ δι' ἐμέτων βουληθείης κενῶσαι, ἐπὶ τὸν στόμαχον πάντα συναγάγῃς, εἰ δὲ διὰ τῆς κάτω γαστρός, ἐπὶ τὰ ἔντερα, εἰ δὲ δι' ἱδρώτων, ἐπὶ τὴν ἐπιφάνειαν προτρέψαι τὰ περιττώματα. ἢ καὶ ἄλλως· ἐφ' ὧν δεῖ σε κάθαρσιν παραλαβεῖν, δεῖ σε εὔροιαν ἐπιτηδεῦσαι, ἡ δὲ εὔροια τὴν ἀκώλυτον δηλοῖ διέξοδον· αὕτη δὲ κατὰ δύο τρόπους γίνεται, κατά τε τὴν λέπτυνσιν τῆς ὕλης καὶ τὴν τῶν μορίων μαλακότητα. δεῖ οὖν καὶ τὰ περιέχοντα χαλάσαι καὶ ἀραιῶσαι καὶ τοὺς πόρους ἀναπετάσαι καὶ τῶν ἀγγείων τὰ στόματα ἀνευρῦναι καὶ τὰ περιεχόμενα τεμεῖν καὶ λεπτῦναι, ἔστιν ὅτε καὶ εὐκρατῶσαι· ἐντεῦθεν γὰρ ῥάστη γίνεται ἡ κάθαρσις. καὶ πῶς ἑκάτερον τούτων ποιήσομεν; τοὺς μὲν πόρους ἀραιοῦμεν καὶ τὰ στόματα τῶν ἀγγείων εὐρύνομεν ἐπὶ λουτρὰ καὶ ἀλοιφὰς καὶ συμμέτρους κινήσεις τε καὶ τρίψεις τοὺς ἀνθρώπους προτρέποντες· τοὺς δὲ χυμοὺς λεπτύνομεν παχεῖς ὄντας καὶ φλεγματικοὺς ἢ καὶ μελαγχολικοὺς διὰ τῶν καταζεμάτων, ἀνήθου φημὶ καὶ σελίνου καὶ γλήχωνος καὶ ὑσσώπου καὶ ἐπιθύμου καὶ χαμαίδρυος, καὶ δι' ὀξυμέλιτος ἁπλοῦ καὶ συνθέτου. εἰ δὲ χολώδεις εἶεν, τῷ τοῦ πολυτρίχου ζέματι χρώμενος πότιζε ἐπικιρνῶν ἠρέμα ὥστε μὴ δῆξιν

6–11] *cf.* Theoph. In Aphor.: II 301,10–14 Dietz 21–25 περιττώματα] *cf.* Gal. In Aphor. II 9: XVII B 464,9–14 K. 25 ἢ – 30 κάθαρσις] *cf.* Gal. In Aphor. II 9: XVII B 465,2–6 K. 25 ἐφ' – 30 εὐκρατῶσαι] *v.* Theoph. In Aphor.: II 301,28–302,5 Dietz

12 ὂν α: *correxi* 14 ἡνίκα *om.* A 15 ἐπ'] ὑπ' P 19 ἄν] *item infra, vol. II, fol. 63ᵛ, Hipp.* C', *Theoph.* SV'': *om. supra, p. 136,9; infra, p. 156,14–15; non hab. Hipp.* MV, *Theoph.* U'' βούληται] *Hipp.* C', *Theoph.* U''V'': βούλεται *supra, p. 136,9; infra, p. 156,15; vol. II, fol. 63ᵛ, Hipp.* MV, *Theoph.* S 20 ποιέει α: *corr.* A[2] 23 συναγάγοις A 24 κάτω *om.* A 27 λέπτωσιν P 30 γὰρ *om.* P

ently been imperfect, and the remainder of the bad humor causes harm to his stomach and spoils his appetite, so that he has no desire for food. Now consider what the art prescribes; and you will find that the remainder of the humor that has stayed behind in the body has to be evacuated, so that the stomach, free from this, can recover its natural appetite.

It should be observed that appetite is one thing and nutrition or digestion another. Appetition is a natural function of the stomach, attended by awareness in the soul, while digestion is an activity of the transformative faculty in each part; and it is quite conceivable that the appetitive faculty may be healthy, while, presumably owing to a cold distemper prevailing in the orifice of the stomach, the other faculties are overburdened by the quantity of food taken.

Some ask the following question: "Since in cases of bodies that are not clean no food should be administered until they have been purged, because otherwise from this food more matter would be added to the bad humor, how is it that we allow food to fever patients, and especially when the fevers are due to humors?" We answer that strictly speaking we do not allow them food, but food in lieu of medication; for barley-water, lettuce, oxymel, etc., serve as medication. Besides, in fever cases we administer food for the sake of resistance, in order to strengthen it so that it can fight and overcome the causes that bring about disease.

II 8. Bodies, where one wants to purge, should be made to flow readily.

He says that the physician who wants to purge should provide for an easy flow, that is to say, he should examine with which parts of the body the humor has the greatest affinity and which way it gravitates, so that, if you want to evacuate by vomiting, you should gather everything in the stomach; if by way of the abdomen, you should collect it in the intestines; if by sweating, you should direct the waste matter toward the surface. Or, alternatively: in cases where you have to apply purging, you must provide for an easy flow, an "easy flow" meaning an unhindered passage; and such a passage is brought about in two ways: by comminution of the matter and by softness of the parts. Accordingly, one must, on the one hand, loosen and rarefy the containing parts, open the pores and widen the orifices of the vessels, on the other hand, fragmentize and comminute the matter contained in them, and sometimes also improve its temperament; in this way the purging becomes easiest. How are we going to achieve these two ends? We open the pores and widen the orifices of the vessels by ordering baths, ointments and moderate exercise and massage; and we comminute the humors, if they are thick and phlegmatic or even atrabiliar, by means of decoctions, namely of dill, celery, pennyroyal, hyssop, epithymum and germander, and by means of simple or composite oxymel. If, however, they are bilious, prescribe a decoction of maidenhair as a potion, slightly diluted so as not to produce irri-

ἐμποιῆσαι τοῖς χωρίοις, δι' ὧν ἐκκρίνονται, ἢ τὰ τῆς δυσκρασίας ἐπιταθῆναι τῷ σώματι, θερμῶν καὶ δριμέων ὑπαρχόντων, οὐ μὴν ἀλλὰ καὶ τὴν τῶν καθαίρειν αὐτοὺς πεπιστευμένων φαρμάκων θερμότητα ὡς μάλιστα χαρακτηριζόντων. δεῖ οὖν τὸν μέλλοντα καθαίρεσθαι πάσης σιτώδους ἀπέχεσθαι τροφῆς καὶ †φθορᾶς† καὶ πάντων τῶν ἐμφράττειν δυναμένων.

II 9 [II 10: IV 472,6–7 L.] Τὰ μὴ καθαρὰ τῶν σωμάτων ὁκόσον ἂν θρέψῃς, μᾶλλον βλάψεις.

Φησὶν ὁ Γαληνός· ἔδει τὸν παρόντα ἀφορισμὸν τῷ μικρὸν πρόσθεν εἰρημένῳ συντάξαι, ἐν ᾧ εἴρηκεν· «ἢν δὲ τροφὴν μὴ λαμβάνοντος τοῦτο γίνηται, σημαίνει, ὅτι κενώσεως τοῦτο δεῖται.» ὥς τινος γὰρ λέγοντος· «Διὰ τί κενώσεως δεῖται;» αὐτὸς ἐπιφέρει· Τὰ μὴ καθαρὰ τῶν σωμάτων ὁκόσον ἂν θρέψῃς, μᾶλλον βλάψεις, διότι κακοχυμίας πεπληρωμένον οὕτως προσίεται τὴν τροφήν. εἶτα μετὰ τοῦτον τὸν ἀφορισμὸν ἔδει συνάψαι τὸν μεταξὺ τῶν δύο τεταγμένον· ἐρωτώμενος γὰρ πάλιν ὁ Ἱπποκράτης, πῶς δεῖ τῇ καθάρσει χρήσασθαι, ἐπήγαγε· «Τὰ σώματα χρή, ὅκου τις βούλεται καθαίρειν, εὔροα ποιέειν.»

II 10 [II 11: IV 472,8 L.] Ῥᾷον πληροῦσθαι ποτοῦ ἢ σιτίου.

Διδάσκει ἡμᾶς, ποῖα τῶν προσφερομένων εὐχερῶς πληροῖ τὸ σῶμα καὶ τὴν διαφορηθεῖσαν ἑτοίμως ἀναπληροῖ οὐσίαν. ποτὸν δὲ ἐνταῦθα οὐ πᾶν ὑγρὸν διὰ στόματος λαμβανόμενον καλεῖ, ἀλλὰ τὸν οἶνον, ὑγρᾶς γὰρ τροφῆς ὄχημα ὁ οἶνος. λοιπὸν δεῖ, φησί, σκοπεῖν, ποία μᾶλλον τοῦ ἡμετέρου σώματος διαπεφόρηται οὐσία. εἰ μὲν γὰρ τὰ στερεὰ ἔπαθε, στερεὰν δεῖ παρέχειν τροφήν, εἰ δὲ τὰ πνεύματα, ἀερώδη διὰ τῶν ὀσφραντῶν, ὑγρᾶς δὲ λειπούσης τοιαύτην ἀντεισάγειν χρεών. ᾧ καὶ ἁρμόζει τὸ παρὰ τοῦ Ἱπποκράτους λεγόμενον· δεῖ γάρ, φησίν, οἶνον παρέχειν τὸν εὐχερῶς ἀναπληρῶσαι τὴν διαφόρησιν δυνάμενον τοῖς ἐπὶ ὑγρᾷ οὐσίᾳ διαφορηθεῖσιν· οὐ γὰρ ἔστιν οἴνου μᾶλλον ἐν τροφαῖς εὐανάδοτον καὶ συναγαγεῖν καὶ ῥῶσαι δύναμιν διασκεδασθεῖσαν δυνάμενον. οὐ μόνον γὰρ εὐανάδοτος, ἀλλὰ καὶ εὐπρόσθετος, καὶ διὰ τοῦτο τροφιμώτατον τῶν διὰ στόματος λαμβανομένων πάντων ὁ οἶνος μεμαρτύρηται. ὥστε τῆς ὑγρᾶς οὐσίας διαφορηθείσης οἶνον δοτέον· οὐ τὸν μέλανα, οὗτος γὰρ ὡς γεώδης ἐν τῇ γαστρὶ μάλιστα χρονίζων οὐκ εὐανάδοτός ἐστιν. οὐδὲ μὴν ὁ ὑδατώδης, εἰ γὰρ καὶ ταχέως οὗτος ἀναδίδοται, ἀλλ' ὅμως ἐλάχιστα τρέφει· τὸ πλεῖον γὰρ δι' οὔρων ἐξέρχεται, διὸ οὐ τρόφιμος ὁ οἶνος οὗτος. ἀλλὰ τὸν μέσον, τοῦτον δὴ τὸν ξανθὸν καὶ κιρρόν, ὁ λόγος αἰνίττεται.

8–15] *v.* Gal. In Aphor. II 8: XVII B 463,13–464,5 K. 9sq. ἢν – δεῖται] Hipp. Aphor. II 8: IV 472,2–3 L. 14sq. Τὰ – ποιέειν] Hipp. Aphor. II 9: IV 472,4–5 L. 18sq. ποτὸν – οἶνος] *v.* Theoph. In Aphor.: II 303,2–4 Dietz 19 ὑγρᾶς – οἶνος] *v.* Hipp. Alim. 55: CMG I 1, p. 84,22 *cf.* Theoph. In Aphor.: II 303,3–4 Dietz 20 λοιπὸν – 22 χρεών] *cf.* Gal. In Aphor. II 11: XVII B 467,4–7 K. Hipp. Alim. 50: CMG I 1, p. 84,12–14 25 οὐ – 27 μεμαρτύρηται] *v.* Theoph. In Aphor.: II 303,5–8 Dietz 28 ὥστε – 32] *cf.* Gal. In Aphor. II 11: XVII B 467, 11–468,2 K. 31sq. ἀλλὰ – αἰνίττεται] *v.* Theoph. In Aphor.: II 303,8–9 Dietz

4 φθορᾶς] *fort.* προσφορᾶς *scribendum est* 6 ὁκόσον] *item infra, lin. 11, Hipp.* C', *Theoph.* U''V'': ὁκόσω *Hipp.* MV, *Theoph.* S 12 τούτων P 13 ἀφορισμῶν P τὸν] τῶν α: *correxi* τῶν *scripsi*: ὄντων A: ὄντα P τεταγμένων A 24 διαφόνησιν P: *corr.* P[2]: διαφώνησιν A 25 εὐανάδοτον *scripsi*: ἀγανάδοτον A: ἀνάδοτον P 31 δὴ *ex* δὲ *corr.* AP 32 κιρρόν] *ras. 1 litt. et* ορρὸν *in* A

tation in the places through which the excretions pass, and so as not to increase the distemper of the body; for these draughts are hot and pungent, and by the hotness of their character as closely as possible resemble the drugs which have the task of purging the patients. The patient about to be purged, then, should abstain from all cereal food and corruption (?) and from anything that can cause stoppage.

II 9. The more you feed bodies that are not clean, the more you will harm them.

Galen says that the present aphorism should be joined to the one a little before it, where it says: "If it happens without his taking food, that is a sign that the body needs evacuation." It is in fact as if somebody asked: "Why does it need evacuation?" and (Hippocrates) himself replies: The more you feed bodies that are not clean, the more you will harm them, because (such a body) receives the food while full of bad humors. Then, after this aphorism, one should append the one placed between the two; for in answer to the next question, how the purging should be done, Hippocrates went on to say: "Bodies, where one wants to purge, should be made to flow readily."

II 10. It is easier to be replenished with drink than with food.

He informs us which kinds of nutriment replenish the body easily and readily supply the dispersed substance. By drink he means here, not any fluid taken through the mouth, but wine, for wine is a carrier of liquid nutriment. What he means, then, is that we must find out, which substance of our body has lost most by dispersal. For if the solids have suffered, we should offer solid food; if the gases have, the food should be airlike, in the form of perfumes to be smelled; if there is a shortage of moisture, we must replace it by food of the same nature. Hippocrates' precept is in accordance with this: to those, he says, who have lost liquid substance by dispersal, we should provide wine, which can easily replace what has been so lost; indeed, there is no food like wine for quick distribution and for power to collect and reinforce dissipated strength. It is not only easily distributed, but also easily absorbed, and for this reason wine is generally recognized as the most nourishing of all foods taken through the mouth. Therefore, when the liquid substance has been dispersed one should give wine; but not the dark red kind, which being earthlike tends to stay in the stomach and is not quickly distributed. Nor the watery kind either, for though this is quickly distributed, yet it is the least nourishing, because most of it is discharged with the urine, and hence this wine is not nutritious. It is the intermediate sort, known as yellow and tawny, which the precept signifies.

Σκόπει δὲ τέχνην Ἱπποκράτους εἰρηκότος· ⟨Ῥᾷον⟩ πληροῦσθαι ποτοῦ ἢ σιτίου, ⟨οὐ πάντως τοῦ πο⟩τοῦ μετὰ τοῦ εὐχεροῦς ἤδη καὶ τὸ βέλτιον ἔχοντος. τί γάρ; ὅτι στερεᾶς οὐσίας διαφορηθείσης ῥᾷον μὲν ὑπὸ τοῦ οἴνου πληροῦται τὸ σῶμα, οὐ μέντοι καὶ πρὸς τὸ βέλτιον ἄγεται· οὐδὲ γὰρ τοῦ λείποντος τὸ τηνικαῦτα ὁ οἶνός ἐστιν ἀναπλήρωσις, τῆς μέντοι ὑγρᾶς οὐσίας ἑτοίμην ὁ οἶνος ποιεῖται τὴν ἀναπλήρωσιν.

II 11 [II 12: IV 472,9–10 L.] Τὰ ἐγκαταλιμπανόμενα ἐν τῇσι νούσοισι μετὰ κρίσιν ὑποστροφὰς ποιέειν εἴωθεν.

Ἐνταῦθα ἀποροῦσί τινες λέγοντες ὅτι «Εἰ κρίσις γέγονε τοῦ νοσήματος, πῶς ἔχει γενέσθαι ὑποστροφὴ πάντα τὰ νοσοποιὰ αἴτια ἐν τῇ κρίσει τῆς φύσεως ἐξοριζούσης;» πρὸς οὓς φαμεν, ὅτι ὁμώνυμός ἐστιν ἡ κρίσις· ἔστι γὰρ καὶ τελεία καὶ ἀτελής, καὶ βεβαία καὶ ἀβέβαιος, καὶ σαφὴς καὶ ἀσαφής. ἐὰν οὖν τελεία γένηται ἡ κρίσις, ἀδύνατον ὑποστροφὴν ἐπακολουθῆσαι· εἰ δὲ ἀτελής, τὸ ἐγκατάλειμμα τῆς ὕλης δύναται ποιῆσαι ὑποτροπιασμόν. περὶ ἀτελοῦς κρίσεως ὁ λόγος τῷ Ἱπποκράτει, ὡς δηλοῖ εἰρηκὼς τὰ ἐγκαταλιμπανόμενα ἐν τῇσι νούσοισιν· ἐπὶ γὰρ τῆς τελείας κρίσεως οὐδὲν ὅλως ἐγκαταλιμπάνεται.

Εἰρηκὼς δὲ ὑποστροφὰς ποιέειν εἴωθε φησὶν ὅσον ἐφ' ἑαυτοῖς τὰ ἐγκαταλιμπανόμενα τὰ νοσοποιὰ ὄντα τῷ εἴδει ἀνατροπὴν ἐμποιεῖν· εἰ μέντοι τὸ τοιοῦτον σῶμα ἐπίκουρον σχοίη τὴν τέχνην σωφρόνως διαιτῶσαν τὸν κάμνοντα καὶ δαπανῶσαν ἐνταῦθα τὸ ἐγκατάλειμμα, οὐ γενήσεται ὑποστροφὴ τῆς τελείας ἀπαλλαγῆς τοῦ νοσήματος προφθανούσης.

Ἀποσῴζει δὲ οὗτος ὁ ἀφορισμὸς συνέχειαν πρὸς τὸν ἀφορισμὸν τὸν λέγοντα· «Ἢν ἐκ νόσου τροφὴν λαμβάνων τις μὴ ἰσχύῃ, σημαίνει, ὅτι πλείονι τροφῇ χρέεται· ἢν δὲ τροφὴν μὴ λαμβάνοντος τοῦτο γίνηται, σημαίνει, ὅτι κενώσεως δεῖται», τουτέστιν, ἐὰν ἐκ νόσου ἀναλαμβάνηταί τις καταβεβλημένην ἔχων τὴν ὀρεκτικὴν δύναμιν, δεῖ καθᾶραι αὐτοῦ τὸ σῶμα, ἐπειδὴ ἐγκατάλειμμα τοῦ νοσοποιοῦ αἰτίου ἐν αὐτῷ ἐμφωλεύει· τὰ γὰρ ἐγκαταλιμπανόμενα ἐν τῇσι νούσοισι μετὰ κρίσιν ὑποστροφὰς ποιέειν εἴωθεν.

II 12 [II 13: IV 472,11–13 L.] Ὁκόσοισι κρίσις γίνηται, τουτέοισι νὺξ δύσφορος ἡ πρὸ τοῦ παροξυσμοῦ, ἡ δὲ ἐπιοῦσα εὐφορωτέρα, ἢ ὡς ἐπὶ τὸ πολύ.

Οὗτος ὁ ἀφορισμὸς συνεχής ἐστι τῷ πρὸ αὐτοῦ· περὶ ἀτελοῦς γὰρ κρίσεως ἐν ἐκείνῳ διαλεγόμενος ὁ Ἱπποκράτης, ὡς ἀπορίαν αὐτῷ λέγοντός τινος· «Πόθεν ὅλως ὀφείλω γνῶναι μέλλουσαν κρίσιν ἔσεσθαι;» φησίν, ὅτι προγινώσκομεν ἐσομένην κρίσιν ἔκ τε τῶν τῆς πέψεως σημείων, ἅτινα ἐν κενουμένοις θεωρεῖται, καὶ τοῦ εἴδους

22–28] *v.* Gal. In Aphor. II 12: XVII B 468,9–469,3 K. *cf.* Theoph. In Aphor.: II 303,22–26 Dietz 23sq. Ἢν – δεῖται] Hipp. Aphor. II 8: IV 472,1–3 L.

1 Ῥᾷον *addidi* 2 οὐ – ποτοῦ] τοῦ α: *supplevi* 3 οἴνου] ὕπνου A 5 μέντι A 9 νοσήματος *scripsi*: σώματος α 23 λαμβάνων τροφὴν A 29 ἡ νὺξ *infra, vol. II, fol. 133ᵛ, Hipp.* 30 ἡ[I]] ἢ α: *corr.* A[2] εὐφορωτέρα, ἢ] εὐφορωτέρα ἤ, α: *correxi*: εὐφορωτέρα *infra, p. 162,4, Hipp.* 31 τὸ] *item infra, p. 162,8, Hipp.*: *om. infra, p. 162,4* 33 αὐτῷ *scripsi*: αὐτ˜ P: αὐτοῦ A 35 ἐν κενουμένοις] ἐκκενουμένης P

Notice Hippocrates' expertise, when he says: It is easier to be replenished with drink than with food, for drink, while easier, is not necessarily better. Why? Because upon dispersal of solid substance the body, though more easily saturated with wine, is none the better for it, since in that case the wine does not replenish what is lacking, but it provides a ready replenishment of the fluid substance.

II 11. Residues in diseases left after the crisis will cause relapses.

Here some make the objection: "If a crisis of the disease has taken place, how can there be a relapse, though in the crisis nature expels all the causes of disease?" We reply that the word crisis is equivocal: there is a perfect and an imperfect, a certain and an uncertain, a distinct and an indistinct crisis. Now if the crisis has been perfect, no relapse can possibly follow; but if it is imperfect, the remainder of the matter may cause recurrence. Hippocrates refers to an imperfect crisis, as appears from the words residues in diseases; for in a case of perfect crisis nothing at all is left.

When he says will cause relapses, he means that, if left to themselves, residues of a disease-producing kind bring about an upheaval; but if such a body finds an ally in medicine, which keeps the patient on a sensible diet and thus disposes of the residue, there will be no relapse, because it will be anticipated by complete recovery.

This aphorism continues the one which says, "If after sickness a person, while taking food, does not gain strength, this is a sign that he receives too much food; if it happens without his taking food, that is a sign that he needs evacuation", in other words, if during recovery a patient's appetitive faculty is low, we must purge his body, because a residue of the cause of the disease is lurking inside; for residues in diseases left after the crisis will cause relapses.

II 12. Patients in a crisis have a restless night before the paroxysm and a more comfortable one after it, at least in most cases.

This aphorism continues the preceding one, in which Hippocrates discussed an imperfect crisis; now, as if somebody asked the question: "How can I tell at all if there is going to be a crisis?" he says that we prognosticate a crisis from the signs of concoction that appear during evacuation, from the kind of

τοῦ νοσήματος ὀξέος τε ὄντος ἢ χρονίου καὶ ἐκ τῶν ἐπιδήλων ἡμερῶν τῶν ἐν ταῖς Κρισίμοις ἡμῖν παραδεδομένων. καὶ μὴ θαυμάσῃς, εἰ κρίσεώς τινος μελετωμένης ἐν δυσφορίᾳ τινὶ καὶ ταραχῇ τὸ σῶμα διατίθεται. οὕτως γὰρ καὶ ἐπὶ τῶν ἐκτὸς ἀγωνιζομένων ἔστι θεάσασθαι· εἴτε γὰρ παλαίστρα εἴτε δρόμος εἴτε ἄλλο τι τῶν γυμνασίων ὁ προκείμενος εἴη ἆθλος, ἐν φροντίδι καὶ ἀγρυπνίᾳ τούς τε ἀγωνοθέτας καὶ τοὺς εἰς τὸν ἀγῶνα παρασκευαζομένους τὸ πᾶν τῆς προηγουμένης νυκτὸς ὄψει διατελοῦντας· πληρωθέντος δὲ τοῦ ἀγῶνος ἠρεμία τοὺς ἀγωνισαμένους διαδέχεται, καὶ μάλιστα τοὺς τὸ τῆς νίκης κράτος διαδεξαμένους. οὕτω γοῦν καὶ ἐπὶ τῆς καθ' ἡμᾶς ἔχει φύσεως· ἡνίκα ὁ τῆς κρίσεως ἐπιστῇ καιρός, δυσφορία κατὰ τὴν προηγουμένην γίνεται νύκτα ἐν ἐκείνῃ τῇ ἡμέρᾳ ἁπάσας τὰς οἰκείας δυνάμεις τῆς φύσεως κατὰ τῶν νοσοποιῶν κινούσης αἰτίων· ἀλλοιωτικὴν μὲν εἰς τὸ τελείως ἐκπέψαι τὰς ὕλας — ἤδη γὰρ σαφῆ πέψεως ἐφάνη σημεῖα, εἴ γε ταῦτα τὴν ἀκμὴν τοῦ νοσήματος χαρακτηρίζει, ἐν γὰρ τῇ ἀκμῇ ἡ κρίσις ἀπαντᾷ —· ἀλλὰ καὶ τῇ διακριτικῇ κέχρηται δυνάμει, χωρίζει γὰρ τὰ ἀναγκαῖα ἀπὸ τῶν περιττῶν, ὥστε τῶν μὲν ἐν κατοχῇ γενέσθαι, τὰ δὲ ἀπορρίψασθαι· ἐπεγείρει δὲ καὶ τὴν ἀποκριτικήν, ὥστε ἀποδιῶξαι τὰ ἄχρηστα καὶ διοχλοῦντα καὶ τὸ ζῷον λυμαίνοντα. ἐν αὐτῇ τοίνυν τῇ κινήσει ἄλλων ἀλλαχόθεν μεταρριπτομένων τοῦ σώματος ὑλῶν πόσην οἴει περὶ τὸν κάμνοντα γίνεσθαι δυσφορίαν· οὐ μόνον δὲ κατὰ τὴν κίνησιν, ἀλλὰ καὶ τῶν ὑλῶν παροδευουσῶν τὸν στόμαχον ἢ τὸ ἧπαρ ἢ τὴν γαστέρα ἤ τι ἕτερον τῶν αἰσθητικῶν μορίων εἰκὸς ῥύσιν ἢ λυγμὸν ἢ στρόφον ἢ βορβορυγμὸν ἤ τι τῶν τοιούτων τοῖς κάμνουσιν ἐπιγίνεσθαι· ἢ καὶ ἀτμοί τινες περὶ τὸν ἐγκέφαλον ἀναγόμενοι παρακοπὰς ἢ βαρυηκοΐας ἢ ἀμβλυωπίας ἐπιφέροντες τοῖς κάμνουσι πολύτροπον τὴν δυσφορίαν ἐργάζονται. καὶ ὁ μὲν ἰδιώτης δεδιὼς τὸν κίνδυνον ταράττεται καὶ ὑπαναχωρεῖ, ὁ δὲ Ἱπποκράτειος ἰατρὸς εὐφραίνεται ταῦτα ὁρῶν. πέψεως γὰρ προεωρακὼς σημεῖα ἀγαθὴν τὴν ἔκβασιν καὶ ἀπαλλαγὴν τοῦ νοσήματος ἐκδέχεται.

Καὶ ἀποροῦσί τινες λέγοντες· «Τί δήποτε μόνην τὴν νύκτα ὑπέθου τὴν πρὸ τῆς κρίσεως δύσφορον ⟨ὡς⟩ πάσης κρίσεως ἐν ἡμέρᾳ γινομένης, οὐχὶ δὲ καὶ ἐν νυκτί; εἰ δὲ καὶ ἐν νυκτὶ γίνεται, ὡς ἐκ τῶν πραγμάτων ἐστὶ δῆλον, διὰ τί μὴ καὶ τὴν ἡμέραν ἔφης τὴν πρὸ τῆς αὐτῆς νυκτὸς δύσφορον γίνεσθαι ἐπὶ τῶν ἐν νυκτὶ μελλόντων κρίνεσθαι;» καὶ λέγομεν πρώτην μὲν λύσιν τοιαύτην· εἰκότως δυσφορίαν βουλόμενος ὑπογράψαι νυκτερινὸν αὐτῆς τὸν χρόνον ἀφώρισεν· ἐν γὰρ τῇ νυκτὶ τῷ λόγῳ τῆς πυκνώσεως τῆς ἐπιφανείας, εἴ γε ἑκάστη νὺξ τῆς ἰδίας ἡμέρας ψυχροτέρα ἐστί, πάχυνσις ἕπεται τῶν χυμῶν, ἐν δὲ τῇ ἡμέρᾳ ἀραίωσις τῶν πόρων καὶ λέπτυνσις τῶν χυμῶν διὰ τὴν τοῦ περιέχοντος ἀλέαν, εἴ γε πᾶσα ἡμέρα τῆς ἰδίας νυκτὸς θερμοτέρα ἐστὶ τῇ τοῦ ἡλίου παρουσίᾳ. ἐν γοῦν τῇ ἡμέρᾳ διαφόρησις τῶν ὑλῶν γίνεται καὶ βοηθεῖται κατὰ τοῦτο καὶ ἡ φύσις, ἐν δὲ τῇ νυκτὶ τῷ ἀδιαφορήτῳ τῆς ὕλης μᾶλλον ἡ φύσις βαρύνεται καὶ τὸ νόσημα βοηθεῖται. διὸ οὐκ εὐχερῶς ἐν ἡμέρᾳ γίνεται ὥσπερ ἐν νυκτὶ δυσφορία. ἑτέραν δὲ τοιαύτην· ὁ ὕπνος ἀνάπαυσις καὶ ἡσυχία τῆς ψυχῆς καὶ λήθη τις τῶν ἐνοχλούντων παθῶν ὑπάρχει. ὅντινα καὶ μάλιστα φυσικῶς ἐν ταῖς νυξὶ παραλαμβάνομεν· τούτου γὰρ ἐν ἡμέρᾳ στερούμενοι οὐδὲν ἀξιόλογον

1 καὶ — 16 λυμαίνοντα] *cf.* Theoph. In Aphor.: II 304,5–11 Dietz 1sq. καὶ — παραδεδομένων] *Stephanus* Gal. De dieb. decr. II 5: IX 871,1–7 K. *explicans* 38 ἑτέραν — 162,3] *cf.* Gal. In Aphor. II 13: XVII B 470,4–9 K.

7 διατελοῦντος α: *correxi* 8 *fort.* δεξαμένους *scribendum est* 18 παρευοδουσῶν α: *correxi* 20 ῥύσιν *scripsi*: οὖσιν α 22 ἐπιφέρονται α: *correxi* πολύτροφον α: *correxi* 27 ὡς *addidi*

disease, acute or chronic, and from the indicative days set forth in the On Critical Days. Do not be surprised if, with a crisis coming on, the body is subject to a certain restlessness and confusion. In daily life we observe the same phenomenon in participants in a contest: whether the forthcoming contest is a wrestling match, a race, or any other form of athletics, you will find both the judges and those who prepare for the match in a state of worry and sleeplessness during the entire preceding night; but when the contest is over, the participants relax, and especially those who have won the victory. Now it is the same with our bodily constitution: when the time of the crisis has come, there is restlessness during the preceding night, for on that day nature mobilizes all its faculties against the causes of the disease; it needs the transformative faculty for complete concoction of the various kinds of matter — distinct signs of concoction have already appeared, since these are characteristic of the acme of the disease, for the crisis takes place during the acme —; but it also uses the separative faculty, segregating the necessary from the superfluous, so as to retain the former and to reject the latter; it activates also the secretory faculty, in order to expel what is useless, troublesome and harmful to the organism. In the course of this commotion, when all kinds of matter are hurled from one part of the body to another, imagine the patient's discomfort; this is not only due to the commotion, but besides, as the matter passes through the stomach, the liver, the belly or another sensitive part, it can easily happen that the patient is further disturbed by flux, hiccup, cramps, rumblings, or similar troubles; or certain vapors, mounting to the brain, may cause delirium, hardness of hearing, or dim sight, and thus harass the patient in many ways. The incompetent man then panics and withdraws in confusion, but the Hippocratic physician is glad when he sees this; for as he observes the signs of concoction, he anticipates a propitious issue and recovery from the sickness.

Some ask the question: "Why did you assume that only the night before the crisis is uncomfortable, as if every crisis occurs in the daytime, and not at night as well? And if it does occur at night too, as the facts prove, why didn't you say also that the day preceding that night is restless for patients who are going to have their crisis in the night?" Our solution is in the first place this: since he wanted to describe a case of discomfort, he had good reason to define it as occurring at night; for at night, owing to the contraction of the surface, because each night is colder than the corresponding day, a thickening of the humors results, while by day there is opening of the pores and comminution of the humors thanks to the warmth of the surrounding air, because each day is warmer than the corresponding night by the presence of the sun. In the daytime, indeed, there is dispersal of matter, and this is helpful to nature, but at night, when the matter remains undispersed, the stress on nature is heavier, and this is helpful to the disease. This is why a state of discomfort does not develop as readily in the daytime as it does at night. Another solution is the following: sleep is rest and quiet for the soul and forgetfulness of disturbing emotions. The most natural time to enjoy it is night; if we have to forgo it in the daytime, we do not consider this a

ζημιοῦσθαι δοκοῦμεν, ἐν δὲ τῇ νυκτὶ ἀγρυπνοῦντες δυσχερῶς καὶ ἐπισφαλῶς φέρομεν. ἐπειδὴ οὖν μείζονα τὴν δυσφορίαν ἡ νὺξ ἀπεργάζεται, διὰ τοῦτο ἐπιτεταμένην δυσφορίαν δηλῶσαι προθέμενος ὁ Ἱπποκράτης νυκτερινῆς αὐτῆς ἐμνημόνευσεν.

Εἶτά φησιν· ἡ δὲ ἐπιοῦσα εὐφορωτέρα ὡς ἐπὶ πολύ. ὡς τινος γὰρ λέγοντος ὅτι «Οὐ πάντως ἡ ἐπιοῦσα νὺξ ἡ μετὰ τὴν κρίσιν εὐφορίαν φέρει, ὦ Ἱππόκρατες· πολλάκις γὰρ γέγονε μὲν ἡ κρίσις ἀτελής, κατεβλήθη δὲ ἐν τῷ κάμνοντι ἡ δύναμις, ὡς παραμεῖναι τὴν δυσφορίαν καὶ μέχρι τῆς ἐπιούσης νυκτός.» ταύτην ἀποκρουόμενος ὁ Ἱπποκράτης τὸ ὡς ἐπὶ τὸ πολὺ ἔφη, τουτέστι τῶν ἐνδεχομένων ἐστὶ καὶ μέχρι τῆς ἐπιούσης νυκτὸς παραμεῖναι τὴν δυσφορίαν διὰ μίαν τῶν εἰρημένων αἰτιῶν. ἀλλὰ τοῦτο σπάνιον, διὸ συγκριτικῶς ἐχρήσατο τῇ φωνῇ εὐφορωτέρη εἰρηκώς· ἢ γὰρ καὶ πρὸς τοὺς ὑγιαίνοντας τὴν παραβολὴν ποιεῖται ἢ καὶ πρὸς τὴν προηγησαμένην τῆς κρίσεως νύκτα, καὶ ἐπὶ ἀνομοίῳ γὰρ ποιεῖται τὴν σύγκρισιν.

II 13 [II 14: IV 474,1–2 L.] Ἐν τῇσι τῆς κοιλίης ῥύσεσιν αἱ μεταβολαὶ τῶν διαχωρημάτων ὠφελέουσιν, ἢν μὴ εἰς πονηρὰ μεταβάλλωσιν.

Διδάσκει ἡμᾶς ὁ Ἱπποκράτης διὰ τῶν προλαβόντων σημεῖα μελλούσης ἔσεσθαι κρίσεως· νῦν δὲ παραδίδωσιν ἕτερα σημεῖα, ἐξ ὧν ἐστι δυνατὸν διαγνῶναι κρίσιν γενομένην, εἴτε τελεία καὶ ἐπ' ἀγαθῷ γίνεται καὶ τὰ τῆς προηγησαμένης δυσφορίας πέπαυται, εἴτε μή, ἀλλὰ προσδοκᾶται ἔτι μένειν ἡ δυσφορία. φησὶ γάρ· Ἐν τῇσι τῆς κοιλίης ῥύσεσιν αἱ μεταβολαὶ τῶν διαχωρημάτων ὠφελέουσιν, ἢν μὴ ἐς πονηρὰ μεταβάλλωσι. καὶ αὐτὸς μὲν τῆς διὰ γαστρὸς γινομένης καὶ μόνης κρίσεως ἐμνημόνευσε, σὲ δὲ ὑπακούειν κελεύει κατὰ τὴν αὐτὴν ἀναλογίαν καὶ τῆς δι' οὔρων καὶ ἱδρώτων καὶ πτυσμάτων καὶ ἐμέτων ἐκκρίσεως. σκόπει οὖν, φησίν, ἐκκρίσεως ἢ ἐκταράξεως κατὰ τὴν γαστέρα γινομένης τὰ διαχωρήματα· καὶ ἐὰν μεταβολὴν ἔχῃ, τῶν μὲν παχέων εἰς λεπτότητα συμμέτρως μεταληφθέντων, τῶν δὲ λεπτῶν εἰς παχέα, καὶ τῶν κακοχύμων εἰς εὐχυμότερα, ἀγαθὴν νόμιζε εἶναι τὴν κρίσιν, σημαίνει γάρ, ὅτι κρατοῦσα ἡ δύναμις τῶν αἰτίων τὴν ἀμυδρὰν πέψιν μείζονα καὶ τελεωτέραν ἐργάζεται. καλῶς δὲ ἔφη ῥύσεσι καὶ οὐκ εἶπεν ἐκκρίσεσι· βούλεται γὰρ κριτικῆς γενομένης τῆς ἐκκρίσεως ἐπιτεταμένην γενέσθαι τὴν κένωσιν, ὅπερ διὰ τῆς ῥύσεως ἐσήμανεν. οὐ μόνον δὲ ἡνίκα κριτικῶς κινοῦνται τὰ κινούμενα τὸ τοιοῦτον ἀγαθὸν δεῖ νομίζειν, ἀλλὰ καὶ ὁπωσοῦν ἄλλως ἐκκρίσεως γινομένης, εἴτε διὰ γαστρός, εἴτε δι' οὔρων, εἴτε διὰ πτυέλων, ἡ ἐπὶ τὴν ἀκριβῆ τῶν κενουμένων πέψιν μεταβολὴ ὠφέλιμός ἐστι καὶ ἀγαθὸν σημεῖον.

Πλὴν ἐπειδὴ μεταβολῆς ἐμνημόνευσεν, ἡ δὲ μεταβολὴ δύναται καὶ ἐπὶ τὸ χεῖρον γενέσθαι, ἡνίκα πεπεμμένα μὲν ἄρχεται κενοῦσθαι, ὀκλάζουσα δὲ ἡ δύναμις καὶ πρὸς τὴν ἔκκρισιν ἀτονοῦσα τῶν χυμῶν ἧττον αὐτῶν τῇ πέψει ἐπιστατεῖ, ἐπήγαγεν· ἢν μὴ εἰς πονηρὰ μεταβάλλῃ, τουτέστιν, ἐὰν μὴ ἀπεψίᾳ ἡ μεταβολὴ γένηται,

16 νῦν – 18 μή] *v.* Theoph. In Aphor.: II 305,8–9 Dietz 20 καὶ – 22 ἐκκρίσεως] *cf.* Theoph. In Aphor.: II 305,17–19 Dietz

1 δυσφερῶς A 10 συγκριτικῆς P 13 ῥύσησιν α: *corr.* A² 14 μεταβάλλωσιν] *item infra, lin. 20*: μεταβάλωσιν P: μεταβάλλῃ (-ει) *infra, pp. 162,36; 164,2; vol. II, fol. 84ʳ, Hipp.* 18 μὴν A 19 ῥύσησιν A 20 μὲν *om.* A 21 κρίσεως *in* ἐκκρίσεως *mut.* A 22 ἐκκρίσεως] *fort.* κρίσεως *scribendum est* 24 ἔχει A μεταληφθέντων] καταβληθέντων A 29 *fort.* κενοῦνται τὰ κενούμενα *scribendum est* 32 μεταβολὴ *scripsi*: μεταβολ' A: μεταβολὴν P 35 ἔκκρισιν *scripsi*: κρίσιν α 36 μεταβάλλωσι A

serious loss, but sleeplessness at night we experience as troublesome and perilous. Therefore, since night makes the discomfort worse, and since Hippocrates' intention was to describe intense discomfort, he referred to it as appearing at night.

He goes on, and a more comfortable one after it in most cases. It is as if somebody had said: "The night after the crisis does not bring relief in every case, Hippocrates; often the crisis has been incomplete, and the patient's resistance has broken down, with the result that the discomfort lasts through the following night." To prevent this objection, Hippocrates added in most cases, that is to say, it is possible for the discomfort to last through the following night for one of the reasons mentioned. This, however, is exceptional, and hence he used the comparative more comfortable, the comparison relating either to healthy persons, or to the night preceding the crisis, for he must be contrasting it with something dissimilar.

II 13. In fluxes of the bowels changes in the excrements are beneficial, if they do not result in bad signs.

In the preceding aphorisms Hippocrates shows us signs of an approaching crisis; here, he deals with other signs which permit us to decide whether a past crisis is perfect and salutary and the discomfort that preceded it is over, or whether this is not so and continuing discomfort is to be expected. His words are: In fluxes of the bowels changes in the excrements are beneficial, if they do not result in bad signs. He himself mentions only the crisis that takes place by way of the bowels, but he wants you to understand, by analogy, excretion by urine, sweating, sputamen and vomiting as well. When there is excretion by, or commotion in, the bowels, he tells you to observe the excrements: when they change, so that the thick become moderately thin, the thin thick, and the kind of humor improves, then you may take it that the crisis is salutary, for it signifies that resistance prevails over the causes and makes the incipient concoction stronger and more complete. He rightly said fluxes, not "excretions"; for he means that if the excretion is critical, evacuation becomes intensive, which he expressed by the word flux. However, not only when the commotion takes place during a crisis should such a thing be regarded as beneficial; whenever there is excretion in any other situation, whether through the bowels, or through urine, or through sputum, the change toward complete concoction of the evacuated matter is helpful and a good sign.

But since he has mentioned change, and change can also be for the worse, when at the beginning the evacuated matter is well concocted, but then resistance gives out, becomes too weak to excrete the humors and loses control of their concoction, he continues, if they do not result in bad signs; this occurs when the change is not due to incomplete concoction, but to the brutal force of a symp-

ἀλλὰ βίᾳ συμπτώματος προπηλακίζοντος αὐτὴν καὶ ἐρεθίζοντος. νόμιζε οὖν διὰ τοῦ εἰπεῖν ἢν μὴ εἰς πονηρὰ μεταβάλλῃ μὴ μόνον τὰ ἄπεπτα σημαίνεσθαι, τυχὸν τὰ παχύτερα ἢ λεπτότερα, ἀλλὰ καὶ τὰ μοχθηρά, ὁποῖά εἰσι τὰ κατὰ τὸ χρῶμα συνεστῶτα, τὰ ἄκρατον ἔχοντα τὸ ξανθόν, τὰ ἄγαν πελιδνά, τὰ μέλανα, οὐ μὴν ἀλλὰ καὶ τὰ ποικίλα, ἡνίκα δὴ καὶ χρωμάτων διαφορὰ ἐμφέρεται τοῖς ἐκκρινομένοις καὶ σύστασις ἀνόμοιος, ὥστε καὶ λεπτὰ καὶ παχέα, καὶ ἀδρομερῆ καὶ λεῖα, καὶ ξανθὰ καὶ πελιδνὰ καὶ μέλανα, καὶ πρασώδη ἢ ἰώδη ἢ λεκιθώδη ἢ τρυγώδη εἶναι τὰ ἐκκρινόμενα, ἅτινα ποικίλῃ τίκτεται δυσκρασίᾳ. τῇ αὐτῇ δὲ διαιρέσει δῆλα καὶ τὰ ὀλέθρια· τὰ αἱματώδη, τὰ ξυσματώδη, τὰ λιπαρά τε καὶ ἐλαιώδη, καὶ τὰ τούτοις παραπλήσια. πᾶσα γὰρ ἡ ἐν τούτοις μεταβολὴ ἐπὶ κακῷ γίνεται, ὥστε ἢ καὶ αὖθις παρεῖναι τὴν προηγησαμένην δυσφορίαν τῆς κρίσεως, ὥσπερ ἐπὶ τῶν ἀπέπτων ὑλῶν, ἢ καὶ ἐπιταθῆναι, ὥσπερ ἐπὶ τῶν ποικίλων καὶ μοχθηρῶν. ἔστι δ' ὅτε καὶ ἐπὶ τῶν ὀλεθρίων τοῦτο συμβαίνει· τούτων γὰρ τὰ μὲν ἁπλῶς ἄπεπτα ἀμυδρὰν τὴν παρὰ φύσιν αἰτίαν ἐνδείκνυται, τὰ δὲ μοχθηρὰ καὶ ποικίλα [καὶ] ἰσχυρὰ καὶ πλείονα τὰ αἴτια δείκνυσι· τὰ γὰρ ὀλέθρια πολλῷ μᾶλλον ἰσχυροτέραν τὴν νοσοποιὸν αἰτίαν ὑποτίθεται.

II 14 [II 15: IV 474,3–6 L.] Ὅκου φάρυγξ νοσέει ἢ φύματα ἐν τῷ σώματι ἐκφύεται, σκέπτεσθαι τὰς ἐκκρίσιας· ἢν γὰρ χολώδεες ἔωσι, τὸ σῶμα συννοσέει, ἢν δὲ ὅμοια τοῖσιν ὑγιαίνουσι γίνονται, ἀσφαλῶς τὸ σῶμα τρέφειν.

Εἴρηται ἡμῖν ἀνωτέρω, ὅτι δεῖ σκοπεῖν ἀτελοῦς γινομένης κρίσεως ὥστε τὸν ἀπολειφθέντα χυμὸν κενῶσαι· μὴ κενούμενος γὰρ ὑποτροπιασμοὺς ποιεῖν εἴωθεν. οὗτος τοίνυν ὁ ἐναπομένων χυμὸς ἢ ἐν ὅλῳ τῷ σώματι περιέχεται ἢ ἐν μέρει. καὶ εἰ μὲν ἐν ὅλῳ τῷ σώματί ἐστιν, ἐπεγειρομένη πολλάκις ἡ φύσις ἀποδιώκει [πολλάκις] αὐτὸν ἐκ τοῦ βάθους εἰς ἐπιφάνειαν· ᾗτινι ὁμιλήσας στεγανῇ οὔσῃ καὶ πυκνῇ ἐσφηνώθη καὶ τῇ δριμύτητι ἀνιᾷ καὶ διεξέρχεται κατά τινα διάβρωσιν, ὡς γίνεσθαι ἑλκύδρια καὶ φύματά τινα. εἰ δὲ ἐν μορίῳ ἐστὶν ἡ ἐγκαταλειφθεῖσα ὕλη αὕτη, ἢ κατὰ τὸν ἐγκέφαλον ὑπόκειται καὶ πέμπεται εἰς τὰ ὑποκείμενα κἀκεῖσε σφηνοῦται, τυχὸν εἰς τὸν φάρυγγα· ἢ κατὰ τὴν καρδίαν πλεονάζει ἢ ἐν τοῖς θρεπτικοῖς καὶ ἀπελαύνεται εἰς τὰ ὑπερκείμενα καὶ εἰς τὸν φάρυγγα σφηνοῦται, ὡς εἴρηται, ὥστε γενέσθαι ἐν αὐτῷ φλεγμονὴν ἢ ἐρυσίπελας ἢ ἄνθρακα ἢ ἕτερόν τι τοιοῦτον. δέχεται γὰρ ὁ φάρυγξ ὑλῶν προσβολὰς καὶ ἀπὸ ἐγκεφάλου ὡς ὑπερκειμένου καὶ ἀπὸ καρδίας καὶ τῶν θρεπτικῶν ὡς ὑποκειμένων.

Καὶ εἰ δοκεῖ, ἐπὶ δυοῖν ὑποθέσεων διευκρινήσωμεν τὰ λεγόμενα. ὑποκείσθωσαν δύο τινὲς κάμνοντες· τὸν μὲν οὖν ἕτερον τούτων εἰσελθὼν εὗρον πολλὰ κατὰ τὴν ἐπιφάνειαν ἔχοντα φύματα, καὶ ἐλογισάμην, ὅτι κακοχυμίας μεστόν ἐστι τοῦτο τὸ σῶμα καὶ δεῖ ταύτην κενῶσαι. εἶτα εἰσελθὼν πρὸς τὸν αὐτὸν καί τις ἀγελαῖος ἰατρὸς

1 νόμιζε – 16] *v.* Hipp. Progn. 11: p. 206,12–207,6 Alexanderson = II 136,7–138,6 L. Steph. In Progn. II 18: CMG XI 1,2, p. 178,14–182,10 21 ἀνωτέρω] *v. supra*, p. 158,7–28 23 καὶ – 29 φάρυγγα] *cf.* Gal. In Aphor. II 15: XVII B 472,5–12 K.

2 μεταβάλη P 8 τίκτεται *scripsi*: τήκεται α 14 καὶ[II] *delevi* 18 χολῶδες *in* χολώδεες *corr.* A[2] 19 ὅμοια] *item infra, p. 166,33, Theoph.* S: ὅμοιαι *Hipp.* ἀσφαλῶς] *item infra, p. 166,21. 35*: ἀσφαλὲς *Hipp.* 24 πολλάκις[II] *delevi* 31 αὐτῇ A γὰρ *om.* A 34 διακρινήσωμεν P 37 τὸν *om.* P

tom which mauls and harasses the power of resistance. It should be clear, then, that when he says, if they do not result in bad signs, he is referring not only to unconcocted excrements, e.g. too thick or too thin, but no less to those that are danger signs, such as, in the case of stools of even color, those that are yellow without admixture, or excessively gray, or black, but also varied ones, when a difference of color appears in the excretions and an unequal consistency, so that the excrements are both thin and thick, both coarse and smooth, yellow and gray and black, the color of leek or verdigris or eggyolk or winelees, which are produced by a variety of distempers. The same classification will also reveal the fatal signs: stools like blood, like scrapings, those fat and oily, etc. For any change in these bodes evil, i.e. either the discomfort that preceded the crisis will reappear, as in the case of unconcocted matter, or it will get even worse, namely when the matter is varied and bad-looking. Sometimes this also happens with those that are deadly signs: if they are simply unconcocted, they indicate that the cause of the abnormal condition is weak, but if they are bad and varied, they point to strong and more numerous causes; for fatal signs presuppose a much stronger disease-producing cause.

> **II 14.** When the throat is diseased or tumors appear on the body, you must examine the excretions: if they are bilious, the body is also affected, but if they are like those of healthy people, it is safe to feed the body.

We said above that, when there is an imperfect crisis, one should plan to evacuate the remaining humor; for if it is not evacuated it frequently causes relapses. Now this residual humor is contained either in the whole body or in a part. If it is in the whole body, often nature will be stirred to action and expel it from the depth to the surface; when reaching the surface, which is compact and dense, (the humor) is wedged in and by its pungency irritates it and passes through by a kind of corrosion, so that small sores and tumors are produced. If, on the other hand, this remaining matter is contained in a part, either it is found on the brain and is dispatched to the underlying parts and is wedged in there, e.g. in the throat; or there is a surplus of it around the heart or in the alimentary organs, and then it is expelled upwards and is wedged in at the throat, as above, so that an inflammation or erysipelas or a carbuncle or something of the sort is formed there. The throat, in fact, receives influxes of matters both from the brain inasmuch as it is above it and from the heart and the alimentary organs inasmuch as they are below it.

If you like, we will illustrate this by two cases. Let us take two patients: when visiting one of them I find that he has a great number of tumors at the surface, and I conclude that this body is full of bad humors and that they must be evacuated. Next, one of those common doctors visiting this same man imme-

εὐθέως ἐχώρησεν ἐπὶ τὴν κάθαρσιν, καὶ ἀπροόπτως κενώσας πλέον ἠδίκησε. τίνι λόγῳ; διὰ τὸ μὴ ἔχειν τὸν νοσοῦντα ὅλον τὸ σῶμα ἔμπλεον τῆς φαινομένης κακοχυμίας· ἥψατο γὰρ τὸ καθάρσιον τῆς ὑγιαινούσης οὐσίας τῶν χυμῶν μὴ εὑρηκὸς ἐκεῖνον, καθ' ὃν ὤφειλεν ἐνεργῆσαι, καὶ τὰς ἐν αὐτῷ τῷ ἀνθρώπῳ δυνάμεις κατέβαλεν. ἅπερ ὁ τεχνίτης σημειούμενος οὐκ ἀπροόπτως ἐκάθηρε τὸν ἄνθρωπον, ἀλλὰ σημειώσασθαι προὔθετο τὰ ⟨ἐκ⟩κρινόμενα, οὖρά φημι καὶ διαχωρήματα, ἵνα, εἰ μὲν εὕροι ταῦτα ὅμοια τοῖς τῶν ὑγιαινόντων, ἀπόσχηται τῆς κενώσεως ὡς δὴ τοῦ βάθους ἐλευθέρου τυγχάνοντος· εἰ δὲ παχύτερα ἢ χολωδέστερα εὑρεθῇ ἐπὶ τούτου τὰ διαχωρήματα, δηλοῦται καὶ τὸ βάθος μετέχον τῆς κακίας τοῦ χυμοῦ καὶ τὴν χρείαν ἐνδείκνυται τῆς καθάρσεως. εἶθ' οὕτως δὲ καὶ εἰς τὸν ἕτερον εἰσέρχομαι ἄρρωστον ἔχοντα ἐν μορίῳ τὸν ἐγκαταλειφθέντα χυμὸν καὶ ὀδυνώμενον τὸν φάρυγγα. καὶ ζητῶ ἐπὶ τούτου τὰ διαχωρήματα· καὶ εἰ μὲν εὑρεθῇ θολερά, λέγω, ὅτι καὶ ὅλον τὸ σῶμα περιττωματικώτερον ὑπάρχει καὶ δεῖ τοῦτο κενῶσαι· εἰ δὲ ὑγιῆ εὑρεθῇ τὰ ἐκκρινόμενα, ὑπερτίθεμαι τὴν κένωσιν, τοῦ λοιποῦ σώματος καθαροῦ ὄντος, τρέπομαι δὲ ἐπὶ τὰ βοηθήματα, ὡς ἐπὶ τοῦ ἐν ὅλῳ τῷ σώματι φύματα ἔχοντος τοῦ βάθους ἐλευθέρου γε ὄντος τοπικοῖς χρῶμαι τοῖς βοηθήμασι.

Διὰ τοῦτο γάρ φησι· δεῖ σκέπτεσθαι τὰς ἐκκρίσεις, τουτέστι τὰ οὖρα καὶ τὰ διαχωρήματα· καὶ εἰ μὲν χολώδη ὦσιν, αὐτὸς μὲν ἐκ τοῦ κατ' ἐξαίρετον εἶπεν, ἐπειδὴ ὡς ἐπὶ πᾶν ἀπὸ χολωδεστέρου αἵματος ἔκβρασις γίνεται· σὺ δὲ σκόπει καὶ σύστασιν, ἤτοι παχύ φημι καὶ θολερὸν καὶ πυρρὸν καὶ τὰ τοιαῦτα· εἰ δὲ μηδὲν τούτων εὕρῃς, ἀσφαλῶς δεῖ τὸ σῶμα τρέφειν καὶ τοπικοῖς χρῆσθαι τοῖς βοηθήμασιν.

Ἀποροῦσι δέ τινες ὅτι «Ἐπὶ μὲν τῶν φυμάτων τῶν καθ' ὅλου τοῦ σώματος βλαστανόντων ἴσως ἔχει λόγον τοῦ νοσεῖν τὸ σῶμα· ἐπὶ δὲ τοῦ φάρυγγος ἑνὸς μορίου πάσχοντος πῶς ἐνδέχεται τὸ ὅλον σῶμα συννοσεῖν; ἴσμεν γάρ, ὅτι ἐνδέχεται τὴν μὲν κεφαλὴν πάσχειν ἢ τοὺς πόδας ἢ ἕτερον μόριον, τὸ δὲ λοιπὸν σῶμα ὑγιαίνειν.» καί φαμεν, ὅτι δυνατὸν τὸν φάρυγγα καὶ ἐκ τῶν ὑπερκειμένων δέχεσθαι ὕλην τινὰ νοσεράν, φημὶ δὴ ἐκ τοῦ ἐγκεφάλου, καὶ ἐκ τῶν ὑποκειμένων, τῶν τε ἀναπνευστικῶν λέγω καὶ τῶν θρεπτικῶν. εἰ οὖν ταῦτα ὑπόκειται μοχθηράν τινα ὕλην ἐπέχοντα, εἰκότως τὸ πᾶν σῶμα νοσεῖν λέγεται, τὰ γὰρ κυρίως ἐπέχοντα ταῦτά εἰσι. τῇ μέντοι συνήθει βραχυλογίᾳ χρώμενος περιφράζει τῶν λεγομένων τὴν ἔννοιαν· εἰρηκὼς γὰρ σκέπτεσθαι τὰς ἐκκρίσιας, ἢν χολώδεες ἔωσιν, ὀφείλων ἐπαγαγεῖν, ὅτι κακοχυμίας πεπλήρωται τὸ σῶμα, ὁ δὲ ἐκ τοῦ ἑπομένου, φημὶ τῆς νόσου, τὸ ἡγούμενον ἐδήλωσεν· εἶτα ἐπαγαγὼν ἢν δὲ ὅμοια τοῖσιν ὑγιαίνουσιν οὐκ εἴρηκε τὸ ἑπόμενον, ὅτι ὑγιὲς καὶ ἀπέριττόν ἐστι τὸ σῶμα, ἀλλὰ τοῦτο παρεὶς τὸ ἐσχάτως ἑπόμενον τέθηκε, φημὶ δὴ τὸ ἀσφαλῶς τὸ σῶμα τρέφειν.

II 15 [II 16: IV 474,7 L.] Ὅκου λιμός, οὐ δεῖ πονέειν.

Οὗτος ὁ ἀφορισμὸς ἐπὶ ὑγιεινῶν εἴρηται παραγγελμάτων. νόμιζε οὖν ἐνταῦθα ταῦτα λέγειν σοι τὸν Ἱπποκράτην, ὅτι ὁ λιμὸς ξηρότητα ἐμποιεῖ τοῖς σώμασι·

29 τῇ – 35] *cf.* Gal. In Aphor. II 15: XVII B 471,14–472,4 K. 37–168,3] *cf.* Theoph. In Aphor.: II 306,22–25 Dietz 37–38 σώμασι] *cf.* Gal. In Aphor. II 16: XVII B 474,1–2 K. Hipp. Aff. 43: VI 252,14–19 L. (?)

4 κατέβαλλεν A 6 κρινόμενα α: *correxi* 12 λέγει P 21 εὕροις A 23 δὲ *om.* A 24 ὅλον τὸ A 27 ἐκ[I] *om.* A 31 χολῶδες *in* χολώδεες *corr.* A[2]

diately proceeds to purging and by imprudent evacuation causes more harm. Why? Because this patient does not have his entire body full of the bad humors that manifest themselves; the purgative attacks the healthy substance of the humors, when it does not find that humor on which it should act, and it impairs the patient's own powers. The experienced physician, observing this, does not purge the man rashly, but makes a point of examining the excretions, i.e. urine and stools; if he finds them similar to those of healthy persons, he will abstain from evacuation, seeing that the inside is clear; but if the man's excretions are found to be too thick or too bilious, this proves that the inside is also affected by the bad humor and it indicates the necessity of purging. Next I visit the other patient, who has the remaining humor in one part, with a sore throat as the result. I ask to see his excretions; and if they are found to be turbid, I say that his entire body suffers from too much surplus matter and that it has to be evacuated; but if the excretions are found to be sound, I abstain from evacuation, the rest of the body being clean, and I proceed to the use of remedies, just as in the case of the patient whose whole body is covered with tumors, provided the inside is clear, I apply local medication.

This is why (Hippocrates) says: You must examine the excretions, i.e. the urine and the stools; then he goes on, if they are bilious, thinking in terms of the prevailing situation, since generally eruptions originate in an excess of bile in the blood; you, however, should also examine the composition, i.e. whether it is thick and turbid and red, etc.; and if you find none of these symptoms, you may safely feed the body and apply local medication.

There are some who object: "In the case of tumors which appear over the entire body, it may make sense to assume that the body is affected; but in the case of the throat, when only one part is sick, how can the whole body be affected with it? Surely we know that it is possible for the head, the feet, or any other part to be ill, while the rest of the body is healthy." We say to this that the throat may receive some kind of diseased matter from the upper parts, i.e. from the brain, as well as from the underlying parts, the respiratory and the alimentary organs. If the situation is such that these contain some corrupted matter, one can say with reason that the whole body is sick, for these are the parts that are vitally affected. (Hippocrates,) however, with his usual conciseness, expresses his thought indirectly; for having told us to examine the excretions, if they are bilious, instead of going on to say, as he should, that the body is full of bad humors, he indicated the preceding cause in terms of the result, i.e. the sickness; then, when he continues, but if they are like those of healthy people, he does not state the conclusion, the body is healthy and free from excess matter, but omitting this he passes on to the final conclusion, that it is safe to feed the body.

II 15. When starved, one should not exert oneself.

This aphorism is concerned with precepts for health. You should look at it this way: Hippocrates tells you here that hunger causes dryness in the body;

σὲ οὖν τὸν ἰατρὸν εἰς τὸ ἐναντίον μετάγειν δεῖ καὶ ὑγραίνειν τὸ σῶμα τὸ κάμνον λιμῷ, τουτέστιν ἡσυχίαν καὶ ἀκινησίαν ἐπιτηδεύειν. ἐπὶ γὰρ τῷ λιμῷ εἰ κινήσεις παραλάβῃς, ἐπιτείνεις τὰ τῆς ξηρότητος τῷ λόγῳ τῆς διαφορήσεως.

Λιμὸν δὲ ἐνταῦθα καλεῖ ὁ Ἱπποκράτης τὴν τῶν σιτίων ἀποχήν. ὁμώνυμον γάρ ἐστι τὸ τοῦ λιμοῦ ὄνομα· λιμὸς γάρ ἐστι καὶ ἡ λεῖψις τοῦ σιτίου· λιμὸς λέγεται καὶ ἡ ἀσιτία, καὶ αὕτη διττῶς· ἢ κατὰ προαίρεσιν, ὡς ὅταν τις διά τινα θρησκείαν νηστεύων ἀπέχηται τῶν βρωμάτων, ἢ ἀπροαιρέτως, καὶ οὕτως ⟨δὲ⟩ διττῶς, ἢ γὰρ κατὰ πρόσταξιν ἄρχοντος ἐν εἱρκτῇ ἀποκλεισθῆναι τὸν ἄνθρωπον καὶ μένειν ἄσιτον, ἢ κατὰ ἰατρικὴν ἀκρίβειαν, ὡς ὅταν πληθωρικὸν ὑπόκειται τὸ σῶμα, τοῦτο γὰρ ἐκτῆξαι βουλόμενοι ἀσιτίαν παραλαμβάνομεν. κατὰ πάντων τῶν σημαινομένων τοῦ λιμοῦ ἁρμόδιός ἐστιν ὁ λόγος τοῦ Ἱπποκράτους· εἰ μή τις εἴποι ἐπὶ τῶν πληθωρικῶν παρὰ τὴν ἀρχὴν τὸ συμμέτρως κινεῖσθαι λυσιτελές τε καὶ οὐκ ἀσύμφορον.

Πόνον δὲ ἐνταῦθα τὸ γυμνάσιον καλεῖ. φησὶ γάρ· Ὅκου λιμός, οὐ δεῖ πονέειν· διὰ τὸ μὴ ἐπιτείνεσθαι τῷ λόγῳ τῶν γυμνασίων τὴν ξηρότητα κακὸν γυμνάζειν τοὺς λιμώττοντας, ἐπὶ μὲν τῶν πληθωρικῶν διὰ τὸ μὴ συγχωρεῖν τὴν ἐκτὸς κίνησιν τῇ φύσει πέττειν τὸν ὠμὸν χυμὸν ἐκεῖνον καὶ εἰς τροφὴν ἑαυτῆς ἀναλίσκειν, ἀλλ' ἐξάγειν αὐτὸν καὶ διαφορεῖν· καὶ ἐπὶ τούτοις δὲ διὰ τὸ ⟨τὸ⟩ ἔμφυτον θερμὸν διαφορεῖσθαι. δεύτερον δέ, ὅτι ἐπὶ τῶν λιμωττόντων ἀσθενοῦσιν αἱ τοῦ σώματος δυνάμεις καὶ καταβέβληνται· ἐπὶ γοῦν ταύτῃ τῇ ἀσθενείᾳ εἰ καὶ γυμνασίοις χρήσαιντο, πολλῷ πλέον καταλυθήσονται. τρίτον ἐπὶ τούτοις κακὴ ἡ ἐπίτασις τῆς ξηρότητος· ὅτι γὰρ διαφορεῖ τὸ σῶμα διὰ ξηρότητα καὶ ἄνικμον ἀπεργάζεται, πρόδηλον παντί.

Ἁρμόζει δὲ καὶ ἐπὶ τῶν νοσούντων τὸ λεγόμενον. πολλάκις γὰρ παραλαμβάνω ἐπὶ πλήθει πυρέττοντα ἄνθρωπον καὶ τοῦτον διὰ πάσης ἄγω ἀσιτίας ὥστε λεπτῦναι τὴν ὕλην καὶ διαφορῆσαι αὐτήν· καὶ οὐ δεῖ ἐφ' ἕτερον κόπον ἤτοι κίνησιν ἄγειν τὸν νοσοῦντα, οὐ τὴν διὰ φλεβοτομίας, οὐ τὴν διὰ καθαρσίου, οὐ τὴν διὰ τρίψεως ἢ λουτροῦ ἢ ἄλλην οἱανοῦν κίνησιν, πολλῷ δὲ πλέον οὐδὲ τὴν κατὰ τόπον· ἀρκούντως γὰρ αὐτῷ ἡ ἀπὸ τῆς ἀσιτίας διαφόρησις ἔχοι ἄν.

II 16 [II 17: IV 474,8–9 L.] Ὅκου ἂν τροφὴ πλείων παρὰ φύσιν εἰσέλθῃ, τοῦτο νόσον ποιέει.

Ἰστέον, ὅτι τὸ τῆς τροφῆς ὄνομα ὁμώνυμόν ἐστι· κατὰ πολλῶν γὰρ φέρεται σημαινομένων, ὡς αὐτὸς ὁ Ἱπποκράτης ἐν τῷ Περὶ τροφῆς ἐδήλωσε, «Τροφὴ» εἰπὼν «τὸ τρέφον, τροφὴ καὶ τὸ οἷον καὶ τὸ μέλλον», εἰς τρία ταύτην διελών. καὶ εἰ

4–11 Ἱπποκράτους] *cf.* Gal. In Aphor. II 16: XVII B 473,11–474,6 K. 5sq. λιμὸς^{II} – ἀσιτία] *v.* Theoph. In Aphor.: II 307,4 Dietz 14 Πόνον – καλεῖ] *v.* Gal. In Aphor. II 16: XVII B 474,8–10 K. 19 δεύτερον – 21 καταλυθήσονται] *cf.* Theoph. In Aphor.: II 306,25–26 Dietz 24–28 τόπον] *cf.* Gal. In Aphor. II 16: XVII B 474,13–475,2 K. Ἁρμόζει – λεγόμενον] *v.* Theoph. In Aphor.: II 307,5–6 Dietz 32–170,14] *cf.* Gal. In Aphor. II 17: XVII B 476,6–477,10 K. 32–170,8 σημαινομένου] *v.* Theoph. In Aphor.: II 307,11–16 Dietz 33sq. Τροφὴ – μέλλον] Hipp. Alim. 8: CMG I 1, p. 79,18 *cf.* Gal. De fac. nat. I 11: Scr. min. III 119,9–24 Helmr. = II 25,14–26,11 K.

2 παραλάβῃς (οι supra ῃ) A 3 ἐπιτείνειν P: ἐπιτείνει *et ras. 1 litt. in* A: *correxi* 7 δὲ *addidi* διττῶς *scripsi*: διττῶν α: διττόν A² 9 τὸ *om.* A 14 καλεῖν A 18 τὸ^{II} *addidi* 26 κένωσιν A 28 ἀρκοῦντος α: *correxi* 29 ἔχει α: *correxi* ἂν] δὲ P 33 Τροφὴ] τροφῆς A

so it is up to you, the physician, to bring about the contrary condition and to provide moisture for the body that is suffering from starvation, in other words, to ensure rest and immobility. For if, in a state of starvation, you prescribe action, you increase the dryness by dispersal.

By starvation Hippocrates here means abstention from food. The word "starvation" has more than one meaning: it is, first, shortage of food; it is also fasting, and this in a twofold sense: either voluntarily, as when a man for some religious reason fasts and abstains from food, or involuntarily, again in two different ways: either the person has been put in prison and is left without food by order of a magistrate, or he is under a strict medical regime, for instance when the body is plethoric, because then we use fasting to reduce it. Hippocrates' rule is applicable to all these meanings of the word "starvation"; unless one wishes to add that in cases of plethora during the initial stage moderate motion is useful and not unprofitable.

By exertion he means athletics here. His words are: "When starved, one should not exert oneself": since we must not increase dryness by exercise, it is dangerous to permit exercise for the hungry, in cases of plethora because the external motion does not allow the constitution to concoct that crude humor and use it for its own nutrition, but drives it out and disperses it; but also in these other cases because the innate heat is dispersed. Secondly because in starvation the faculties of the body are weak and low; if in addition to this weakness patients should also take exercise, the breakdown will be much worse. Thirdly, the increased dryness is bad; for it goes without saying that (exercise) disperses the body by dryness and dehydrates it.

The rule holds also for the sick. Often I treat a person for fever due to excess matter and I put him on a strict fast so as to comminute and disperse the matter; then one should not expose the patient to other kinds of fatigue or commotion, not by bleeding, not by purging, not by massage or bathing or any other action whatsoever, and least of all by locomotion; we may take it that the dispersal by fasting is sufficient for him.

II 16. When an abnormal abundance of food is taken, this causes disease.

The word food is equivocal; for it has several meanings, as Hippocrates himself pointed out in Nutriment, when he says: "Food is what does nourish, it is also what can nourish, and it is what will nourish", thus making a threefold

δοκεῖ, ἕκαστον σαφηνίσωμεν. ὄντως μὲν τροφή ἐστιν ἡ προστεθεῖσα τῷ σώματι, καθ' ἣν τὸ προστεθὲν τῷ νεύρῳ γίνεται νεῦρον καὶ ἐν μυῒ μῦς καὶ ἐν φλεβὶ φλὲψ καὶ ἐν ὀστῷ ὀστοῦν καὶ ἐπὶ τῶν λοιπῶν ὁμοίως. οἷον δὲ τροφή ἐστι τὸ μέλλον ἀναδίδοσθαι ἐξ ἥπατος καθ' ὅλον τὸ σῶμα διὰ τῶν φλεβῶν αἷμα. διὰ τοῦτο δὲ οἷον τροφὴ λέγεται, ἐπειδὴ πολλάκις φλεβοτομίας γενομένης κενοῦται μήπω διασπαρὲν ὥστε γενέσθαι καὶ πρόσφυσιν καὶ ἐξομοίωσιν. μέλλουσα δὲ τροφὴ λέγεται τὰ σιτία· χρόνῳ γάρ τινι μέλλει ταῦτα χυλοποιεῖσθαι καὶ προστίθεσθαι καὶ ἐξομοιοῦσθαι. ἔστιν οὖν ὁ λόγος ἐνταῦθα τῷ Ἱπποκράτει περὶ παντὸς σημαινομένου. καὶ ἡ μέλλουσα γὰρ τροφή, ἥτις ἐστὶ τὰ σιτία, πολλὴ παραληφθεῖσα καὶ διὰ τοῦτο ἀπεπτηθεῖσα νόσον ποιεῖ· καὶ ἡ οἷον τροφή, φημὶ δὴ τὸ αἷμα, πλεονάσαν οὐδὲν ἧττον νόσον ἐμποιεῖ τῷ σώματι, κατὰ τὸ εἰρημένον ἀνωτέρω ὑπ' αὐτοῦ· «αἱ ἐς ἄκρον εὐεξίαι σφαλεραί»· οὐ μὴν ἀλλὰ καὶ ἡ ὄντως τροφὴ οἶδε βλάπτειν τὸ σῶμα πολλὴ καὶ ἀθρόα ἐπὶ τῶν μερῶν ἐνεχθεῖσα, ἐμφράξεις τε γὰρ καὶ φλεγμονὰς ἐρυσιπέλατά τε καὶ ἕρπητας καὶ τὰ τοιαῦτα ἀπεργάζεται.

Παρὰ φύσιν δὲ λέγει τὸ ὑπὲρ τὴν δύναμιν. λέγουσι δέ τινες· «Τί δήποτε εἰρηκὼς τὸ παρὰ φύσιν ἐπήγαγε καὶ τὸ πλέον εἶναι, εἰ τὸ παρὰ φύσιν πάντως ἄμετρόν ἐστι;» καί φαμεν, ὅτι διττὸν τὸ πλῆθος· ἢ γὰρ πρὸς τὴν εὐρυχωρίαν τῶν ἀγγείων γίνεται ἢ πρὸς τὴν δύναμιν τῆς ἀλλοιωτικῆς ἢ τῆς καθεκτικῆς. διὰ μὲν οὖν τὴν ἀσθένειαν τῆς ἀλλοιωτικῆς ἢ τῆς καθεκτικῆς ἀπεπτεῖται τὸ προσφερόμενον καὶ τυχὸν ἢ δι' ἐμέτων ἢ διὰ γαστρὸς ἐκκρίνεται, καθ' ἑαυτὸ μὲν ἴσως ὀλίγον ὑπάρχον, πλεῖον δὲ τῆς δυνάμεως ὑπαντῆσαν, ᾗ προσενήνεκται, ἀσθενούσης πρὸς τὸ κατεργάσασθαι τὸ ταύτῃ προσενεχθέν. λέγεται δὲ πλῆθος καὶ τὸ πρὸς τὴν τῶν ἀγγείων εὐρυχωρίαν συγκρινόμενον, ὁπότε ἡ μὲν δύναμις ἔρρωται, τὰ δὲ σιτία τὴν εὐρυχωρίαν τῶν ἀγγείων καὶ τὸ τῆς γαστρὸς ὑπερβάλλοι κύτος, ἥτις ταῦτα λαμβάνουσα ἀχθοφορεῖν ἀναγκάζεται. καλῶς οὖν εἴρηται τῷ Ἱπποκράτει· Ὅκου ἂν τροφὴ πλείων ⟨παρὰ φύσιν⟩ εἰσέλθῃ, τουτέστι τὸ πολὺ εἴτε πρὸς τὴν εὐρυχωρίαν τῶν ἀγγείων θεωρούμενον εἴτε πρὸς τὴν δύναμιν τοῦ λαμβάνοντος παρὰ φύσιν ἐστὶ καὶ νόσον οἶδε ποιεῖν· διὰ μὲν γὰρ τοῦ παρὰ φύσιν τὴν δύναμιν, διὰ δὲ τοῦ πλείων τὴν τῶν ἀγγείων εὐρυχωρίαν ἐδήλωσεν. ἢ εἰπὲ καὶ τοῦτο, ὅτι τὸ ἄμετρον οὐ μόνον κατὰ ποιότητα λέγεται, ἀλλὰ καὶ κατὰ ποσότητα· οὐδὲ γὰρ μόνον τὸ πολὺ καὶ ὀλίγον ἀσύμμετρόν φαμεν, ἀλλὰ καὶ τὸ θερμότερον ἢ ψυχρότερον, ἢ ξηρότερον ἢ ὑγρότερον τοῦ προσήκοντος. νόμιζε οὖν τὸν Ἱπποκράτην διὰ μὲν τοῦ εἰπεῖν παρὰ φύσιν τὸ κατὰ ποιότητα ἄμετρον δηλοῦν, διὰ δὲ τοῦ πλέον τὸ κατὰ ποσότητα. καὶ ἄλλως· διὰ μὲν τοῦ παρὰ φύσιν τὴν διττὴν ἀμετρίαν νόμιζε αὐτὸν λέγειν, καὶ τὴν κατὰ ποιότητα καὶ τὴν κατὰ ποσότητα, διὰ δὲ τοῦ πλέον τὸ μέγεθος τῆς ἐκτροπῆς, γινώσκοντα, ὅτι ἡ καθ' ἑκάτερον παρατροπὴ παρὰ φύσιν μέν ἐστιν, οὐ πάντως δὲ καὶ νόσον ποιεῖν δύναται.

11 αἱ – σφαλεραί] Hipp. Aphor. I 3: IV 458,11 L. 17 καί – 25 ἀναγκάζεται] *v.* Gal. In Aphor. II 17: XVII B 476,3–15 K. 30 ἢ – 34 ποσότητα] *v.* Theoph. In Aphor.: II 307,16–308,2 Dietz

2 τῷ] τὸ A 7 *post* προστίθεσθαι *add.* καὶ φύεσθαι P 9 παραλειφθεῖσα A 17 τὴν *om.* P 19 οὖν *om.* A 21 ᾗ] εἰ A 26 πλεῖον A παρὰ φύσιν *ex Hipp. addidi (cf. supra, p. 168,30)* 30sq. ποιότητα . . . ποσότητα] *immo* ποσότητα . . . ποιότητα 31 μόνον *om.* A 34 δηλοῖ A

distinction. Let us comment on each of these. Real food is what has been absorbed by the body, so that what is absorbed by nerve becomes nerve, by muscle, muscle, by vein, vein, by bone, bone, etc. "What can nourish" is the blood which will be distributed from the liver over the entire body through the veins. It is called "what can nourish", because often it is evacuated by bleeding, before it has spread so that there can be adhesion and assimilation. "What will nourish" is the food taken, which eventually will be turned into chyle and be absorbed and be assimilated. *Hippocrates* here refers to all the meanings: what will nourish, i.e. the food, if taken in quantity and therefore not digested, causes disease; what can feed, i.e. blood, if it is superabundant, will no less cause disease in the body, in accordance with what he said above, "A top condition is dangerous"; finally, that which does feed will harm the body, when it rushes to the organs in sudden large quantities, for then it has consequences such as stoppings, inflammations, erysipelas and shingles.

By *abnormal* he means what exceeds one's strength. There are some who ask: "Why, after saying *abnormal*, did he add that it is *abundant*, when the abnormal is inevitably disproportionate?" We answer that the notion of abundance is twofold, according as it is viewed in reference to the width of the vessels, or to the strength of the transformative or the retentive faculty. Weakness of the transformative or the retentive faculty prevents digestion of the food taken, so that it is excreted either by vomiting or through the bowels; in itself it may be little, but it comes in a quantity too large for the strength of the person to whom it is administered, which is too weak to digest what it receives. On the other hand, there can be question of superabundance also in comparison to the width of the vessels, when the strength is unimpaired, but the volume of the food exceeds the width of the vessels and of the abdominal cavity, which is forced to receive and carry its burden. Therefore *Hippocrates* is right in saying *When an abnormal abundance of food is taken*, implying that excess, whether in view of the width of the vessels or of the strength of the person taking it, is abnormal and will cause disease: the *abnormal* relates to strength, the *abundance* to the width of the vessels. An alternative solution: the notion "disproportionate" applies not only to quantity, but to quality as well: disproportionate we call not only what is too much and too little, but also what is hotter or colder, drier or moister than it ought to be. You may assume, then, that *Hippocrates*, when he says *abnormal*, designates qualitative disproportion, and when he says *abundance*, quantitative disproportion. Or again, you can think that by *abnormal* he means both kinds of disproportion, qualitative and quantitative, and by *abundance* the degree of the deviation, as he is aware that a deviation in either respect, though abnormal, does not necessarily result in sickness.

II 17 [II 17: IV 474,9 L.] Δηλοῖ δὲ ἡ ἴησις.

Ὅτι δὲ τοῦτο ἀληθές, φησίν, ἐκ τῆς ἰάσεως δῆλον, τουτέστιν ἐκ τῆς θεραπείας. οἷον εἰσελθὼν καὶ ἄρρωστον εὑρὼν χυλὸν πτισάνης ἢ ἄρτον πεπλυμένον λαμβάνοντα καὶ τοῦτον ὀλίγον καὶ πέψαι μὴ δυνάμενον εἰς ἔννοιαν ἔρχομαι, ὅτι ἄτονος αὐτῷ ἐστι καὶ ἀσθενὴς ἡ καθεκτικὴ τῆς γαστρὸς δύναμις· καὶ κέχρημαι ἐμβροχῇ τῇ διὰ τοῦ ἀψινθίου καὶ οἴνου καὶ ἐλαίου καὶ μηλίνου καὶ γλευκίνου, δι' ὧν αἱ δυνάμεις αὐτῆς τονοῦνται· καὶ τούτου γενομένου ὁ μὴ δυνάμενος πρὸ τούτου χυλὸν πτισάνης πέψαι νῦν τονωθεὶς καὶ δυσκατεργαστοτέραν τροφὴν ἀλλοιῶσαι δύναται. καὶ δῆλον γέγονεν ἐκ τῆς θεραπείας, ὅτι πολλὴ ἦν ἡ προσφερομένη τροφή, ἤγουν παρὰ φύσιν, πρὸς τὴν δύναμιν παραλαμβανομένη τὴν τοῦ λαμβάνοντος. εἶτα καὶ εἰς ἕτερον ἐλθὼν ἄρρωστον εὗρον αὐτὸν πολλὰ λαμβάνοντα καὶ τῷ πλήθει δυσφοροῦντα, καὶ ἀφελὼν τοῦ ποσοῦ τὴν πέψιν ἀνεκαλεσάμην· ὡς δῆλον ἐντεῦθεν εἶναι, ὅτι περὶ τὴν εὐρυχωρίαν τῶν ἀγγείων τὰ τῆς πέψεως ἡμαρτάνετο. οὐ μόνον δὲ ἐκ τῆς ἰάσεως ἀκριβοῦται τὰ ἐπὶ πλήθει βλάπτοντα, ἀλλὰ καθόλου καὶ ἐπὶ τῆς κατὰ ποσότητα παρατροπῆς καὶ ἐπὶ τῆς κατὰ ποιότητα ἡ διὰ τῆς ἐναντίας ἀγωγῆς ἐπὶ τὸ κατὰ φύσιν ἐπανάκλησις βεβαίαν καὶ ἀσφαλῆ παραδίδωσι τὴν τῶν βλαπτόντων αἰτίων σημείωσιν.

II 18 [II 18: IV 474,10–11 L.] Τῶν τρεφόντων ἀθρόως καὶ ταχέως ταχεῖαι καὶ αἱ διαχωρήσιες γίνονται.

Φησίν, ὅτι ἐκ τοῦ τάχους ἢ τῆς βραδυτῆτος τῶν διαχωρουμένων περιττωμάτων ἔστι [τὸ] τεκμήρασθαι τὸ τάχος τῆς τῶν τροφῶν προσθέσεώς τε καὶ ἀναπληρώσεως. καὶ ἐπειδὴ τρεῖς εἰσιν ἐν ἡμῖν πέψεις, ἡ ἐν γαστρί, ἧς περίττωμα ἡ κόπρος, ἡ ἐν ἥπατι τοῦ χυλοῦ μεταβολή, ἥτις καὶ ἐξαιμάτωσις ὀνομάζεται, ποιοῦσα περίττωμα τὸ οὖρον, ἡ τοῦ παντὸς σώματος καθ' ἕκαστον μόριον μεταβολή, περίττωμα ἔχουσα τοὺς ἱδρῶτας, εἴτε ἡ κόπρος οὐ μετὰ πολὺ τοῦ τὴν τροφὴν παρασχεθῆναι ἐκκριθῇ, ταχεῖαν τὴν ἐν γαστρὶ πέψιν σημαίνει· εἴτε τὸ οὖρον ταχέως διεξέλθῃ μετὰ τὴν ἀνάδοσιν τοῦ χυλοῦ, ταχεῖαν τὴν ἐξαιμάτωσιν ἐνδείκνυται· ὥσπερ οὖν καὶ ἱδρῶτες τῆς εἰς τὸ σῶμα τοῦ αἵματος διασπορᾶς προστάξαντες ταχεῖαν τὴν τῶν ἐν ἡμῖν μορίων ὑπεμφαίνουσι πέψιν.

Καὶ τὸ μὲν ταχέως τέθηκεν ἐπὶ τοῦ τῆς πέψεως καιροῦ, τὸ δὲ ἀθρόως ἐπὶ τοῦ τῆς προσθέσεως. εἰ γὰρ καὶ ἑκάτερον χρόνῳ περιμετρεῖται, ἀλλὰ κατὰ τὸ μᾶλλον καὶ τὸ ἧττον ἑκάτερον ἔχει τινὰ διαφοράν. ἐπειγόμενον γὰρ τάχος δηλοῖ τὸ ἀθρόως, ὡς εἶναι τὸ λεγόμενον τοιοῦτον· «Τῶν ταχέως πεττομένων καὶ ἀθρόως προστιθεμένων ταχεῖαι καὶ αἱ διαχωρήσιες γίνονται», τουτέστιν αἱ διὰ γαστρός.

Τινὲς δὲ τῷ χαρακτῆρι τῶν λέξεων πειθόμενοι ἁρμόζειν ἔφασαν τὸν λόγον ἐπὶ τῆς τρίτης πέψεως καὶ ἐκκρίσεως ἐκ τοῦ εἰπεῖν τὸν Ἱπποκράτην τῶν τρεφόντων ἀθρόως καὶ ταχέως, οὐ μὴν «τῶν πεττομένων»· εἰ γὰρ ἑκάτερον καθ' ἑκάστην γίνεται τῶν πέψεων, λέγω δὴ θρέψις καὶ πέψις, ἀλλ' οὖν ἐν τῇ πρώτῃ καὶ δευτέρᾳ

14 ἀλλὰ – 16] *v.* Theoph. In Aphor.: II 308,3–7 Dietz 34–174,7 τάξιν] *cf.* Gal. In Aphor. II 18: XVII B 488,4–17 K.

1 ἴασις A 9 ἦν A 10 παραλαμβανομένη] *fort.* παραβαλλομένη *scribendum est (cf. infra, p. 184,3)* 12 περὶ] *fort.* παρὰ *scribendum est* 14 καθόλου *sec. Theoph. scripsi*: καθὸ α 20 τὸ^I *delevi* 25 διεξέλθῃ *scripsi*: διεξέλθ *(ambig.)* α 30 ἑκάτερον *scripsi*: ἑκάτρ A: ἑκατέρω P 31 τὸ^I *om.* A ἑκάτερον *scripsi*: ἑκάτρ α

II 17. The cure makes this clear.

That this is true, he says, is proved by the cure, i.e. by the treatment. For instance, when I visit a patient and find he is taking barley-water or fine bread in small quantity and is yet unable to digest it, it occurs to me that the retentive faculty of his stomach is atonic and weak; I then apply an infusion of absinthe, wine, oil, apple-juice and grape-juice, to stimulate its strength; after which the man who until now could not digest barley-water, is strong enough to convert even less digestible food. Thus it has become clear from the treatment that the food taken was too much, i.e. abnormal, in comparison to the strength of the person who received it. Next I come to another patient and find him eating a great deal and troubled by the bulk of it, so I reduce the quantity and thus restore his digestion; which proves that the width of the vessels caused his digestion to fail. From the cure we derive exact information not only as to harm through overindulgence, but we can say generally that in cases both of quantitative and of qualitative deviation, restoration of the normal state by an opposite regime affords us a reliable and safe indication as regards the causes of the harm.

II 18. What nourishes instantaneously and quickly is also quickly excreted.

(Hippocrates) says that from the speed or slowness with which surplus matter is evacuated, we can infer the speed with which foods are absorbed and provide replenishment. Now we have three kinds of digestion: that in the stomach, the surplus matter of which are the feces; the mutation of the chyle in the liver, also called conversion into blood, which produces urine as its surplus matter; and the mutation in each part of the whole body, with sweat as its surplus matter; accordingly, if the feces are excreted not long after the food has been administered, this indicates quick digestion in the stomach; if the urine is passed quickly after the distribution of the chyle, this points to quick conversion into blood; similarly, when sweat begins to drip as the result of the spreading of the blood through the body, it reveals a quick digestion by the different parts of our body.

He uses the word quickly in reference to the time of digestion, and instantaneously in reference to the time of absorption. For though both are limited by time, yet there is a certain difference in degree between the two: instantaneously denotes heightened speed, so that the sense is, "What is digested quickly and absorbed instantaneously is also quickly excreted", namely by way of the stomach.

Some, guided by the expressions used, have said that the rule applies to the third kind of digestion and excretion, on the ground that Hippocrates says What nourishes instantaneously and quickly, but not "what is digested"; for though both nutrition and digestion play a part in each of the kinds of digestion, still in the first and in the second kind of digestion there is more matter

πέψει τὸ πεττόμενον ἐπὶ πλέον ἐστὶ τῶν τρεφομένων. ἐν μὲν γὰρ τῇ πρώτῃ πέψει χυλοῦ γενομένου ἡ γαστὴρ καὶ μόνη τρέφεται, καὶ οὐδὲ αὐτὴ καθ' ὅλην ἑαυτήν, ἀλλὰ κατὰ τὸν ἔνδον χιτῶνα καὶ μόνον· ἐν δὲ τῇ δευτέρᾳ πέψει ἡ κοιλότης καὶ μόνη τοῦ ἥπατος τρέφεται, ἐν ᾗ καὶ ἡ ἐξαιμάτωσις γίνεται· ἐν μέντοι τῇ τρίτῃ πέψει οὐ τοσαύτη ἐστὶν ἡ πεττομένη ὕλη ἐν ἑκάστῳ τῶν μορίων ὡς καὶ ἄλλοις χορηγηθῆναι, ἀλλὰ τοσοῦτον μεταβάλλει, ὑφ' οὗ δὴ καὶ πάντα τραφήσεται, τὸ δὲ λοιπὸν ἅπαν περιττώματος ἔχει τάξιν. ἐπειδὴ οὖν πλεονάζει πως ἢ ἐξισάζει ἐπὶ τῆς τρίτης πέψεως ἡ θρέψις, ἐπὶ δὲ τῶν ἄλλων ὑπεναντίως ἔχει, εὔλογον ὑπονοῆσαι τὸν Ἱπποκράτην περὶ ταύτης διαλαμβάνειν ἐκ τοῦ εἰπεῖν τῶν ἀθρόως καὶ ταχέως τρεφόντων καὶ οὐχὶ «πεττομένων». τοιαῦτα δέ ἐστιν, ὅσα λεπτομερῆ φύσει καὶ θερμὰ ἐν τροφαῖς, ὧν κυριώτατον καὶ πρώτιστόν ἐστιν ὁ οἶνος· οὗτος γὰρ ὡς μὲν θερμὸς ἑτοιμότατα πέττεται, ὡς δὲ λεπτομερὴς καὶ χρηστὴν τροφὴν παρέχων ταχέως ἀναδίδοται καὶ ἀθρόως τρέφει, δηλονότι ταχέως, καὶ διεξέρχεται ἱδρωτοειδῶς διὰ τῶν πόρων τὸ αὐτοῦ περίττωμα. τά τε ταχέως μεταβαλλόμενα καὶ πεττόμενα ταχεῖαν ποιεῖται τὴν διαφόρησιν, τὰ δὲ βραδέως τοὐναντίον.

Δεῖται δὲ πλειόνων διορισμῶν, εἰ μέλλει ἀληθὴς εἶναι, ὁ παρὼν ἀφορισμός. οὐδὲ γὰρ ἐπειδὴ τὸ ταχέως καὶ ἀθρόως τρέφον ταχέως καὶ διεξέρχεται, τὸ ταχίστην ἐπάγον τὴν διαχώρησιν ἤδη καὶ θρέψις ταχεῖα ἐγένετο. πολλάκις γὰρ τὰ προσενεχθέντα ῥυπτικήν τινα καὶ ὑπαγωγὸν ἔχοντα δύναμιν, καθάπερ κράμβαι καὶ τεῦτλα καὶ φακὸς καὶ πτισάνη καὶ τὰ τοιαῦτα, ταχεῖαν μὲν ἐπάγει τὴν ἔκκρισιν, οὐκ ἤδη δὲ καὶ ταχεῖαν τὴν πέψιν ἐποιήσατο. δεύτερος προσδιορισμός ἐστιν, ὅστις λαμβάνεται πρὸς τῆς καρυκείας ἤτοι ἀρτύσεως τῶν ὄψων· ἡμεῖς γὰρ αὐτοὶ πολλάκις ψυχρούς τινας καὶ φλεγματικοὺς χυμοὺς εἰς τὰ περὶ τὴν γαστέρα καὶ τὰ ἔντερα χωρία ἀθροιζομένους ὑπονοοῦντες ἁλυκώτερα τὰ ὄψα παρασκευάζομεν ἅλας ἢ γάρον ἤ τι τῶν ταριχερῶν ἐμβάλλοντες ἐν αὐτοῖς· ἔστι δ' ὅτε καί τινα δριμεῖαν ἢ καθαρτικὴν ἐπιπλέκομεν τούτοις ποιότητα σκορόδοις καὶ πράσοις καὶ πεπέρεϊ καὶ τοῖς τοιούτοις χρώμενοι, ὑφ' ὧν τὴν ἔκκρισιν ταχίστην συμβαίνει γίνεσθαι μαστιζομένης ὑπὸ τούτων τῆς ἀποκριτικῆς δυνάμεως. λάχανα γοῦν ἐκζεστὰ καὶ ᾠὰ τρομητὰ σὺν ἐλαιογάρῳ ἤ τι τοιοῦτον ὁ παρέχων ταχίστην τὴν διαχώρησιν τῆς γαστρὸς ἀπεργάζεται. τρίτος προσδιορισμός ἐστιν ἀπὸ τοῦ τρόπου τῆς ἑψήσεως. δεδόσθωσαν γάρ, εἰ τύχοι, ὄρνιθες δυσὶν ἀνθρώποις, τῷ μὲν ὀπτηθεῖσα, τῷ δὲ ζωμῷ παρασκευασθεῖσα. τούτων ὁ μὲν ταχέως καὶ πέττει καὶ διαχωρεῖ, ὁ τὴν ζωμευθεῖσαν ὄρνιν ἐδηδοκώς, ὁ δὲ τὴν ὀπτὴν τοὔμπαλιν. τέταρτος προσδιορισμός ἐστιν ἀπὸ τῆς κράσεως τῶν τρεφομένων σωμάτων. τῆς γὰρ αὐτῆς πολλάκις παρεχομένης τροφῆς τὸν μὲν συμβαίνει ταχέως καὶ πέψαι καὶ τραφῆναι, τὸν δὲ βραδέως, τῷ διαφέροντι λόγῳ τῆς κράσεως, τοῦ μὲν θερμοῦ ὑπάρχοντος καὶ ταχέως διὰ τοῦτο πέττοντος, τοῦ δὲ ψυχροῦ καὶ διὰ τοῦτο ὑστεροῦντος.

II 19 [II 19: IV 474,12–13 L.] Τῶν ὀξέων νοσημάτων οὐ πάμπαν ἀσφαλέες αἱ προαγορεύσιες.

11 ὧν – 14 περίττωμα] *cf.* Gal. In Aphor. II 18: XVII B 485,13–486,12 K. Theoph. In Aphor.: II 309,5–9 Dietz

1 τὸ *om.* P   2 *fort.* αὕτη *scribendum est*   7 ἅπαν] ἅμα P   21 προδιορισμός P   22 ἀρτήσεως α: *correxi*   24 *post* ἅλας *add.* γὰρ A   31 τύχῃ P   35 διαφοροῦντι α: *correxi*   39 προσαγορεύσιες P

digested than organs nourished. In the first digestion, when chyle is formed, only the stomach is nourished, and not even all of it, but only its inner lining; in the second digestion only the cavity of the liver is nourished, in which the conversion into blood takes place; in the third digestion, however, the matter digested in each part is not sufficient to be passed on to other parts, but only so much is converted as is needed to nourish all the parts, while all the rest has the character of surplus matter. Since, then, in the third digestion, nutrition somehow plays the prevalent or at least an equal part, whereas in the other (two) the contrary is the case, it is a probable supposition that Hippocrates refers to the third, because he says, What nourishes instantaneously and quickly, and not "what is digested". Now such are all kinds of nourishment which are naturally fine and hot, of which wine is the first and the most important; for insofar as it is hot, it is easily digested, and insofar as it is fine and provides wholesome nutrition it is quickly distributed and nourishes instantaneously, i.e. fast, and its surplus matter passes through the pores in the form of sweat. What is quickly converted and digested is also quickly dispersed, and when conversion is slow, the contrary is the case.

The present aphorism needs several qualifications, if it is to hold good. From the fact that food which nourishes quickly and instantaneously also passes through quickly, it does not follow that food which brings about excretion soonest, has also provided quick nourishment. Often, indeed, food with a certain cleansing and laxative power, such as cabbages, beets, lentil-soup, barley-water, etc., while causing quick excretion, is not necessarily digested quickly. A second qualification is to be derived from the spicing or seasoning of the dishes: often, when we suspect that certain cold and phlegmatic humors are collecting in the region of the stomach and the intestines, we make the dishes saltier ourselves by adding salt or fish-sauce or pickled fish to them; sometimes, too, we give them a sort of pungent or purgative quality by the use of garlic, leek, pepper and similar ingredients, which cause very quick excretion, by stimulating the secretory faculty. If, for example, you administer boiled vegetables or soft-boiled eggs with fish preserved in oil, etc., the result is very fast excretion. A third qualification has to do with the manner of cooking. Suppose two persons are given chicken to eat, the one fried, the other boiled in soup. The second, who has eaten the boiled chicken, has quick digestion and excretion, but with the one who ate it fried, the contrary is the case. A fourth qualification is necessary in view of the temperament of the bodies nourished. Often when the same food is provided, digestion and nutrition will be fast for one person, slow for the other, depending on their different temperaments, the one being hot-tempered and therefore digesting quickly, the other cold-tempered and for this reason slower.

II 19. In acute diseases predictions are not very safe.

Παρακελεύεται ἡμῖν ὁ Ἱπποκράτης μὴ προπετῶς ἐπὶ τῶν ὀξέων ἀποφαίνεσθαι νοσημάτων. ὀξέα δὲ νῦν ἀκουστέον νοσήματα τοὺς συνεχεῖς πυρετούς, μεγάλους τε καὶ σφοδροὺς ἐπὶ θερμῇ καὶ λεπτῇ καὶ δριμείᾳ ὕλῃ ἀναπτομένους, εἴτε ἐν τοῖς ἀγγείοις περιέχεται εἴτε ἐν μορίῳ περιγράφεται ἡ ὕλη.

Ἐφ' οἷς ζητητέον, διὰ τί ἐπὶ τῶν ὀξέων νοσημάτων εὐλαβεῖται τὴν ἀποφαντικὴν πρόρρησιν. καὶ λέγομεν ὅτι διὰ τὸ λεπτὸν καὶ εὔοργον τῆς ὕλης, ἐπειδὴ πολλάκις ἀπὸ κυρίων μορίων ἐπὶ ἄκυρα μέτεισιν ἢ τοὔμπαλιν. καὶ ὅσον μὲν ἐπὶ τῇ νῦν θεωρουμένῃ καταστάσει τοῦ νοσοῦντος, εἰσερχόμενος, εἰ τύχοι, παρὰ τὸν ἄρρωστον εὑρίσκεις ὀξύτατον πυρετὸν καὶ χαλεπὰ τὰ συμπτώματα καὶ κύριον τὸ πάσχον μόριον. καὶ προλέγεις, ὅτι τεθνήξεται ὁ ἄνθρωπος διά τε τὸ μέγεθος τοῦ νοσήματος διά τε τὸ ἀξίωμα τοῦ πάσχοντος τόπου, τυχὸν ἥπατος, καὶ ταῦτα ἀποφηνάμενος ὑποχωρεῖς. καὶ ἐν τοσούτῳ διὰ τὸ λεπτὸν τῆς ὕλης καὶ εὐκίνητον ἔστιν ὅτε γίνεται μετάστασις, διεξερχομένης αὐτῆς ἀπὸ τοῦ κυρίου μορίου καὶ ἐπὶ τὰ ἄκυρα τρεπομένης, τυχὸν ἐπὶ γαστέρα ἢ ἔντερα ἢ νεφροὺς ἢ οὐρητῆρας· εἰ γὰρ καὶ μὴ πάντῃ ἄτιμά ἐστι τὰ τοιαῦτα μόρια, ἀλλ' οὖν ὡς πρὸς ἧπαρ ἄκυρά εἰσιν. οὕτινος γενομένου ἐκκλίνει τὸν θάνατον ὁ κάμνων. ὡσαύτως πάλιν ἕτερον ὁρᾷς νοσοῦντα νόσημα ὀξύ, τὸ δὲ πάσχον μόριον ἀκυρότερον, στόμαχον ἴσως ὑπὸ χολῆς ἐνοχλούμενον, ὅστις, εἰ καὶ μὴ τῶν ἀκύρων ἐστίν, ἀλλὰ πρὸς καρδίαν καὶ ἧπαρ ἀκυρότερος πέφυκε· καὶ ὅσον ἐπὶ τούτῳ ἀπηλλάγης εἰρηκὼς μὴ ἔχειν κίνδυνον τὸ νόσημα. εἶτα σοῦ ἀναχωρήσαντος μεταχώρησις τῆς ὕλης γέγονε διὰ λεπτότητα ἐπὶ κύριον μόριον, λέγω δὴ ἀναπνοήν, καὶ δι' αὐτῆς ἐπὶ τὴν καρδίαν, καὶ συγκοπῆς ἀθρόας γινομένης κατελύθη ἡ δύναμις καὶ ἀπώλετο ὁ ἄνθρωπος.

II 20 [II 20: IV 476,1–2 L.] Ὁκόσοισι νέοισιν ἐοῦσιν αἱ κοιλίαι ὑγραί εἰσι, τουτέοισιν ἀπογηράσκουσι ξηραίνονται.

Νῦν περὶ ἡλικιῶν βούλεται διαλεχθῆναι καὶ τούτων διαφορὰς ἡμῖν παραδοῦναι, οὐκ ἐν ὀλίγῳ χρόνῳ θεωρουμένας, ἐνὶ τυχὸν ἢ δυσὶν ἢ τρισίν, ἀλλ' ἐν τριάκοντα ἔτεσι. λέγει γὰρ οὕτως· «Ὅσοι νέοι ὄντες τὰς κοιλίας ὑγρὰς ἔχουσιν, οὗτοι ἐν γήρᾳ ἐρχόμενοι ξηρὰς αὐτὰς ἔχουσι, καὶ τοὔμπαλιν.»

Κοιλίαν δὲ τὴν σιτοδόχον λέγει γαστέρα. προσκείσθω δὲ τὸ «ἐπὶ πολύ», εἰ μὴ μέλλοι ψευδὴς εἶναι ὁ λόγος.

Δεῖ δὲ καὶ τοῦτο εἰδέναι, ὅτι ἀέναός ἐστι τοῦ ἡμετέρου σώματος ἡ διαφόρησις· καὶ πρῶτον μὲν ἡ ἐπιφάνεια διαφορεῖται ὡς καὶ τῷ ἐκτὸς ἀέρι ἀμέσως ὁμιλοῦσα, ἐφεξῆς δὲ καὶ τὰ λοιπὰ κατὰ τάξιν ἐκ τῶν παρακειμένων ἑκάστου ἕλκοντος, τῆς μὲν ἐπιφανείας ἐκ τῶν σαρκῶν, τῶν δὲ σαρκῶν ἐκ τῶν φλεβῶν τῶν εἰς ὅλον τὸ σῶμα διανενεμημένων, φημὶ δὴ τῶν πρὸ τῆς κοίλης φλεβός, τῶν δὲ φλεβῶν ἐκ τοῦ ἥπατος, τοῦ δὲ ἥπατος ἐκ τῶν μεσαραίων, τῶν δὲ μεσαραίων ἐκ τῆς γαστρός, ⟨τῆς δὲ γαστρὸς⟩ ἐκ τοῦ στομάχου. καὶ πᾶσα αὕτη ἡ ὄρεξις φυσικὴ λέγεται, ἡ μέχρι τῆς γα-

2 ὀξέα – 4] *cf.* Gal. In Aphor. II 19: XVII B 490,6–12 K. 5–7 τοὔμπαλιν] *cf.* Gal. In Aphor. II 19: XVII B 491,16–492,2 K. 29sq.] *v.* Gal. In Aphor. II 20: XVII B 492,8 K. Theoph. In Aphor.: II 315,26–27 Dietz

8 τύχη P 13 ἄκυρα] ἄκρα P 14 ἄτιμά] ἄκυρα P 15 *post* πρὸς *add.* τὸ A ἐκκλίνει] ἐκλύει P 19 ἀπηλλάγη P 29 προκείσθω P 35 φλεβός] φλεβῶν A 36 τῆς δὲ γαστρὸς *addidi*

Hippocrates counsels us not to be rash in our statements about acute diseases. By acute diseases we must here understand non-intermittent fevers, strong and violent and kindled upon hot, thin and pungent matter, whether the matter is contained in the vessels or limited to one part.

The question is now why in acute diseases (Hippocrates) is chary of a positive prediction. This is, we say, because the matter is thin and easily commoved: it will often shift from vital parts to unimportant ones or conversely. As far as the momentary condition of the patient is concerned, you may find, for example, when you visit him, very high fever, grave symptoms and a vital part affected. You then predict the man's death on the ground of the seriousness of the disease and the importance of the affected organ, let us say the liver, and after making this statement you leave. Meanwhile, thanks to the thinness and mobility of the matter, a metastasis sometimes occurs: the matter passes out of the vital organ and shifts to less important parts, such as the stomach, the intestines, the kidneys or the ureters, parts which, though not entirely unimportant, are of less account as compared to the liver. When this happens, the patient escapes death. Again, you visit another patient suffering from an acute disease, but the affected part is less important, perhaps a stomach troubled by bile, which, without being unimportant, is yet of less consequence in comparison to the heart and the liver; and guided by this fact you take your leave after saying that the disease is not dangerous. After your departure the matter, thin as it is, shifts to a vital part, let us say the respiratory organs, and through them to the heart, there is a sudden collapse, resistance breaks down and the patient dies.

II 20. In those who have wet cavities when young, they dry up as they grow old.

His intention is now to discuss age groups and to explain their differences to us, viewed not over a short period, for instance one, two or three years, but over a space of thirty years. What he says is: "Those who have wet cavities when young, have them dry as they approach old age, and conversely."

By cavity he means the belly as receptacle of food. We should add, "on the whole", if the statement is to hold true.

It should further be observed that the dispersal of our body is continuous: first the surface is dispersed, inasmuch as it is in immediate contact with the air outside, then the other parts successively, each drawing upon the adjoining parts, the surface upon the flesh, the flesh upon the veins which are distributed over the entire body – i.e. those in front of the vena cava –, the veins upon the liver, the liver upon the mesenteries, the mesenteries upon the belly, the belly upon the stomach. This whole (system of) appetition is called "natural", as far as the stomach;

στρὸς γινομένη· τὸ μέντοι στόμα τῆς γαστρὸς μετὰ συναισθήσεως προαιρετικῆς τοῦ λείποντος ἐφιέμενον τὴν κυρίως ποιεῖ ὄρεξιν, ἥτις καὶ πεῖνα προσαγορεύεται. αὕτη οὖν ψυχική ἐστιν ὄρεξις, καθ' ἣν ἐφιέμεθα τῶν σιτίων· ἅτινα λαμβάνοντες πέττομεν, καὶ πάλιν καὶ πολλάκις, ἐπειδὴ ἡ διαφόρησις ἀεννάως γίνεται. ἔστι δὲ ὅτε καὶ διὰ ψυχρὸν καὶ ὀξώδη χυμὸν ὑποτραφέντα ἐν τῷ στόματι τῆς γαστρὸς γίνεται ὄρεξις, ἥτις καὶ παρὰ φύσιν ἐστί.

Τούτων οὕτως ἐχόντων ἰστέον, ὅτι κατὰ δύο αἰτίας ἡ διάρροια γίνεται τῆς γαστρός, ἢ διὰ πλῆθος σιτίων ἢ δι' ἐνδεῆ ἀνάδοσιν. καὶ διὰ μὲν πλῆθος σιτίων τριχῶς· πρῶτον μὲν ὅτι πολλῶν δεδομένων καὶ καλῶς μὴ πεττομένων διαφθείρεσθαι αὐτὰ συμβαίνει, κἀντεῦθεν τὰ διαχωρήματα ⟨ὑγρὰ⟩ ἐκκρίνεται· εἴρηται γάρ, ὅτι ψυχρὰ γαστὴρ ὀρεχθῆναι μὲν ἀγαθή, πέψαι δὲ οὐκ ἀγαθή. δεύτερον δὲ ὅτι ἀσθενεῖν συμβαίνει τὴν καθεκτικὴν δύναμιν καὶ οἷον ἐκλύεσθαι τὸν τόνον αὐτῆς τῇ ὑγρότητι, ὡς μὴ κατέχειν τὰ σιτία, ἀλλ' ἐᾶν αὐτὰ φέρεσθαι ὑγρὰ καὶ ἀμετάβλητα, ξηρότητι γὰρ αὐτὴν χαίρειν μεμαθήκαμεν· ὥσπερ οὖν ἀσθενεῖν συμβαίνει καὶ τὴν ἀποκριτικήν, διύγρου γὰρ καὶ πλαδαροῦ γινομένου τοῦ στόματος τῆς γαστρὸς καὶ μὴ ἰσχυούσης περιστεῖλαι αὐτὴν τῆς καθεκτικῆς δυνάμεως ἀφίεται ἄπεπτα τὰ σιτία, ἀφ' οὗ πάλιν ὑγρὰ γίνεται διαχώρησις. συμβαίνει δὲ πάλιν τοῦτο αὐτὸ καὶ διὰ ῥώμην τῆς ἀποκριτικῆς δυνάμεως πρὸ ὥρας ἐπανισταμένης καὶ ἐξωθούσης τὰ σιτία· κἀντεῦθεν γὰρ πάλιν ὑγρὰ γίνεται διαχώρησις διὰ τὴν ἐνδεῆ ἀνάδοσιν.

Διχῶς οὖν ὑγραίνεται ἡ γαστήρ, ἢ διὰ ψυχρότερον ἧπαρ ἢ διὰ θερμότερον. διὰ μὲν ψυχρότερον, ὅτι μὴ ἐρρωμένως ἕλκει τὸν χυλὸν ἀπὸ τῆς γαστρός, θερμότητι γὰρ συμμέτρῳ τὴν ἑλκτικὴν εἶπον δύναμιν ἐνεργεῖν. ἐντεῦθεν οὖν μένων ὁ χυλὸς εἰς τὴν γαστέρα ὡς φορτικὸς καὶ ἀλλότριος ἐπὶ ἔντερα ἐκκρίνεται καὶ ὑγρὰν ποιεῖται τὴν διαχώρησιν. διὰ δὲ θερμότερον· ἡνίκα ἂν τὸ θερμὸν ἐκκαίῃ τὸ αἷμα καὶ πολὺν τὸν ξανθοχολικὸν γεννᾷ χυμόν, ἐπὶ τῶν ἐντέρων αὐτὸν δαψιλῆ ἀπεργάζεται· ὅστις μαστίζει συνεχέστερον τὴν ἀποκριτικὴν δύναμιν, κἀκείνη διὰ παντὸς ἐπεγειρομένη ἀπωθεῖται τάχιστα τὰ σιτία, κἀκεῖθεν ὑγροτέρα γίνεται ἡ διαχώρησις.

Ξηραίνεται δὲ πάλιν ἡ γαστὴρ κατὰ δύο αἰτίας, ἢ διὰ τὴν ὀλιγότητα τῶν σιτίων ἢ διὰ πολλὴν ἀνάδοσιν. καὶ διὰ μὲν τὴν ὀλιγότητα τῶν σιτίων τριχῶς· πρῶτον μὲν ὅτι ταχέως πέττονται ὀλίγα ὄντα καὶ ῥᾷον ἀναδίδονται καὶ οὐδὲν ἐν τῇ γαστρὶ καταλιμπάνεται. δεύτερον δὲ διὰ ῥώμην τῆς καθεκτικῆς· ξηροτέρας γὰρ καὶ ἀνίκμου τῆς γαστρὸς γινομένης ἰσχυρῶς καὶ ἐπιτεταμένως αὕτη ἐνεργεῖν δύναται. καὶ τρίτον διὰ τὴν τῆς ἀποκριτικῆς ἀσθένειαν· αὕτη γὰρ ἀσθενοῦσα οὐκ ἐπεγείρεται εἰς τὸ ἀποδιῶξαι, καὶ ξηρὰ διὰ τοῦτο εὑρίσκεται ἡ διαχώρησις. διὰ δὲ πολλὴν ἀνάδοσιν, ἢ θερμοτέρου ὄντος τοῦ ἥπατος καὶ τοῦ ὅλου σώματος καὶ ὅλον ἀνέλκοντος τοῦ μὲν τὸν χυλόν, τοῦ δὲ τὸ αἷμα· ἢ διὰ τὸ μὴ καταρρεῖν ἐν τοῖς ἐντέροις χολήν, μὴ μαστίζεσθαι τὰ ἔντερα καὶ πρὸς ἔκκρισιν ἐπεγείρεσθαι.

Οὐκοῦν, εἰ δοκεῖ, ὡς ἐξ ὑποθέσεως ἐπὶ τῶν ἡλικιῶν τὸν λόγον γυμνάσωμεν. ὑποκείσθω νέος τις ἔχων ὑγρὰν τὴν γαστέρα διὰ πλῆθος θερμότητος καὶ ὄρεξιν

7–37] *cf.* Gal. In Aphor. II 20: XVII B 494,4–495,6 K. 7–27] *cf.* Theoph. In Aphor.: II 315,5–8 Dietz 10 εἴρηται] *v. supra*, p. 154,6–11 14 μεμαθήκαμεν] *locum non inveni* 22 εἶπον] *locum non inveni* 28–37] *cf.* Theoph. In Aphor.: II 315,14–17 Dietz 39 ὑποκείσθω – 180,34] *cf.* Theoph. In Aphor.: II 315,8–14 Dietz ὑποκείσθω – 180,12] *cf.* Gal. In Aphor. II 20: XVII B 494,7–9; 495,6–10 K.

2 ἐφιεμένη α: *corr. Dietz* 5 ὑπογραφέντα P 10 ὑγρὰ *addidi* 24 δὲ] μὲν (δὲ *supra*) A θερμό-τ(η)τ(α) A 39 νέος *om.* A

the orifice of the stomach, however, which consciously and voluntarily strives to supply what is missing, causes appetite properly so called, also described as hunger. This is psychic appetition, by which we desire food; we take and digest it, and this happens again and again, since the dispersal is continuous. Sometimes appetite is also due to a cold and acid humor formed in the orifice of the stomach, but this is abnormal.

This being so, let it be stated that diarrhoea can result from two causes, either from an excess of food, or from defective distribution. As regards excess of food there are three possibilities: first, too much has been administered, and because it is not well digested, it spoils in consequence, and this explains the watery excretion of the feces; for, as we said already, a cold stomach means a good appetite, but not a good digestion. Second, the retentive faculty is weak, its vigor having been dissolved, so to speak, by the moisture, so that it cannot retain the food, but lets it pass watery and unconverted, since as we have seen this faculty thrives on dryness. Similarly, the secretory faculty becomes weak in consequence, for when the orifice of the stomach becomes watery and splashy and the retentive faculty is not strong enough to block it, the food escapes undigested, and the result is again a watery discharge. Again, the same effect may be brought about by a strong secretory faculty, which is activated before its time and expels the food; this, too, produces a watery discharge because of deficient distribution.

Now there are two causes of wet bowels: either a liver that is too cold, or one that is too hot. When it is too cold, there is no vigorous attraction of chyle from the stomach, for as I said before, the attractive faculty operates by means of moderate heat. Hence the chyle remains in the stomach, then, as troublesome and incompatible, it is excreted into the intestines and makes the excrements watery. As for a liver that is too hot: when the heat burns the blood and produces a large quantity of bilious humor, this leads to a surplus of it in the intestines, which incessantly stimulates the secretory faculty; owing to this continual activation it very soon expels the food, and the outcome is a watery discharge.

There are again two causes of dryness of the bowels: either scarcity of food, or excessive distribution. In the case of scarcity of food there are three possibilities: first, because there is so little of it, it is quickly digested and easily distributed, so that nothing remains in the bowels. A second cause is strength of the retentive faculty; for when the bowels become too dry and lack moisture, this faculty can operate forcefully and intensively. The third is weakness of the secretory faculty; for when it is too weak, it does not come into action to expel matter, and thus stools are found to be dry. In the case of excessive distribution, either the liver and the whole body are too hot and absorb, respectively, all the chyle and all the blood; or, because no bile flows into the bowels, the bowels are not stimulated and activated to excretion.

So now, if you wish, let us take some hypothetical cases to apply this rule to age groups. Suppose we have a young man with wet bowels due to abundant heat

ἐπιτεταμένην. καὶ μὴ ἀπορήσῃς ὅτι «Πῶς ἐνδέχεται ἐπὶ νέας ἡλικίας, ἐφ' ἧς τὸ θερμὸν δυναστεύει, ἐπιτεταμένην εἶναι τὴν ὄρεξιν; τοῦτο γὰρ ψυχροῦ στομάχου σημεῖον.» δυνατὸν γὰρ ἐν τοῖς μορίοις ἡμῶν εἶναι κρᾶσιν ἀνώμαλον, καὶ τὸ μὲν ἧπαρ τυχὸν θερμὸν ὑπάρχειν, τὸ δὲ στόμα τῆς γαστρὸς ψυχρόν, κἀντεῦθεν ἐπιτεταμένην γίνεσθαι ὄρεξιν· ἢ καὶ χυμόν τινα περιέχοντος τούτου καὶ πλῆθος σιτίων μεταλαμβάνοντος, ταῦτα δὲ μὴ πεττόμενα τὰ σιτία ὑγροτέραν ἐξ ἀνάγκης ἀπεργάζονται τὴν γαστέρα. τῆς ψύξεως γοῦν μενούσης καὶ μέχρι τῆς γεροντικῆς ἡλικίας μᾶλλον αὐτοῖς τὰ τῆς ὀρέξεως ἐπιτείνεται, καὶ πλέον ἢ πρόσθεν αἱρούμενοι τὰ σιτία καὶ μὴ πέττοντες αὐτὰ μένουσι κἀν τῇ γεροντικῇ ἡλικίᾳ ὑγρὰν ἔχοντες τὴν γαστέρα· εἰ δέ γε ἐπιταθῇ ἡ ψῦξις τῷ λόγῳ τῆς γεροντικῆς ἡλικίας, ὡς τελείως ναρκῶσαι τὸν στόμαχον καὶ καταλῦσαι τὴν ὄρεξιν, οὐ προσίεται τὸ τηνικαῦτα τὰ σιτία, τῆς δὲ ὕλης ἐνδεῶς ἐχούσης ἀνάγκη ἀπέριττον καὶ ξηρὰν αὐτοῖς ἐν γήρᾳ γενέσθαι τὴν γαστέρα.

Πάλιν ὑποκείσθω ἕτερος νέος ὑγρὰν ἔχων τὴν γαστέρα ἐπὶ ἀσθενείᾳ τῆς καθεκτικῆς δυνάμεως, ἥτις ἐπὶ ὑγρότητι καταλύεται. ἐπὶ τούτου φημὶ πάντως ἐν γήρᾳ ξηρὰν ἔσεσθαι τὴν γαστέρα διὰ τὸ τὴν ὑγρότητα δαπανᾶσθαι καὶ εἰς ξηροτάτην μεταπίπτειν κρᾶσιν ἐπὶ τῶν γερόντων, ἥτις ῥώννυσι τὴν καθεκτικὴν δύναμιν, ταύτης δὲ κατεχούσης ἐξ ἀνάγκης ξηραίνεται ἡ γαστήρ.

Ἕτερος πάλιν νέος ὑγρὰν ἔχων τὴν γαστέρα ἐπὶ ῥώμῃ τῆς ἀποκριτικῆς δυνάμεως ὑποκείσθω, ἥτις ξηρότητι ἕπεται. καὶ ἐνταῦθα τοίνυν, εἰ τὰ αὐτὰ μέτρα μείνωσι τῆς ξηρότητος, ὑγρὰν ἕξει ὁ τοιοῦτος καὶ ἐν γήρᾳ τὴν γαστέρα· εἰ δὲ ἐπιταθῶσι τῷ λόγῳ τῆς γεροντικῆς ἡλικίας, ὡς καταλῦσαι τῇ ἀμετρίᾳ τὴν ἀποκριτικὴν δύναμιν, ταύτης ἀσθενούσης οὐδὲν ἀποκρίνεται καὶ γίνεται ξηρὰ ἡ γαστήρ. ἔχει οὖν καὶ οὗτος ὁ λόγος τὸ ἐνδεχόμενον, ὁ δὲ δεύτερος τὸ ἀληθές.

Πάλιν ὑποκείσθω ἕτερος νέος ὑγρὰν ἔχων τὴν γαστέρα διὰ ψυχρότερον ἧπαρ. ἐφ' οὗ λέγω, ὅτι, εἰ ἐν τῇ νέᾳ ἡλικίᾳ ψυχρὸν ἔχει τὸ ἧπαρ, πολλῷ μᾶλλον ἐν τῷ γήρᾳ ψυχρότερον αὐτὸ ἕξει· τοιοῦτον δὲ ὂν οὐχ ἑλκύσει ἐφ' ἑαυτὸ τὸν χυλόν, μὴ γινομένης δὲ ἀναδόσεως ἐκχεῖται οὗτος εἰς τὰ ἔντερα καὶ ὑγραίνει τὴν διαχώρησιν· ὥστε οὖν καὶ γηράσας ὁ τοιοῦτος οὐδὲν ἧττον ὑγρὰν ἔχει τὴν γαστέρα. καὶ ἔψευσται ὁ λόγος οὗτος πάντῃ.

Πάλιν ἕτερος ὑποκείσθω ὑγρὰν ἔχων τὴν γαστέρα χολώδους περὶ τὰ ἔντερα φερομένου περιττώματος καὶ συνεχῶς αὐτὴν ἐπεγείροντος πρὸς ἔκκρισιν. ἐνταῦθα ἀποφαίνομαι, ὅτι ὁ τοιοῦτος ἐν τῷ γήρᾳ ξηρὰν ἕξει τὴν γαστέρα ψυχρᾶς οὔσης τῆς ἡλικίας· οὐ γὰρ γεννᾶται τοσαύτη χολὴ ὥστε πέμπεσθαι δαψιλῶς αὐτὴν εἰς τὰ ἔντερα καὶ τὴν ἀπόκρισιν συνεχῆ ἀπεργάζεσθαι. ὅστις λόγος ἔχει τὸ ἀληθές.

Τρέψωμεν δὴ οὖν τὸν λόγον καὶ ἐπὶ τοῦ ἑτέρου. προκείσθω τις νέος ξηρὰν ἔχων τὴν γαστέρα· καὶ ζητῶν εὑρίσκω, ὅτι δι' ἔνδειαν σιτίων τοῦτο ὑφίσταται, ἐνδεῶς μεταλαμβάνων τροφῆς διὰ τὸ ἐσβέσθαι αὐτῷ τὴν ὄρεξιν ἐπὶ θερμοτέρᾳ τῇ τοῦ στομάχου κράσει. ἐπὶ τούτου τοίνυν λέγω, ὅτι πάντως ἐν γήρᾳ ὑγροτέρα γενήσεται ἡ διαχώρησις· τῷ ψυχρῷ γὰρ τῆς ἡλικίας ἐπεγείρεται ἡ ἔφεσις ὡς πλείονα προσφέρε-

13–17] *cf.* Gal. In Aphor. II 20: XVII B 494,16–17; 495,13–496,8 K. 18–23] *cf.* Gal. In Aphor. II 20: XVII B 494,17–18 K. 30–34] *cf.* Gal. In Aphor. II 20: XVII B 494,13–15; 495, 10–13 K. 35–182,26] *cf.* Theoph. In Aphor.: II 315,17–24 Dietz 35–182,3] *cf.* Gal. In Aphor. II 20: XVII B 496,12–13; 496,16–497,1 K.

7 γοῦν μενούσης *scripsi*: γουνούσις P: γοῦνούσης P²: μενούσης A αὐτῆς P 14 ὑγρότητι *scripsi*: ὑγρότ^τ α 19 ξηρότητι *scripsi*: ξηρότ^τ α 25 ἀφ' α: *correxi (cf. infra, p. 182,22)* εἰ] ἡ P 30 χολῶδες A 32 ἔχει P

and a strong appetite. Do not ask how it is possible at an early age, when heat prevails, for the appetite to be strong, though this is a sign of a cold stomach. For the temperament in the several parts may be uneven, so that for instance the liver is hot, but the orifice of the stomach cold, with a strong appetite as the result; or else, if the orifice contains a certain humor and if (the person) takes a large quantity of food, the food will not be digested and thus inevitably make the bowels wetter. Now if such coldness lasts into their old age, the appetite of these persons increases even more, and by consuming still more food than before without digesting it, they continue to have wet bowels even in old age; if, however, the coldness is so increased by old age as to numb the stomach completely and to destroy the appetite, then (the stomach) no longer accepts the food, and for want of matter these people in old age will necessarily have their bowels free from waste matter and dry.

Suppose another young man has wet bowels as a result of weakness of the retentive faculty, which is enfeebled by moisture. I contend that in this case the bowels will certainly be dry in old age, because in old men the moisture is spent and changes into an extremely dry temperament, which strengthens the retentive faculty, and when this prevails, the bowels necessarily dry up.

Take another young man who has wet bowels as a result of strength of the secretory faculty, itself a result of dryness. So in this case too, if dryness persists in the same proportion, the person will have wet bowels in old age too; but if it increases owing to old age, so that by its excess it breaks down the secretory faculty, the weakening of this faculty causes nothing to be excreted and the bowels become dry. Here, once more, the rule may or may not hold true, whereas in the second case it does.

Let us suppose another young man who has wet bowels, because his liver is too cold. With regard to him I say that if he has a cold liver at an early age, he will have it even colder in old age; being such it will not attract the chyle, and when distribution fails, the chyle flows into the intestines and moistens the feces; consequently this person will have wet bowels even in old age. Here the rule completely fails to apply.

Suppose another (young) man has wet bowels because bilious waste matter is conveyed to the intestines and continually stimulates the bowels to excretion. In this case I declare that the person will have dry bowels in old age, because that age is cold, so that not enough bile is produced to be dispatched to the intestines in quantity and cause continual excretion. Here the rule holds good.

Let us now pass on to the discussion of the other process. Let there be a young man with dry bowels; and upon inquiry I find that his condition is due to lack of food, for he takes insufficient food because his appetite has been stifled by an excessively hot temperament of the stomach. In this case I say that the feces will inevitably become moister in old age; for owing to the coldness of that age the appetite is stimulated so that he will take more food, no doubt by the natural

σθαι τὰ σιτία διὰ τὴν φυσικὴν πάντως ἀντιπεπόνθησιν· πλειόνων δὲ προσφερομένων καὶ μὴ κατὰ λόγον πεττομένων διὰ τὴν ψυχρότητα, ὑγροτέρα ἐξ ἀνάγκης ἡ διαχώρησις γίνεται.

Εἶτα ἐφ' ἑτέρου νέου ξηροτέραν εὑρίσκω τὴν γαστέρα διὰ ῥώμην τῆς καθεκτικῆς δυνάμεως· καί φημι ἐπὶ τούτου, ὅτι, ἐὰν τὰ αὐτὰ μέτρα μείνῃ τῆς ξηρότητος καὶ ἐν τῇ πρεσβυτικῇ ἡλικίᾳ, καὶ ἡ γαστὴρ μενεῖ ξηροτέραν ποιουμένη τὴν διαχώρησιν· εἰ δὲ πλεονάσει τὰ [αὐτὰ] μέτρα τῆς ξηρότητος ἐν τῷ γήρᾳ, ὡς καταλῦσαι τὴν καθεκτικὴν καὶ ἀσθενῆ αὐτὴν ἀπεργάσασθαι, τὸ τηνικαῦτα ὑγρὰ ἐκ μεταπτώσεως ἐν γήρᾳ ἡ διαχώρησις γίνεται. καὶ ἔχει ὁ λόγος τὸ ἐνδεχόμενον.

Ἄλλος πάλιν νέος ἐχέτω ξηροτέραν γαστέρα ἐπὶ ἀσθενείᾳ τῆς ἀποκριτικῆς δυνάμεως ὑγρότητος αὐτὴν βλαπτούσης. ἐπὶ τούτου ἐν τῷ γήρᾳ ξηροτέρας γινομένης τῆς κράσεως ῥωμαλεωτέρα ἡ ἀποκριτικὴ ἀπεργάζεται δύναμις καὶ ὑγροτέραν ποιεῖται τὴν διαχώρησιν.

Ἕτερος πάλιν ἔστω νέος ξηρὰν ἔχων τὴν γαστέρα τῷ λόγῳ τῆς ἐπιτεταμένης ἀναδόσεως θερμοῦ αὐτῷ ὑποκειμένου τοῦ ἥπατος. καὶ ἐπειδὴ πᾶς ὁ χυλὸς ἀνειλκυσμένος ἄνικμον καταλιμπάνει τὴν γαστέρα, τὸ τῆς ξηρότητος κατὰ τὴν διαχώρησιν ἡ γαστὴρ ὑφίσταται πάθημα. ἐπὶ τούτου οὖν ἀποφαίνομαι, ὅτι γηράσκων ὑγρὰν σχοίη τὴν διαχώρησιν διὰ τὸ ἐπὶ τὸ ψυχρότερον τῆς κράσεως μεταβαλλομένης τοῦ ἥπατος τὸν χυλὸν εἰς τὴν γαστέρα καταλιμπάνεσθαι κἀντεῦθεν ὑγρὰν ἐξ ἀνάγκης τὴν διαχώρησιν γίνεσθαι.

Εἶτα καὶ ἕτερος ὑποκείσθω ξηρὰν ἔχων τὴν γαστέρα διὰ τὸ μὴ πλείστην χολὴν ἐπιρρεῖν ἐν τοῖς ἐντέροις καὶ μαστίζειν αὐτὰ πρὸς ἔκκρισιν. ἐφ' οὗ λέγω, ὅτι οὐδὲν ἧττον ἐπὶ τούτου καὶ ἐν πρεσβυτικῇ ἡλικίᾳ ἐξηραμμένη ἔσται ἡ γαστήρ· εἰ γὰρ ἐν νεότητι οὐ τοιαύτης εὐπορεῖ ὕλης δυναμένης μαστίζειν τὰ ἔντερα καὶ ἐπεγείρειν αὐτὰ εἰς ἀπόκρισιν, πολλῷ μᾶλλον ἐν τῇ πρεσβυτικῇ ἡλικίᾳ γενόμενος τοιούτου χυμοῦ ἀπορήσει. ὥστε οὖν κἀνταῦθα ἔψευσται πάντῃ ὁ Ἱπποκράτειος λόγος.

Ἐπεὶ δὲ εἰρήκαμεν, ὅτι διὰ τὸ ἀένναον τῆς διαφορήσεως ξηρὰ πολλάκις γίνεται ἡ γαστήρ, ἐάν ποτε ἐν νέᾳ ἡλικίᾳ τοῦτο φανῇ, λέγω δὴ ξηραινομένη κατὰ διαφόρησιν ἡ γαστήρ, προλέγειν ἐπὶ τῶν τοιούτων εἰκός, ὅτι γηράσκοντες ὑγρὰν ἕξουσι πάντως τὴν γαστέρα διὰ τὸ ἐν γεροντικῇ ἡλικίᾳ πυκνο⟨υ⟩μένης τῆς ἐπιφανείας ἐπέχεσθαι τὴν διαφόρησιν· ἧστινος μὴ γενομένης τὰ εἰωθότα διαφορεῖσθαι ὑγρὰ ἐπὶ γαστέρα ἀντικαταρρεύσαντα ὑγροτέραν ποιεῖται τὴν διαχώρησιν.

II 21 [II 21: IV 476,5 L.] Λιμὸν θώρηξις λύει.

Εἴρηται ἡμῖν, ὅτι ψυχρὰ πολλάκις ὕλη καταλαβοῦσα τὸν στόμαχον παρὰ φύσιν ὄρεξιν ἐπιτεταμένην ἐργάζεται. ταύτην τοίνυν τὴν διάθεσιν διὰ τοῦ νυνὶ ῥησειδίου θεραπεύει ὁ Ἱπποκράτης ἀκρατοποσίᾳ χρώμενος· φησὶ γὰρ οὕτως· Λιμὸν θώρηξις λύει. ὁ δὲ οἶνος οὔτε μέλας, διὰ τὸ παχυμερὲς καὶ γεῶδες, οὔτε μὴν

4–9] *cf.* Gal. In Aphor. II 20: XVII B 496,14–15; 497,5–7 K. 14–20] *cf.* Gal. In Aphor. II 20: XVII B 496,13; 497,1–3 K. 21–26] *cf.* Gal. In Aphor. II 20: XVII B 496,14; 497, 3–5 K. 34 Εἴρηται] *v. supra*, p. 154,6–11 37 ὁ – 184,6] *cf.* Gal. In Aphor. II 21: XVII B 500,2–6 K. *supra*, p. 156,28–32

7 αὐτὰ *delevi* 11 ὑγρότητος *scripsi*: ὑγρότ[τ] A: ὑγρότητι P 14 τὴν *om.* A 24 δύναμις P 27 Ἐπεὶ] ἐπειδὴ A 30 πυκνομένης α: *corr. Dietz* 36 οὕτως] ὄντως P

counteraction; and when more food is taken and not adequately digested because of coldness, the discharge inevitably becomes moister.

Next, in another young man I find the bowels too dry owing to the strength of the retentive faculty; with regard to him I declare that if dryness persists in the same proportion in old age, his bowels too will continue to produce an excessively dry discharge; but if the degree of dryness increases in old age, so that it breaks down the retentive faculty and makes it weak, then the feces in old age will change to moist. Here the rule may be valid or not.

Let us take another young man whose bowels are too dry in consequence of the weakness of the secretory faculty, which is harmed by moisture. As this person's temperament grows drier with age, his secretory faculty becomes stronger and excretion moister.

Again, suppose another young man has dry bowels on account of intensive distribution, due to the fact that his liver is hot. So, since all the chyle is absorbed and leaves the bowels without moisture, the bowels suffer from dryness in excretion. In this case I declare that when he grows old he will have wet excretion, because, as the temperament of the liver changes to colder, the chyle is left behind in the bowels and the feces inevitably become moist as a result.

Finally, let us take another (young) man whose bowels are dry because there is not very much bile flowing to the intestines and stimulating them to excretion. In his case I say that even in old age his bowels will nevertheless remain dry; for if in youth he lacks sufficient matter of the kind that can stimulate the intestines and activate them toward excretion, the shortage of this humor will become even greater when he has reached old age. So that in this instance, too, Hippocrates' rule is entirely false.

We said already that it is often owing to the continuity of dispersal that the bowels become dry; if ever this – i.e. drying up of the bowels by dispersal – occurs at an early age, one may reasonably predict for these cases that upon growing old they will doubtless have wet bowels, because in old age dispersal is checked by the tightening of the surface; and when there is no dispersal, the fluids that used to be dispersed flow down into the bowels instead and make the excretion moister.

II 21. A stiff drink dispels hunger.

We said above that often cold matter which has settled abnormally in the stomach brings about a violent appetite. It is this condition which Hippocrates treats in the present maxim by means of a drink of unmixed wine: A stiff drink, he says, dispels hunger. The wine should be neither dark red, because of its thick and earthy quality, nor thin and white, because this wine is easily distributed

λεπτὸς εἴη καὶ λευκός, διὰ τὸ εὐανάδοτος εἶναι καὶ μὴ χρονίζειν ἐν τῇ γαστρί, ἀλλὰ κιρρὸς ἢ ξανθὸς καὶ θερμός· οὐχ ὅτι ἔστι ψυχρὸς οἶνος, ἀλλ' ὅτι οἶνος πρὸς οἶνον παραβαλλόμενος ἧττον θερμὸς εὑρίσκεται. ὁ τοιοῦτος τοίνυν οἶνος, ὁ θερμὸς λέγω καὶ κιρρός, ἄκρατος παρεχόμενος χρονίζει περὶ τὸ στόμα τῆς γαστρὸς καὶ τῇ οἰκείᾳ θερμασίᾳ λεπτύνει καὶ ἀναλύει καὶ διαφορεῖ τὸν ὀξώδη χυμὸν τὸν ποιοῦντα τὴν ἐπιτεταμένην ἤγουν κυνώδη ὄρεξιν.

Ὥστε οὖν συνεχὴς ὑπάρχει ὁ ἀφορισμὸς οὗτος τῷ πρὸ αὐτοῦ προσεχῶς εἰρημένῳ, ὅτι ὑγρὰ γίνεται ἡ γαστὴρ πολλάκις καὶ διὰ προσφορὰν πολλῶν σιτίων, ἥτις ψυχρᾷ στομάχου ἕπεται κράσει. προὔθετο δὲ τὴν τοιαύτην διάθεσιν θεραπεῦσαι, ἄτοπον ἡγησάμενος τὸ τεσσαράκοντα χρόνους ἀναμεῖναι τὸν οὕτω πάσχοντα ὥστε φυσικῶς θεραπευθῆναι, καὶ ἴσως μηδὲ τούτου τυχεῖν, ὥσπερ τὸ «ὡς ἐπὶ πολὺ» ἔδειξε.

Τινὲς δὲ λιμὸν λέγουσιν ἐνταῦθα καλεῖν τὸν Ἱπποκράτην τὴν σιτοδείαν, τουτέστι τὴν λεῖψιν τοῦ σιτίου, ὅτι, ἐὰν τυχὸν ἀπορία ἐστὶ σίτου, παρακελεύεται οἶνον παρέχειν διὰ τὸ τρόφιμον αὐτοῦ. ἔστι δὲ τοῦτο πιθανόν.

Ἕτεροι δέ φασιν, ὅτι λιμὸν τὸ⟨ν⟩ βούλιμον καλεῖ· δεῖ γάρ, φησί, τὸ τηνικαῦτα οἶνον διδόναι τοῖς παντελῆ ἀνορεξίαν ἔχουσιν. ὅπερ οὐκ εὔλογον· ἅπαξ γὰρ καταβληθείσης εἰς ἄκρον τῆς ὀρέξεως ὑπὸ τῆς ἀμέτρου ψύξεως δηλητήριον καθίσταται ἡ τοῦ ἀκράτου οἰνοποσία, πολλῷ πλέον αὐτὴν καταλύουσα, νικηθήσεται γὰρ ἡ θερμότης τοῦ οἴνου τῇ ἀμετρίᾳ τῆς ἐν τῷ στομάχῳ ψύξεως. διὸ τὸ τηνικαῦτα τοῖς ἔτι μᾶλλον δυναμένοις θάλψαι χρώμεθα βοηθήμασι, φαρμάκοις τε θερμοῖς καὶ δριμέσι, καὶ οὐ τροφαῖς ἀμυδρῶς τοῦτο ποιῆσαι δυναμέναις. βούλιμος δέ ἐστιν ὁ μέγας λιμὸς ἤτοι ἡ παντελὴς ἀνορεξία. λιμὸν οὖν ἀκουστέον νῦν τὴν κυνώδη ὄρεξιν, ἥτις γίνεται ὀξώδους χυμοῦ τὸν στόμαχον καταλαβόντος καὶ δάκνοντος καὶ διαφθείροντος πᾶσαν αὐτοῦ τὴν ἰκμάδα.

II 22 [II 22: IV 476,6–7 L.] Ἀπὸ πλησμονῆς ὁκόσα ἂν νοσήματα γένωνται, κένωσις ἰῆται.

Ἐνταῦθά φησιν ὁ Ἱπποκράτης ὅτι «Σκόπει· εἰ μὲν ἐπὶ πλησμονῇ τὸ νόσημα γέγονε, τῇ ἐναντιότητι θεράπευσον κένωσιν παραλαμβάνων· ἐὰν δὲ δι' ἔνδειαν τροφῆς καταλέλυται», φησίν, «ἡ δύναμις, ἀντεισάγαγε σὺ πλῆθος τροφῆς· τὰ γὰρ ἐναντία τῶν ἐναντίων ἰάματα.» μὴ ὡς ἔτυχε δὲ τοῦτο διαπράττου· ἐὰν γὰρ ἀμέτρως χρήσῃ τῇ ἐναντιώσει, εἰς ἀμετρίαν πάλιν ὑπαγάγῃς τὸν κάμνοντα.

Οὐ μόνον δὲ ἐπὶ ταύτῃ τῇ ἀντιθέσει ἁρμόζει τὸ λεγόμενον, λέγω δὴ τῇ κατὰ ποσότητα, ἀλλὰ καὶ κατὰ πᾶσαν ἀντίθεσιν ἐν ποιότητι θεωρουμένην. ἐὰν γὰρ

3 ὁ[I] – 6] *cf.* Theoph. In Aphor.: II 317,10–12 Dietz 7 τῷ – εἰρημένῳ] *v.* Hipp. Aphor. II 20: IV 476,1–4 L. 11 ὡς ἐπὶ πολὺ] *cf. supra*, p. 176,29–30 13–15] *v.* Gal. In Aphor. II 21: XVII B 499,6–7 K. 16–20 ψύξεως] *v.* Gal. In Aphor. II 21: XVII B 501,2–8 K. 23 λιμὸν – ὄρεξιν] *v.* Gal. In Aphor. II 21: XVII B 499,7–10 K. τὴν – 25] *v.* Gal. In Aphor. II 21: XVII B 500,15–18 K. 30sq. τὰ – ἰάματα] *v.* Hipp. Flat. 1: CMG I 1, p. 92,8 33–186,4] *cf.* Gal. In Aphor. II 22: XVII B 502,2–5. 11–16 K.

1 λεπτὸς] λευκὸς A μὴ *om.* A 3 παραλαμβανόμενος A 7 τῷ . . . εἰρημένῳ] τὰ . . . εἰρημένα P προσεχῶς] συνεχῶς A 8 πολλὴν P 16 ἕτερον P τὸν *scripsi*: τὸ α φησί] *fort.* φασί *scribendum est* 27 γίνονται *Hipp.* C′: γίγνεται *vel* γένηται *al.*: γίγνηται *Theoph.* 31 τούτου α: *corr.* A[2] 33 λέγω] λέγει P 34 ποσότητα] ποσότ[τ] P: ποσότητι A

and does not linger in the stomach, but it should be tawny or yellow, and hot; not that cold wine exists, but one wine as compared to another is found to be less hot. This kind of wine, then, hot and tawny, if administered unmixed, lingers around the orifice of the stomach and by the heat that is proper to it comminutes, dissolves and disperses the acid humor which causes the violent or canine hunger.

It follows that this aphorism is a sequel to the one immediately preceding it, namely that the bowels often become moist, among other causes, by the consumption of a great quantity of food combined with a cold temperament of the stomach. (Hippocrates) proposed to treat this condition, because he considered it absurd for the patient to wait forty years for the natural cure, and even then perhaps fail to get it, as the words "in most cases" implied.

Some say that by hunger Hippocrates here means famine, i.e. shortage of food, in other words, if for example grain is not available, he advises you to administer wine because of its nourishing quality. This seems plausible.

Others hold that hunger stands for bulimia; if so, (Hippocrates) tells us to give wine, in that situation, to patients whose appetite has failed completely. This does not make sense: once the appetite has been utterly repressed by immoderate coldness, a drink of unmixed wine becomes poison, for it will destroy the appetite even further, since the hotness of the wine will be defeated by the immoderate coldness in the stomach. In this condition, therefore, we use remedies that can provide still more heat, hot and pungent medicines, not nutriments which can have this effect only in a weak degree. Bulimia is intense hunger, that is to say, a total absence of appetite. By hunger, then, we should here understand the canine appetite which results when an acid humor has settled in the stomach, corroding it and corrupting all its moisture.

II 22. All diseases caused by repletion are cured by evacuation.

What Hippocrates says here is: "Pay attention: if the disease is the result of repletion, you must treat it by means of its opposite and apply evacuation; but if resistance", he says, "has failed through lack of food, make it up by abundant feeding; for opposites cure opposites." However, you should not do this at random; for by excessive application of the opposite you will bring the patient to the other extreme.

The statement fits not only this particular — I mean, quantitative — antithesis, but also every kind of qualitative antithesis. If the disease is hot, you must pro-

θερμὸν εἴη τὸ νόσημα, δεῖ ψύχειν, ἂν δὲ ψυχρόν, θερμαίνειν, ὁμοίως καὶ τὸ ὑγρὸν ξηραίνειν καὶ τὸ ξηρὸν ὑγραίνειν. ταῦτα γὰρ πάντα εὐμεθοδεύτου ἰατροῦ ἐστιν ἐπιζητεῖν· ἅτινα διὰ μιᾶς λέξεως ὁ Ἱπποκράτης ἐσήμανεν εἰρηκώς· [II 22: IV 476, 7–8 L.] καὶ τῶν ἄλλων ἡ ὑπεναντίωσις.

Ἐφ' οἷς ζητήσωμεν, εἰ δοκεῖ, εἰ γενικὸς ὁ λόγος οὗτος. ἰστέον τοίνυν, ὅτι καταβάλλεται ἡ ἐν ἡμῖν φύσις ὑπὸ τῆς τριμερείας τῶν παρὰ φύσιν· τρία γάρ εἰσι τὰ παρὰ φύσιν πάντα, οἷς ἡ ἡμετέρα φύσις ὑποβέβληται, αἴτια, νοσήματα καὶ συμπτώματα. καὶ πρῶτον ζητήσωμεν ἐπὶ τῶν αἰτίων, εἰ ἀληθὲς τὸ λεγόμενον. καί φαμεν, ὅτι, ἐὰν [τὸ] πλῆθος ᾖ, δεῖ κενοῦν, καὶ τούτου μάρτυς ὁ Ἱπποκράτειος λόγος. προσεχῶς γὰρ περὶ αἰτίων ἡμῖν διαλέγεται, ἡ γὰρ πλησμονὴ καὶ ἡ ἔνδεια αἰτιά εἰσι νοσημάτων ποιητικά· ταῦτα δὲ δι' ἐναντιώσεως θεραπεύεται, ὥστε ἀληθεύει ὁ παρὼν ἀφορισμὸς ἐπὶ τῷ κατὰ τὰ αἴτια λόγῳ, εἴ γε καὶ τὰ παχέα λεπτύνομεν καὶ τὰ λεπτὰ παχύνομεν καὶ τὰ γλίσχρα τέμνομεν καὶ τὰ ἐμφράττοντα ἐκφράττομεν.

Ἐφ' οἷς ζητήσωμεν, εἰ καὶ ἐπὶ τῶν νοσημάτων οὕτως ἔχει. καί φαμεν, ὅτι προδήλως τῇ ἐναντιώσει ἐξάγει τὰ νοσήματα καὶ ταύτῃ θεραπεύεται τὸ νοσοῦν σῶμα. ἀλλ' ἴσως ἀπορήσει τις· «Πῶς ἐπί τινων πυρετῶν ζέμασι βοτανῶν χρώμεθα, ἀνήθου φημὶ καὶ σελίνου καὶ ἀψινθίου καὶ τῶν τοιούτων, εἴ γε καὶ ὁ πυρετὸς θερμὸν χρῆμά ἐστι;» πρὸς ὃ ῥητέον, ὅτι διττή ἐστιν ἡ θεραπεία, ἡ μὲν καθ' ἑαυτὸ καὶ πρώτως, ἡ δὲ κατὰ συμβεβηκός. καὶ πρώτως μὲν θεραπεύειν λεγόμεθα πυρετὸν χυλῷ πτισάνης καὶ θριδακίνῃ καὶ ὑδρομέλιτι καὶ τοιούτοις χρώμενοι, ψύχουσι γὰρ τὰ τοιαῦτα. κατὰ συμβεβηκὸς δὲ θεραπεύομεν τὸν πυρετόν, ἡνίκα μὴ ἀμέσως τοῖς ψύχουσι χρώμεθα, ἀλλὰ διὰ μέσου ἑτέρου τινός. οὕτω γοῦν ἀπόζεμα ἀνήθου παρέχοντες ἢ ἀννήσου καὶ τῶν τοιούτων λεπτύνομεν τὴν ὕλην τοῦ πυρετοῦ καὶ ἐξάγομεν αὐτήν· ἧς κενουμένης σβέννυται ὁ πυρετὸς μὴ ἔχων τὸ ὑλικὸν αἴτιον. ἔστιν οὖν καὶ ἡ τοιαύτη θεραπεία κατ' ἐναντίωσιν· τὸ γὰρ θερμὸν ἐψύξαμεν, ⟨οὐ⟩ κατὰ πρῶτον μέντοι λόγον – τοὐναντίον δὲ θερμοῖς ἐδόξαμεν κεχρῆσθαι –, ἀλλὰ κατὰ συμβεβηκὸς τοῦτο ἀπειργασάμεθα.

Ἐφ' οἷς ζητήσωμεν, εἰ ἐπὶ τῶν συμπτωμάτων οὕτως ἔχει. ἐφ' ὧν οὐδὲ κυρίως ἐστὶν ὀνομάσαι ἴασιν, παρηγορικοὶ γὰρ λεγόμεθα κατὰ τοῦ σφοδροῦ συμπτώματος ἐνιστάμενοι· πλὴν ὅτι ἐστὶν ἀναλογίαν τινὰ καὶ ἐνταῦθα θεωρῆσαι, ὡς διὰ τῆς ἐναντιώσεως καὶ τὸ σφοδρὸν τῶν συμπτωμάτων κολάζομεν, καὶ φρενῖτιν κίνησιν οὖσαν τῆς ψυχῆς ἄμετρον διὰ τῆς ἠρεμίας παραμυθούμεθα.

Ἀλλ' ἴσως ἀπορεῖς ὅτι «Πῶς ὀδύνην κώλου, καὶ ταῦτα ἐπὶ ψυχρῷ χυμῷ γενομένην, διὰ τῶν ναρκούντων παύομεν;» ⟨καὶ λέγομεν⟩, ὅτι οὐκ ἔστι τοῦτο θεραπεία, ἀλλὰ παραμυθία· οὐδὲ γὰρ ἐξάγομεν τὴν ὕλην, ἥτις ἐμποιεῖ τὴν ὀδύνην τῷ σώματι, ἀλλ' αὕτη μὲν ἐν αὐτῷ μένει, τὸ δὲ κρῖνον τέως τῆς αἰσθήσεως παύεται ἐπὶ συμφέροντι ἀναισθητότερον τοῦτο ἀπεργαζομένων ἡμῶν τοῖς ναρκωτικοῖς βοηθήμασι. διὸ καὶ συντόμως πάλιν ἡ ὀδύνη ἐπανακάμπτει, ὅπερ ἐπὶ τῶν τελέως θεραπευομένων, τῆς ὕλης δηλονότι κενωθείσης, οὐ γίνεται. ταύτην δὲ κενῶσαι βουλόμενοι τοῖς λεπτύνουσι καὶ τέμνουσι καὶ ἑλκύουσι χρώμεθα βοηθήμασιν, ἅτινα πάντα θερμά ἐστι τῇ φύσει. εἴρηται οὖν, ὅτι καὶ ἐπὶ τῶν συμπτωμάτων ἁρμόζει ὁ λόγος καὶ γενικός ἐστι.

1 ἂν] ἐὰν A   6 τὰ] τῶν A   9 τὸ *delevi*   10 αἰτιά *scripsi*: ἅτινα α   12 λεπτυνόμενα P   13 ἐμφράττομεν A   15 εἰσάγει α: *correxi (cf. infra, lin. 24 et 35)*   20 χυλὸν α: *corr.* A[2]   θριδακίνης P   25 οὐ *addidi*   29 *fort.* παρηγορεῖν *scribendum est*   συμπτωμάτου P   33 ἀπορῇ P   34 καὶ λέγομεν *addidi*

vide cold, if it is cold, you must provide heat, and similarly you must provide dryness for the wet and wetness for the dry. All these further questions can be left to a doctor well versed in the method; Hippocrates expressed all this in the single phrase and all the rest by their contraries.

Let us inquire next, if you wish, whether this rule is of general application. It should be known, then, that our natural condition is overthrown by the abnormal in its threefold aspects: there are three forms of the abnormal to which our nature is subject, to wit, causes, diseases, and symptoms. We will examine first whether the statement is applicable to causes. As to this we say that any surplus should be evacuated, as testified by the Hippocratic maxim. Causes, indeed, are its immediate subject, for repletion and shortage are causes which bring about diseases; they are cured by their contraries, so that the present aphorism holds good as regards causes: we make thin what is thick and thick what is thin, we fragmentize what is sticky and we remove what blocks the passages.

Let us see next if it is also true of diseases. We state that he manifestly expels diseases by their contraries and that by this method the ailing body is cured. But perhaps somebody will ask: "How is it that for certain fevers we use decoctions of herbs such as dill, celery, absinthe, etc., when the fever itself is also a hot thing?" The answer to this is that treatment is twofold, either direct and primary, or indirect. We are said to treat fever directly by means of barley-water, lettuce, hydromel, etc., i.e. cooling remedies. On the other hand, we treat fever indirectly, when we use remedies that do not cool immediately, but through something else. Thus by administering a decoction of dill or anise, etc., we comminute and eliminate the matter of the fever; and when this has been evacuated, the fever, deprived of its material cause, is quenched. So this is also a cure by contraries: we have cooled the hot, not, however, immediately – on the contrary, we seemed to use hot remedies –, but we achieved this result indirectly.

Finally let us see if it also applies to symptoms. Here the word "cure" is strictly speaking out of place, for we are said to provide "relief", when we take action against a violent symptom; yet even here a certain analogy can be observed: we check the violence of symptoms by means of contrary treatment; phrenitis, which is an immoderate commotion of the soul, is relieved by quiet.

Perhaps you will wonder why colic pain, though due to a cold humor, is allayed by narcotics. Our answer is that this is not a cure, but alleviation; we do not eliminate the matter that causes the pain in the body, but it remains there, only the judging faculty of perception is suspended for the moment, because for the (patient's) benefit we make the pain less noticeable with the help of narcotics. This explains why the pain soon returns, a thing which does not happen to those who are completely cured, i. e. by evacuation of the matter. To achieve this evacuation we apply comminuting, fragmentizing and drawing remedies, all of which are naturally hot. We conclude that the rule is also true of symptoms and is of universal validity.

II 23 [II 23. 24: IV 476,9–12 L.] Τὰ ὀξέα τῶν νοσημάτων κρίνεται ἐν τεσσαρεσκαίδεκα ἡμέρῃσι· τῶν ἑπτὰ ἡ τετάρτη ἐπίδηλος· ἑτέρης ἑβδομάδος ἡ η̄ ἀρχή, θεωρητικὴ δὲ ἡ ἑνδεκάτη.

Παραδοὺς ἀνωτέρω τὴν δίαιταν τῶν ὀξέων νοσημάτων νῦν παραδίδωσι καὶ τὴν κρίσιν· ἥστινος κρίσεως τὸν ἀριθμὸν τῶν ἡμερῶν βούλεται διαγράψαι. ἰστέον οὖν, ὅτι ἡ κρίσις διττή· ἢ γὰρ τελεία ἐστὶν ἢ ἀτελής, καὶ ἑκατέρα ἢ ἀγαθὴ ἢ κακή· καὶ οὐκ ἔστιν ἔξω τούτων γενέσθαι κρίσιν. μὴ μέντοι νομίσῃς, ὅτι ἐν τῇ ι̅δ̅ ἡμέρᾳ πάντως δεῖ τὰ ὀξέα κρίνεσθαι, πολλάκις γὰρ καὶ ἡ δ̅ κρίνει καὶ ἡ ζ̅ καὶ ἡ ι̅α̅· ἀλλὰ τὴν ι̅δ̅ εἶπε κρίσιμον τῶν ὀξέων ὡς ἔσχατον αὐτὴν ὅρον λαβὼν τῆς τῶν ὀξέων κρίσεως, οὐ γὰρ ἐνδέχεταί ποτε ὀξὺ νόσημα τὴν ι̅δ̅ ὑπερβῆναι. τὰ γὰρ ὀξέα νοσήματα ἐπὶ λεπτοτάτῃ καὶ κούφῃ καὶ δριμείᾳ γίνεται ὕλῃ, ἥτις διὰ μὲν τὴν σύστασιν ἔχει τὸ εὐδιαφόρητον, διὰ δὲ τὴν δριμύτητα τὸ εὔκριτον. δάκνουσα γὰρ καὶ ἀνιῶσα τὴν φύσιν ἐπεγείρει αὐτήν, ὥστε ἀποδιῶξαι τὸ λυποῦν τοῦ σώματος καὶ ταχέως ἐπιστῆναι τὴν κρίσιν.

Εἰ δέ τις εἴποι· «Καὶ μήν τινα τῶν ὀξέων ὁρῶμεν εἰς τὴν ι̅ζ̅ καὶ εἰς τὴν κ̅ ἡμέραν κρινόμενα», λέγομεν, ὅτι περὶ τῶν ὡς ἐπὶ πᾶν καὶ ὡς ἐπὶ τὸ πολὺ ὀξέων νοσημάτων τὴν μνήμην ἐνταῦθα ποιεῖται ὁ Ἱπποκράτης, ἡ δὲ ι̅ζ̅ καὶ κ̅ ἡμέρα τῶν σπανίως κρινουσῶν εἰσιν. ἄλλως τε εἰ καὶ ἡ ι̅ζ̅ καὶ κ̅ κρίνουσαι φαίνονται ἐπὶ τῶν ὀξέων νοσημάτων, ἀλλά γε τοῖς ἀκριβῶς τὸν νοῦν προσέχουσιν ἡ ι̅δ̅ καὶ ἐνταῦθα εὑρίσκεται κρίσιμος. οὐδὲν γὰρ ἄτοπον μέχρι μὲν τῆς δ̅ ἡμέρας ἀργοτέρως πως κινηθῆναι τὸ νόσημα διὰ φλεγματικὴν ὕλην καὶ προσεχῆ ἀπεψίαν καὶ πλήρωσιν στομάχου ἢ γαστρὸς ἢ ἐντέρων, ἀπὸ δὲ τῆς δ̅ αὐτὸ λοιπὸν σφοδρότερον καὶ ὀξύτερον γενέσθαι καὶ τῇ ι̅δ̅ κριθῆναι ἀπὸ τῆς δ̅. ὁμοίως καὶ ἐπὶ τῆς κ̅ ἔστιν εἰπεῖν, ὅτι ἀπὸ μὲν τῆς πρώτης ἡμέρας μέχρι τῆς ζ̅ ἀργότερον ἐκινήθη τὸ νόσημα, ἀπὸ δὲ τῆς ζ̅ τῶν ὠμοτέρων καὶ παχυμερῶν ἤδη δαπανηθέντων ὀξέως κινεῖσθαι ἤρξατο καὶ ἐκρίθη τῇ κ̅· πάλιν οὖν ἡ ι̅δ̅ εὑρίσκεται κρίσιμος ἀπὸ τῆς ζ̅ ἡμῶν ἀριθμούντων τὰς τοῦ νοσήματος ἡμέρας, ἀφ' ἧς καὶ ὀξέως ἤρξατο κινεῖσθαι. πᾶσαν δὲ τὴν ἀπορίαν προαπεκρούσατο ὁ Ἱπποκράτης μνησθεὶς τῆς ι̅δ̅ ἡμέρας.

Ἡ δὲ αἰτία τοῦ ἀργότερόν ποτε κινηθῆναι τὸ νόσημα καὶ τοῦ ὅσον οὔπω ὀξέως μέλλειν κινεῖσθαι αἱ προσεχεῖς εἰσιν ἀπεψίαι καὶ τὸ ἐν τῇ γαστρὶ ἀθροιζόμενον κατὰ τὸν στόμαχον φλέγμα, ὅπερ δεῖται δαπάνης, ἀναλώσεως ὑφαπτομένης, καὶ μέχρις ὅτου τὸ πᾶν διαφορηθῇ, ἐκλύειν δοκεῖ τὸν τόνον τοῦ ὀξέος νοσήματος· ὅπερ παρὰ τὸ μᾶλλον καὶ ἧττον ἢ μέχρι τῆς ζ̅ ἢ μέχρι τῆς δ̅ διαρκεῖ. δαπανηθέντος δὲ αὐτοῦ περὶ τὴν δ̅ ἢ τὴν ζ̅ ἡμέραν ἐφάπτεται λοιπὸν ἡ χολὴ τοῦ παντὸς κυριεύουσα νοσήματος καὶ ὀξὺ αὐτὸ ἐντεῦθεν ἀπεργαζομένη.

Καλῶς δὲ εἶπε κρίνεται καὶ οὐ «παύεται» διὰ τὸ τὴν κρίσιν ἢ τελείαν εἶναι ἢ ἀτελῆ, ἢ ἀγαθὴν ἢ κακήν.

4 Παραδοὺς – νοσημάτων] *v.* Hipp. Aphor. I 4–11: IV 460,7–464,13 L. 6 ἢ[I] – κακή] *cf.* Gal. In Aphor. II 23: XVII B 505,10–506,3 K. 7 μὴ – 10 ὑπερβῆναι] *v.* Gal. In Aphor. II 23: XVII B 506,10–14 K. 8 ἀλλὰ – 13] *v.* Theoph. In Aphor.: II 318,15–22 Dietz

3 ἡ η̄ *scripsi*: ἣν P: ἡ ὀγδόη A θεωρητικὴ] *item infra, p. 190,1. 2*: θεωρεῖται *infra, vol. II, fol. 96*ʳ: θεωρητὴ *Hipp.* 5 τῶν ἀριθμῶν A 6 *post* καὶ[II] *add.* ὡς A 17 εἰ *om.* A 22 τῆς[II]] τὴν P 33 *fort.* ὑφάπτεται *scribendum est*

II 23. Acute diseases reach their crisis in fourteen days; of the seven, the fourth is indicative; the 8th is the beginning of another week, and the eleventh is significant.

After dealing above with regimen in acute diseases he now discusses their crisis; of which crisis he proposes to define the number of days. Let us state first that crisis is twofold: either it is perfect or imperfect, and each of these may be good or bad; no other kind of crisis besides these is possible. Do not think, however, that acute diseases necessarily have their crisis on the 14th day; often the 4th, the 7th and the 11th are critical also; when (Hippocrates) said the 14th is critical in acute diseases, he meant that for the crisis in acute diseases it is the last possible limit, for an acute disease can never exceed the 14th day. This is because acute diseases result from very thin, light and pungent matter, which owing to its degree of consistency is easily dispersed, and owing to its pungency leads to a speedy crisis. By stinging and irritating the constitution, such matter stimulates it to expel the cause of the trouble from the body, so that the crisis is soon reached.

If someone should remark, "Yet we see that some acute diseases reach their crisis on the 17th and on the 20th day", we reply that Hippocrates here refers to acute diseases in their common and current form, whereas the 17th and the 20th day are rarely critical. Furthermore, even though the 17th and the 20th day appear to be critical in acute diseases, yet on close inspection it is the 14th which is critical even in those cases. It is quite conceivable, indeed, that until the 4th day the disease somehow moves slower because of phlegmatic matter, previous indigestion and fullness of the stomach, the belly or the intestines, while from the 4th day onward it becomes more violent and acute, so that the crisis takes place on the 14th day counting from the 4th. As regards the 20th day one can argue similarly that from the first to the 7th day the disease moved slower, but from the 7th onward, when the cruder and coarser matter had at last been spent, it began to move quicker and arrived at its crisis on the 20th; so once more the 14th is found to be critical, if we count from the 7th day of the disease, when it began to move fast. Hippocrates has disposed of the whole objection in advance by his reference to the 14th day.

The reason why the disease was slow in starting and will very soon move fast, are the preceding indigestions and the phlegm collecting in the belly in the region of the stomach, which has to be disposed of by the kindling of a consuming factor, and until all of it has been dispersed, it seems to paralyze the force of the acute disease; depending on intensity, it may hold out until the 7th or until the 4th day. When about the 4th or the 7th day it is spent, bile takes over as the dominating force in the entire disease, and from that point onward makes it an acute one.

It rightly says reach their crisis, not "reach their end", because the crisis can be perfect or imperfect, good or bad.

Ῥητέον δὲ καὶ περὶ τῆς ἐπιδήλου καὶ θεωρητικῆς ἡμέρας· ἑνὸς οὖν σαφηνισθέντος καὶ τὸ λοιπὸν δῆλον γενήσεται. θεωρητικὴν ἡμέραν ἐκείνην λέγομεν, ἥτις κρίσιμος μέν ἐστι καὶ αὐτὴ τῷ οἰκείῳ λόγῳ, διὰ δὲ τὸ ἀπαρασκεύαστον εἶναι τὴν ὕλην οὐ κρίνει μέν, σημεῖον δέ τι ὑποφαίνει κρίσεως. οἷόν τι τὸ λεγόμενον· ἡ δ̄ κρίσιμός ἐστιν ἡμέρα, ὑποκείσθω γὰρ κάτοξυ νόσημα προσδοκώμενον ἐν ταύτῃ κρίνεσθαι· ἥστινος ἐπιστάσης οὐκ ἐκρίθη μὲν τὸ νόσημα, σημεῖα δὲ ἡμῖν ἐφάνη κρίσεως ἐν αὐτῇ, ἢ ἀπὸ οὔρων ἢ ἀπὸ διαχωρήσεως ἢ ἀφ' ἑτέρων τινῶν· δῆλον οὖν, ὡς τῇ ζ̄ κρίσις γενήσεται.

II 24 [II 25: IV 478,1–3 L.] Οἱ θερινοὶ τεταρταῖοι ὡς τὰ πολλὰ γίνονται βραχέες, οἱ δὲ φθινοπωρινοὶ μακροί, καὶ μάλιστα οἱ πρὸς τὸν χειμῶνα συνάπτοντες.

Περὶ τῶν χρονίων νῦν διαλέγεται νοσημάτων· ὁ γὰρ τεταρταῖος τῶν χρονίων ὑπάρχει διὰ τὸ τὴν ὕλην, ὑφ' ἧς γίνεται, παχεῖαν εἶναι καὶ γεώδη καὶ δυσδιαφόρητον. οἱ θερινοὶ οὖν φησι τεταρταῖοι ὡς τὰ πολλὰ γίνονται βραχέες. διὰ τί; διότι τὰ ἐν τῷ θέρει συνιστάμενα νοσήματα ὀλιγοχρόνιά εἰσι διὰ τὴν τοῦ περιέχοντος ἐπικουρίαν πολλῆς γινομένης ὑπὸ τῆς ἀλέας τῆς τοῦ ἀέρος διαφορήσεως· τὰ δὲ ἐν τῷ χειμῶνι χρονιώτερα γίνονται διὰ τὴν πύκνωσιν τοῦ σώματος καὶ τὸ δυσδιαφόρητον τοῦ περιέχοντος. ἐν γὰρ τῷ θέρει ἀναλύονται οἱ χυμοὶ καὶ λεπτύνονται· ἀραιοῦται γὰρ ἡ ἐπιφάνεια καὶ διαφορεῖται τὰ περιττά, καὶ ταύτην ἔχων τὴν ἐπικουρίαν ὁ νοσῶν, κἂν χρονίῳ περιπέσῃ νοσήματι, ἐν ὀλίγῳ χρόνῳ αὐτοῦ ἀπαλλάσσεται. οἱ δὲ ἐν τῷ φθινοπώρῳ γινόμενοι ἢ χειμῶνι μακροχρόνιοί εἰσι· πρῶτον μὲν ὅτι ἐν τῷ φθινοπώρῳ τίκτεται ὁ χυμός, ὑφ' οὗ γεννᾶται ὁ τεταρταῖος, λέγω δὴ ὁ μελαγχολικός, ἔπειτα δὲ καὶ ἡ φύσις αὐτοῦ δυσκίνητός ἐστι καὶ παχυμερής. οἷστισι συλλαμβάνουσα καὶ ἡ τοῦ περιέχοντος ψῦξις χρονιώτερον ἀπεργάζεται τὸ νόσημα, καὶ μᾶλλον τοῦ χειμῶνος ἐπικαταλαμβάνοντος διὰ τὸ ἐπὶ πλέον παχυνομένην τὴν ὕλην ὡς μᾶλλον πιλουμένην δυσκίνητον εἶναι· οὐδέποτε γὰρ ἡ τοιαύτη τῶν ὑλῶν κατάστασις προπηλακίζει τὴν φύσιν καὶ οἱονεὶ ἐρεθίζει πρὸς ἔκκρισιν. ἔχει δὲ καὶ πολὺ τὸ ἐν τῷ μέσῳ διάστημα καὶ τὴν ἀνάπαυλαν, ὅπερ τῷ δυσκινήτῳ τοῦ χυμοῦ παρέπεται· ὃ δὴ καὶ αὐτὸ χρονιωτέραν τὴν ἀπαλλαγὴν ἀπεργάζεται. ἐπὶ δὲ τῶν ὀξέων τῷ μήτε ἀνακωχὴν ἔχειν τὴν δύναμιν ἐπὶ πολλῷ διαστήματι, ἀλλὰ καὶ προπηλακίζεσθαι τὴν φύσιν διά τε τὸ θερμὸν καὶ εὐκίνητον τῶν ὑλῶν ὀξεῖα γίνεται καὶ εὐκίνητος ἡ ἀπαλλαγή, ἐφ' ὁπότερον ἂν ῥέψῃ τὰ τῆς ἐκβάσεως.

«Ἀλλ' ἐνταῦθα ἀνατρέπεται ὁ κανὼν ⟨ὁ⟩ λέγων· "Ἐν τῇσι νούσοισιν ἧσσον κινδυνεύουσιν οἱ νοσέοντες, οἷς ἂν οἰκείη τῆς φύσιος καὶ τῆς ἕξιος καὶ τῆς ὥρης ἡ νοῦσος ὑπάρχει"· εἰ τοίνυν τὰ ἐν ταῖς οἰκείαις ὥραις γινόμενα νοσήματα οὐκ ἐπάγουσι

1–4 κρίσεως] *v.* Gal. In Aphor. II 24: XVII B 510,9–11 K. 4 ἡ – 8] *cf.* Gal. In Aphor. II 24: XVII B 510,13–14 K. 12–13 ὑπάρχει] *cf.* Theoph. In Aphor.: II 320,1–3 Dietz 14 οἱ – 16 διαφορήσεως] *v.* Theoph. In Aphor.: II 320,3–7 Dietz 14 διότι – 20 ἀπαλλάσσεται] *cf.* Gal. In Aphor. II 25: XVII B 513,8–514,8 K. 20 οἱ – 26 εἶναι] *cf.* Theoph. In Aphor.: II 320,7–11 Dietz 33 Ἐν – 35 ὑπάρχει] Hipp. Aphor. II 34: IV 480,7–9 L.

1 θεωρη^{ικ}τῆς A 4 κρίνη P 6 ἡμῖν *om.* P 9 ὡς] *item infra, lin. 14; p. 192,10, Hipp. pauci, Theoph.: non hab. Hipp. plerique* 13 γεώδη *(?) in* θολώδη *mut.* A 14 διὰ τί *om.* A 22 τίκτεται] τήκεται A 29 δὲ *om.* P τῷ *scripsi*: τὸ α 33 ὁ^{II} *addidi* τῇσι] τοῖσι α: *correxi*

A word about the indicative and significant day; if the one is explained, the other will also be clear. Significant we call a day which is properly critical in itself, but owing to the unprepared state of the matter does not bring the crisis, but only shows some sign of a crisis. To take an example: the 4th day is a critical one, if we take the case of a very acute disease, of which the crisis is expected on that day; but when it has come, there is no crisis; however, we observe signs of crisis that day, either in the urine or in the stools or in something else, so that it is evident that the crisis will come on the 7th.

II 24. Quartan fevers in summer are generally short, those in autumn long, especially those extending into winter.

The subject is now chronic diseases, to which quartan fever belongs because the matter which produces it is thick, earthy and difficult to disperse. (Hippocrates) says, then: Quartan fevers in summer are generally short. Why? Because diseases originating in summer are of short duration thanks to the beneficial influence of the surrounding air, for there is much dispersal of air owing to the warmth of the sun; those in winter, on the other hand, last longer, because of the closing of the pores of the body and the slow dispersal of the surrounding air. In summer the humors dissolve and become thinner; for the pores of the surface widen, waste matter is dispersed, and with this support the patient, even if he has contracted a chronic disease, needs little time to recover from it. Quartans starting in autumn or in winter, however, last long; first, because it is in autumn that the humor which generates quartan fever – to wit, the atrabiliar humor – is produced, secondly because by its own nature it is slow-moving and coarse. In conjunction with these the chilling effect of the surrounding air helps to make the disease last longer, especially if in the meantime winter sets in, since then the matter, being further compressed, becomes still thicker and more difficult to move; matter so structured never harasses the constitution and thus, in a manner of speaking, spurs it on to excretion. (The constitution) also gets a long interval of rest, which is incidental to the slowness of the humor; this, too, helps to delay the end of the illness. In acute diseases, on the contrary, where resistance has no long period of reprieve, but the constitution is constantly harassed by the hotness and the quick motion of the matter, the end is also sudden and quick, whichever turn the final issue may take.

"But this upsets the rule which says, 'In diseases there is less danger for patients, when the disease has more affinity with their nature and disposition and with the season'; consequently, if diseases incurred in their own season cause

κίνδυνον, δῆλον, ὅτι τὰ τοὐναντίον μὴ ἐν ταῖς οἰκείαις ὥραις γινόμενα μᾶλλον ἔσονται κινδυνώδη. ὁ οὖν ἐν θέρει τεταρταῖος, καθ' ὅσον ἀσυμφώνως ἔχει πρὸς τὴν ὥραν, κινδυνώδης ἔσται μᾶλλον ἤπερ ἐν φθινοπώρῳ· ἐκεῖνος γὰρ οἰκείως ἔχει πρὸς τὴν ὥραν.» πρὸς ὅ φαμεν, ὅτι οὐ τὸ σωτήριον ἢ κινδυνῶδες τοῦ τεταρταίου διὰ τῶν λεχθέντων ὑπέγραψεν ὁ Ἱπποκράτης, ἀλλὰ τὸ βραχὺ καὶ χρόνιον. σὸν τοίνυν ἐστὶ τοῦ τεχνικοῦ ἐκ τῶν συνεδρευόντων συμπτωμάτων τὸ κινδυνῶδες ἢ περιεστηκὸς τοῦ νοσήματος κρῖναι. ἴσμεν γάρ, ὅτι κίνδυνον πολλάκις φέρει καὶ τὸ ὀλιγοχρόνιον, οἷον ὁ τεταρταῖος, τῷ τὴν δύναμιν ἀτονωτέραν καὶ ἀδρανῆ τὸ τηνικαῦτα ὑπάρχειν ἀμετρότερον διαφορουμένου τοῦ σώματος τῇ τοῦ περιέχοντος θερμοῦ ὁμιλίᾳ.

Καλῶς δὲ πρόσκειται τὸ ὡς τὰ πολλά· οὐδὲν γὰρ ἄτοπον ἀπὸ μὲν τοῦ ἔαρος γεννηθῆναι τὸν μελαγχολικὸν χυμόν, ἐν δὲ τῷ θέρει ἐκφανθῆναι, κἀντεῦθεν τὴν φυσικὴν ἔχοντα κατάστασιν, λέγω δὴ τὸ πάχος καὶ τὸ δυσκίνητον, χρονιώτερον ἐργάσασθαι καὶ τὸ νόσημα, ὡς μὴ παύσασθαι ἐν τῷ θέρει.

Ἀλλ' ἴσως ἀπορεῖ τις λέγων· «Καὶ πῶς δυνατὸν ἐν τῷ θέρει γενέσθαι τεταρταῖον χολῆς ξανθῆς γεννητικῆς ὑπαρχούσης τῆς ὥρας;» φαμὲν οὖν, ὅτι οὐδὲν ἄτοπον ἐπιτηδείως ἔχειν τὸ σῶμα πρὸς τὸ γεννῆσαι τὸν μελαγχολικὸν χυμόν, ὥσπερ ἐπὶ τῶν ἰσχνοτέρων καὶ μελαντέρων καὶ παρακμαστικῶν ὁρᾶται. ἔπειτα δὲ καὶ χρῆσις μελαγχολικωτέρων διαιτημάτων γεννῆσαι δύναται ἐν θέρει χυμὸν μελαγχολικόν, ὀσπρίων φημὶ καὶ τυρῶν καὶ χοιρείων κρεῶν καὶ ταρίχων καὶ ὅσων τοιούτων. διὰ τοῦτο οὖν δυνατὸν ἐν τῷ θέρει γεννηθῆναι μελαγχολικὸν χυμὸν καὶ εἰδοποιηθῆναι τεταρταῖον πυρετόν.

II 25 [II 26: IV 478,4–5 L.] Πυρετὸν ἐπὶ σπασμῷ βέλτιον γενέσθαι ἢ σπασμὸν ἐπὶ πυρετῷ.

Ὁ λόγος νυνὶ τῷ Ἱπποκράτει περὶ ἐπιγεννημάτων ἐστὶ τῶν ἑτέρῳ τινὶ προϋποκειμένῳ παθήματι ἐπιγενομένων. ἔστι δὲ ἡ τῶν ἐπιγεννημάτων φύσις τριττή. ἐπιγίνεται γὰρ ἢ νόσημα νοσήματι· ἢ σύμπτωμα νοσήματι – οὐ τὸ παθογνωμονικὸν σύμπτωμα, ὅπερ πάντως ἐπιγίνεται τῷ οἰκείῳ νοσήματι, λέγω δὴ ἡ βλάβη τῆς ἐνεργείας· εἰ γὰρ καὶ ἐπιγίνεται αὕτη καὶ κατὰ τοῦτο δοκεῖ ἐπιγεννήματος λόγον ἔχειν, ἀλλ' οὖν ὡς αἰτίῳ αὐτῷ ἐπακολουθεῖ τρόπον τινά· οὐ περὶ τοιούτου οὖν ὁ λόγος τῷ Ἱπποκράτει συμπτώματος, ἀλλὰ τοῦ ἔξωθεν ἐπιγενομένου ξένου καὶ παρ' ἐλπίδα καὶ μὴ ὄντος παθογνωμονικοῦ –· ἐπιγίνεται δὲ καὶ σύμπτωμα συμπτώματι.

Οὐ μάτην δέ μοι εἴρηται τοῦτο, ἀλλ' ὅτι βούλεται γυμνάσαι ὁ Ἱπποκράτης ἐν νοσήματι ἕτερον νόσημα ἐπιγενόμενον. φησὶ γὰρ οὕτως· ὑποκείσθω πυρετός, ὅπερ ἐστὶ θερμὸν καὶ ξηρὸν πάθος, καὶ μάλιστα διακαὴς ὑπάρχων· ἔστω δὲ ἀραιόπορον τὸ σῶμα· καὶ ἡ ὥρα μᾶλλον ὑποκείσθω θερινή. ἐὰν οὖν ἐπὶ τῷ σώματι τῷ οὕτως διακειμένῳ σπασμὸς γένηται, κακὸν ⟨τὸ⟩ τοιοῦτον. μεμαθήκαμεν γάρ, ὅτι σπασμὸς ἢ ἐπὶ κενώσει γίνεται ἢ ἐπὶ πληρώσει. ἐνταῦθα οὖν πυρετοῦ διακαοῦς ὑποκειμένου καὶ πληρώσεως πολλῆς οὔσης ἐν τῷ σώματι, ἐὰν σπασμὸς γένηται, δεῖ

14–21] *cf.* Theoph. In Aphor.: II 320,11–17 Dietz 24–32] *cf. infra*, vol. III, fol. 213r 37sq. μεμαθήκαμεν – πληρώσει] *v.* Hipp. Aphor. VI 39: IV 572,8 L. Gal. In Aphor. II 26: XVII B 514,12–13 K. De loc. aff. III 8: VIII 170,11–173,4 K. Steph. Ad Glauc.: I 311,16–20 Dietz

8 τῷ] τὸ A 9 ἀμετρότερον *scripsi*: ἀμετρώτρ A: ἀμετρωτέρου P 16 τὸν *om.* A 26 νοσήματι[II]] συμπτώματι A 28 ἐπιγενήματος P 35 ἀραιοπόρου P 37 τὸ *addidi*

no danger, it is obvious that, conversely, those that occur out of their own season will be more dangerous. So a quartan in summer, inasmuch as it disagrees with the season, will be more dangerous than one in autumn, which is related to the season." To answer this objection we say that it is not the benign or dangerous character of the quartan which Hippocrates described in this passage, but its short or long duration. It is therefore up to you as a well-trained physician to judge the dangerous or benign nature of the disease on the ground of the attending symptoms. We know that even a short disease, e.g. a quartan, is often dangerous, because resistance at that time is weaker and ineffectual, when there is disproportionate dispersal of the body by the contact with the surrounding hot air.

There is good reason to add generally; for it is quite conceivable that the atrabiliar humor may have been produced already in the spring, to become manifest only in the summer; hence, since it would have its natural condition, i.e. thickness and slow motion, it would also cause the disease to last longer, so that it does not end in the summer.

Somebody may wonder how a quartan can begin in summer, though this season naturally produces yellow bile. We say that there is nothing unusual in a predisposition of the body to produce the atrabiliar humor, as we observe in those who are too meager, those with a dark complexion, and those past their prime. Besides, the use of a preponderantly atrabilious diet can generate atrabiliar humor in summer, for example pulse, cheese, pork and dried fish. For this reason atrabiliar humor can be produced, and quartan fever can form, in summer.

II 25. Fever upon convulsion is better than convulsion upon fever.

Hippocrates here deals with secondary affections supervening upon another already existing ailment. The nature of secondary affections is threefold. A disease may supervene upon a disease; or a symptom upon a disease – not the distinctive symptom, which necessarily supervenes upon the disease to which it is proper, in other words, impairment of the function; for though this supervenes also and to that extent seems to have the character of a secondary affection, yet it accompanies the disease in the sense that the disease is somehow its cause; so Hippocrates is not referring to that kind of symptom, but to a strange one that supervenes from outside and is unpredictable and not distinctive –; finally, a symptom may supervene upon a symptom.

I have not mentioned this without reason, but to point out that Hippocrates intends to discuss a practical example of a disease supervening upon another disease. What he says is this: Suppose we have a fever, which is a hot and dry affection, and especially so if it is a burning one; suppose the pores of the body are wide; and let the season be summer or thereabouts. Now if a body in this condition becomes subject to convulsion, this is a bad sign. We have learned that convulsion occurs either in a state of evacuation or in one of repletion. Now in our case, when there is burning fever to begin with and when there is a high degree of repletion in the body, we can have good hope if convulsion occurs, because the disposition in

ἐλπίσαι ἀγαθόν· ἐφ' ὑγρότητι γὰρ αὐτὸν συμβαίνει γενέσθαι. ἔνθα δὲ ἐπὶ κενώσει συμβῇ ξηροῦ μὲν ὑπάρχοντος τοῦ νοσήματος, ἐπὶ τοσοῦτον δὲ τὸ σῶμα ξηράναντος ὥστε καὶ ἕτερον ἀπεργάσασθαι νόσημα ξηρόν, τουτέστι τὸν σπασμόν, πῶς οὐκ ἀπειλεῖ κινδύνου ὀξυτάτου φοράν; καὶ γὰρ τὸ μὲν ὑγρὸν σῶμα ξηρὸν ἀπεργάσασθαι δυνατόν, ξηρὸν δὲ ὑγρᾶναι σχεδὸν ἀδύνατον.

Εἰ δέ γε πυρετὸς ἐπὶ πληθωρικῷ σώματι συστῇ ἢ σπασμώδη διάθεσιν ἔχοντι, οὐ δεῖ τὸ τηνικαῦτα ταράττεσθαι, ἀλλὰ μᾶλλον εὐφραίνεσθαι, ἄν τε προϋπόκειται ὁ σπασμός, ἄν τε καὶ ἐπιγένηται. σημεῖον γὰρ οὗτος τοῦ ἀναλύεσθαι καὶ διαχεῖσθαι τὴν ὕλην καὶ φέρεσθαι ⟨εἰς⟩ τοὺς μύας καὶ τὰ προαιρετικὰ νεῦρα, ὥστε σπασμώδη αὐτοῖς ἐντεθῆναι διάθεσιν. ὅσον γὰρ οὔπω διαφορηθήσεται καὶ καταδαπανηθήσεται τῷ λόγῳ τῆς θερμασίας, καὶ οὕτως ἀπαλλαγήσεται τοῦ σπασμοῦ ὁ κάμνων.

Εἰ δὲ πληθωρικὸν ὑπάρχει τὸ σῶμα, ἔστι δὲ καὶ δυσδιαφόρητον, καὶ γένηται σπασμός, λόγῳ πληρώσεως γίνεται. δεῖ γὰρ εἰδέναι, ὅτι, ὅθεν τρέφεται ἕκαστον μόριον, ἐκ τούτου καὶ βλάπτεται λόγῳ ἀμετρίας. τὰ γοῦν νεῦρα, ὑπὸ φλεγματικοῦ καὶ παχέος καὶ γλίσχρου τρεφόμενα χυμοῦ, ὑπὸ τούτου πλεονάζοντος ἐμφράττονται καὶ πληρούμενα καὶ διατεινόμενα τὸν σπασμὸν ὑφίστανται. οὐδὲν γὰρ ἕτερόν ἐστι σπασμὸς ἢ κίνησις ἀπροαίρετος ἐν προαιρετικοῖς μορίοις συνισταμένη. οὗτος οὖν ὁ σπασμὸς ἐπὶ πληρώσει γινόμενος καὶ ψυχρῷ αἰτίῳ συνιστάμενος διὰ τῆς ἐναντιώσεως θεραπεύεται, λέγω δὴ διὰ τῶν θερμαινόντων. ἀναλύεται γὰρ τὸ τηνικαῦτα καὶ λεπτύνεται ἡ ὕλη, καὶ οὕτως κενοῦται ἀραιουμένου τοῦ δέρματος. οὐδὲν δὲ τοιοῦτον ἔχομεν βοήθημα κάλλιον τοῦ πυρετοῦ ὥστε τὰ εἰρημένα ἐργάσασθαι· οὗτος γὰρ διὰ πάντων διήκει τῶν μορίων τοῦ σώματος καὶ πάντων ἅπτεται ὁμοτίμως, τῶν τε ἐπιπολῆς καὶ τῶν διὰ βάθους, καὶ διαχεῖ καὶ λεπτύνει τὴν ὕλην καὶ πρὸς διαφόρησιν παρασκευάζει.

Δεῖ δὲ καὶ τοῦτο γινώσκειν, ὅτι αἱ πέψεις τῶν χυμῶν οὐ τῷ παρὰ φύσιν θερμῷ γίνονται. δόξειε γὰρ ἄν τις ἀπορεῖν ἐνταῦθα ὅτι «Πῶς ὁ πυρετὸς παρὰ φύσιν ὢν θερμὸς ἀγαθὰ τοσαῦτα ἀπεργάσασθαι δύναται;» πρὸς οὓς φαμεν, ὅτι οὐ τῷ συμπέττειν τὴν ὕλην ταῦτα ποιεῖ, ἀλλὰ τῷ λεπτύνειν καὶ διαφορεῖν αὐτὴν ἀραιουμένων τῶν πόρων ὑπὸ τῆς †δυνάμεως†. ὥστε σὺν τῷ πυρετῷ χρεία καὶ δυνάμεως ἐρρωμένης, τῷ οὐ κατὰ πρῶτον λόγον ⟨ἀγαθὸν⟩ εἶναι τὸν πυρετόν, ἀλλὰ κατὰ συμβεβηκός, τῷ λόγῳ τοῦ κενοῦν τὴν ὕλην. διὸ καλῶς ὁ Ἱπποκράτης ἀπεφήνατο ὅτι Καλὸν ἐπὶ σπασμῷ πυρετὸν γενέσθαι ἢ σπασμὸν ἐπὶ πυρετῷ, ἵνα ἡ πολλὴ θερμασία καταναλώσῃ τὴν ὑγρότητα· ἄμφω γὰρ ξηρῶν ὄντων τῶν παθημάτων καταλύεται ἡ δύναμις τῇ ἀμετρίᾳ τῆς δυσκρασίας καὶ ἀνίατος καὶ μαρασμώδης ἕξις ἀποτελεῖται τοῦ σώματος.

II 26 [II 27: IV 478,6–8 L.] Τοῖσι μὴ κατὰ λόγον κουφίζουσιν οὐ δεῖ πιστεύειν οὐδὲ φοβέεσθαι λίην τὰ μοχθηρὰ γινόμενα παραλόγως· τὰ γὰρ πολλὰ τῶν τοιουτέων ἐστὶν ἀβέβαια.

1 ἔνθα – 5] *cf.* Gal. In Aphor. II 26: XVII B 515,4–10 K. 6–11] *cf.* Gal. In Aphor. II 26: XVII B 514,13–515,4 K. 13sq. δεῖ – ἀμετρίας] *cf. infra,* vol. II, fol. 30ᵛ (ἐν τῇ Φυσικῇ)

3 *ante* νόσημα *add.* τὸ A 6 ἔχοντα α: *correxi* 9 εἰς *addidi* 18 ψυχρᾷ αἰτίᾳ P 29 δυνάμεως] *fort.* θερμασίας *scribendum est* 30 τῷ οὐ *scripsi*: οὐ τῷ P: οὐ τὸ A ἀγαθὸν *addidi* 32 Καλὸν *om.* A

which it occurs is one of moisture. When, however, it happens in a state of evacuation, while the disease is a dry one and has dehydrated the body to the extent of producing another dry disease, the convulsion, what else can it mean than the threat of a very acute danger on its way? For to make a moist body dry is possible, but to moisten a dry one is next to impossible.

However, if fever manifests itself in a body that is plethoric or predisposed to convulsions, one should not be afraid in this case, but rather happy, no matter whether the convulsion precedes or supervenes. It signifies that the matter is being dissolved and diffused and that it moves toward the muscles and the motor nerves, causing a convulsive disposition in them. Very soon it will be dispersed and spent thanks to the heat, and thus the patient will cease having convulsions.

If the body is plethoric and dispersal is also difficult, then if convulsion occurs, it is due to repletion. You should know that the source from which each part is nourished can also be a source of harm due to disproportion. Thus the nerves, which are fed by a phlegmatic, thick and sticky humor, are blocked, filled and distended by a surplus of it, and the result is convulsion. Convulsion, indeed, is nothing but involuntary motion in motor parts. This convulsion, then, if it occurs in a state of repletion and results from a cold cause, is cured by contrary treatment, i.e. by heating remedies. In that way the matter is dissolved and comminuted, so that it can be evacuated when the pores of the skin are widened. Now there is no remedy like fever to effect this; it penetrates all the parts of the body and attains them all and sundry, those at the surface as well as those inside, and it spreads and comminutes the matter and prepares it for dispersal.

It must also be observed that concoction of humors is not brought about by abnormal heat. Indeed, there might seem to be reason to wonder here, how fever, with its abnormal heat, can cause such benefits. Our answer is that it does not do so by concocting the matter, but by comminuting and dispersing it, when the pores are widened by the warming effect (?)[1]. Consequently, besides the fever, a strong resistance is also needed, because the fever is not beneficial in itself, but incidentally, by evacuating the matter. Hippocrates rightly declared, therefore, that Fever upon convulsion is better than convulsion upon fever, so that the abundance of heat can consume the moisture; for if both the affections are dry, resistance is broken down by the excessive distemper and an incurable marasmic disposition of the body results.

II 26. One should not trust signs of relief which are not regular, nor be overly afraid of unaccountable bad signs; most of such indications are unreliable.

[1] See the app. crit.

Τὸ λεγόμενον, εἰ δοκεῖ, ἐξ ὑποθέσεως σαφηνίσωμεν. ὑποκείσθω τις πυρέττων πυρετὸν διακαέστατον ἐν ἀγρυπνίᾳ καὶ δυσφορίᾳ πολλῇ καὶ δίψῃ καὶ ἀθυμίᾳ. ταύτῃ αὐτοῦ ἔχοντος αἰφνίδιον ῥᾳστώνη τις παρ' αὐτῷ ἐπακολουθησάτω, καὶ εἰσιόντι τῷ ἰατρῷ ἀποκρινέσθω οὗτος· «Οὐδέν μοι νυνὶ παρενοχλεῖ καὶ καλῶς ἔχω.» ὁ γοῦν ἰατρός, εἰ τύχοι ἰδιώτης, διορίζεται πρὸς αὐτὸν ὅτι «Ἐὰν ἐπαύσατο ὁ πυρετὸς καὶ ἡ δυσφορία ἐκείνη, ἄπελθε λοῦσαι.» λουσάμενος οὖν χεῖρον ἔσχεν, οὔπω γὰρ ἦν τὸ σῶμα λυθὲν τοῦ νοσήματος, καὶ διὰ τοῦτο ὑπονοστησάσης ἐν τῷ βάθει τῆς ὕλης διὰ τὴν ἰδίαν κακίαν φαύλη καὶ ψευδὴς ἡ ῥᾳστώνη γέγονεν. ὁ δὲ Ἱπποκράτειος ἰατρὸς εἰσελθὼν παρὰ τὸν ἄρρωστον καὶ εὑρηκὼς ἐξαίφνης παυσάμενον τὸν πυρετὸν καὶ τὴν δυσφορίαν, ἐρωτᾷ τὸν κάμνοντα, μή τις κένωσις ἐγένετο διὰ γαστρὸς ἢ δι' οὔρων ἢ δι' ἱδρώτων ἢ δι' αἱμορραγίας ἢ δι' ἐμέτων, μή τι βουβὼν ἐγένετο μέγας ἢ παρωτὶς ἢ ἐν ἑτέρῳ τινὶ μορίῳ ἀπόστασις. κἂν μέν τι τοιοῦτον εὕρῃ γενόμενον καὶ ἐπὶ κενώσει τυχὸν πυνθανόμενος τὰ συμπτώματα, ἀδεῶς καὶ οὗτος ἐπὶ λουτρὸν τὸν τοιοῦτον ἄρρωστον πέμπει εἰδώς, ὅτι ἀπήλλακται τοῦ νοσοποιοῦ αἰτίου τὸ σῶμα. εἰ δὲ μηδὲν τούτων παρηκολούθησε, ταράττεται ὁ ἰατρὸς λέγων ὅτι «Τίνι λόγῳ τῆς ὕλης μὴ ἐκκριθείσης μηδ' εἰς ἀπόσκηψιν τραπείσης οὕτως αἰφνίδιον ῥᾳστώνη γέγονεν; ἢ δῆλον ὅτι μέγα κακὸν τὸ τοιοῦτον· ἐμφωλεύει γὰρ ἡ ὕλη καὶ ὅσον οὔπω τὰ οἰκεῖα πάλιν κακὰ ἀπεργάσεται.» καὶ ταῦτα ἐννοήσας ἐμμένει ἔτι τῇ λεπτῇ διαίτῃ ὡς τῶν αὐτῶν καὶ νῦν ἔτι παρενοχλούντων αἰτίων νοσοποιῶν. πάλιν εἰσερχέσθωσαν πρός τινα ἄρρωστον δύο ἰατροί, ὁ μὲν ἰδιώτης, ὁ δὲ Ἱπποκράτειος, καὶ εὑρέτωσαν αὐτὸν δυσφοροῦντα καὶ μαρμαρυγὰς καὶ ὀρφνώδη φαντάσματα ὁρῶντα καὶ ἀναπηδῶντα ἀπὸ τῆς κλίνης. ὁρῶν οὖν ταῦτα ὁ ἰδιώτης ταράττεται καὶ νομίζων αὐτὰ μοχθηρὰ εἶναι ἀπηλλάγη τοῦ κάμνοντος· ὁ δὲ τεχνίτης ἰατρὸς βλέπων ταῦτα εὐφραίνεται, γινώσκει γάρ, ὅτι κρίσις ὅσον οὔπω ἔσεσθαι μέλλει τοῦ νοσήματος. πέψεως γὰρ προηγησαμένης ταῦτα ἐπηκολούθησε· κενουμένης οὖν ὅσον οὔπω τῆς ὕλης, ἢ δι' ἐμέτων ἢ διὰ ῥινῶν αἱμορραγίας, ἀπαλλαγήσεται ὁ κάμνων τοῦ νοσήματος.

Τὸ δὲ κατὰ λόγον πρὸς τὴν τέχνην εἴρηκεν, οἷον ἐφ' ὧν μὴ κατὰ ἀναλογίαν τοῦ νοσήματος ἡ κένωσις ἢ ἡ ῥᾳστώνη γέγονεν, οὐ δεῖ τοῖς τοιούτοις νοσήμασι πιστεύειν περὶ τῆς εὐφορίας.

Καλῶς δὲ εἶπε κουφίζουσι, τοιαύτῃ φαντασίᾳ· κουφισμὸς μέν τις εἶναι δοκεῖ, οὐκ ἀπαλλαγὴ δὲ τοῦ νοσήματος. ἄξιον δὲ ζητῆσαι, πῶς γίνεται κουφισμός· καί φαμεν, ὅτι οὐδὲν ἄτοπον κινουμένης τῆς ὕλης ἀτμούς τινας καὶ πνεύματα γεννηθῆναι, ἅτινα τῇ λεπτομερείᾳ διαφορούμενα μετρίας τινὸς ῥᾳστώνης ἔμφασιν ὑποφαίνει.

Τὰ δὲ παρὰ λόγον γινόμενα πρὸς τὸν ἰδιώτην εἴρηκεν, ἐκείνῳ γὰρ νομίζεται παρὰ λόγον γίνεσθαι καὶ μοχθηρὰ εἶναι τὰ τὴν κρίσιν ὅσον οὔπω προδηλοῦντα συμπτώματα.

Προσέθηκε δὲ τὸ λίην, ὅτι ποτὲ ἐν τῷ μέσῳ ὀκλάζουσα ἡ φύσις καταπίπτει

1–19 νοσοποιῶν] *cf.* Gal. In Aphor. II 27: XVII B 516,1–7 K. Theoph. In Aphor.: II 321, 25–29 Dietz 21sq. μαρμαρυγὰς – ὁρῶντα] *cf.* Hipp. Progn. 24: p. 229,1–3 Alexanderson = II 184,13–15 L. 36–38] *cf.* Theoph. In Aphor.: II 321,33–322,3 Dietz

1 σαφηνίσομεν A 2 δίψει A 5 τύχη P 8 ἱπποκράτης P: *corr.* P²: ἱπποκράτ *(ambig.)* A 11 τις A 12 μέν τι] μέντοι A 13 πυνθανόμενα α: *correxi* 15 παρακολουθήσει A 32 οὐκ ἀπαλλαγὴ] οὐ καταλλαγὴ P 37 παράλογον P

Let us explain the meaning by a hypothetical case. Suppose we have a patient suffering from an extremely burning fever, with sleeplessness, great discomfort, thirst and dejection. While he is in this condition, suppose an unexpected alleviation follows, and when the doctor comes to see him, he says: "Nothing troubles me now and I am fine." The doctor, if he happens to be an amateur, gives him his directions: "If the fever is over and that discomfort is gone, go and take a bath." After the bath the patient gets worse, because his body was not yet free from the disease, and therefore, the matter having retreated deep inside by its own malignancy, the relief was a bad and deceptive sign. But when the Hippocratic physician visits this patient and finds the fever and the discomfort suddenly gone, he questions the patient if perhaps there has been some kind of evacuation, through the bowels or through urine or through sweating or through hemorrhage or through vomiting, if perhaps there has been a large bubo, a parotid tumor or an abscess in any other part. If he finds that such a thing has occurred and that the symptoms have resulted, for instance, from evacuation, he too confidently sends such a patient to his bath, knowing that his body has been freed from the disease-producing cause. If, on the other hand, nothing of the kind has happened, the doctor is worried and asks himself: "Since the matter has neither been excreted nor deflected, how to account for this sudden relief? Obviously this is a very bad thing: the matter is still lurking deep down and very soon it will return to its work of destruction." On the ground of this consideration he maintains the light diet, believing that the same disease-producing causes are even now troubling (the patient). Again, let us suppose that a patient is visited by two doctors, the one ignorant, the other Hippocratic, and that they find him restless, seeing flashes of light and dark spots, and jumping up from his bed. When the ignorant doctor sees this, he is worried, and he leaves the patient in the belief that these are bad signs; but the able doctor is glad to see them, for he knows that the crisis of the disease is close at hand. This is because these signs are the consequence of preceding concoction, so that very soon the matter will be evacuated, either by vomiting or by nosebleeding, and the patient will get rid of the disease.

The word regular is used with respect to the art, as if to say: Where evacuation or alleviation are not proportionate to the disease, one should not trust such diseases on the point of euphoria.

He rightly said relief, because the way he sees it is this: there seems to be a sort of relief, but not recovery from the disease. The question must be asked, however, how there can be relief; we reply that it is quite plausible, once the matter is in motion, that certain vapors and gases develop, which thanks to their fineness are dispersed and produce the appearance of a moderate alleviation.

He used the word unaccountable in view of the incompetent doctor, who regards the symptoms that predict the imminent crisis as unaccountable and unfavorable.

Overly is added because sometimes in the middle (of the process) the con-

καὶ διαφορεῖται καὶ ἡ δύναμις σὺν τοῖς αἰτίοις, ὥστε καὶ κίνδυνον θανάτου παρακολουθῆσαι. διὰ τοῦτο ἔφη· πάνυ μὲν οὐ δεῖ φοβεῖσθαι, πλὴν οὐδὲ παντάπασιν ἄφοβον εἶναι ἐπὶ τῶν κριτικῶς κινουμένων, ἀλλ' εὐλαβεῖσθαι, μήποτε ἐν τῷ μέσῳ ἀπείπῃ ἡ φύσις, ἢ διὰ τὴν ποιότητα ἢ διὰ τὴν ποσότητα τῶν κενουμένων.

II 27 [II 28: IV 478,10–12 L.] Τῶν πυρεσσόντων μὴ παντάπασιν ἐπιπολαίως τὸ διαμένειν καὶ μηδὲν ἐνδιδόναι τὸ σῶμα ἢ καὶ συντήκεσθαι μᾶλλον τοῦ κατὰ λόγον μοχθηρόν.

Καὶ οὗτος ὁ ἀφορισμὸς σημειωτικός ἐστιν, ἀπὸ τοῦ ὅλου σώματος ποιούμενος τὴν διάγνωσιν, πρός τε τῆς ἰσχνότητος αὐτοῦ καὶ πρὸς ⟨τοῦ⟩ ἀσυμπτώτου. καί τινα δύο ἡμῖν δηλοῖ ἡ τοιαύτη σημείωσις, ἦθος νοσήματος καὶ χρόνον· ἦθος μέν, εἰ κακόηθες, χρόνον δέ, εἰ μακροχρόνιον.

Λοιπόν, εἰ δοκεῖ, ὑποκείσθω ἄρρωστος ἔχων διακαῆ πυρετὸν καὶ ἀσύμπτωτον σῶμα. ὁ μὲν οὖν ἰδιώτης ἰατρὸς ὁρῶν ἀσύμπτωτον χαίρει καὶ ἀποφαίνεται μηδὲν κακὸν ἔχειν, «'Ιδοὺ γάρ» φησι «καὶ τὸ πρόσωπον καὶ ἡ ἕξις τοῦ σώματος εὐθαλὴς καὶ ὑγιεινή ἐστιν.» ὁ δὲ τεχνίτης ταράττεται ὁρῶν τὸ τοιοῦτον· συλλογίζεται γὰρ οὕτος· «Τί δήποτε ὁ πυρετὸς οὗτος διακαὴς ὢν καὶ ὀφείλων δαπανῆσαι πᾶσαν ὑγρότητα καὶ ἐκτῆξαι τοὺς χυμοὺς οὐδὲν τούτων ἔδρασεν, ἀλλὰ τοὐναντίον καὶ παχύτερον ἑαυτοῦ τὸ σῶμα ἀπέδειξεν; ἀλλ' ἢ δῆλον ὅτι πλῆθος ὕλης περιττωματικῆς ἔν τινι τόπῳ ἐστί, περὶ ἣν ἀσχολεῖται ὁ πυρετός· εἰ γὰρ μὴ τοῦτο ἦν, τοῦ παντὸς ἂν εἶχεν ἅψασθαι σώματος καὶ σύντηξιν ἀπεργάσασθαι τῶν ὠμῶν καὶ παχέων χυμῶν.» διὸ ἀποφαίνεται, ὅτι, ὅπου πυρετὸς διακαὴς καὶ ἀσύμπτωτον σῶμα, πολλῆς ὑγρότητος δείκνυται περιουσία, καὶ τὸ τοιοῦτον νόσημα πάντως εἰς μῆκος χρόνου ἐκταθήσεται.

'Αλλὰ δεῖ προσδιορίσαι ὅτι «ἐὰν καὶ ⟨ἡ⟩ δύναμις ἔρρωται»· οὐδὲν γὰρ ἄτοπον τὴν μὲν φύσιν τοῦ νοσήματος χρονίαν εἶναι, τῆς δυνάμεως δὲ ἀσθενούσης μὴ ἐκταθῆναι εἰς χρόνον, ἀλλὰ καὶ ὀκλάσαι τὴν φύσιν καὶ ἀπειπεῖν καὶ θάνατον ὀξὺν ἐπακολουθῆσαι. δυοῖν γὰρ τούτων δεῖται τὸ χρόνιον νόσημα, πέψεως ὕλης καὶ δυνάμεως ἐρρωμένης, ὑφ' ἧς ἡ πέψις γενήσεται.

Πολλάκις δὲ καὶ πυρετὸς διακαὴς ὑπόκειται καὶ ἀσύμπτωτον σῶμα, καὶ οὐκ ἔστι πλῆθος ὑγρότητος. τί γάρ; ὅτι ψυχροῦ ὄντος τοῦ περιέχοντος, μὴ διαφορουμένων τῶν περιττωμάτων διὰ τὴν πύκνωσιν τῆς ἐπιφανείας ἀσύμπτωτον δείκνυται τὸ σῶμα. οὐ γὰρ ἂν διὰ πλῆθος ὕλης εἴη τοῦτο, ἀλλὰ διὰ τὸ τοῦ περιέχοντος δυσδιαφόρητον, ἐφ' ᾧ οὐδὲ χρόνιον ἔσται τὸ νόσημα.

Πάλιν ὑποκείσθω ἕτερος ἄρρωστος μὴ πάνυ ὀξὺν καὶ διακαῆ πυρετὸν ἔχων, τὸ ἐπιεικέστερον· ἰσχνανθήτω δὲ τὸ σῶμα ὑπὲρ ἀναλογίαν τῆς θερμασίας. ἐφ' ᾧ ζητητέον, μή τις κένωσις παρηκολούθησε διὰ γαστρὸς ἢ δι' ἱδρώτων ἢ δι' ἐμέτων. εἰ μὲν γάρ τι τοιοῦτον γέγονεν, οὐδὲν φαῦλον ὑπονοήσομεν· δῆλον γάρ, ὅτι τῆς ὑγρότητος δαπανηθείσης τῷ λόγῳ τῆς κενώσεως διὰ ξηρότητα ἴσχνανσις τῷ σώματι

18 ἀλλ' – 23] *cf.* Gal. In Aphor. II 28: XVII B 521,8–13 K. Theoph. In Aphor.: II 322, 18–20 Dietz 35 ἐφ' – 200,1 παρηκολούθησεν] *cf.* Gal. In Aphor. II 28: XVII B 519,9–13 K.

1 διαφορεῖται καὶ *scripsi*: διαφορητικὴ α 4 ἀπείπῃ] ἀπήτει A 9 τοῦ *addidi* 18 παχυτέρου P 24 προδιορίσαι P ἡ *addidi* 26 ἀποπτεῖν A 34 ὀξὺ A 37 ἀπονοήσομεν P 38 ἰσχνανσία α: *correxi*

stitution gives way and breaks down, and resistance is dispersed along with the causes (of the disease), so that even life may be endangered. That is why he said: There is no need to worry too much, but neither should we be entirely unconcerned about patients in the process of crisis; we must remain aware of the danger that in the middle of it the constitution may give way, owing to either the quality or the quantity of the matter evacuated.

II 27. In fever cases, unless altogether superficial, for the body to remain intact and to lose no weight at all, or again to be emaciated beyond proportion, is a bad sign.

This is another semiotic aphorism, which derives a diagnosis from the condition of the whole body, according as it is emaciated or intact. This kind of indication teaches us two things, the nature of the disease and its duration: its nature, whether it is malignant, its duration, whether it will last long.

Suppose then we take the case of a patient with burning fever and an intact body. The incompetent doctor, seeing that there is no loss of volume, is satisfied and declares that nothing is seriously wrong: "You can see", he says, "how fresh and healthy his face and the condition of his body are." The able physician, on the contrary, is worried when he sees this; for he argues: "A fever as burning as this is should use up all the moisture and consume the humors; why, then, has it done nothing of the kind, but actually made the body heavier than it was? Evidently because somewhere there is a large quantity of surplus matter, on which the force of the fever spends itself; otherwise it would affect the whole body and reduce the crude and thick humors." He declares accordingly that when there is a burning fever and an intact body, we have evidence of a great superfluity of moisture, and an illness of this kind will necessarily extend over a long period of time.

We must, however, add the restriction, "if resistance is strong enough"; for quite possibly the disease may be chronic as far as its own nature is concerned, but owing to weak resistance it may not last long: the constitution may fail and give way and sudden death may be the result. A chronic disease, in fact, requires two things: concoction of the matter and a resistance strong enough to achieve the concoction.

Often, too, we have a case of burning fever without loss of weight, and yet there is no excess of moisture. Why? Because the surrounding air is cold, and as the surplus matter fails to be dispersed owing to the tightening of the surface, no loss of weight is observed. Here the cause would not be an excessive quantity of matter, but prevention of dispersal by the surrounding air, in which case the sickness need not even be long.

Let us now take the case of another patient whose fever is not very acute or burning, which is a less serious situation; and let us assume that his body has emaciated out of proportion to the heat (of the fever). We must examine him for a possible evacuation by way of the bowels or by sweating or vomiting. If something of the kind has occurred, we need not suspect anything wrong: obviously, the moisture has been exhausted by evacuation, and dryness is the cause of the emacia-

παρηκολούθησεν· εἰ δὲ μηδὲν τούτων γέγονε μήτε μὴν τῷ λόγῳ τοῦ περιέχοντος ἰσχνάνθη – οἶδε γὰρ τὰ θερμὰ καὶ τὰ θερινὰ καταστήματα πολλὴν τοῦ σώματος ἀπάγειν ὑγρότητα – καὶ ἁπλῶς εἰπεῖν, ἐὰν μήτε ἐπὶ προηγουμένῃ αἰτίᾳ μήτε ἐπὶ προκαταρκτικῇ τὸ τοιοῦτον ἰσχνάνθη σῶμα, φαῦλον καὶ κάκιστον ὑπάρχει τὸ τῆς ἰσχνάνσεως σημεῖον καὶ κακοήθειαν πολλὴν ἐνδείκνυται τοῦ νοσήματος. ἀσθένειαν γὰρ τῶν δυνάμεων ὑπογράφει, αἵτινες ὀχοῦσαι τὸ σῶμα ἐν τῷ ἐρρῶσθαι στηρίζουσι τὰ ὑγρὰ καὶ τὸν πρέποντα ὄγκον αὐτῷ παρέχουσι. τούτων οὖν ἀσθενουσῶν μὴ κραταιουμένη καὶ οἷον ἑδραιουμένη ὑπὸ τούτων ἡ τῶν ὑγρῶν οὐσία ἔξω φέρεται καὶ δαπανᾶται, κἀντεῦθεν κάτισχνον τὸ σῶμα γίνεται ὑπὲρ τὴν ποιότητα τῆς θερμασίας τὴν διαφόρησιν τῶν ὑγρῶν ὑφιστάμενον. ὥστε ἡ μὲν πρώτη ὑπόθεσις ἡ ἀσύμπτωτον ἔχουσα τὸ σῶμα ἐπιφανοῦς ὑπάρχοντος τοῦ πυρετοῦ χρόνιον δηλοῖ τὸ νόσημα· ἡ δὲ δευτέρα, ἐν ᾗ ἄμετρος ἴσχνανσις ὑπόκειται ἐπιπολαιοτέρας οὔσης τῆς θερμασίας, ὀξὺ καὶ ὀλιγοχρόνιον δηλοῖ τὸ νόσημα.

Ὡς τινος δὲ μέλλοντος ἀπορεῖν· «Πῶς, ὦ Ἱππόκρατες, ἐὰν ἀσύμπτωτον ᾖ τὸ σῶμα πυρετοῦ ὑποτεθέντος, κακὸν λέγεις εἶναι τὸ τοιοῦτον; καὶ μὴν ἐπὶ τῶν πυρεσσόντων ἐφήμερον πυρετὸν ἀσύμπτωτον μὲν ὡς ἐπὶ τὸ πολὺ εὑρίσκεται τὸ σῶμα, οὐκ ἔστι δὲ κακόν», τούτου χάριν προσέθηκε τὸ μὴ παντάπασιν ἐπιπολαίως, διὰ τὸ τοὺς ἐφημέρους πυρετοὺς ἐπιπολαίους πως εἶναι καὶ τοῦ βάθους μὴ ἅπτεσθαι μήτε μὴν τὰ ὑγρὰ ἐξαναλίσκειν ὅσα τε ἐπὶ πνεύμασιν ἔχουσι τὴν ὑπόστασιν. ἐπὶ τούτων οὖν καὶ τῶν τοιούτων παντάπασιν ἐπιπολαίων ὑπαρχόντων οὐδὲν ἄτοπον τὸ ἀσύμπτωτον μένειν τὸ σῶμα· κακὸν δὲ τὸ τοιοῦτον, ἡνίκα τοῦ βάθους ἅπτεται ἡ θερμασία. ἐπὶ τούτων γὰρ τῶν χυμῶν δηλονότι πασχόντων, ἢν μὴ τοῦ σώματος ὁ ὄγκος πρεπόντως ἰσχνανθῇ, χρόνιον δηλοῦται τὸ νόσημα. τὸ δὲ τῆς ἰσχνότητος σύμπτωμα οὐκ ἀπὸ πρώτης ἢ δευτέρας ἡμέρας χρὴ ζητεῖν ἐπακολουθοῦν, ἀλλ' ὅταν γένηται πέμπτη ἢ ἕκτη ἡμέρα καὶ μέχρι τῆς ἑβδομάδος· τὸ τηνικαῦτα γὰρ ἀσύμπτωτον μένον τὸ σῶμα χρόνιον ὑποφαίνει τὸ νόσημα.

Ἢ καὶ συντήκεσθαι φησὶ μᾶλλον τοῦ κατὰ λόγον μοχθηρόν. ἐπὶ τούτου τοῦ νοσήματος ὑπετέθη ⟨ὁ⟩ δεύτερος ἄρρωστος, ὑπὲρ τὴν ἀναλογίαν καὶ τὴν ζέσιν τοῦ πυρετοῦ τὴν σύντηξιν ὑφιστάμενος. ἰστέον δέ, ὅτι οὐ περὶ ἑκτικοῦ πυρετοῦ εἴρηται αὐτῷ ὁ λόγος, ὅσον ἐκ τοῦ εἰπεῖν ἢ καὶ συντήκεσθαι, ἀλλὰ περὶ συντήξεως σαρκῶν καὶ μόνων. οἱ γὰρ ἑκτικοὶ πυρετοὶ τὸ πᾶν συντήκοντες σῶμα ὅλου τοῦ βάθους ἅπτονται, καὶ οὐδεὶς ἂν φαίη ἑκτικὸν ἐπιπολαιοτέραν ἔχειν τὴν ζέσιν.

II 28 [II 29: IV 478,14–15 L.] Ἀρχομένων τῶν νούσων ἤν τι δοκέῃ κινεῖν, κίνει· ἀκμαζουσῶν δὲ ἡσυχίην ἄγειν βέλτιον.

Λέγει, ὅτι ἐπὶ τῶν ὀξέων νοσημάτων ἐν ἀρχῇ δεῖ παραλαμβάνειν τὴν κένωσιν· λεπτὸς γὰρ ἐπ' αὐτῶν ὑπόκειται ὁ χυμὸς καὶ εὔοργος καὶ εὐκίνητος, καὶ δεῖ αὐτὸν

1 εἰ – 3 ὑγρότητα] *cf.* Gal. In Aphor. II 28: XVII B 519,6–9 K. 3 καὶ – 10 ὑφιστάμενον] *cf.* Gal. In Aphor. II 28: XVII B 520,11–13 K. 14–21 σῶμα] *cf.* Gal. In Aphor. II 28: XVII B 517,3–10 K. 36 Λέγει – κένωσιν] *v.* Theoph. In Aphor.: II 323,5 Dietz 37 λεπτὸς – 202,2 ἀπεργάσεται] *v.* Theoph. In Aphor.: II 323,14–19 Dietz

2 πολλῇ A 3 ὑγρότητα *scripsi*: ὑγρότ^τ α 15 εἶναι λέγεις A 23 ἰσχναθῇ A 27 μοχθηροῦ A 28 ὁ *addidi* 31 μόνον P 35 ἡσυχίαν P ἄγειν] ἔχειν *infra, p. 202,22, Hipp.* *post* βέλτιον *hab.* ἐστι(ν) *infra, p. 202,22, Hipp.* 37 λεπτῶς α: *correxi*

tion of the body; but if nothing like this has happened, and if the emaciation is not due to the surrounding air either – hot summery weather will usually withdraw a great deal of moisture from the body –; if, in a word, there is neither an antecedent nor an immediate cause for the emaciation of this body, then the meagerness is a bad and most serious sign, and it shows that the disease is utterly malignant. It points, indeed, to weakness of the faculties, which sustain the body in health by lending consistency to its moist components and by ensuring that it has the right volume. Now if these faculties are too weak, the moist substances are no longer supported and as it were stabilized by them, so that they escape and are lost; the result is extreme emaciation, since the body is subjected to dispersal of moisture which exceeds the quality of its heat. The first case, then, in which the body preserves its bulk in spite of considerable fever, indicates a chronic disease; while the second, in which we have disproportionate emaciation, though the heat is more superficial, points to an acute and short illness.

But he feels as if somebody will ask: "How can you say, *Hippocrates*, when the body remains intact in a case of fever, that this is a bad sign? Surely in cases of ephemeral fever the body is usually found to lose no weight, without this being a bad sign." For this reason he added, *unless altogether superficial*, for ephemeral fevers are in a way superficial, they do not reach the depths nor consume moisture or whatever depends on gases for its existence. Therefore in these and similar fevers, which are *altogether superficial*, it is not surprising that the body should lose no weight; but it is bad, when the heat reaches the depths. In that kind of fever the humors are evidently affected, and if the mass of the body is not reduced proportionately, it proves that the disease will be long. The symptom of emaciation should not be expected to occur from the first or second day, but when the fifth or sixth day has come, and up to the seventh; by that time, if the body does not lose weight, this indicates that the disease is a chronic one.

Or again to be emaciated beyond proportion, he says, *is a bad sign*. This is the disease of which the second patient was supposed to suffer, emaciation out of proportion to the seething of the fever. Note that the aphorism does not refer to hectic fever, as you might think going by the words, *or again to be emaciated*, which, however, have to do with wasting away of the flesh only. As for hectic fevers, they consume the entire body, affecting even the depths, and nobody could say that in hectic fever the seething is more superficial.

II 28. *At the beginning of diseases, if you think some motion is required, provide it; during the acme, rest is preferable.*

In acute diseases, he says, evacuation should be applied at the beginning; for in these diseases the underlying humor is thin, easily commoved and easily

ταχέως ἀπελάσαι τοῦ σώματος, ὥστε μὴ τῇ ἀτάκτῳ κινήσει ἐπὶ κύρια ῥεύσει μόρια καὶ μεγάλα κακὰ ἀπεργάσεται. εἰ δὲ μὴ ἐν τῇ ἀρχῇ τὴν κένωσιν παραλάβῃς, οὐ δεῖ σε ἐν τῇ ἀκμῇ τῷ κενωτικῷ φαρμάκῳ χρήσασθαι· τότε γὰρ ζέων καὶ διακαὴς ὑπόκειται πυρετὸς καὶ ξηρότητος πολλῆς τῷ σώματι γέγονεν αἴτιος. ἔστι δὲ καὶ τὸ διδόμενον φάρμακον θερμὸν καὶ ξηρόν, καὶ δέος μήποτε πολλαπλασιασθείσης τῆς ξηρότητος καὶ δριμυτέρας καὶ καυσωδεστέρας τῆς πυρεκτικῆς ζέσεως γενομένης πολλὰ χαλεπὰ ἐπακολουθήσει τῷ κάμνοντι. ἄλλως τε δὲ τίς χρεία ἐν τῇ ἀκμῇ διδόναι τὸ κενωτικὸν φάρμακον καὶ ταράττειν τὴν φύσιν μετὰ τοσοῦτον κάματον, ὅτε ἤδη προέκοψε τὰ τοῦ πάθους καὶ ἐλεπτύνθη καὶ ἐπέφθη ὁ χυμὸς καὶ μέλλει λοιπὸν φυσικῶς διαφορεῖσθαι;

Οὐ δεῖ δὲ ἐπὶ μόνης φαρμακοποσίας ἐκλαβεῖν τὸ λεγόμενον, ἀλλὰ καὶ ἐπὶ φλεβοτομίας. εἰ γὰρ ἐν τῇ ἀκμῇ τὸ πολὺ μέρος τῶν περιττωμάτων διεφορήθη, παραλαμβάνεις δὲ σὺ κένωσιν διὰ φλεβοτομίας, χρηστὴν ὕλην εὑρίσκει κενοῦν, κἀντεῦθεν καταβολὴ γίνεται τῆς δυνάμεως.

Τί δέ ἐστιν ἤν τι δοκέῃ; ῥητέον, ὅτι περὶ τοῦ εἴδους αὐτὸς τῆς κενώσεως ἐν τούτῳ διαλαμβάνει· εἴτε καθάρσει, φησίν, εἴτε φλεβοτομίᾳ δοκεῖ χρήσασθαι, κέχρησο. καὶ ἄλλως δέ· σκόπει, ἂν ὀργᾷ ἡ ὕλη, καὶ τότε κένωσον, τοῦτο γὰρ δοκεῖ· ἢν δὲ μὴ ὀργᾷ, μὴ κενώσῃς, ὅπερ οὐ δοκεῖ.

Κίνησιν δὲ οὐ μόνον τὴν διὰ κενώσεως λέγει, ἀλλὰ καὶ τὴν ἀπὸ τόπου εἰς τόπον κίνησιν. δεῖ γὰρ ἐν τῇ ἀκμῇ καὶ ταύτην ὑποστέλλεσθαι διὰ τὸ τὴν φύσιν τὸ τηνικαῦτα περὶ τὰ νοσοποιὰ αἴτια ἀπασχολεῖσθαι. καὶ τοῦτο δῆλον ἐκ τοῦ εἰπεῖν ἀκμαζουσῶν δὲ ἡσυχίην ἔχειν βέλτιόν ἐστι. τὸ γὰρ εἰρημένον ὑπ' αὐτοῦ ὅτι «Πέπονα φαρμακεύειν καὶ κινέειν, μὴ ὠμά», περὶ χρονίων λέλεκται, οὐ περὶ ὀξέων.

II 29 [II 30: IV 478,16–17 L.] Περὶ τὰς ἀρχὰς καὶ τὰ τέλη πάντα ἀσθενέστερα, περὶ δὲ τὰς ἀκμὰς ἰσχυρότερα.

Εἰπὼν ἀνωτέρω ὅτι «Ἀρχομένων τῶν νούσων ἤν τι δοκέῃ κινεῖν, κίνει» καὶ τὰ ἑξῆς, ὥς τινος ἀπορεῖν μέλλοντος· «Τί δήποτε ἐν τῇ ἀρχῇ δεῖ κινεῖν τὴν ὕλην, ἐν δὲ τῇ ἀκμῇ ἡσυχίην ἐπιτηδεύειν;» ἐπήγαγεν ὅτι διὰ τοῦτο ἐν ταῖς ἀρχαῖς παρακελεύομαι ἐπὶ τῶν ὀξέων νοσημάτων τῇ κενώσει κεχρῆσθαι, ἐπειδὴ περὶ τὰς ἀρχὰς καὶ τὰ τέλη πάντα ἀσθενέστερα, περὶ δὲ τὰς ἀκμὰς ἰσχυρότερα. ἀρχὴν δὲ λέγει οὐ τὴν ἀκαριαίαν οὐδὲ μὴν τὴν ἐν τρισὶν ἡμέραις, ἀλλὰ τὴν διαστελλομένην τοῖς λοιποῖς καιροῖς, ἀναβάσει καὶ ἀκμῇ καὶ παρακμῇ· τέλος δὲ λέγει τὴν παρακμήν.

Δεῖ δὲ καὶ τοῦτο εἰδέναι, ὅτι ἐπὶ τῶν νοσούντων δύο τινά εἰσιν ἐν τῷ σώματι θεωρούμενα, τὰ μὲν κατὰ φύσιν, τὰ δὲ παρὰ φύσιν. καὶ κατὰ φύσιν μέν εἰσιν αἱ

7 ἄλλως – 10] *cf.* Theoph. In Aphor.: II 323,12–14 Dietz   11–14] *v.* Gal. In Aphor. II 29: XVII B 523,14–16 K.   Οὐ – φλεβοτομίας] *v.* Theoph. In Aphor.: II 323,8–9 Dietz   17 σκόπει – 18] *v.* Theoph. In Aphor.: II 323,6–8 Dietz   23 Πέπονα – ὠμά] Hipp. Aphor. I 22: IV 468, 13 L.   26–30 ἰσχυρότερα] *v.* Gal. In Aphor. II 29: XVII B 522,9–14 K. Theoph. In Aphor.: II 324,1–5 Dietz   Ἀρχομένων – κίνει] Hipp. Aphor. II 29: IV 478,14 L.   30 ἀρχὴν – 32] *cf. supra*, p. 38,21–22 Theoph. In Aphor.: II 324,5–9 Dietz   34 καὶ – 204,3 ἀποκριτική] *cf. supra*, p. 36,16–21

1 παχέως P   ῥεῦσαι A   2 ἀπεργάσασθαι A   8 ταράττειν *scripsi*: πράττειν α   κάματον] φάρμακον A   13 *fort.* εὑρίσκῃ κενῶν *scribendum est*   20 τόπον] τόπου P   22 δὲ *om.* A   ὅτι *om.* A   25 ἀσθενέστερα ... ἰσχυρότερα] *item infra, p. 242,34 (cf. vol. II, fol. 62ʳ), Hipp.* C'V, *Theoph.* SV'': ἀσθενέστατα ... ἰσχυρότατα *Hipp.* M, *Theoph.* U''

disturbed, and one has to chase it quickly from the body, so that it will not, by its disorderly motion, flow to vital parts and cause great harm. But if you have not applied evacuation at the beginning, do not use the evacuant during the acme, when there is seething, burning fever, which is the cause of extreme dryness in the body. The medicine that is administered is also hot and dry, and it is to be feared that if the dryness is multiplied and the seething of the fever becomes more pungent and more scorching, there will be a great many evil consequences for the patient. Besides, what is the use of administering the evacuant during the acme and upsetting the constitution after so much exhaustion, when the disease is already well on its way and the humor has already been comminuted and concocted and will further be dispersed in the natural way?

The statement should not be taken to refer to purging only, but to bleeding as well. If during the acme the greater part of the surplus matter has been dispersed, and you apply evacuation by bleeding, it will be found that you are evacuating healthy matter, and the result is loss of strength.

What is the meaning of the words, if you think some motion is required? The answer is that (Hippocrates) himself here deals with the kind of evacuation, saying: Whether you think you should purge, or bleed, do so. Or otherwise: Watch if the matter is in commotion, and then evacuate it, for that is required; if it is not in commotion, do not evacuate, since it is not required.

By motion he means not only evacuation, but also (bodily) motion from place to place. This motion too should be avoided in the acme, because then the constitution is occupied with the disease-producing causes. This appears from the words, during the acme, rest is preferable. As for his rule, "Purge and disturb humors, when ripe, not while crude", this refers to chronic, not to acute diseases.

II 29. About the beginning and the end everything is weaker, about the acme stronger.

Just above, he has said, "At the beginning of diseases, if you think some motion is required, provide it", etc.; now, as if he expected the question, "Why ever should we disturb the matter at the beginning and provide rest during the acme?" he continued: The reason why I recommend evacuation at the beginning of acute diseases, is that about the beginning and the end everything is weaker, about the acme stronger. By beginning he does not mean the initial moment, nor the first three days, but the beginning as opposed to the other stages, the increase, the acme and the decrease; by end he means the decrease.

It should further be known that with regard to sick people there are two kinds of phenomena to be observed in the body, the normal and the abnormal.

δυνάμεις αἱ ψυχικαὶ καὶ φυσικαὶ καὶ ζωτικαί. καὶ ψυχικαὶ μὲν εἰσιν αἵ τε αἰσθητικαὶ καὶ λογιστικαί· κινητικαὶ δὲ ἤγουν ζωτικαὶ ἥ τε σφυγμικὴ καὶ ἡ ἀναπνευστική· φυσικαὶ δὲ ἑλκτική, καθεκτική, ἀλλοιωτική, ἀποκριτική. καὶ τὰ παρὰ φύσιν δὲ τρία εἰσίν· αἴτια, συμπτώματα, νοσήματα. τούτων οὖν οὕτως ἐχόντων ἰστέον, ὅτι ἐν τῇ ἀρχῇ ἀσθενεῖς ὑπάρχουσιν αἱ δυνάμεις αἱ φυσικαὶ διὰ τὸ ἄπεπτον τῶν χυμῶν· καὶ γὰρ ἐν οὔροις καὶ ἐν πτυέλοις καὶ διαχωρήμασι καὶ ἐμουμένοις ἡ ἀρχὴ τὰ τῆς ἀπεψίας ἔχει γνωρίσματα, οἷστισι καὶ περιγράφεσθαι πέφυκεν. ἰσχυραὶ δέ εἰσιν αἵ τε ψυχικαὶ καὶ ζωτικαὶ δυνάμεις· οὔτε γὰρ ἡ σφυγμικὴ δύναμις ἀξιόλογόν τι ἐν τῇ ἀρχῇ πέπονθεν· ἀλλὰ καὶ λογιζόμεθα καὶ αἰσθανόμεθα δεόντως. ἐπὶ μέντοι τῶν παρὰ φύσιν ἐν τῇ ἀρχῇ ἀσθενῆ εἰσι τὰ νοσήματα, οὔτε γὰρ εὐθέως σφοδρῶς εἰσβάλλει ὁ πυρετὸς πρὸς τὴν οἰκείαν ἀκμὴν συγκρινόμενος· οὔτε μὴν τὰ συμπτώματα πάνυ κατεπείγει, ἀγρυπνίαν λέγω ἐπιτεταμένην ἢ κεφαλαλγίαν ἢ παραφορὰν ἢ τὰ τοιαῦτα, ἀλλὰ προκόπτοντος τοῦ χρόνου τὸ μέγεθος προσλαμβάνει. ὁρμώμενα δέ εἰσι τὰ αἴτια, ταῦτα γὰρ εἰ μὴ τὴν οἰκείαν ἀκμὴν προσλάβωσιν, οὐ δύνανται δρᾶσαι ἐν τῷ σώματι ἡμῶν νόσημα, ἀλλὰ τοῦ δυνάμει πρῶτα τυχόντα, ἐπειδὰν ἀκμάσῃ, προσλαμβάνει τὸ ἐνεργείᾳ.

Ἐν τοίνυν τῇ ἀκμῇ αἱ φυσικαὶ δυνάμεις ἐρρωμέναι εἰσί, τότε γὰρ πέψεις γίνονται ἐν τοῖς οὔροις καὶ τοῖς διαχωρήμασι, καὶ ἁπλῶς εἰπεῖν ἐν τοῖς ἐκκρινομένοις τὰ τέλεια τῆς πέψεως διαφαίνεται σημεῖα. ἰσχυρὰ γοῦν εἰσι τότε τὰ νοσήματα καὶ τὰ συμπτώματα, ὅτι προπέπονθεν ἥ τε ψυχικὴ καὶ ζωτικὴ δύναμις καὶ ὅτι λεπτυνθείσης τῆς ὕλης σφοδρότερον ἡ φύσις τοῖς παροξυσμοῖς ὑποτίθεται· διὸ καὶ συμβαίνει δυνατωτέρους γίνεσθαι τοὺς παροξυσμούς. εἰσὶ δὲ τὸ τηνικαῦτα συμπτώματα ἰσχυρότερα· τῶν γὰρ νοσημάτων ἰσχυρῶν γενομένων καὶ τῆς ὕλης λεπτοποιουμένης καὶ τῶν φυσικῶν δυνάμεων ῥωννυμένων καὶ πλείονα ἐξάπτεσθαι περιττώματα ὡς λεπτότερα καὶ δριμύτερα καὶ πρὸς τὴν δαπάνην τῶν ὑλῶν ἐπείγεσθαι τὴν φύσιν, ἀνάγκη τήν τε ἀγρυπνίαν καὶ τὴν κεφαλαλγίαν καὶ τὴν δίψαν ἢ παραφοράν, εἰ τύχοι, καὶ τὰς ὀδύνας καὶ τὰ τοιαῦτα κατεπείγειν. εἴρηται οὖν ἐνταῦθα, ποῖά εἰσιν ἰσχυρὰ ἐν τῇ ἀκμῇ τῶν τε κατὰ φύσιν καὶ παρὰ φύσιν, ὅτι αἱ φυσικαὶ δυνάμεις καὶ τὰ νοσήματα καὶ τὰ συμπτώματα. ἀλλὰ καὶ ὁ πυρετὸς ἐν τῇ ἀκμῇ ἰσχυρότερός ἐστι κατὰ φαντασίαν, οὐ μὴν τῇ δυνάμει, ὅσον γὰρ οὔπω καὶ κρίσις καὶ ἀπαλλαγὴ αὐτοῦ γενήσεται. ἀσθενοῦσι δὲ ἐν τῇ ἀκμῇ αἱ ψυχικαὶ δυνάμεις· οὔτε γὰρ κινεῖσθαι τὸ τηνικαῦτα ἀμέμπτως δύνανται οὔτε μὴν φαντάζεσθαι καὶ διαλέγεσθαι. ἀλλὰ μὴν καὶ αἱ ζωτικαὶ πάσχουσιν ἐν τῇ ἀκμῇ· ἀμυδρότεροι γὰρ πάντως οἱ σφυγμοὶ εὑρίσκονται χρόνῳ καταβαλλομένων τῶν τοιούτων δυνάμεων ὑπὸ τῆς νόσου. ἐν δὲ τοῖς παρὰ φύσιν τὰ αἴτιά εἰσιν ἀσθενῆ καὶ ἐξίτηλα κατὰ τὰς ἀκμάς, ὡς οἷον παρηκμακότα· δηλοῖ δὲ τὸ πεφθῆναι καὶ λεπτυνθῆναι τὴν ὕλην καὶ τὸ πολὺ αὐτῆς δαπανηθῆναι διὰ τῶν κατὰ μέρος παροξυσμῶν, οὐ μὴν ἀλλὰ καὶ τὸ λοιπὸν

9 ἐπὶ – 13 προσλαμβάνει] *v.* Theoph. In Aphor.: II 324,9–16 Dietz 11 οὔτε – 13 προσλαμβάνει *et* 19 ἰσχυρὰ – 27 κατεπείγειν] *cf.* Gal. In Aphor. II 30: XVII B 524,11–14 K. 34 ἐν – 36 παρηκμακότα] *cf.* Gal. In Aphor. II 30: XVII B 524,14–15 K.

2 *fort.* λογιστικαὶ ⟨καὶ⟩ κινητικαὶ [δὲ] ἤγουν ⟨προαιρετικαί⟩· ζωτικαὶ ⟨δὲ⟩ *scribendum est* 3 *ante* ἀποκριτική *add.* καὶ A 6 διαχωρήματα A τὰ *om.* P 11 κατεπεγείρει α: *correxi (cf. lin. 27)* 12 περιφορὰν α: *correxi* 15 *fort.* πρῶτον *scribendum est* τυγχάνοντα A 21 σφοδροτέρα P 24 καί[II]] *fort.* ὡς *vel* ὥστε *scribendum est* 25 ὡς] *fort.* καὶ *scribendum est* 33 πάντως] πως A

Normal are the faculties, psychic, natural and vital. Psychic faculties are the sensory and the ratiocinative ones; motive or vital faculties the pulsatory and the respiratory; natural faculties the attractive, retentive, transformative and secretory. Abnormal phenomena are also three in number: causes, symptoms, and diseases. This being so, you must know that in the beginning the natural faculties are weak owing to the unconcocted state of the humors: the urine, the sputum, the stools and the vomit show in the beginning the signs of absence of concoction, and it is by these that the beginning can be described. The psychic and vital faculties, on the other hand, are strong: the pulsatory faculty is not seriously affected at the outset, and we reason and perceive as we should. As regards the abnormal phenomena, diseases are weak in the beginning, fever for instance does not assail with violence right at the start, as compared to the same fever in its acme; nor are the symptoms very urgent, such as prolonged insomnia, headache, delirium, etc., but in the course of time they gain strength. Only the causes are fully active, for if they have not attained their acme, they cannot bring about disease in the body; while only potentially present at first, they pass to actuality when they have reached their high point.

In the acme, then, the natural faculties are strong, for it is then that concoction takes place in the urine and the stools, and generally speaking the signs of complete concoction appear in the excretions. The diseases and the symptoms are strong at that stage, because the psychic and the vital faculty have already been affected, and because owing to the comminution of the matter the constitution is more susceptible to paroxysms, with the result that paroxysms gain in strength. Symptoms at that time are stronger; for as diseases have become strong, as the matter is comminuted and the natural faculties are vigorous, so that more waste matter is kindled – owing to its thin and pungent quality – and the constitution is impatient to get rid of the matter, it is inevitable that insomnia, headache, thirst, delirium in some cases, pains etc. should become disturbing. So now it has been made clear which phenomena, normal as well as abnormal, are strong during the acme: the natural faculties, the diseases and the symptoms. As for fever, in appearance it is also stronger during the acme, but in effect it is not, for very soon the crisis will come and it will be gone. The psychic faculties, on the other hand, are weak in the acme; (patients) in that stage can no longer move, imagine or speak properly. But the vital faculties as well are affected during the acme; pulses are necessarily found to be weaker, as these faculties are gradually worn down by the disease. Of abnormal phenomena, the causes are weak and fading away during the acme, as if they were past their prime; this is proved by the fact that the matter has been concocted and comminuted, and the greater part of it has been eliminated by partial paroxysms, while

πρὸς διαφόρησιν ἢ πρὸς ἔκκρισιν ἐπείγεσθαι ἅτε κρατηθὲν καὶ κυριευθὲν ὑπὸ τῆς φύσεως καὶ τῶν φυσικῶν δυνάμεων.

Ἐν δὲ τῷ τέλει ἤγουν παρακμῇ ἀσθενέστερά ἐστι τὰ παρὰ φύσιν, τὰ αἴτια λέγω καὶ τὰ νοσήματα καὶ τὰ συμπτώματα. ἤδη γὰρ πέπαυται ὁ ἀγών· καὶ γὰρ ἐπέφθησαν αἱ ὕλαι καὶ ἐξεκρίθησαν καὶ ὅσον ἤδη ἀπομαραίνονται πάντα καὶ ἀποσβέννυνται· ἔρρωνται δὲ τὸ τηνικαῦτα αἵ τε φυσικαὶ καὶ ζωτικαὶ δυνάμεις. κἂν γὰρ μὴ παραχρῆμα ἀμέμπτως τὰ οἰκεῖα ἐπιτελῶσιν, ἀλλ' οὖν τὸ λοιπὸν ἀνενόχλητοι ὑπὸ τῶν παρὰ φύσιν καταστᾶσαι καὶ ἐπὶ ὑγείαν ὁδεύουσαι ἔτι καὶ μᾶλλον ἀμέμπτους τὰς ἐνεργείας προβάλλονται.

Καλῶς οὖν ἔφη ὁ Ἱπποκράτης· δεῖ ἐν τῇ ἀρχῇ ποιεῖσθαι τὰς κενώσεις ἐπὶ τῶν ὀξέων νοσημάτων, ἐφ' ὧν ὀργᾷ ἡ ὕλη, ὅτε ἐρρωμέναι τυγχάνουσιν αἱ φυσικαὶ δυνάμεις ⟨καὶ⟩ αἱ ψυχικαί, καὶ τὰ αἴτια ἀκμάζουσι· τοῦτο γὰρ οὕτως γίνεται, καὶ τῆς αἰτίας ἐκκοπτομένης οὐ λαμβάνει ἐπίδοσιν τὸ νόσημα. ἐν δὲ τῇ ἀκμῇ, ἐπειδὴ τὸ αἴτιον ἀσθενέστερόν ἐστιν, οὐ μὴν ἀλλὰ καὶ αἱ ψυχικαὶ καὶ ζωτικαὶ δυνάμεις, τὰ δὲ συμπτώματα καὶ τὰ νοσήματα ἰσχυρά, οὐ δεῖ παραλαμβάνειν κένωσιν, ἐπεί τοί γε ἐπιτείνεται ταῦτα καὶ χαλεπώτερα γίνονται.

II 30 [II 31: IV 478,18 L.] Τῷ ἐξ ἀρρωστίης εὖ σιτεύοντι μηδὲν ἐπιδιδόναι.

Ὁ παρὼν ἀφορισμὸς ἀναληπτικός ἐστιν, ἔχων συνέχειαν πρὸς τὸν ἀφορισμὸν τὸν λέγοντα· «Ἢν ἐκ νόσου τροφὴν λαμβάνων τις μὴ ἰσχύῃ, σημαίνει τὸ σῶμα ὅτι πλείονι τροφῇ χρέεται». ἀλλ' ἐκεῖ μὲν περὶ δυνάμεως ἔλεγε ταῦτα, ἐνταῦθα δὲ περὶ φυσικοῦ ὄγκου τοῦ σώματός φησι. καὶ ἐκεῖνος μὲν ὁ ἀφορισμὸς μερικώτερός ἐστιν, οὗτος δὲ καθολικώτερος. τί γάρ φησιν ἐνταῦθα; ἐὰν μετὰ κρίσιν μὴ τελείαν γενομένην τροφὴν προσαίρηται καὶ μὴ λαμβάνῃ ἐπίδοσιν τὸ σῶμα, τουτέστι μὴ παχύνηται καὶ ἀνατρέφηται, κακὸν τὸ τοιοῦτον. κἀκεῖ μὲν βιαστὴν ὄρεξιν ἔφη, ἐνταῦθα δὲ οὐ τῇ αὐτῇ ἐχρήσατο λέξει, ἀλλὰ τῷ εἰπεῖν εὖ σιτεύοντι ἐδήλωσε τὸ καλῶς ὀρέγεσθαι, τουτέστι τὴν κατὰ φύσιν ὄρεξιν. εἰσερχόμενος οὖν καὶ εὑρίσκων τινὰ μετὰ τὴν νόσον καλῶς ὀρεγόμενον καὶ πολλῆς τροφῆς μεταλαμβάνοντα, τῷ δὲ φυσικῷ τοῦ σώματος ὄγκῳ ἐπίδοσίν τινα μὴ λαμβάνοντα, συλλογίζομαι, ὅτι κακοχυμία τις, ὡς ἔοικεν, ἐν τῷ σώματί ἐστιν ἐλλιποῦς τῆς κρίσεως γενομένης, ὑφ' ἧς διαφθείρεται ἡ τροφή, κἀντεῦθεν οὐ προστίθεται τῷ σώματι, ἵνα διαθρέψῃ αὐτοῦ τὸν ὄγκον.

II 31 [II 32: IV 480,1–4 L.] Ὡς τὰ πολλὰ πάντες οἱ φαύλως ἔχοντες κατ'

3–4 συμπτώματα] *cf.* Gal. In Aphor. II 30: XVII B 524,11–12 K. 19–27 ὄρεξιν] *v.* Gal. In Aphor. II 31: XVII B 525,4–15 K. 20sq. Ἢν – χρέεται] Hipp. Aphor. II 8: IV 472,1–2 L. *v.* Theoph. In Aphor.: II 324,1 Dietz 29sq. συλλογίζομαι – γενομένης] *v.* Gal. In Aphor. II 31: XVII B 526,2 K.

2 φυσικῶν] ψυχικῶν A 3 εἰσι A 5 ἀπομαραίνεται A 7 ἐπιτελοῦσιν A 12 καὶ[I] *addidi* 16 ἐπιτείνεται *scripsi*: ἐπιγίνεται α 17 εὖ σιτεύοντι] *item infra, lin. 26*: εὐσιτέοντι *Hipp.* 24 προσερηται P: προσαιρεῖται A: *correxi* λαμβάνει A 30 ἐλλιποῦσα P: ἐλλειπούσης A: *correxi*

the dispersal or excretion of the remainder is imminent, since it is mastered and dominated by nature and the natural faculties.

At the end, i.e. during the decrease, the abnormal factors, causes, diseases and symptoms, are weaker. By now the struggle is over; the matter has been concocted and excreted and all the abnormal factors are almost immediately decaying and waning; at the same time the natural and vital faculties are strong. Though they may not at once perform their functions faultlessly, at least they are now safe from annoyance by the abnormal phenomena, and as they progress toward health, they exercise their functions with increasing perfection.

Hippocrates is therefore right when he prescribes that in acute diseases, in which the matter is in a state of disturbance, we should evacuate at the beginning, when the natural and the psychic faculties are strong and the causes are at their peak: when things are handled in this way, the cause is extirpated and the disease does not gain ground. During the acme, on the other hand, when the cause is weaker, but so are the psychic and vital faculties, whereas the symptoms and the diseases are strong, one should not apply evacuation, because then they are intensified and become worse.

II 30. For a convalescent who eats well to gain nothing.

The present aphorism deals with the subject of convalescence; it continues the one that said: "If after sickness a person, while taking food, does not gain strength, this is a sign that his body receives too much food". But while there he dealt with resistance, he is speaking here of the natural bulk of the body. Also, the other aphorism is more particular, this one more general. What, indeed, does he say here? If after an imperfect crisis (a patient) takes food and the body gains nothing, i.e., does not get fatter and healthier, this is a bad sign. In the other one he spoke of immoderate appetite, here he did not express himself in the same terms, but by the words who eats well, he described a good, that is a normal, appetite. So when I visit a patient and find that after his disease he has a good appetite and eats well, but without regaining the normal bulk of his body, I infer that there seems to be some bad humor in the body as a result of an incomplete crisis; this humor corrupts the food, hence it is not absorbed by the body, so as to restore its weight.

II 31. As a general rule, all sickly persons who at the beginning

ἀρχὰς μὲν εὖ σιτεύοντες, μὴ ἐπιδιδόντες δὲ πρὸς τῷ τέλει πάλιν ἀσιτεύουσιν, ⟨...⟩ ὕστερον εὖ σιτεύουσιν.

Φησὶν ὅτι ὁρῶ ἄρρωστον ἐκ νόσου ἀνακομιζόμενον καὶ πολλῶν τροφῶν ὀρεγόμενον, οὐ κατὰ φύσιν δέ, ἀλλὰ διὰ τὸ χυμὸν ὀξώδη ἐν τῷ στόματι τῆς γαστρὸς περιέχεσθαι· ὅστις κἂν πλείστην ὄρεξιν ἔχῃ, οὐδεμίαν ἐπίδοσιν ἴσχει κατὰ τὸ σῶμα. ἐντεῦθεν ἀποφαίνεται, ὅτι πρὸς τῷ τέλει ἀσιτήσει πάλιν οὗτος ἐξ ἀνάγκης διὰ τὸ προϊόντος τοῦ χρόνου πληθυνόμενον ἐκεῖνον τὸν ὀξώδη χυμὸν καταλύει⟨ν⟩ τῇ ἀμετρίᾳ τὴν ὀρεκτικὴν δύναμιν. τὸ τοιοῦτον οὖν διαβάλλει, εἶτά φησιν ὅτι ὁρῶ ἕτερον ἄρρωστον ἀναλαμβανόμενον καὶ ἀσιτοῦντα, καὶ λέγω, ὡς οὗτος πρὸς τῷ τέλει εὖ σιτήσει. ἐπειδὴ γὰρ ἡ νόσος κατέβαλεν αὐτοῦ τὴν ὀρεκτικὴν δύναμιν, διὰ τοῦτο ἐν τῇ ἀρχῇ τῆς ἀνακομιδῆς οὐκ ὀρέγεται τροφῆς· προϊόντος δὲ τοῦ χρόνου ἀναλαμβάνουσα ἑαυτὴν ἡ ὀρεκτικὴ δύναμις καὶ ἐρρωμενεστέρα γενομένη ἐφίεται τοῦ οἰκείου ἔργου· ὅπερ ἀποδέχεται ὁ Ἱπποκράτης.

Καλῶς δὲ εἶπεν· Ὡς τὰ πολλά· οὐδὲν γὰρ ἄτοπον εὐθέως κατ' ἀρχὰς τῆς ἀνακομιδῆς διὰ φυσικὴν ῥώμην τῆς ὀρεκτικῆς δυνάμεως καὶ πολλῶν ὀρέγεσθαι τὸν ἀνακομιζόμενον καὶ πρὸς τῷ τέλει μὴ ἀσιτῆσαι, ἐπειδὴ κατὰ φύσιν προϋποκειμένης τῆς ὀρέξεως καὶ μὴ ὑπό τινος ἀλλοκότου χυμοῦ ἐπιτελουμένης οὐχ ἕπεται παράλυσις αὐτῇ τῷ χρόνῳ εἰς ἀμετρίαν τοῦ τοιούτου χυμοῦ ἐκτρεπομένου.

Φαύλως δὲ ἀντὶ τοῦ «μὴ κατὰ φύσιν ὀρεγόμενοι, ἀλλ' ὑπὸ τοῦ ὀξώδους χυμοῦ πρὸς τοῦτο ἐπεγειρόμενοι».

Ἀρχὴν δὲ ἐνταῦθα οὐ τὴν τοῦ νοσήματος ἀκουστέον, ἀλλὰ τὴν ἐκ νόσου ἐπὶ τὴν ὑγείαν, τουτέστι τὴν τῆς ἀναλήψεως.

Τὸ δὲ ἰσχυρῶς πρόσκειται οὐ διὰ τὸ ἐκ χυμῶν ἀλλοκότων τοῦτο γίνεσθαι, ἐπεί τοί γε οὐκ ἂν ἀπήλλακτο τηνικαῦτα τὸ σῶμα τηλικαύτης βλάβης ὑποκειμένης, ἀλλὰ διὰ τὴν ἐκ νόσου ἀσθένειαν τῆς ὀρεκτικῆς δυνάμεως, ἥτις ὅσον οὔπω ἀνακομισθήσεται ὑπὸ μηδενὸς τῶν παρὰ φύσιν ὀχλουμένη.

II 32 [II 33: IV 480,5–6 L.] Ἐν πάσῃ νούσῳ τὸ ἐρρῶσθαι τὴν διάνοιαν καὶ εὖ ἔχειν πρὸς τὰς προσφορὰς ἀγαθόν, τὸ δὲ ἐναντίον κακόν.

Νόμιζε τὸν Ἱπποκράτην ταῦτά σοι λέγειν, ὅτι εἰσερχόμενος πρὸς τὸν ἄρρωστον σκόπει, εἰ ὑγιεινῶς ἔχουσιν αἱ ψυχικαὶ δυνάμεις, αἰσθητικαί φημι, κινητικαί, ἡγεμονικαί· τούτων γὰρ ἐρρωμένων ἐν ταῖς νόσοις καλὸν σημεῖον· δηλοῦται γὰρ ἡ πρώτη ἀρχὴ ὑγιῶς ἔχουσα. ὁ γὰρ ἐγκέφαλος ἢ ἑτέροις μορίοις συμπάσχει ἢ αὐτὸς οἰκεῖον ἔχει πάθος, εἴρηται δὲ καὶ τοῦτο τῷ Ἱπποκράτει, ὅτι «Ἡ κοιλία τῇ κεφαλῇ καὶ ἡ κεφαλὴ τῇ κοιλίᾳ» τῶν οἰκείων παθῶν μεταδιδόασιν. ἐρρωμένων οὖν οὐσῶν τῶν τε ἡγεμονικῶν καὶ αἰσθητικῶν καὶ κινητικῶν ἤγουν προαιρετικῶν δυνάμεων οὔτε αὐτὸς ἔχει ἴδιον πάθος οὔτε μὴν ἑτέροις συμπάσχει μορίοις· τούτου δὲ

3 Φησὶν – ἀνακομιζόμενον] *cf.* Gal. In Aphor. II 32: XVII B 526,8–9 K. 19sq.] *cf.* Theoph. In Aphor.: II 325,17–19 Dietz 31sq. τούτων – ἔχουσα] *cf.* Gal. In Aphor. II 33: XVII B 528, 17–529,4 K. 33sq. Ἡ – μεταδιδόασιν] *v.* Hipp. Loc. hom. 1: VI 276,10–13 L.

1 μὲν *non hab. Hipp. plerique* (C'), *Theoph.* U'' εὐσιτέοντες *Hipp.* μὴ ἐπιδιδόντες δὲ] καὶ μηδὲν ἐπιδιδόντες *Hipp.* ἀσιτέουσιν *Hipp. plerique* 2 *lac. indicavi*: οἱ δὲ κατ' ἀρχὰς μὲν ἀσιτέοντες ἰσχυρῶς *Hipp. (cf. infra, lin. 23)* εὖ σιτεύουσιν] δὲ εὐσιτέοντες βέλτιον ἀπαλλάσσουσιν *Hipp.* 5 ἔχει A ἴσχει] ἔχει A 7 καταλύει α: *corr.* A[2] 8sq. ὁρῶ ἕτερον] ὁρῶμεν P 11 τροφῆς *om.* A 35 τε *om.* A 36 μη *(sic)* P

eat well, but without gaining, end eating badly, $^{+}$while those who strongly dislike food at first, but^{+} eat well later, $^{+}$fare better^{+}[1].

(Hippocrates) says: I visit a patient who is recovering from an illness, and who has a great appetite for food, not a normal appetite, however, but one due to an acid humor contained in the orifice of the stomach; in spite of his strong appetite the patient does not gain weight at all. On the ground of this he declares that toward the end this person will necessarily be again without appetite, for in the course of time that acid humor will increase and by its excessive quantity will paralyze the appetitive faculty. He warns against this, then goes on: I visit another convalescent who has no appetite, and I say that this one will end by eating well. For because the disease has weakened his appetitive faculty, he has no taste for food at the beginning of his recovery; as time goes on, however, and the appetitive faculty recovers its strength, it longs to resume its work; and Hippocrates considers this a welcome sign.

He rightly said, As a general rule, since it is quite conceivable that immediately at the beginning of convalescence, thanks to a naturally robust appetite, the recovering patient wants much food and yet does not end eating badly; the appetite was then normal to begin with, not brought about by some unwholesome humor, and so it does not fail later, when eventually this humor becomes disproportionate.

Sickly means those who have no normal appetite, but are stimulated to eat by the acid humor.

The beginning here is not to be understood as that of the illness, but of the transition from illness to health, i.e. of convalescence.

The qualification strongly does not imply that this results from unwholesome humors, otherwise the body would not be free from disease, with such a harmful force still present; rather, the appetitive faculty is still weak from the disease, but very soon it will be restored, since there is now no abnormal influence to disturb it.

II 32. In any disease soundness of reason and a good appetite is a favorable sign, and the contrary a bad one.

What Hippocratès tells you, you may consider to be this: When visiting your patient, you should see if the psychic faculties are healthy, i.e. the sensory, the motor and the governing faculties; if these are sound in sickness, this is a good sign; for it proves that the first principle is unimpaired. The brain, indeed, is affected either simultaneously with other parts, or by itself alone, as Hippocrates also says: "The belly passes on its affections to the head, and the head to the belly." Now as long as the governing, the sensory, and the motor or voluntary faculties are sound, the brain is affected neither by itself nor together with

[1] $^{+}$while – but^{+} and $^{+}$fare better^{+}: see the app. crit.

ἀλύπως ἐνεργοῦντος δῆλον, ὅτι καὶ ἡ γαστὴρ καλῶς ἔχει καὶ αἱ φυσικαὶ δυνάμεις καλῶς διάκεινται. τῆς μέντοι τιμιωτέρας τοῦ ἐγκεφάλου ἐνεργείας μνημονεύσας, λέγω δὴ τῆς διανοίας, σοὶ προσυπακούειν ἐκέλευσε καὶ τῶν ἄλλων ἁπασῶν, φαντασίας καὶ μνήμης καὶ αἰσθήσεως καὶ κινήσεως.

Εἶτά φησι· καὶ τὸ εὖ ἔχειν πρὸς τὰς προσφορὰς ἀγαθόν, ἐκ τοῦ τιμιωτέρου καὶ νῦν ποιούμενος τὴν σημείωσιν· τιμιωτέρα γὰρ πασῶν τῶν φυσικῶν δυνάμεων ἡ ὀρεκτική ἐστιν. ὡς δὲ καὶ πρῶτον, καὶ διὰ τούτου ὑποτίθεται καὶ ἑτέραν ἀρχὴν ἐρρωμένην εἶναι. ἰστέον γάρ, ὅτι ἡ τῶν σιτίων προσαγωγὴ ἐπιθυμία τίς ἐστι καὶ ἔφεσις· εἰ γὰρ μὴ ἐφιέμεθα, οὐκ ἄν ποτε τροφὴν λάβοιμεν. εἰ τοίνυν ἐν τῇ ἐπιθυμίᾳ κεῖται ἡ τῶν σιτίων προσφορά, ἡ δὲ ἐπιθυμία ἐν τῷ ἥπατί ἐστι, δῆλον, ὅτι καὶ τὸ ἧπαρ εὖ ἔχον πρὸς τὰς ὑποφορὰς τῶν νούσων ὑγιὲς ὑπάρχει.

Μὴ προπετῶς δὲ εἴπῃς, ὅτι τὸ ἐρρῶσθαι τὴν διάνοιαν τῶν ἀνθρώπων καὶ εὖ ἔχειν πρὸς τὰς προσφορὰς σωτήριόν ἐστιν· οὐδὲν γὰρ ἄτοπον τούτων ὑγιῶς ἐχόντων, ἐγκεφάλου φημί, ἥπατος καὶ στομάχου καὶ γαστρός, ἐν ἀλλοτρίῳ ὑποστῆναι τὴν ὕλην καὶ θάνατον ἀπεργάσασθαι. τί γάρ; ὅτι τὰ ἔντερα ἔχουσι διάθεσιν, ἐπικρατεῖ δὲ καὶ μεγεθύνεται ἡ ἐν τοῖς ἐντέροις διάθεσις ὡς θάνατον ἀπεργάσασθαι. ἢ πολλάκις περὶ τὸν θώρακα ὑφίσταται νοσοποιὸς ὕλη ἀνελεῖν δυναμένη νοσοῦντα. λοιπὸν διὰ τοῦτο οὐκ εἶπεν ὁ Ἱπποκράτης «σωτήριον», ἀλλ' ἀγαθὸν καὶ οὐ φαῦλον ἐπιστάμενος, ὅτι πολλάκις τούτων καλῶς διακειμένων θάνατος ἕπεται τῷ νοσοῦντι ἐν ἄλλοις μορίοις, πνεύμονι τυχὸν ἢ ὑπεζωκότι ἢ ἑτέρῳ τινί, τῆς νοσοποιοῦ ὕλης ἐνεργούσης. εἰ δέ γε πρὸς τούτοις καὶ αἱ ψυχικαὶ καὶ αἱ φυσικαὶ ὑπέκειντο πεπονθυῖαι, χαλεπώτατον ἂν ἦν τὸ τοιοῦτον.

Εἰ δέ γέ ποτε ἐν νοσήματι εὕροις τὸ ἐναντίον, τάς τε ψυχικὰς καὶ τὰς φυσικὰς ἀσθενεῖς, κακὸν νόμιζε τὸ τοιοῦτον, οὐ μὴν πάντως ὀλέθριον. οἶδε γάρ, ὅτι καὶ τῶν ψυχικῶν πολλάκις καὶ τῶν φυσικῶν δυνάμεων κακῶς διακειμένων ἡ ζωτικὴ δύναμις ἐρρωμένη ὑπάρχουσα ὑγείαν ἐποίη⟨σεν⟩.

II 33 [II 34: IV 480,7–9 L.] Ἐν τῇσι νούσοισιν ἧσσον κινδυνεύουσιν οἱ νοσέοντες, οἷς ἂν οἰκείη τῆς φύσιος καὶ τῆς ἕξιος καὶ τῆς ἡλικίης ἡ νοῦσος ὑπάρχῃ, μᾶλλον ἢ οἷσιν ἂν μὴ οἰκεί⟨η⟩ κατά τι τουτέων.

Λέγει, ὅτι ὅσα νοσήματα τοῖς ἰδίοις συμφωνεῖ συστοίχοις ἧττονα ἔχει τὸν κίνδυνον. καὶ ἀπορεῖ ὁ Διοκλῆς πρὸς τὸν Ἱπποκράτην λέγων· «Τί φῄς, ὦ Ἱππόκρατες; ὁ καῦσος, ᾧτινι ἕπεται ζέσις διὰ τὴν ποιότητα τῆς ὕλης καὶ δίψος ἀφόρητον καὶ ἀγρυπνία καὶ τὰ τοιαῦτα, ὅσα ἐν θέρει ἐστίν, ἐπιεικέστερος διὰ τὴν σύστοιχον

5–8 εἶναι] *cf.* Gal. In Aphor. II 33: XVII B 529,4–6 K. 12–13 ἐστιν] *cf.* Gal. In Aphor. II 33: XVII B 528,1–2 K. 23–24 ὀλέθριον] *cf.* Gal. In Aphor. II 33: XVII B 528,2–3 K. 30 Λέγει – κίνδυνον] *v.* Theoph. In Aphor.: II 326,25–327,1 Dietz 31 Τί – 212,3 καθίσταται] Diocl. fr. 34 Wellmann *v.* Gal. In Aphor. II 34: XVII B 530,9–16 K.

1 ἀλήπτως P 7 πρῶτον *scripsi*: πρώτ *(ambig.)* A: πρώτη P τοῦτο α: *correxi* 11 ὑποφορὰς τῶν νούσων] *fort.* προσφορὰς [τῶν νούσων] *scribendum est* 14 ἐγκέφαλον P ἀλλοτρίῳ] *fort.* ἄλλῳ μορίῳ *scribendum est* 16 ὡς] καὶ P 17 περὶ τὸν θώρακα *om.* A δυναμένην P 25 καλῶς α: *correxi* 26 ἐποίη α: *supplevi* 28 οἱ νοσέοντες] *item supra, p. 190,34, Hipp.* C′ *et al.*: *non hab. Hipp. plerique, Theoph.* καὶ τῆς ἡλικίης *om. supra, p. 190,34* *post* ἡλικίης *hab.* καὶ τῆς ὥρης *Hipp.* 29 ὑπάρχει A ἢ – τουτέων *om.* A οἰκείη *scripsi*: οἰκεί *et spat. 2 litt.* P τουτέως P: *correxi* *post* τουτέων *hab.* ἢ *Hipp. quidam, Theoph.* U′′ 33 ὅσα] *fort.* ὅταν *scribendum est* τὴν] τῶν, *ante* τῶν *inser.* τὴν A συστοίχων α: *correxi*

other parts; and when it functions without trouble, it is clear that the stomach is also healthy and that the natural faculties are in good condition. Though (Hippocrates) mentioned only the most precious function of the brain, reason, he wanted you to include with it all the others, imagination, memory, sense-perception and motion.

He goes on: And a good appetite is a favorable sign, another inference drawn from the most precious function, since the most precious of all the natural faculties is the appetitive. And as before, here too he supposes that another principle is sound. For we should be aware that the partaking of food is a kind of desire and a craving; if we felt no desire, we would never take food. Since, then, the partaking of food depends on desire, and desire is seated in the liver, it is evident that the liver, too, if capable of enduring diseases, must be healthy.

But do not draw the rash conclusion that soundness of reason in people and a good appetite guarantee recovery: it is still possible, when these are sound, the brain, the liver, the stomach and the belly, that the matter forms in a different place and causes death. For instance because there is an affection of the intestines, and this affection of the intestines prevails and increases to the point that it brings about death. Often, too, in the region of the chest, disease-producing matter forms which is strong enough to kill a patient. It is for this reason, then, that Hippocrates did not say, "a sign of recovery"; but a favorable, not a bad sign, because he knew that often, though these are in good condition, the patient succumbs to disease-producing matter that is active elsewhere, for example in the lungs, the undergirding membrane, or another part. If, in addition to these, the psychic and natural faculties were already diseased also, this would be the worst of all.

If, however, in a disease, you should sometimes find the contrary case, i.e., a weak condition of the psychic and natural faculties, this is to be considered a bad sign, but not necessarily a deadly one. (Hippocrates) knows that often when the psychic and natural faculties were in a poor state, soundness of the vital faculty has restored health.

II 33. In diseases there is less danger for patients, when the disease has more affinity with their nature and disposition and age, than for those with whom it has no affinity in one of these respects.

He says that those diseases which coincide with the corresponding correlative factors are less dangerous. So Diocles asks Hippocrates this question: "What do you mean, Hippocrates? Is a causus, which owing to the quality of the matter is attended with scalding heat, intolerable thirst, sleeplessness, and whatever else goes with summer, more benign on account of the correlative

ὥραν ἐστίν, ὅτε πάντα τὰ κακὰ ἐπιτείνεται, ἢ ἐν τῷ χειμῶνι, ἡνίκα τὸ σφοδρὸν τῆς κινήσεως κολάζεται καὶ φλογώσεως καὶ ἀμαυρότερον γίνεται καὶ τὸ δριμὺ ἀμβλύνεται καὶ τὸ ὅλον νόσημα ἠπιώτερον καθίσταται;» καὶ λέγομεν, ὅτι ἐν τῷ θέρει ἡ θερμασία ἐστὶ τοῦ περιέχοντος ἐπικρατής, καὶ χολὴν τὸ τηνικαῦτα γεννᾶσθαι συμβαίνει· ἐὰν οὖν ἐν τῇ ὥρᾳ ταύτῃ καῦσον ἢ τριταῖον συμβαίη γενέσθαι, οὐ δηλοῦται μεγάλη ἡ ποιήσασα αἰτία, ἐπὶ τὸ ὅμοιον γὰρ ἡ θερμὴ ποιότης τὴν ἐκτροπὴν ἐδέξατο, ἥτις εὐχερῶς γίνεται, κἂν μὴ σφοδρὸν εἴη τὸ τὴν ἐκτροπὴν ἐργαζόμενον αἴτιον. εἰ δὲ ἐν τῷ χειμῶνι, ὃς ψυχρότατος τῇ φύσει ὑπάρχει, συμβῇ καῦσος, χαλεπὸν τὸ τοιοῦτον, μεγάλην γὰρ καὶ δραστικὴν σημαίνει τὴν αἰτίαν ἐπὶ τὸ ἀνόμοιον τῆς ἐκτροπῆς γενομένης, ὡς ἐκβιάσασθαι τὸ ἐναντίον, λέγω δὴ τὴν ψῦξιν, καὶ κινῆσαι αὐτὴν εἰς τὸ ἐναντίον, τὴν ζέσιν λέγω καὶ καῦσιν. οὐ μόνον γὰρ τὴν ὑποκειμένην ἐν τῇ ὥρᾳ ψῦξιν ἐνίκησεν, ἀλλὰ καὶ θερμασίαν ὑφῆψεν.

Ὡσαύτως καὶ ἐπὶ ἡλικιῶν δεῖ λαβεῖν τὸν λόγον καὶ ἐπὶ τῶν ἄλλων πάντων συστοίχων. ἐὰν γὰρ ἐν ἀκμαστικῇ ἡλικίᾳ γένηται τριταῖος, οὐδὲν φαῦλον, θερμῆς γὰρ φύσει οὔσης τῆς ἡλικίας οὐ δηλοῦται δραστικὸν τὸ αἴτιον τὸ ἐργασάμενον τὸ νόσημα· εἰ δέ γε ἐπὶ γεροντικῇ ἡλικίᾳ γενήσεται τριταῖος, κακὸν τὸ τοιοῦτον, δηλοῖ γὰρ ἰσχυρὰν τὴν ἐκβιασαμένην αἰτίαν, ἥτις οὐ μόνον τὴν τῆς ἡλικίας ψῦξιν ἐνίκησεν, ἀλλὰ καὶ παρὰ φύσιν θερμασίαν ἐδημιούργησε.

Καὶ ἔστιν ἀπορῆσαι· «Πῶς ὁ Ἱπποκράτης παρακατιὼν εἴρηκε· 'Βράγχοι καὶ κόρυζαι τοῖσι σφόδρα πρεσβυτέροισιν οὐ πεπαίνονται'; ἰδοὺ ἡλικία γεροντικὴ καὶ νόσημα σύμφωνον – ψυχρὸν γάρ –, ἀλλ' ὅμως ἔφη 'οὐ πεπαίνονται'.» πρὸς ὃ λέγομεν, ὅτι αὐτὸς ἑαυτὸν ἐπελύσατο εἰπὼν «τοῖσι σφόδρα πρεσβυτέροισι», τουτέστι τοῖς πάνυ γεγηρακόσιν· οὗτοι γὰρ διὰ τὴν τῆς δυνάμεως ὑπερβάλλουσαν ἀσθένειαν οὐδὲ τὰ σύμφωνα νοσήματα καταγωνίσασθαι δύνανται.

II 34 [II 35: IV 480,10–12 L.] Ἐν πάσῃ νούσῳ τὰ περὶ τὸν ὀμφαλὸν καὶ τὸ ἦτρον πάχος ἔχειν βέλτιόν ἐστι, τὸ δὲ σφόδρα λεπτὸν καὶ ἐκτετηκὸς μοχθηρὸν καὶ ἐπισφαλές.

Σκόπει, φησίν, ἐπὶ τῶν νοσημάτων τὰ περὶ τὸν ὀμφαλὸν καὶ τὸ ἦτρον· καὶ εἰ μὲν πάχος ἔχει ταῦτα, καλόν ἐστι – πάχος δὲ ἁπλῶς εἰπεῖν ἀντὶ τοῦ σύμμετρον –, εἰ δὲ κάτισχνά ἐστι καὶ ἐκτετηκότα, μοχθηρόν. πόθεν δὲ δῆλον, ὡς οὐκ εἶπε τὸ εἰς ἄκρον πάχος, ἀλλὰ τὸ σύμμετρον; ἢ δῆλον ὅτι ἐκ τοῦ ἐπαγαγεῖν τὸ δὲ σφόδρα λεπτὸν καὶ ἐκτετηκὸς μοχθηρόν, γινώσκων, ὅτι καὶ τὸ ἄκρως παχὺ καὶ τὸ ἄκρως λεπτὸν κακόν, ἀσύμμετρα γὰρ ἄμφω.

Ἰστέον δέ, ὅτι ἀπὸ τοῦ ξιφοειδοῦς χόνδρου μέχρι τοῦ περιτοναίου, ὅπερ καὶ κτένα καλοῦμεν, ἐπιγάστριον τὸ πᾶν ὀνομάζεται· διαιρεῖται δὲ τοῦτο εἰς δύο, εἰς αὐτό

3 καὶ[II] – 12] *cf.* Gal. In Aphor. II 34: XVII B 530,16–531,4 K. 14 ἐὰν – 18] *v.* Theoph. In Aphor.: II 327,3–6 Dietz 19–24] *v.* Gal. In Aphor. II 34: XVII B 531,12–532,3 K. 19sq. Βράγχοι – πεπαίνονται] Hipp. Aphor. II 40: IV 482,3–4 L. 28–30 μοχθηρόν] *v.* Theoph. In Aphor.: II 328,9–12 Dietz 34–214,2] *cf.* Gal. In Aphor. II 35: XVII B 534,11–15 K. Theoph. In Aphor.: II 328,12–16 Dietz

4 γενέσθαι A 15 οὐ *om.* A 16 γέννηται A 17 ἐνίκησεν *scripsi (cf. lin. 12)*: ἐκίνησεν α 22 ἀπελύσατο P 25 πάσῃ νούσῳ *Hipp. pauci*: πάσῃσι τῇσι νούσοισι *Hipp. cett., Theoph.* 27 καὶ ἐπισφαλές] ἐπισφαλὲς δὲ τὸ τοιοῦτο καὶ πρὸς τὰς κάτω καθάρσιας *Hipp. (cf. infra, p. 214,30–31)* 29 καλόν] βέλτιον A 30 δὲ *om.* P 32 ἄκρος *(bis)* P 35 ἐπὶ γαστέρα A

season, when all the evils are intensified, or in winter, when the violence of its motion and of its ardor is curbed and weakened, when its pungency is blunted and the whole disease becomes milder?" We reply that in summer heat prevails in the surrounding air, and consequently bile is then produced; now if in that season a causus or a tertian occurs, this does not indicate great force of the cause which brought it about, for the hot quality has deviated toward its own kind, and such a deviation can easily happen, even if its cause is not violent. But if the causus occurs in winter, which by its nature is very cold, this is serious, since it points to a strong and active cause; the deviation is now toward the dissimilar, so that it forces out its contrary, the cold, and changes it into its opposite, seething and burning heat. Not only has it overcome the cold which is the fundamental quality of the season, but it has even kindled heat.

The same reasoning should be applied to ages and to all the other correlative factors. If a tertian fever occurs in the prime of life, this is not grave, for inasmuch as this age is naturally hot, there is no indication that the cause which brought about the disease is an active one; if, on the other hand, a tertian occurs in old age, this is bad, for it shows that the cause which has prevailed is a strong one, since it has not only overcome the coldness proper to that age, but has also created abnormal heat.

This raises the question: "Why did Hippocrates say later on: 'Sore throats and running noses in extremely old people do not ripen'? Here you have a case of old age and a corresponding, i.e. cold, disease, and yet he said, 'they do not ripen'." Our answer is that he has solved the problem himself by saying "in extremely old people", i.e. in those far gone in years, who owing to the utter weakness of their resistance cannot even overcome diseases corresponding (to their own age).

II 34. In any disease it is better for the region about the navel and the abdomen to be fleshy, while extreme thinness and emaciation is a bad and dangerous sign.

In cases of sickness you must, he says, examine the region of the navel and the abdomen; and if it is fleshy, this is all right – taking "fleshy" in the loose sense of "normal" –, but if it is too thin and emaciated, that is bad. How can we tell that he did not mean excessive, but normal fleshiness? From the words that follow, while extreme thinness and emaciation is a bad sign; he knows that extreme thickness as well as extreme thinness is bad, for both are disproportionate.

Note that the entire region from the ensiform cartilage down to the peritoneum, also named pubes, is called the epigastrium; it is divided into two parts,

τε τὸ ἐπιγάστριον, ὅπερ καὶ ὀμφαλὸν καλοῦμεν, καὶ εἰς τὸ ὑπογάστριον, ὅπερ ἐστὶ τὸ κάτω τῆς γαστρός, ὃ δὴ καὶ ἦτρον προσαγορεύεται.

Δεῖ οὖν εἰδέναι, ὅτι πολλὴν τοῦ ἐν ἡμῖν θερμοῦ φροντίδα ποιουμένη ἡ φύσις δυσὶ μορίοις ἐχρήσατο πρὸς τοῦτο, καρδίᾳ φημὶ καὶ ἥπατι, καὶ μάλιστα καρδίᾳ· αὕτη γὰρ ἐξ ἀρχῆς ἐργαστήριον καὶ πηγὴ τοῦ ἐν ἡμῖν ἐμφύτου θερμοῦ ὑπὸ τῆς φύσεως κατεσκευάσθη. ἐκ τούτων οὖν τὰ λοιπὰ γεγένηται μόρια τῆς ἐμφύτου θερμασίας, ἑκάστου πρὸς τὸ μέγεθος καὶ τὸ ἀξίωμα τῆς ἐνεργείας καὶ τῆς χρείας αὐτοῦ μεταλαμβάνοντος. πῇ μὲν γὰρ πλέον, πῇ δὲ ἧττον ἡ ταύτης μετάληψις γίνεται· αὐτίκα γοῦν γαστρὶ μὲν πολὺ παρέχεται τὸ θερμόν, κύστει δὲ ἐλάχιστον, διότι ἡ μὲν πεπτικόν ἐστιν ὄργανον, καθάπερ ἔκ τινος ταμείου ἥπατί τε καὶ τῷ παντὶ σώματι τὴν τροφὴν παρασκευάζουσα, ἡ δὲ χωρητικὸν ἤτοι ἀγγεῖον δεκτικὸν τοῦ ὀρώδους περιττώματος. διὰ τοῦτο τοίνυν καὶ τὴν καρδίαν ἀγχοῦ γαστρὸς ἔταξεν ἡ φύσις, ὥστε ἄφθονον αὐτῇ τὴν τοῦ θερμοῦ χορηγίαν οἷον ἐκ πρώτης ἀφετηρίας χορηγεῖσθαι· οὐ μὴν ἀλλὰ καὶ τὸ ἧπαρ ἐκ δεξιῶν προτέθηκεν αὐτῆς, ἵνα καὶ ὑπ' αὐτοῦ δεόντως θάλπηται· ἔταξε δὲ καὶ ἐν τοῖς ἀριστεροῖς τὸν σπλῆνα, οὕτω καὶ αὐτὸν θερμασίας αἴτιον αὐτῇ γενήσεσθαι, ψυχρὸν γὰρ τοῦτο κατ' οὐσίαν τὸ σπλάγχνον, ἀλλὰ διὰ τῶν ἐν αὐτῷ φερομένων ἀρτηριῶν τε καὶ φλεβῶν οὐδὲν ἧττον ἐπιτηδεύσασα κἀκείνῳ τῷ μέρει θερμασίας τὴν γαστέρα παραπολαύειν. ἀλλὰ καὶ φυλακῆς οὐ τὴν τυχοῦσαν ἐποιήσατο πρόνοιαν τοῦ ἐν γαστρὶ πολυτρόπως †ἐπινοουμένου† θερμοῦ. περιεφρούρησε γὰρ αὐτὴν τῷ καλουμένῳ ἐπίπλῳ πανταχόθεν αὐτῇ περικειμένῳ, ὥστε μὴ διαπνεῖσθαι τὸ ἐν αὐτῇ θερμὸν κἀντεῦθεν τὸ ἔργον τῆς πέψεως τῇ καταψύξει ἀποτυγχάνειν.

Λοιπὸν οὖν, ἐὰν ἐπὶ τῶν νοσημάτων ἐν τοῖς περὶ τὸν ὀμφαλὸν καὶ τὸ ἦτρον ἴσχνανσις γίνηται, κακόν· χηρεύει γὰρ ἡ γαστὴρ τῶν οἰκείων σκεπασμάτων καὶ φυλαττόντων τὸ ἔμφυτον θερμόν, ὧνπερ ἀμοιροῦν ἑτοίμως διαφορηθήσεται, τούτου δὲ διαφορουμένου ἡ πέψις τῆς τροφῆς βλαβήσεται. οὐ μὴν ἀλλ' οὐδὲ ἡ τῶν χυμῶν γενήσεται πέψις· οἱ γὰρ χυμοὶ οἵ τε ἄπεπτοι καὶ ἀλλόκοτοι τῷ κατὰ φύσιν θερμῷ μεταβάλλονται καὶ πέττονται· τούτων δὲ μὴ πεττομένων, τῆς τε τροφῆς καὶ τῶν χυμῶν, καταλύεται ἡ δύναμις. ἐφ' οἷς τί δεῖ ἀγαθὸν ἐλπίσαι ἐπὶ τῶν οὕτως νοσούντων;

Πρόσθες δὲ καὶ τοῦτο, ὅτι πολλάκις χρεία ἐστὶν ἐπὶ τῶν τοιούτων νοσημάτων καὶ καθᾶραι τὸ σῶμα, ὅπερ οὐδενὶ λόγῳ τολμητέον διαπράξασθαι. λεπτοῦ γὰρ καὶ ἀβαθοῦς ὑπάρχοντος τοῦ κατὰ τὸν ὀμφαλὸν καὶ τὸ ἦτρον τόπου ἐρεθιζόμενοι καὶ ἑλκόμενοι ἀπὸ τοῦ καθαρσίου φαρμάκου οἱ χυμοὶ ἐπὶ τὰ στερρὰ σώματα δριμεῖς τυγχάνοντες τῇ παρόδῳ χωροῦσι καὶ ἑλκοῦσιν αὐτά — ὅπερ παχυτέρων αὐτῶν ὑποκειμένων οὐδέποτε γενήσεται — διὰ τὸ οἰκείᾳ ὑγρότητι ἐπιτείνειν αὐτὰ καὶ [μὴ] διπλασιάζειν τὸ δριμὺ καὶ δακνῶδες τῶν πρὸς ἔκκρισιν ἐπειγομένων χυμῶν. κάλλιον οὖν ἐστιν ἐν τοῖς νοσήμασι τούτοις τὴν διὰ τῆς ἀσιτίας τῶν χυμῶν πέψιν παραλαμβάνειν, ὥστε μὴ κακωθῆναι τὰ κάτισχνα ἐκεῖνα μέρη τοῦ σώματος.

24sq. ὧνπερ – βλαβήσεται] *cf.* Gal. In Aphor. II 35: XVII B 533,14–534,2 K.

6 *fort. post* μόρια *addendum est* μέτοχα 9 πεττικόν A 15 οὕτω] *fort.* ὥστε *scribendum est* 18 παραπολαβεῖν α: *correxi* 19 ἐπινοημένου P: *fort.* ἐπιναομένου *scribendum est (cf. Steph., In Progn. I 16: CMG XI 1,2, p. 68,6)* περιεφόρησε A 21 τῷ ... θερμῷ A 32 τὸ *om.* A 34 ἕλκουσιν A 35 μὴ *delevi*

the epigastrium itself, which we also call the navel, and the hypogastrium, which is the lower part of the belly, also named abdomen.

Now you must know that Nature, having great concern for our internal heat, has made use of two organs to this end, namely the heart and the liver, and especially the heart, which was from the first produced by Nature as the workshop and fountainhead of our innate heat. From these the other parts derive (?) their innate heat, each sharing in it according to its size, the importance of its function, and its usefulness. There is more participation of it in one place, less in another: thus, much heat is provided for the stomach, but very little for the bladder, because the former is a digestive organ, which furnishes food, as if from a storeroom, for the liver and the entire body, while the latter is a container, i.e. a vessel serving to receive the whey-like surplus matter. For this reason Nature has placed the heart near the stomach, so that the stomach should have its heat supplied abundantly and as it were at first hand; further she placed the liver in front of it to the right, so that it should receive from that part too the warmth it needs; and on its left she placed the spleen, which thus would also become a source of heat for it; it is true that this organ is essentially a cold one, but by means of the arteries and veins that run through it, Nature nevertheless contrived for the stomach to receive a certain measure of heat on that side too. She also bestowed considerable care on the preservation of the heat which is supplied to the stomach by a variety of devices. She protected it by the so-called omentum, which envelops it on all sides, so that the heat in it cannot be dissipated and the digestive process fail through cooling.

Hence, if in diseases there is emaciation in the region of the navel and the abdomen, this is bad, because then the stomach is deprived of its natural coverings which protect the innate heat, and without which it will readily disperse, by which dispersal the digestion of food will suffer. Nor will concoction of humors take place; for unconcocted and unwholesome humors are transformed and concocted by the natural heat; but when neither the food is digested nor the humors are concocted, the power of resistance breaks down. After this, what hope is there for such patients?

In addition to this, there is often need for a purge in this kind of diseases, but you must on no account take this risk. The region of the navel and the abdomen is now thin and without substance; and the humors, provoked and drawn out by the purgative, during their passage assail the solid parts of the body with their pungency and ulcerate them – which will never happen as long as these parts are thicker –, for by their own moistness they intensify and double the pungent and biting quality of the humors on their way to excretion. It is better, therefore, in these diseases, to proceed to concoction of the humors by fasting, so that those emaciated parts of the body do not suffer.

II 35 [II 36: IV 480,14–15 L.] Οἱ ὑγιεινὰ τὰ σώματα ἔχοντες ἐν τῇσι φαρμακείῃσι καθαιρόμενοι ἐκλύονται ταχέως καὶ οἱ πονηρᾷ τροφῇ χρεόμενοι.

Πολλοὶ πολλάκις διὰ βάρος τοῦ σώματος ὑπαντῶσι τοῖς ἰατροῖς βούλεσθαι φάσκοντες καθαρθῆναι. ὁ δὲ ἰατρὸς πάντα περιελθὼν εὑρίσκει κακοχυμίαν ἐν τῷ σώματι καὶ ὑπαγορεύει, ὅτι δεῖ παρέχειν τὴν κάθαρσιν· καὶ καλῶς πέρας τοῦτον διαδέχεται κενουμένου τοῦ λυποῦντος χυμοῦ. ὑποκείσθω δὲ ἕτερος ὑγιῶς μὲν ἔχων τοῦ σώματος, λαβὼν δὲ καθάρσιον παρά τινος ἰατροῦ ἰδιώτου, ὅπερ ἐπὶ λύμῃ γίνεται. ἀρίστη γὰρ ἦν ἐν αὐτῷ ἡ ὑγεία, ἡ δὲ ἀρίστη ὑγεία συμμετρία ἐστὶ καὶ εὐκρασία τοῦ σώματος· ἔνθα δὲ συμμετρία καὶ εὐκρασία τοῦ σώματος, οὐδὲν περιττόν. ἀπέριττος οὖν ὑπάρχων ἔλαβε τὸ καθάρσιον· τοῦτο ἐν τῇ γαστρὶ γενόμενον περινοστεῖ ὃν ὤφειλε κενῶσαι χυμόν· ὃν μὴ εὑρίσκον κατὰ τοῦ σώματος αὐτοῦ χωρεῖ καὶ ἀναστοιχειοῖ αὐτοῦ τὴν ἕξιν, καὶ ἅπτεται πνευμάτων, ἅπτεται ὑγρῶν, ἅπτεται καὶ τῶν στερεῶν, καὶ τὰ μὲν σκεδαννύει καὶ διαφορεῖ, τὰ δὲ συντήκει ἤτοι ἀναβιβρώσκει. γίνεται τοίνυν ἐν τοῖς τοιούτοις λιποθυμία καὶ συγκοπὴ τῆς οὐσίας αὐτῆς ἀναλυομένης.

Τὸ δὲ ταχέως πρόσκειται, ἐπειδὴ καὶ οἱ διὰ κακοχυμίαν καθαιρόμενοι λιποθυμοῦσι πολλάκις ἀπὸ ἀμετρίας, ἀλλὰ βραδέως· διὰ τοῦτο οὖν ἐπὶ τῶν τοιούτων τὸ ταχέως ἔταξεν, ἐπειδὴ ὑγιεῖς ὑπόκεινται.

Εἶτά φησι· καὶ οἱ πονηρᾷ τροφῇ χρεόμενοι. τροφὴν ἐνταῦθα λέγει τὴν κατὰ ποιότητα βλάπτουσαν. οἷον μέλλων τις καθαρθῆναι καὶ προδιαιτηθῆναι κελευσθεὶς ἐχρήσατο κρομμύοις ἢ φακῷ ἤ τισι τοιούτοις εἰς τροφὴν μεταξύ. ἐν γοῦν τῷ ἄρχεσθαι καθαίρεσθαι ἐκλύεται· τοῦτο δὲ γίνεται ἐκ τῆς προσφάτως ἀθροισθείσης αὐτῷ μοχθηρᾶς ποιότητος, ἥτις παριοῦσα διὰ τῶν αἰσθητικῶν μορίων δριμεῖα καὶ δακνώδης τυγχάνουσα τῇ ἀνίᾳ καὶ δήξει τὴν ἔκ[κ]λυσιν ἐπιφέρει. ὥστε οὖν ἐν ταῖς μεταξὺ πρὸ τοῦ καθαρσίου ἡμέραις δεῖ τὸν τοιοῦτον ἀποζέματι χρήσασθαι τῷ διὰ γλήχωνος καὶ ἀνήθου καὶ σελίνου καὶ ἀνίσου καὶ τῶν τοιούτων, ὅσα λεπτύνειν εἴωθε καὶ τέμνειν καὶ συμπέττειν τοὺς παχεῖς τε καὶ ὠμοὺς χυμοὺς καὶ ἐπιτηδείους παρασκευάσαι πρὸς ἔκκρισιν· εὐθὺς δὲ καὶ ὅπου τις δριμεῖα ποιότης εὑρεθῇ ἐκ τῶν προηγησαμένων τροφῶν, ταύτην καταπραΰνει καὶ μεταβάλλει. καὶ τοῦτό ἐστι τὸ «προεξευκρινήσαντας ποιέειν».

II 36 [II 37: IV 480,16 L.] Τοῖς εὖ τὸ σῶμα ἔχουσι τὸ φαρμακεύεσθαι ἐργῶδες.

Ἔδει τὸν παρόντα ἀφορισμὸν προταγῆναι τοῦ προσεχῶς εἰρημένου. φησὶ γὰρ ὁ Ἱπποκράτης, ὅτι οἱ εὖ τὰ σώματα ἔχοντες ἔργα ἑαυτοῖς τε καὶ τῷ ἰατρῷ παρ-

11 ἀπέριττος – 15 συγκοπὴ] *v.* Theoph. In Aphor.: II 329,14–20 Dietz τοῦτο – 15 ἀναβιβρώσκει] *cf.* Gal. In Aphor. II 37: XVII B 536,12–537,2 K. 22 ἐν – 25 ἐπιφέρει] *v.* Theoph. In Aphor.: II 329,21–26 Dietz 31 προεξευκρινήσαντας ποιέειν] Hipp. Aphor. I 24: IV 470,5 L. 34–218,4] *cf.* Gal. In Aphor. II 37: XVII B 536,5–9 K.

1 ὑγιεινὰ] *item infra, p. 218,4*: ὑγιεινῶς *Hipp.* ἔχοντες τὰ σώματα *infra, p. 218,4, Hipp.* 2 οἱ] ἡ P 5 φάσκοντες *scripsi*: πάσχοντες α 6 *fort.* καλὸν *scribendum est* 12 εὑρίσκων α: *correxi* 13 ἀναστοιχοῖ A 14 *ante* καὶ[I] *add.* δὲ A 16 αὐτοῖς *(e corr.)* A 18 τὸ *om.* P 25 ἀνοία A ἔκκλυσιν α: *correxi* 28 τε *om.* P 32sq. Οἱ εὖ τὰ σώματα ἔχοντες φαρμακεύεσθαι ἐργώδεες *Hipp.*

II 35. Those with healthy bodies will quickly collapse during purging, as well as those who take the wrong kind of food.

Many people come to see their doctors because of overweight, requesting to be purged. The doctor, after a thorough examination, finds a bad humor in the body, and declares that a purge should be applied; and he gets a good result, for the troublesome humor is evacuated. But let us take the case of another man, who, while in good health, is given a purgative by an incompetent doctor; this leads to serious damage. For his health was excellent, and excellent health is due proportion and a well-tempered condition of the body; and where there is due proportion and a well-tempered condition of the body, there is no excess matter. So he took the purgative while free from excess matter; the purgative, upon reaching the stomach, searches for the humor which it is supposed to evacuate, and finding none, it assails the body itself and decomposes its constitution: it sets upon the gases, the fluids, even the solids, dissipating and dispersing the former, dissolving or corroding the latter. The result in such cases is fainting and collapse, because the substance itself is disintegrated.

Quickly is added because often those who are purged for a bad humor will also faint owing to an overdose, but slowly; hence the quickly in reference to these cases, since they were healthy to begin with.

He goes on, as well as those who take the wrong kind of food. He is referring here to food that causes harm by its quality. For instance, someone who is going to have a purge and who has been told to observe a diet before the cure, eats onions or lentils or similar food in the meantime. So he collapses at the beginning of the purge; this is due to humor of bad quality which he has just collected in himself: its passage through the sensitive parts, pungent and corrosive as it is, brings about the prostration through soreness and irritation. Therefore in the intervening days before the purge such a person should take a decoction of pennyroyal, dill, celery, anise, and similar herbs, which comminute, fragmentize and concoct the thick and crude humors and prepare them for excretion; at the same time, wherever some pungent quality is found as the result of food taken earlier, they soothe and transform it. This is the sense of "after thorough preparation".

II 36. With those in good condition purging is laborious.

The present aphorism ought to be placed before the one immediately preceding it. Hippocrates says purging those in good condition means trouble for

ἔχουσι φαρμακευόμενοι. εἶθ' ὥς τινος ἀποροῦντος ὅτι «Τίνος ἕνεκεν οὗτοι ἔργα παρέχουσιν ἑαυτοῖς καὶ τῷ ἰατρῷ;» νόησον ἐπαγόμενον τὸν προλεχθέντα ἀφορισμόν, «Ἐπειδὴ ταχέως λιποθυμοῦσι», τουτέστιν «ἐκλύονται»· ἔφη γὰρ ἐν ἐκείνῳ ὅτι «Οἱ ὑγιεινὰ ἔχοντες τὰ σώματα ἐν τῇσι φαρμακείῃσι καθαιρόμενοι ἐκλύονται ταχέως».

II 37 [II 38: IV 480,17–18 L.] Τὸ σμικρὸν χεῖρον καὶ πόμα καὶ σιτίον, ἥδιον δέ, τῶν βελτιόνων μέν, ἀηδεστέρων δέ, μᾶλλον αἱρετέον.

Ὅπερ νῦν φησι, καὶ ἐν τῇ ἕκτῃ Ἐπιδημίᾳ εἶπεν· «Αἱ χάριτες τοῖς νοσέουσι» καὶ τὰ ἑξῆς· «χάριτάς» φησι τὰς ἐκ τῶν ἰατρικῶν δώρων χαριζομένας τοῖς νοσοῦσιν· εἰσὶ δὲ αὗται τὸ τὸ σμικρόν τι χεῖρον τῇ τοῦ κάμνοντος ἐπιθυμίᾳ χαρίσασθαι. οἷον ὑποκείσθω τις διακαῆ καὶ ζέοντα πυρετὸν πυρέττων, ἐφ' οὗ κέχρημαι μέχρι τρίτης ἡμέρας μελικράτῳ. εἶτα εἰσερχόμενος ἐν τῇ τετάρτῃ ἡμέρᾳ καὶ εὑρίσκων αὐτὸν λιχνευόμενον μεταλαβεῖν ὕδατος περιέρχομαι πάντα ζητῶν τὰ περὶ αὐτὸν καὶ ἐν αὐτῷ θεωρούμενα, μὴ ὑπόκειται φλεγμαῖνον ἧπαρ ἢ ὑποχόνδρια ἢ στόμαχος ἀσθενὴς ἢ κῶλον ἢ νεφρὸς φλεγμονὴν ἔχων. καὶ εὑρηκὼς πάντα ταῦτα ὑγιῶς διακείμενα ἀνακρίνω ἔτι, εἰ ἔθος ἐστὶ ψυχροποσίας τῷ κάμνοντι, καὶ τυχὸν εὑρίσκω. εἶτα λαμβάνω καὶ τὴν χώραν καὶ τὴν ὥραν καὶ τὴν ἡλικίαν συμφώνως ἔχοντα, καὶ ἐπὶ τῇ συμφωνίᾳ τούτων πάντων δίδωμι κατὰ τέχνην μὲν τὸ ὕδωρ, χαριζόμενος δὲ τὸ δοκεῖν τῇ ἐπιθυμίᾳ τοῦ νοσοῦντος. ὅπερ ὡς ἡδὺ καὶ ἐράσμιον ληφθὲν τῷ κάμνοντι ἠγκαλίσατο ἡ φύσις τῇ καθεκτικῇ δυνάμει χρωμένη ἠλλοίωσέ τε αὐτὸ καὶ ἐκέρδησε τὴν ἐξ αὐτοῦ εὐκρασίαν, καὶ τοσοῦτον ὥστε καὶ τὸ νόσημα παύσασθαι.

Τοῦτο γοῦν ἐστι τὸ σμικρὸν χεῖρον. εἰ γὰρ μὴ ἐπιδῶμεν τῆς ἐπιθυμίας περὶ τοῦτο κινουμένης, καὶ ἐν ἑτέρῳ καιρῷ τῆς νόσου ἀπεπτούσης χρείαν ἔχομεν παρασχεῖν αὐτὸ ἀνηδόνως καὶ ἀνορέκτως λαμβανόμενον καὶ μηδὲ τὸ οἰκεῖον ἐνταῦθα ποιῆσαι δυνάμενον. τούτου οὖν χάριν δοτέον τοῖς ἐπιθυμοῦσι καὶ ὑπερθετέον τὴν ἐπίδοσιν ἐν τῷ καιρῷ τῆς ἐπιθυμίας. ὥσπερ γὰρ ἐπὶ τῶν ὑγιαινόντων πολλὰ λαμβανόμενα τὰ σιτία ἀνήδονα καὶ ἀπροσηνῆ τῇ φύσει λογίζεται, τὰ δὲ ὀλίγα καὶ μέτρια προσηνῶς καὶ μεθ' ἡδονῆς ἡ φύσις ἐναγκαλίζεται, οὕτω καὶ ἐπὶ τῶν νοσούντων τὴν μὲν πολλὴν τοῦ μελικράτου χύσιν τυχόν τις ὡς ἀηδῆ ἀπεστράφη, τὸ δὲ ὀλίγον ὕδωρ ἐρασμίως ὑπεδέξατο, ὡς εὑρεθῆναι τὴν τούτου χρῆσιν μᾶλλον τῆς τροφῆς χρησιμεύσασαν.

Ὡσαύτως δὲ καὶ ἐπὶ τῆς τροφῆς δεῖ ποιεῖν· ἐὰν γὰρ τῇ πολλῇ χρώμενος πτισάνῃ πυρέττων εἴπῃ σοι τῷ ἰατρῷ ἀκηδιάσας· «Μετέλθοιμι λοιπὸν ἐφ' ἑτέραν τροφήν, ἐπὶ ἄρτον τυχὸν ὕδατι δεδευμένον», πάρεχε αὐτῷ, κἂν χρεία πτισάνης ἐστίν. ἡδύτερον γὰρ τοῦτο λαμβάνει, ὅπερ μέγα δύναται ἐπὶ τῶν νοσούντων, τὸ μετά τινος ἡδονῆς λαμβάνεσθαι τὰς τροφάς. ὅπερ καὶ ἀνωτέρω ἔφη· «καὶ εὖ ἔχειν πρὸς τὰς προσφορὰς ἀγαθόν».

3 ἐκλύονται] Hipp. Aphor. II 36: IV 480,15 L. 3sq. Οἱ – ταχέως] Hipp. Aphor. II 36: IV 480,14–15 L. 7 Αἱ – νοσέουσι] Hipp. Epid. VI 4,7: V 308,13–15 L. *cf.* Theoph. In Aphor.: II 330,18–19 Dietz 9 οἷον – 18 νοσοῦντος] *cf. supra*, p. 116,10–18 17 χαριζόμενος – 20] *cf.* Gal. In Aphor. II 38: XVII B 537,6–9 K. 34sq. καὶ[II] – ἀγαθόν] Hipp. Aphor. II 33: IV 480,5–6 L.

3 ὅτι *om.* P 4 τοῦ σώματος α: *sec. Hipp. correxi* 5 σμικρὸν] *item supra, p. 78,24; infra, lin. 21, Hipp.* V, *Theoph.* U'': σμικρῷ *Hipp. plerique* 6 τῶν] τὸ P 9 χαρίσασθαι *scripsi*: χρήσασθαι α 13 ὑποχόνδρ *(ambig.)* P 14 νεφροὶ P ταῦτα πάντα A 17 τὸ[II]] *fort.* τῷ *scribendum est* 26 λογίζονται A 31 εἴπει A μετέλθοιμε P 32 ἄρτου A

the patients themselves and for the physician. Then, as if somebody had asked: "Why does it mean trouble for the patients themselves and for the physician?", the preceding aphorism should be read as the sequel: "Because they quickly faint", i.e., "collapse"; for that other one ran: "Those with healthy bodies will quickly collapse during purging".

II 37. Drink and food which, though slightly less good, are tastier, should be preferred to those which are better, but less palatable.

What he says here, is also expressed in Epidemics VI: "Favors to patients", etc., meaning those favors which it is in the doctor's power to bestow upon patients, that is to say, allowing something slightly less good in order to fall in with the patient's wish. Let us take, for instance, a patient with a burning, seething fever, whom I have treated with honey-and-water until the third day. Then, when I visit him on the fourth and find that he is longing for a drink of water, I thoroughly examine every circumstance around him and in him, if there is no inflammation of the liver or the hypochondria, no weak stomach, no inflamed colum or kidney. Having found that all this is sound, I inquire if the patient has the habit of drinking cold water, and let us say I find it to be the case; next I make sure that the region, the season and the patient's age also agree, and on the ground of the agreement between all these, I let him have the water, in accordance with the rules of the art, though apparently to comply with the patient's wish. Since it is received by the patient as something nice and pleasant, his constitution accepts it through the retentive faculty, then transforms it and derives from it the benefit of a well-tempered condition, to the extent that even the sickness comes to an end.

This then is the sense of slightly less good. For if we do not yield to the desire for it, when it is stirred, we will yet have to give it at another stage of the disease, when there is no concoction, when it is taken without pleasure and without desire, and thus cannot even do its work. Therefore we should give it to those who want it and put off giving it until the moment when it is wanted. Just as, in the case of healthy people, food taken in great quantity is considered unappetizing and unsuitable to the constitution, while a small, moderate quantity is accepted with joy by the constitution, so a sick man too may turn away from a liberal supply of honey-and-water as distasteful to him, while he eagerly accepts that little drink of water, so that it proves more useful to him than the food.

With regard to food you should act on the same lines: if a fever patient, tired of all the barley-water, says to you, his doctor: "I should like to change to something else now, for example bread soaked in water", let him have it, even though barley-water is indicated. For he takes it with more pleasure, and this is an important thing for sick people, to take their food with a certain pleasure. He said this already above: "a good appetite is a favorable sign".

II 38 [II 39: IV 480,19–482,2 L.] Οἱ πρεσβῦται τῶν νέων τὰ μὲν πλεῖστα νοσέουσιν ἧσσον· ὁκόσα δὲ αὐτοῖς χρόνια νοσήματα γίνεται, τὰ πολλὰ ξυναποθνήσκει.

Φησίν, ὅτι δύο συζυγίαι εἰσὶ καθ' ἑκατέραν ἡλικίαν, φημὶ δὴ γεροντικὴν καὶ ἀκμαστικήν· πλεονασμὸς καὶ ἧττα, νόσος καὶ θάνατος. καὶ ἐπὶ μὲν τῶν ἀκμαζόντων πλεονάζει τὰ νοσήματα, ἡττᾶται δὲ ὁ θάνατος· ἐπὶ δὲ τῶν γερόντων ἡττᾶται τὰ νοσήματα, νικᾷ δὲ ὁ θάνατος, εἰ γάρ ποτε γένωνται ἐπ' αὐτῶν, θάνατον ἀπεργάζονται. τοῦτο δὲ γίνεται, ἐπειδὴ οἱ γέροντες βεβηκότα καὶ καθεστηκότα ἔχουσι τὸν λογισμὸν καὶ φείδονται ἀδηφαγίας, ἐφ' ἧς πλῆθος γεννᾶται περιττωμάτων· ἀπέριττοι δὲ τὰ πολλὰ τυγχάνοντες ἧττον νοσοῦσιν. οἱ δὲ νέοι διὰ τὸ τοῦ λογισμοῦ ἄστατον καὶ μετέωρον καὶ διὰ τὴν τῶν σιτίων ἀπληστοτέραν προσαγωγὴν ἀπεψίαις ἑτοιμότατα περιπίπτοντες εὐχερῶς καὶ ὡς ἐπὶ πᾶν νοσοῦσιν. ἢ καὶ διὰ τὰς πράξεις, ἃς ἑκάτεροι μεταχειρίζονται, τὸ τοιοῦτον συμβαίνει. οἱ γὰρ νεώτεροι καὶ γυμνασίοις κέχρηνται καὶ κυνηγεσίοις καὶ ἐν πολέμοις ἐκστρατείαις καὶ τοῖς τοιούτοις· ἐφ' οἷς ἄμετρα κινούμενοι κοπιῶσι, κἀντεῦθεν πολλὰ συμβαίνειν τούτοις νοσήματα εἴωθεν. οἱ δὲ πρεσβῦται οἰκουροῦσιν ἐν ἡσυχίᾳ καὶ ἀνέσει ὡς τὰ πολλὰ διάγοντες, κἀντεῦθεν τὰ πολλὰ τῶν νοσημάτων διαφεύγουσι.

Τῇ μὲν οὖν γεροντικῇ ἡλικίᾳ ἀσυμφώνως ἡ ἐπιληψία προσγίνεται, τῇ δὲ ἀκμαστικῇ συμφώνως. καλῶς τοιγαροῦν ὁ Ἱπποκράτης φησίν· Οἱ πρεσβῦται τῶν νέων τὰ μὲν πλεῖστα νοσέουσιν ἧσσον· ὁκόσα δὲ αὐτέοισι χρόνια νοσήματα γίνονται, τὰ πολλὰ ξυναποθνήσκει. τὰ γὰρ γινόμενα σφίσι χρόνια νοσήματα διὰ τὴν ἡλικίαν ὡς ἐπὶ πᾶν γίνεται, χηρεύουσι τοῦ κατὰ φύσιν θερμοῦ, ὑφ' οὗ ἡ τῶν ὑλῶν πέψις γίνεται· κἀντεῦθεν εἰς χρόνον πλείονα παρεκτεινόμενα ἐπὶ αὐτῶν τὰ νοσήματα ἔστιν ὅτε καὶ συναποθνήσκει διὰ τὴν τῆς δυνάμεως ἀσθένειαν, τῷ χρόνῳ συμπαρομαρτοῦντος δὴ τοῦ νοσήματος.

Καλῶς δὲ πρόσκειται τὰ πολλὰ ξυναποθνήσκει· οὐδὲν γὰρ ἄτοπον ἐπιπολαιοτέραν εἶναι τὴν νόσον, ὥστε τὴν ἐν αὐτοῖς δύναμιν ἐρρωμενεστέραν εἶναι ὡς πρὸς τὴν νόσον καὶ μὴ συγχωρῆσαι γενέσθαι θάνατον.

II 39 [II 40: IV 482,3–4 L.] Βράγχοι καὶ βῆχες καὶ κόρυζαι τοῖσι σφόδρα πρεσβυτέροισιν οὐ πεπαίνονται.

Οὗτος ὁ ἀφορισμὸς τὸν γοῦν προσλαβὼν σύνδεσμον συνεχὴς τῷ πρὸ αὐτοῦ εὑρεθήσεται. εἰρηκὼς γὰρ ἀνωτέρω ὅτι «ὅσα γίνεται τοῖς πρεσβύταις νοσήματα, χρόνια γίνεται καὶ τὰ πολλὰ ξυναποθνήσκει», ὥς τινος τὴν αἰτίαν τούτου πυθομένου

8 τοῦτο – 12 νοσοῦσιν] *v.* Theoph. In Aphor.: II 331,4–10 Dietz 21 τὰ[II] – 25] *v.* Gal. In Aphor. II 39: XVII B 538,8–12 K. 31–222,2 πεπαίνονται] *v.* Gal. In Aphor. II 40: XVII B 539,1–7 K. 32 εἰρηκὼς – 222,3] *v.* Theoph. In Aphor.: II 331,21–26 Dietz 32sq. ὅσα – ξυναποθνήσκει] Hipp. Aphor. II 39: IV 482,1–2 L.

1 πλεῖστα] *item infra, lin. 20, Hipp.* C′: πολλὰ *Hipp. plerique, Theoph.* 2 ὁκόσα] *item infra, lin. 20, Theoph.*: ὅσα *Hipp. plerique* δὲ] *item infra, lin. 20, Hipp.* C′, *Theoph.* V′′: δ' ἂν *Hipp. plerique, Theoph.* SU′′ 7 γένονται A: γένοιται P: *correxi* 11 τὴν *om.* P 12 ἢ *scripsi*: οἱ α 14 κυνηγεσίαις A 21 συναποθνήσκει A 29 καὶ βῆχες *Hipp. perpauci*: *om. supra, p. 212,19; infra, p. 222,1; non hab. Hipp. cett.* 30 πρεσβυτέροισιν] *item supra, p. 212,20. 22; infra, p. 222,2; vol. II, fol. 23*v, *Hipp.* C′, *Theoph.* U′′: πρεσβύτῃσιν *Hipp.* MV, *Theoph.* SV′′ 31 προλαβὼν P 33 τούτου *scripsi*: τοῦ P: γοῦν A πειθομένου A

II 38. Old men on the whole are less often ill than young men; but such chronic diseases as they contract usually die with them.

He says that there are two pairs of possibilities in each of the two age groups, old age and the prime of life: namely, prevailing and yielding, disease and death. With those in their prime, diseases prevail, but death yields; in the case of old men, diseases yield, but death prevails, for if they ever catch a disease, it causes death. The explanation of this is that old men have staid and sober minds and refrain from overeating, which produces a great quantity of waste matter; so, being usually free from waste matter, they are less often ill. Young men, on the other hand, owing to the instability and levity of their reason and to the gluttony with which they consume their food, fall easy victims to indigestions, and so it happens easily and commonly for them to be ill. Or it may be a consequence of the way in which each group is occupied. The business of younger men is athletics, hunting, military campaigns, etc.; these entail excessive and exhausting exercise, which leads to many illnesses. Old men, on the other hand, stay at home and spend most of their time in rest and relaxation, and in this way they escape most diseases.

Now epilepsy is a disease which is not conformable to old age, but is conformable to the prime of life. Therefore Hippocrates says rightly: Old men on the whole are less often ill than young men; but such chronic diseases as they contract usually die with them. The chronic diseases, indeed, which befall them, are for the most part due to their age, because they lack the natural heat which causes the concoction of matter of various kinds; hence their diseases extend over a longer period of time, and sometimes die with them, because of the weakness of their resistance, the course of the disease obviously following the course of time.

The restriction usually die with them is made for good reason; for it is quite common for the disease to be of a more superficial type, so that their resistance is too strong for the disease and prevents death.

II 39. Sore throats, coughs and running noses in extremely old people do not ripen.

If the conjunction "for" is prefixed to this aphorism, it will be found to be a sequel to its predecessor. Having said above, "Such diseases as old men contract become chronic and usually die with them", he seems to expect somebody to inquire after the cause of this, and so he continues with the present aphorism,

ἐπάγει τὸν παρόντα ἀφορισμὸν ἔχοντα οὕτως· Βράγχοι γοῦν καὶ κόρυζαι τοῖσι σφόδρα πρεσβυτέροισιν οὐ πεπαίνονται, ἐπειδὴ ἀσθενεῖ τὸ ἐν αὐτοῖς ἔμφυτον θερμὸν καὶ οὐ δύνανται ἐκπέψαι καὶ ἀπολεπτῦναι τὰς τοιαύτας ὕλας.

Αἵτινες γίνονται τρόπῳ τοιούτῳ· τὸ λόγῳ τῆς τροφῆς ἐν τῷ ἐγκεφάλῳ φερόμενον ἀσθενούσης ἐν αὐτῷ τῆς ἀλλοιωτικῆς δυνάμεως ἀπεπτεῖται καὶ ψύχεται καὶ οἷον ἀποφλεγματοῦται· ὅπερ πλημμυροῦν ἀντικαταρρεῖ καὶ ἓν ὑπάρχον ποικίλα ἀπεργάζεται νοσήματα παρὰ τοὺς ὑποδεχομένους αὐτὸ διαφόρους τόπους. ἐπὶ ῥῖνας μὲν γὰρ ἐνεχθὲν τὴν καλουμένην ἀπεργάζεται κόρυζαν· ἐπὶ δὲ τὴν ὑπερῴαν καὶ τὴν τραχεῖαν ἀρτηρίαν, τοὺς λεγομένους βράγχους καὶ τὸν κατάρρουν· εἰ δὲ κάτω εἰς τὸν θώρακα ἐμπέσοι, τὴν καλουμένην βῆχα ποιεῖ. καὶ ἐπειδὴ ὑπόκειται ἥ τε δύναμις ἐπὶ τῶν γερόντων ἀσθενὴς τό τε ἔμφυτον θερμὸν ὀλίγον καὶ ἀδρανές, μὴ πεττομένης τῆς ὕλης, ἀλλὰ χρονιζόντων ἐπ' αὐτῶν τῶν εἰρημένων παθῶν θάνατος ἕπεται· σφόδρα γάρ εἰσι γέροντες.

II 40 [II 41: IV 482,5–6 L.] Οἱ ἐκλυόμενοι πολλάκις καὶ ἰσχυρῶς ἄνευ φανερῆς προφάσιος ἐξαπίνης τελευτῶσιν.

Σημειωτικός ἐστιν ὁ παρὼν ἀφορισμὸς τοῦ μέλλοντος, τὸν μὲν θάνατον δηλῶν, οὐ μήν γε κατὰ τὸν σύνεγγυς χρόνον, ἀλλὰ τὸν πόρρω. δεῖ τοίνυν εἰδέναι, ὅτι πάθος, ἵνα μᾶλλον γένηται πάθος, ἀπὸ τοῦ δρῶντος ἐπὶ τὸ ἐνεργούμενον ἔρχεται. τριῶν τοίνυν ἐστὶ χρεία, ἐπιτηδειότητος τοῦ κάμνοντος, μεγέθους τοῦ δρῶντος καὶ τῆς μεταξὺ τοῦ χρόνου δαψιλείας· ἑνὸς δὲ τούτων ἀπόντος ἀδύνατον γενέσθαι πάθος. πρὸς σαφήνειαν δὲ τῶν λεγομένων ὑποκείσθω τὸ ποιοῦν δραστήριον, οἷον σίδηρος ἠκονημένος καὶ τμητικώτατος· ἀνεπιτήδειον δὲ τὸ πάσχον, οἷον ἀδάμας· καὶ χρόνος πολύς, ἐν ᾧ περὶ τὸ ὑποκείμενον δοκεῖ δρᾶν τὸ ποιοῦν. δῆλον οὖν, ὡς ἀδύνατον πάθος τὸ τηνικαῦτα ἐν τῷ ἀδάμαντι γενέσθαι διὰ τὸ μὴ πεφυκέναι αὐτὸν ἐνδαμάζεσθαι σιδήρῳ. πάλιν ὑποκείσθω τὸ μὲν πάσχον ἐπιτήδειον, οἷον κηρὸς μαλακὸς ἢ ἕτερόν τι σῶμα, ἄρτος τυχὸν ἢ κρέας, εὔλυτον τοῖς τέμνουσι· καὶ ὁ ἐν τῷ μεταξὺ χρόνος τῆς τοῦ δρῶντος ἐνεργείας ἐν τῷ πάσχοντι πολύς· τὸ ποιοῦν δὲ ἀνεπιτηδείως ἔχον πρὸς τὸ τέμνειν, οἷον σίδηρος μὴ σχηματισθεὶς τμητικῶς ἢ ξύλον ἢ λίθος. ἐνταῦθα οὖν πάλιν οὐ τμηθήσεται τὸ ὑποκείμενον διὰ τὴν ἀνεπιτηδειότητα τοῦ δρῶντος. ὡσαύτως δὲ καί, εἰ τὸ ποιοῦν δραστήριον ὑποτεθῇ, οἷον πῦρ, καὶ τὸ πάσχον ἐπιτήδειον, οἷον στυβὴ ἢ στυππίον, ἐλάχιστος δὲ ὁ ἐν τῷ μεταξὺ τοῦ δρῶντος πρὸς τὸ ἐνεργούμενον χρόνος, οὐδ' οὕτως γενήσεται πάθος ἐν τῷ ὑποκειμένῳ. οὕτω γοῦν διὰ φλογὸς τὴν χεῖρα πολλάκις ἐν ἀκαριαίῳ χρόνῳ παροδεύοντες οὐδὲν ὑπὸ τοῦ πυρὸς πάσχομεν· εἰ μέντοι καὶ χρόνον ἀξιόλογον ἔχοι τὸ δρῶν, ἐνεργεῖ πρὸς τὴν τοῦ ὑποκειμένου ἐπιτηδειότητα. τούτων οὕτως ἐχόντων ἔλθωμεν ἐπὶ τὴν ἐξήγησιν.

Οἱ ἐκλυόμενοι πολλάκις καὶ ἰσχυρῶς. ἔκλυσιν δὲ νοητέον τὴν λιποθυμίαν, ἥτις δι' ἀσθένειαν τοῦ ζωτικοῦ γίνεται. καὶ ἰδοὺ τὰ μὲν δύο κατασκευάζει, τό τε ποιοῦν καὶ τὸν χρόνον· τὴν δὲ τοῦ πάσχοντος ἐπιτηδειότητα ὡς ὁμολογουμένην

13 σφόδρα – γέροντες] *cf. supra*, p. 212,22–23 17 δεῖ – 35] *cf.* Gal. De temp. III 4: p. 104,8–20 Helmr. = I 675,11–676,7 K.

2 πρεσβυτέροις P 4 λόγῳ] λεῖον A 7 αὐτῶ A 15 προφάσεως P 16 τὸν *scripsi:* τὰ α δηλοῦντος α: *correxi* 18 ἐπὶ] πρὸς A 19 κάμνοντος] *fort.* πάσχοντος *scribendum est* 25 ἐπικείσθω A 27 πάσχοντι] κάμνοντι A ἀνεπιτηδείους P 28 τέμνον A τμητικὸς α: *correxi* 31 στυπτίον A (?) P: *correxi* 34 τοῦ *om.* A 37 ζωτικοῦ] ζώου A

which runs as follows: For sore throats and running noses in extremely old people do not ripen, their innate heat being too weak to concoct and comminute such kinds of matter.

This matter is formed in the following manner: That which is conveyed to the brain by way of food remains unconcocted, owing to weakness of its transformative faculty, and it becomes cold and is as it were converted into phlegm; running over, it flows back downward, where, though being one and the same, it brings about a variety of diseases according to the different parts of the body that receive it. Conveyed to the nose, it causes the so-called running nose; to the palate and the windpipe, so-called sore throats and catarrh; if it sinks low and invades the chest, it causes what we call cough. And since in the case of old men resistance is already weak and their innate heat slight and ineffectual, if the matter is not concocted and the affections mentioned above linger with them, death must follow; for they are extremely old.

II 40. Those who have frequent and violent collapses without any visible cause, die suddenly.

This aphorism deals with a sign indicative of the future, which forecasts death, not, however, in the near, but in a remote future. It should be understood, then, that an affection, if it is to be an affection in the stricter sense, proceeds from the agent toward the object acted upon. Thus, three things are needed: receptivity of the patient, adequate magnitude of the agent, and plenty of intervening time; if one of these is lacking, there can be no affection. To illustrate this, let us assume an effective agent, for instance, a whetted, very sharp steel knife; an unreceptive object, such as a diamond; and a long time during which we suppose the agent is acting upon the object. It is evident that in this case the diamond cannot possibly be affected, because it is naturally proof against steel. Again, let us assume a receptive object, for instance soft wax, or some other body, let us say bread or meat, which is easy to cut with an edged tool; and a lengthy period of time during which the agent acts upon the object; but an agent unsuitable for the purpose of cutting, such as iron without an edge, or wood or stone. In this case the object will once more fail to be cut, owing to the unsuitability of the agent. Similarly, if the agent is assumed to be effective, e.g. fire, and the object receptive, e.g. tow or oakum, but the time during which the agent acts upon the object minimal, the object will not be affected either. Thus if we repeatedly pass our hand through a flame in an indivisible moment, we are not affected by the fire in any way; but if the agent also disposes of an appreciable period of time, it acts in proportion to the receptivity of the object. This having been settled, let us pass on to the interpretation.

Those who have frequent and violent collapses. By collapse we must understand a fainting fit, which is due to weakness of the vital force. As you see, he lays down two (of the three) requirements, the agent and the time; as for the receptivity of the object, this is tacitly taken for granted, for we have

παρεσιώπησε, σῶμα γὰρ ὑπόκειται ἀνθρώπινον, δεκτικὸν πάντων ⟨τῶν⟩ παρὰ φύσιν. τὸν μὲν οὖν χρόνον κατασκευάζει διὰ τοῦ εἰπεῖν πολλάκις· οὐδὲν γὰρ ἄτοπον ἅπαξ γενέσθαι λιποθυμίαν ἐπ' εὐλόγῳ αἰτίᾳ, κενώσει τυχὸν ὑπερβαλλούσῃ ἢ ἀσιτίᾳ ἢ ἀμέτρῳ διαφορήσει, καὶ μὴ ἐπακολουθῆσαι θάνατον. διὰ δὲ τοῦ εἰπεῖν ἰσχυρῶς τὸ μέγεθος ἤτοι τὴν σφοδρότητα τοῦ αἰτίου ἐδήλωσεν. ὥστε ἐὰν ὑποπέσῃ τις πολλάκις καὶ ἰσχυρῶς λιποθυμῶν, θαρρούντως πρόλεγε, ὅτι οὗτος ὁ ἄνθρωπος ἀθρόον τεθνήξεται.

Δεῖται δὲ ἑνὸς προ⟨σ⟩διορισμοῦ τὸ λεγόμενον, ἵνα ἀληθὲς ᾖ. τοῦτο γοῦν φησιν ὁ Γαληνός· «Προσῆλθέ μοι γύναιον λιποθυμίαν χρονίαν αἰτιώμενον. καὶ πολλὰ περιελθὼν καὶ ἀνακρίνας ἠρόμην τὸν χρόνον, καθ' ὃν αὐτῇ τὸ σύμπτωμα συμβαίνει τῆς ἐκλύσεως, ἡ δὲ ἔφη μετὰ λουτρὸν ἀεὶ τοῦτο ὑφίστασθαι. καὶ τότε», φησί, «πολυπραγμονήσας εὗρον τὴν αἰτίαν, ὅτι ὑπὸ μοχθηρᾶς ὕλης τὸ λουτρὸν ὑπεκαίετο· οὐδὲ γὰρ μόνη αὕτη ἐφαίνετο πάσχουσα, ἀλλὰ καὶ πλεῖσται τῶν ἐν τῷ λουτρῷ λουομένων.» καὶ ἄλλο πάλιν γύναιον συνεχῶς λιποθυμοῦν, ὅπερ ἐπὶ ὑστερικοῖς ἀλγήμασιν ἔπασχε τὴν λιποθυμίαν. ἕτερος δὲ πάλιν ἅμα τῷ εἰσελθεῖν ἐν τῷ θερμῷ τοῦ βαλανείου ἀέρι παραχρῆμα ἐλιποθύμει, καὶ τοῦτο διηνεκῶς συνέβαινεν αὐτῷ, καὶ εἰ πολλάκις τῆς ἡμέρας ἐπετήδευσε λούσασθαι, εἰ μὴ προειληφὼς ἦν ἄρτου τι μέρος μέτριον ἐν οἴνῳ βεβρεγμένον. τούτων οὖν καὶ τῶν τοιούτων φανεραὶ αἱ τῆς λιποθυμίας αἰτίαι· αἵτινες προκαταρκτικαὶ ὡς ἐπὶ πᾶν οὖσαι οὐδὲ κίνδυνον ἐπιφέρουσι. τοῦτο οὖν γινώσκων ὁ Ἱπποκράτης προ⟨σ⟩διορισμὸν ἐν τῷ λόγῳ ἔθετο ἄνευ φανερῆς προφάσιος φάμενος, τουτέστιν ἡνίκα μὴ ἐπὶ προκαταρκτικῇ αἰτίᾳ ἡ ἔκλυσις γίνεται· δήλου γὰρ ὄντος τοῦ ποιοῦντος αἰτίου εὔπορος καὶ ἡ τῆς θεραπείας δεῖξις γίνεται.

Ἡ μέντοι λιποθυμία εἰ καὶ πολλάκις γίνεται καὶ ἰσχυρῶς καὶ ἄνευ φανερᾶς αἰτίας, δεῖ προλέγειν θάνατον ἐσόμενον. τίς δὲ ἡ τούτου αἰτία; ἐπειδὴ ἡ λιποθυμία, λεῖψις θυμοῦ τις οὖσα, εἰκὼν ὑπάρχει θανάτου. πολλάκις οὖν λιποθυμοῦντες καὶ ἀεὶ διάλειψίν τινα καὶ διαφόρησιν τοῦ ζωτικοῦ τόνου ὑφιστάμενοι ἥττονες ἑαυτῶν καὶ ἀσθενέστεροι καθ' ἑκάστην γίνονται· εἶτα τούτου πάλιν συμβαίνοντος καὶ τοῦ ἐμφύτου θερμοῦ δι' ὀλιγότητα καὶ ἀσθένειαν τῷ χρόνῳ ἀποσβεννυμένου καὶ σκεδαννυμένου ἐξαίφνης αὐτοῖς ὁ θάνατος ἐπιγίνεται τῶν παρεστώτων ὑπολαμβανόντων, ὅτι κατὰ τὸ εἰωθὸς μετὰ τὴν λιποθυμίαν πάλιν εἰς ἑαυτοὺς ἐπανέρχονται.

Ζητῶν δὲ τὴν αἰτίαν, ὥς φησιν ὁ Γαληνός, πόθεν ἡ συνεχὴς αὕτη τοῖς οὕτω πάσχουσι λιποθυμία, ἥτις τῷ χρόνῳ καὶ εἰς θάνατον ἀποτελευτᾷ, εὗρεν, ὅτι πολλὰ τῶν ζῴων ἀνατμηθέντα τρόπῳ τοιούτῳ ἀδοκήτως πως τεθνηκότα εὕρηνται ἐν ταῖς κοιλίαις τῆς καρδίας χιτῶνά τινα περικείμενον ἔχοντα πεπληρωμένον ὑγροῦ δυσώδους· ὅπερ ὑγρὸν τῇ μοχθηρᾷ ἐκείνῃ ποιότητι διέφθειρεν ἀεὶ καὶ ἐλυμαίνετο

2 τὸν – 7] *cf.* Gal. In Aphor. II 41: XVII B 540,1–3 K. De loc. aff. V 1: VIII 301,1–9 K. 9 Προσῆλθέ – 15 λιποθυμίαν] *v.* Gal. In Aphor. II 41: XVII B 540,4–9 K. Theoph. In Aphor.: II 332,6–9 Dietz 15 ἕτερος – 18 βεβρεγμένον] *v.* Gal. In Aphor. II 41: XVII B 540,10–12 K. 20sq. ἄνευ – φάμενος] *cf.* Gal. In Aphor. II 41: XVII B 540,3–4 K. 25sq. ἐπειδὴ – θανάτου] *cf. supra*, p. 134,6–7 *infra*, vol. III, fol. 169v 32–226,8 αἰσθάνονται] *v.* Gal. De loc. aff. V 2: VIII 303,3–304,5 K. 32–226,1 ἐποίει] *v.* Theoph. In Aphor.: II 332,9–14 Dietz

1 τῶν *addidi* 6 λυποθυμεῖν A θαρροῦντος α: *corr.* P² 8 προδιορισμοῦ α: *correxi* 11 ἀεὶ] αὐτῇ A 13 γὰρ *om.* A 20 προδιορισμὸν α: *correxi* 20sq. φανερᾶς προφάσεως A 22 δῆλον A ὄντος] οὗτος A 29 τοῦ χρόνου P 34 πως *scripsi*: πρὸς P: προσ A

to do with a human body, subject to all abnormal influences. He lays down the time by saying frequent; for a fainting fit may quite well occur just once for an understandable reason, for example excessive evacuation or fasting, or disproportionate dispersal, without resulting in death. By the word violent he expressed the magnitude or intensity of the cause. Consequently, if somebody is subject to frequent deep swoons, you may predict with confidence that this person will die suddenly.

One restriction should be made, if the statement is to hold true. Galen tells us: "I was visited by a woman, who complained of fainting fits spread over a long period. Having questioned her from many angles, I asked the time at which this symptom of fainting happened to her, and she said that it always occurred after a bath. Then", he says, "I inquired into the matter, and found out the cause, namely that the bath-house was heated by unsound fuel; for it turned out that she was not the only victim, but a great many other women who used that bath." There was another woman who fainted constantly, and in her case the fainting was due to uterine pains. Another patient, again, would faint as soon as he entered the hot air of the bath-house, and this happened to him regularly, even if he bathed several times a day, unless he had first eaten a small piece of bread soaked in wine. In these and similar cases the causes of the fainting are obvious; since they are mostly immediate ones, they do not involve any danger. As Hippocrates was aware of this, he qualified his rule by adding, without any visible cause, i.e. when the collapse is not due to an immediate cause; for when the efficient cause is obvious, the cure is also easy to indicate.

However, if the fainting is not only frequent and violent, but also without any visible cause, one must forecast death. What is the reason for this? The fact that fainting – (etymologically) a "failing of life" – is an image of death. Therefore if people faint often and are each time subjected to an interruption and a dispersal of the vital strength, they become daily weaker and less resistant than they were; then, when this happens again and their innate heat, scanty and weak as it was, is finally quenched and dissipated, death suddenly overtakes them, while the bystanders still believe that they will come to themselves after the fit as usual.

Galen says that searching for the origin of the constant fainting of these patients, which finally ends in death, he found by section upon a great number of animals which had died a similar unexpected death, that they proved to have a sort of enveloping membrane in the chambers of the heart, filled with a malodorous fluid; this fluid, by its foul quality, would corrupt and ravage the vital

τὸν ζωτικὸν τόνον καὶ τὸ πάθος τῆς ἐκλύσεως ἐποίει. πάλιν δὲ ἀναφέρεται τὰ τοιαῦτα ζῷα ἀτελῶς ἔτι ἐχούσης τῆς τοιαύτης ὑγρότητος πρὸς τὸ καταπνῖξαι καὶ ἀποσβέσαι τὸ ἔμφυτον θερμόν· ἡνίκα μέντοι μέτρον πλημύρας ἀναδεξαμένη τῷ χρόνῳ ἡ ὑγρότης περιγένηται, ὥστε ἀποσβέσαι τὸ ἐν τῇ καρδίᾳ θερμὸν τελείως, καὶ τὸν θάνατον τηνικαῦτα ἐπ' ἐσχάτῃ λιποθυμίᾳ εἰργάσατο. τοῦτο οὖν καὶ ἐπὶ τῶν ἀνθρώπων συμβαίνει, κατ' ἀρχὰς μὲν πολλὰς ἐπάγον τὰς λιποθυμίας τῷ ἐπικειμένῳ ὑγρῷ· οὗ πλεονάζοντος καὶ ἰσχυρῶς πλημμυροῦντος ὁ θάνατος ἐπάγεται. διὸ οἱ τοιοῦτοι καὶ παλμοῦ τινος κατὰ τὴν καρδίαν αὐτῶν γινομένου αἰσθάνονται· ὅπερ καὶ Ἀντιπάτρῳ συνέβαινε τῷ ἰατρῷ, ὅστις ἐπὶ πολλαῖς λιποθυμίαις λιποθυμήσας ἐξαίφνης ἐτελεύτησεν.

II 41 [II 42: IV 482,7–8 L.] Λύειν ἀποπληξίην ἰσχυρὴν μὲν ἀδύνατον, ἀσθενέα δὲ οὐ ῥηΐδιον.

Ζητήσωμεν τί ἐστιν ἀποπληξία καὶ τὴν διάθεσιν αὐτῆς, καὶ τί τὸ αἴτιον τῆς ἀποπληξίας καὶ τίς ὁ πεπονθὼς τόπος. καὶ ἀποπληξία μέν ἐστιν ἀναισθησία καὶ ἀκινησία τοῦ παντὸς σώματος μετὰ βλάβης τῶν ἡγεμονικῶν ἐνεργειῶν· ἡ δὲ διάθεσις ἔμφραξίς ἐστι τῶν κοιλιῶν τοῦ ἐγκεφάλου· τὸ δὲ αἴτιον παχὺς καὶ γλίσχρος χυμός, λέγω δὴ φλέγμα.

Ἀποροῦσι δὲ οἱ διαλεκτικοὶ λέγοντες· «Εἰ στέρησίς ἐστιν ἡ ἀποπληξία, ἀναισθησία καὶ ἀκινησία τυγχάνουσα τοῦ παντὸς σώματος, πῶς τὸ μᾶλλον καὶ ἧττον ἐπιδέχεται; ἡ γὰρ στέρησις παντελής ἐστιν ἀναίρεσις τῆς ἐνεργείας· ἐνταῦθα οὖν ἐπὶ τῆς ἀποπληξίας πῶς ἐνδέχεται τὴν μὲν ἀσθενῆ εἶναι, τὴν δὲ ἰσχυράν; οὐδεὶς λέγει καὶ γάρ, ὅτι οὗτος τυφλότερός ἐστιν ἐκείνου.» φαμὲν οὖν, ὅτι ἡ πήρωσις οὐκ ἐπιδέχεται τὸ μᾶλλον καὶ ἧττον, ἡ δὲ φαινομένη στέρησις δύναται τοῦτο ἐπιδέξασθαι. φαινομένη δὲ στέρησίς ἐστιν, ἡνίκα ἡμῖν μὲν ἕτερον εἶναι δοκεῖ, τῇ δὲ φύσει καὶ αὐτῇ τῇ δυνάμει μή ἐστι παντελὴς ἡ βλάβη, ἀλλ' ἀτελής. μηδὲ γὰρ ὑπολάβῃς, ὅταν λέγωμεν ἀκινησίαν καὶ ἀναισθησίαν ἐπὶ τῆς ἀποπληξίας, ὅτι παντοίως μηδὲ αἰσθάνεσθαι μηδὲ κινεῖσθαι τὸν οὕτως πάσχοντα ὑποτιθέμεθα, ἀλλ' ὅτι αἰσθάνεται μὲν καὶ κινεῖται, ἀνεπαισθήτως δὲ ἡμῖν τοῦτο γίνεται. οὕτω γοῦν καὶ ἀ⟨σ⟩φύκτους καλοῦμεν οὐ τοὺς μηδεμίαν σφυγμικὴν ἀποσῴζοντας κίνησιν, ἀλλ' ἐφ' ὧν ἡμῖν ἡ αἰσθητικὴ κίνησις οὐ γίνεται. αὕτη δὲ ἡ στέρησις ἐπιδέχεται τὸ μᾶλλον καὶ ἧττον.

Διαγινώσκεται δὲ ἐκ τῆς ἀναπνοῆς ἤγουν ἐκ τῆς τοῦ θώρακος κινήσεως, εἴτε ἰσχυρά ἐστιν εἴτε ἀσθενὴς ἡ ἀποπληξία. καὶ μή τις ὡς ἀδίκου κατηγορείτω τῆς

8 διὸ – 10] *cf.* Gal. In Aphor. II 41: XVII B 540,16–541,2 K. 9 ὅπερ – 10] *v.* Gal. De loc. aff. IV 11: VIII 293,8–296,6 K. 13–17] *cf.* [Gal.] Def. med. 264: XIX 415,13–14 K. Gal. De sympt. diff. 3: VII 59,2–4 K. Steph. Ad Glauc.: I 316,19–20 Dietz Theoph. In Aphor.: II 333,13–16 Dietz 14sq. καὶ^{II} – σώματος] *cf.* Gal. In Aphor. II 42: XVII B 541,6–7 K. 15 ἡ – 17] *cf.* Gal. In Aphor. II 42: XVII B 541,15–542,4 K. 18 – 28 γίνεται] *v.* Theoph. In Aphor.: II 334,9–16 Dietz 18–20 ἐνεργείας] *aliter* Aristot. Categ. 10: 13 a 3–13 *et comm. ad loc.; cf. etiam* Eliae In categ.: CAG XVIII 1, p. 244,23–25 32 καὶ – 228,22 διαφαίνεσθαι] *cf.* Gal. In Aphor. II 42: XVII B 542,6–18 K.

3 μέτρον *scripsi*: μέτρ *(ambig.)* α 4 παραγένηται A 6 ἐπάγον *scripsi*: ἐπάγοντα P: ἐπάγοντ *(ambig.)* A 9 λειποθυμίας P 14sq. ἀκινησία καὶ ἀναισθησία A 24 ἑτέρου P: *fort.* στέρησις *vel* ἐστερημένον *scribendum est* 26 λέγομεν A *fort.* παντελῶς *scribendum est* 28 ἀφύκτους α: *correxi* 29sq. ἡ αἰσθητικὴ] *fort.* αἰσθητὴ ἡ *scribendum est* 32 ἀδίκον *(sic)* P

strength and it caused the condition of collapse. Such animals recover again as long as the fluid still has insufficient force to smother and extinguish the innate heat; but when at length the fluid has reached the point of overflowing and won the fight, so that it completely extinguishes the heat in the heart, then it brings about death in a last fainting fit. The same thing happens also to men: at first it causes frequent fainting fits by the pressure of the fluid; but when it prevails and there is a violent overflow, death follows. This is why these patients feel a kind of palpitation of the heart; this was also the case of the physician Antipater, who after many fainting fits suddenly died in such a fit.

II 41. To undo a strong apoplexy is impossible, a weak one not easy.

Let us ask the questions what apoplexy is, what the condition is that leads to it, what its cause is and what the affected organ. Apoplexy is insensibility and immobility of the whole body with damage to the governing functions; the condition that leads to it is a stoppage of the cavities of the brain; the cause is a thick and sticky humor, I mean phlegm.

Dialecticians raise the objection: "If apoplexy is a privation, being insensitivity and immobility of the whole body, how can it admit of degrees? Privation, indeed, is the total removal of a function; so here, in the case of apoplexy, how is it possible for it to be either weak or strong? Nobody says that this man is blinder than that one." Our reply is that mutilation does not admit of degrees, but apparent privation may. There is apparent privation when, though we think otherwise, the damage is not total but incomplete as far as nature and the faculty itself are concerned. For you should not think, when we speak of immobility and insensibility in apoplexy, that we assume the patient to have no sensation or motion at all; he has sensation and motion, but in a way that is imperceptible to us. Thus we also say that "the pulse is gone", not to describe patients who have no pulsation left at all, but those in whom this motion is not perceptible (?) to us. This kind of privation admits of degrees.

We can diagnose from the breathing, i.e. the motion of the chest, whether the apoplexy is strong or weak. And let us not accuse Nature of injustice for

φύσεως, τὸν μὲν ϑώρακα κινούσης, οὐ τὸ ἄλλο δὲ σῶμα. καὶ πάντων μὲν γὰρ τῶν μορίων καὶ μερῶν προνοητικῶς λόγον τινὰ πεποίηται, πολλῷ δὲ πλέον ἐκείνων τῶν μορίων, ὧν ἐνεργούντων ἡ ζωὴ διατηρεῖται καὶ δι' ὧν ἡ ζωτικὴ δύναμις ἐπὶ τὸ πᾶν ἀφικνεῖται σῶμα. δεῖ γὰρ εἰδέναι, ὅτι κινεῖται τυχὸν δάκτυλος ὑπὸ μυὸς ἑνὸς τῇ καλουμένῃ κάμψει· ὅστις μῦς ὑπὸ νεύρου πάντως κινεῖται, τοῦ νεύρου δύναμιν ἔχοντος κινητικήν. καὶ ἐπειδὴ εἷς ἐστι μῦς ὁ τὴν εἰρημένην κάμψιν τοῦ δακτύλου ποιούμενος, ἐλαχίστη δέ ἐστιν ἡ χορηγουμένη αὐτῷ κινητικὴ δύναμις, διὰ τοῦτο ἐπὶ τοῦ δακτύλου οὐ γίνεται αἰσϑητικὴ κίνησις ἀποπληξίας ὑποκειμένης. ἐπὶ δὲ τοῦ ϑώρακος, ἐπειδὴ μόριόν ἐστιν, ἐν ᾧ τὸ περιέχον τὴν ζωήν ἐστι, λέγω δὴ τὸ ἔμφυτον ϑερμόν, οὕτινος ἐργαστήριον πέφυκεν ἡ καρδία, τοῦτο δὲ ἀεὶ χρεία, ἔστ' ἂν ἡ ζωὴ διαφυλάττηται, ῥιπίζεσϑαί τε καὶ ἀναρρώννυσϑαι, ὅπερ γίνεται διὰ τῆς εἰσπνοῆς καϑαροῦ εἰσιόντος ἀέρος· ὅπερ οὐδέποτε ἐνεργηϑήσεται μὴ τῆς εἰσπνοῆς καὶ ἐκπνοῆς ἐπιτελουμένης, τοῦτο δὲ οὐδὲν ἕτερόν ἐστιν ἢ διαστολὴ καὶ συστολὴ τοῦ ϑώρακος, αἱ δὲ τοιαῦται κινήσεις ὑπὸ μυῶν τελοῦνται, καὶ τούτων πλείστων· τούτου χάριν ἡ φύσις ὡς περιεκτικὸν τὸν ϑώρακα τῆς ἐν ἡμῖν ζωῆς πολλοῖς μυσὶν ἐτίμησέ τε καὶ συνεστήσατο – καὶ γὰρ καὶ τοῦ ϑώρακός εἰσιν οἵ τε ὑψηλοὶ καλούμενοι καὶ οἱ μεσόπλευροι καὶ τὸ διάφραγμα –, καὶ τούτων πάντων κινούντων αὐτὸν τὸ τῆς εἰσπνοῆς καὶ ἐκπνοῆς ἀποτελεῖται ἔργον. καὶ ἐπειδὴ πολλοί εἰσιν οἱ μύες οἱ κινοῦντες αὐτόν, δῆλον ὅτι πολλά εἰσι καὶ τὰ νεῦρα τὰ χορηγοῦντα αὐτοῖς τὴν κινητικὴν δύναμιν· ὥστε κἂν ἐλαχίστη καϑ' ἕκαστον χορηγῆται ἡ δύναμις, τῇ τῶν πολλῶν συνδρομῇ μᾶλλον τῶν ἄλλων ἁπάντων μορίων ἐν τῷ ϑώρακι τὴν κίνησιν ἐπὶ τῶν ἀποπλήκτων διαφαίνεσϑαι. ἐνταῦϑα οὖν, λέγω δὴ ἐκ τῆς ἀναπνοῆς, εἴτε ἰσχυρὰ εἴτε ἀσϑενὴς ἡ ἀποπληξία, γνωρίζεται. εἰ μὲν γὰρ μηδ' ὅλως αἴσϑησις ἡμῖν γίνεται τῆς τοῦ ϑώρακος κινήσεως, κακὸν τὸ τοιοῦτον· ἰσχυρὰν γὰρ δηλοῖ τὴν αἰτίαν καὶ αὐτὴν τὴν οὐσίαν τοῦ ἐγκεφάλου ἐμφραγεῖσαν ἐπὶ τοσοῦτον ὡς μήτε ἀκτινοειδῶς ἐργάζεσϑαι διὰ τῶν νεύρων καὶ χορηγεῖσϑαι τοῖς μυσὶ τὴν ψυχικὴν δύναμιν. εἰ δὲ μετρία τις ὑποπέσοι ἡ ἀναπνοή, ἀσϑενεστέρα δηλοῦται ἡ ἀποπληξία καὶ ἀτελὴς ἡ διάϑεσις· τὰς κοιλίας γὰρ τοῦ ἐγκεφάλου τὸ τηνικαῦτα κατειλήφει τὸ αἴτιον καὶ αὗται μόναι τὴν ἔμφραξιν πεπόνϑασιν, ὡς δύνασϑαι μόλις ποτὲ ὀλίγης οὔσης εὐρυχωρίας ἐν αὐταῖς τὸ ψυχικὸν πνεῦμα ἀκτινοειδῶς ἐκπέμπειν τὸν ἐγκέφαλον τοῖς νεύροις καὶ τοῖς μυσὶ τοῖς τὸν ϑώρακα κινοῦσιν, ὑφ' ὧν ἡ ἀναπνοὴ γίνεται. μετρία γοῦν, ὡς ἔφην, ἐνταῦϑα δοκεῖ σωτηρίας ἐλπίς.

Ἔστι δὲ καὶ ἄλλοϑεν χαρακτηρίσαι, εἴτε ἀσϑενὴς εἴτε ἰσχυρά ἐστιν ἡ ἀποπληξία. ἰστέον γάρ, ὅτι ἀναισϑησία καὶ ἀκινησία τοῦ παντὸς ὑπάρχουσα σώματος μᾶλλον ἐν ἀκινησίᾳ, ἧττον δὲ ἐν δυσαισϑησίᾳ ϑεωρεῖται, ὥστε αἰσϑάνεσϑαι μὲν μετρίως τοὺς τοιούτους, κινεῖσϑαι δὲ οὐδαμῶς. φησὶ γὰρ ὁ Γαληνός, ὅτι ὑπὸ μείζονος δυνάμεως ἡ κίνησις ἐπιτελεῖται, ἡ δὲ αἴσϑησις ὑπὸ ἥττονος. ἐνταῦϑα οὖν πολλὴ μὲν ἡ δύναμις διικνεῖσϑαι καὶ διαλανϑάνειν τὴν ἐν τῷ ἐγκεφάλῳ ἔμφραξιν οὐχ οἵα τέ ἐστιν, ὑφ' ἧς ἡ κίνησις ἐπιτελεῖται· ἐλαχίστη δὲ καὶ μετρία διεξέρχεται, ὑφ' ἧς ὁ τῆς αἰσϑήσεως λόγος εἰ καὶ ἀμυδρῶς γοῦν συντηρεῖται ὁ ἐν τοῖς μορίοις. καὶ διὰ

22 ἐνταῦϑα – 32] *cf.* Gal. In Aphor. II 42: XVII B 541,6–15 K. 36sq. φησὶ – ἥττονος] *v.* Gal. De loc. aff. I 6: VIII 58,16–59,2 K.

1 οὐ – σῶμα] τὸ δὲ ἄλλο σῶμα, οὐχὶ A καὶ *om.* A 8 *fort.* αἰσϑητὴ *scribendum est* 10 τούτου P 12sq. καϑαροῦ – εἰσπνοῆς *om.* A 17 οἱ μεσόπλευροι] τὸ μεσόπλευρον A 18 αὐτῶν A ἀποτελεῖ A ἐπεὶ A 19 οἱ[I]] αἱ A οἱ[II]] αἱ A δῆλον ὅτι *om.* A 20 χορηγεῖται A 39 ἧς[I]] οἷς P

allowing the chest to move, but not the rest of the body. She has provided in some way for all the organs and parts, but more especially for those organs by whose functioning life is preserved and by way of which the vital faculty pervades the entire body. You should be aware that for instance a finger, in so-called "bending", is moved by one muscle; this muscle is of course moved by a nerve, for it is the nerve that has the power to move. Now since there is only one muscle that causes the bending of the finger to which we referred and since the motive power provided for it is very slight, therefore there is no perceptible (?) motion in the finger in a case of apoplexy. It is otherwise with the chest, because in this part is found that which contains life, i.e. the innate heat, of which the heart is the factory, and as long as life is preserved, it is necessary for this heat to be continually fanned and reinforced, and this is brought about by inhalation, in which pure air comes in; this, in turn, can never be accomplished if there is no process of inhalation and exhalation, in other words, expansion and contraction of the chest, motions which are effected by a great number of muscles; this is why Nature has privileged the chest, as the container of our life, to be composed of a great number of muscles – to the chest belong the so-called "high" muscles, the intercostal muscles, and the diaphragm –, and by the joint motive force of all these the process of inhalation and exhalation is kept going. And because there are so many muscles that keep it moving, there are obviously also many nerves that provide them with their motive power, so that, however small the power provided for each, the concurrent activity of so great a number causes motion, in cases of apoplexy, to be more apparent in the chest than in all the other parts. Therefore it is here, that is, in breathing, that the strength or weakness of the attack can be discerned. If we notice no motion of the chest at all, this is a bad sign; for it indicates that the cause is a strong one and that the very substance of the brain has been blocked up to such an extent that it does not even operate in a diffuse way through the nerves, so that the psychic power is passed on to the muscles. But if we feel moderate breathing, this indicates that the stroke is weaker, and the condition incomplete: in this case the cause has affected the cavities of the brain and only these have been obstructed, so that, though with great difficulty, through what little space there is in them, the brain can send the psychic pneuma diffusely to the nerves and the muscles that move the chest and to which respiration is due. So, as I said, here we seem to have a modest chance of survival.

There is another sign by which we can determine whether the stroke is weak or strong. The point is that, though (apoplexy) is insensitivity and immobility of the whole body, it is characterized preponderantly by immobility and only to a lesser degree by diminished sensitivity, so that patients have a certain amount of perception, but cannot move at all. This is, as Galen says, because it needs a greater force to achieve motion, and only a lesser one to achieve perception. In this case, then, power cannot pass through and escape the obstruction in the brain in great quantity so as to accomplish motion; but a very small, modest quantity does pass through, by which the principle of perception in the members is preserved, however dimly. It is because of this that the symptom of apoplexy con-

τοῦτο τὸ τῆς ἀποπληξίας σύμπτωμα μᾶλλον ἐν ἀκινησίᾳ ἢ ἐν ἀναισθησίᾳ θεωρεῖται. σκόπει οὖν ἐπὶ τῶν ἀποπλήκτων σὺν τῇ ἀναπνοῇ καὶ τὴν κατὰ τὴν ἁφὴν αἴσθησιν· καὶ ἐὰν εὕρῃς αὐτὸν ἀναίσθητον παντελῶς γενόμενον, γίνωσκε, ὅτι χαλεπωτάτη ἐστὶν ἡ ἀποπληξία· εἰ δὲ αἰσθάνεται μετρίως, ἀσθενεστέρα ὑπάρχει. καὶ ἐπὶ μὲν τῆς ἰσχυρᾶς συνεισάγεται ἡ ἀπόγνωσις καὶ τὸ τῆς θεραπείας ἀδύνατον, ἐπὶ δὲ τῆς μετριωτέρας δεῖ ἐγχειρεῖν, προλέγοντας μέντοι, ὅτι οὐ πάντως σωθήσεται. ὅμως μέντοι ἐγχειρεῖν δεῖ τῇ θεραπείᾳ· ἐὰν γὰρ ἐπιτάσσουσαν σχοίης καὶ τὴν ὑπερτέραν δύναμιν καὶ τὴν τύχην ἐπιλάμπουσαν, δυνατὸν ἴσως περιγενέσθαι τοῦ τοιούτου παθήματος.

Λύειν δὲ εἶπε καὶ οὐ «θεραπεύειν» εἰδώς, ὅτι ὥσπερ ὑπό τινων δεσμῶν ἐπὶ τῶν ἀποπλήκτων κατέχεται ὁ ἐγκέφαλος ὑπὸ τοῦ αἰτίου· τῇ ἐναντιώσει οὖν χρώμενος τὴν ἀπαλλαγὴν εἴρηκεν.

II 42 [II 43: IV 482,9–10 L.] Τῶν ἀπαγχομένων καὶ καταλυομένων, μήπω δὲ τεθνηκότων, οὐκ ἀναφέρουσιν οἷς ἂν ἀφρὸς ᾖ περὶ τὸ στόμα.

Φησίν, ὅτι πολλάκις τις ἀπαγχονεῖται ἢ ὑπὸ κελεύσεως ἄρχοντος ἢ βασιλέως ἢ ὑπό τινος τῶν τοιούτων. ἐπὶ γοῦν τῶν τοιούτων ἐὰν ἀφρὸς εὑρεθῇ ἐν τῷ στόματι ἀπαγχονεῖσθαι μέλλοντος ἀνθρώπου μετὰ τὸ κατενεχθῆναι αὐτόν, πάντως τεθνήξεται. τίς δὲ ἡ γένεσις τοῦ ἀφροῦ καὶ διὰ τί ἐπιγενόμενος θανάτου γίνεται σημεῖον, καλὸν διεξελθεῖν. ἀφρός ἐστι μάχη ὑγροῦ καὶ πνεύματος ἢ ἄθροισμα πλειόνων πομφολύγων· πομφόλυξ δέ ἐστιν ὑγρότης λεπτὴ καὶ ὑμενώδης περιεκτικὴ πνεύματος. γίνεται δὲ ὁ ἀφρὸς ἢ διὰ κίνησιν ἢ διὰ θερμασίαν ἢ διὰ τὸ συναμφότερον. διὰ μὲν τὴν κίνησιν, ὅπερ ἐπὶ ταῖς ἀκταῖς ὁρῶμεν γινόμενον τοῦ ὕδατος ταῖς πέτραις προσαρασσομένου· ἀφρὸν γὰρ τὸ τηνικαῦτα ἀποτίκτει ἡ θάλασσα. διὰ δὲ θερμασίαν, ὡς ἐπὶ τῶν ἑψομένων κρεῶν ἐπὶ ζωμοῖς ἔστι θεάσασθαι· ἀναλύουσα γὰρ τὸ πιμελῶδες τῶν κρεῶν ἡ πυρὰ καὶ λιπαράν τινα ὑγρότητα ἀπογεννῶσα ὑμενώδη ταύτην ὑπὸ τῶν περιεχομένων πνευμάτων ἐργάζεται, ὅπερ ἐστὶν ἀφρὸς ἤγουν πομφόλυγες. διὰ δὲ τὸ συναμφότερον, ὡς ἐπὶ τῶν τρεχόντων ἵππων ὁρῶμεν, ὅτι μετὰ τὸν δρόμον ἀφρὸς ἐν τῷ στόματι αὐτῶν γίνεται διά τε τὴν κίνησιν ἅμα καὶ τὴν θερμασίαν. τούτων οὕτως ἐχόντων ἔλθωμεν ἐπὶ τὸ ζητούμενον.

Ἐάν τις ληφθῇ τῇ ἀγχόνῃ, πίλησιν ὑφίσταται τῶν περὶ τὸν τράχηλον ἀγγείων· τούτων δὲ πιλουμένων ἀποκλείονται δηλονότι καὶ οἱ πόροι· τούτων ἀποκλειομένων ἀὴρ οὐκ εἰσάγεται· τούτου μὴ εἰσαγομένου τὸ ἔμφυτον θερμὸν οὐ ῥιπίζεται· τούτου μὴ ῥιπιζομένου κίνδυνος πνιγμοῦ ἀπειλεῖται. κἀντεῦθεν ἐπείγεται ὡς ἐπὶ τὰ ἔξω τὸ θερμόν, εἶτα περιτυγχάνει τοῖς πόροις πεπιλημένοις καὶ πάλιν ὑπονοστεῖ ἐπὶ τὰ ἐντός, εἶτα πάλιν ἐπὶ τὰ ἔξω ὁρμᾷ. κἀντεῦθεν πολυειδῶς κινούμενον, ἅμα δὲ καὶ θερμότερον ἑαυτοῦ γινόμενον, τὸν ἀφρὸν ἀπεργάζεται πνευμάτων τινῶν ἐν τῇ τοιαύτῃ κινήσει τικτομένων καὶ ὑμενούντων τὴν παρατυγχάνουσαν ἐκεῖσε ὑγρότητα. ἄλλως τε δὲ τὸ ἔμφυτον θερμὸν μὴ εὑρίσκον τὸν τρέφοντα αὐτὸ ἀέρα χωρεῖ κατὰ

10–11 αἰτίου] *cf. infra*, vol. II, fol. 52[v] 18 τίς – 29] *v.* Gal. In Aphor. II 43: XVII B 543, 8–544,12 K. 30–37 ὑγρότητα] *v.* Theoph. In Aphor.: II 335,3–15 Dietz

4 εἰ] ἡ P 14 μήπω *Hipp.* C′ *et al.*, *Theoph.* U′′: μηδέπω *Hipp. plerique*, *Theoph.* SV′′ 16 τῷ *om.* A 21 ὁ *om.* P 33 ἀπολεῖται P 34 πεπιλημένοις *sec. Theoph. scripsi*: ἢ πεπιλημένοις P: ἀπειλημμένοις A ἐπινοστεῖ P 37 κινήσει *sec. Theoph. scripsi*: κρίσει α

sists in immobility rather than in insensitivity. Therefore, in victims of stroke, you should examine not only their breathing, but also their sense of touch; and if you find that the patient has become totally feelingless, you may infer that the stroke is very severe; but if he has a certain measure of perception, it is lighter. A severe stroke is by implication hopeless, and no cure is possible, while in the lighter case one must make an attempt, though with the caution that (the patient) will not necessarily survive. Yet you must attempt the cure; for if it is the will of the Higher Power and if chance is favorable, he may perhaps recover from this disease.

He said to undo instead of "to cure", because he knew that in cases of apoplexy the cause is like a fetter that impedes the brain; so he used the opposite term to describe recovery.

II 42. People hanged and cut down, but not yet dead, do not get up again if they foam at the mouth.

(Hippocrates) discusses the common event of a man hanged by order of a magistrate, a king, or someone in a similar position. In such cases, if foam is found in the mouth of a man condemned to death by hanging after he has been taken down, he will inevitably die. It is useful to explain the origin of the foam and why its appearance is a sign of death. Foam is a fight between moisture and gas, or an aggregate of bubbles, a bubble being moisture in the form of a thin membrane which contains gas. Foam is produced either by motion or by heating or by both. By motion, as we see it happen on the seashore, when the water crashes against the rocks; then the sea generates foam. By heat, as we can see when meat is boiled for soup: the heat of the fire dissolves the fattish matter of the meat and produces a sort of greasy moisture, which it makes membrane-like by the gases contained in it, and this is foam or bubbles. Or by both together, as we see it in running horses: after the race they foam at the mouth as a result of both motion and heat. This being settled, let us come to the point.

When a man is hanged, he is subjected to compression of the vessels of the neck; when these are compressed, the pores are naturally closed also; when they are closed, no air is taken in; when no air is taken in, the innate heat is not fanned; when this is not fanned, it is in danger of being smothered. Hence the heat tries to rush outside, then finds the pores stopped up and returns inside, then once more tries to make its way outside. By the resulting complicated motion, during which it also becomes hotter than normal, it produces the foam, when certain gases are generated in the course of that motion and form bubbles from the moisture that happens to be there. Besides, when the innate heat does not find the air to feed it, it turns against the body; it cannot assail the heart, because

τοῦ σώματος· καὶ κατὰ μὲν τῆς καρδίας οὐχ οἷόν τέ ἐστι χωρῆσαι, στερεὸν γὰρ αὐτῆς ὑπάρχει τὸ σῶμα, κατὰ δὲ τῶν ὑγροτέρων χωρεῖ· τοιαύτης δὲ φύσεως ὄντος τοῦ πνεύμονος, ἐν τούτῳ χωρεῖ καὶ ἀναλύει καὶ ἀναστοιχειοῖ τὴν οὐσίαν αὐτοῦ – μεμαθήκαμεν γάρ, ὅτι ἐξ ἀερώδους αἵματος γίνεται τρεφόμενος ὁ πνεύμων – καὶ λεπτοποιῶν αὐτὸν τὸν ἀφρὸν ἀπεργάζεται.

Τινὲς δὲ ἔφασαν τὴν ἀφρώδη ὑγρότητα ἐκ τῆς γαστρὸς καὶ τῆς περὶ τὸν στόμαχον οὐσίας ἀνάγεσθαι. πρὸς οὓς ῥητέον, ὅτι, εἰ ἐκ τοῦ στομάχου ἀνήγετο, ἔδει αὐτὴν δι' ἐμέτου ἀνάγεσθαι. ἀλλὰ καὶ αὖθις οὗτοί φασιν· «Εἰ διὰ τοῦ θώρακος ἀνήγετο, ἔδει αὐτὴν βῆχα ποιῆσαι.» πρὸς οὓς φαμεν· βῆχα οὐ ποιεῖ διὰ τοιαύτην αἰτίαν· ἡ βὴξ μάχη ὑγροῦ τυγχάνει καὶ πνεύματος· τοῦτο γοῦν τὸ ἀναγόμενον οὐκ ἔχει τοσαύτην σύστασιν ὑγροῦ ὥστε ποιῆσαι βῆχα, ἀλλ' ἀτμωδέστερον ὂν ἀφρὸν μὲν ποιῆσαι δύναται, βῆχα δὲ οὐχί.

Ἐπὰν οὖν ἐπὶ τῶν τοιούτων ἀφρὸν εὕρωμεν περὶ τὸ στόμα, τὸν θάνατον δεῖ προλέγειν, ἐπειδὴ δηλοῦται πολλὴ τοῦ ἐμφύτου θερμοῦ κατάλυσις καὶ συγκοπή· εἰ δὲ μὴ εὕρῃς ἀφρόν, ἔλπιζε τὴν σωτηρίαν, δηλοῦται γὰρ μὴ πολλῇ συντονίᾳ τὸ ἔμφυτον θερμὸν περὶ τὴν κίνησιν χρήσασθαι.

Καταλυομένων δέ φησιν ἀντὶ τοῦ «καταφερομένων ἀπὸ τῆς ἀγχόνης».

Οὐκ ἀναφέρουσι δὲ τουτέστιν οὐκέτι φέρεται ἡ ζωὴ ἐπὶ τούτων. ἐπειδὴ γὰρ ἡ μὲν ζωὴ ἄνωθέν ἐστιν, ὁ δὲ θάνατος κάτωθεν, διὰ τοῦτό φησιν οὐκ ἀναφέρουσιν.

II 43 [II 44: IV 482,11–12 L.] Οἱ παχέες σφόδρα κατὰ φύσιν ταχυθάνατοι γίνονται τῶν ἰσχνῶν μᾶλλον.

Βλέπε, πῶς πανταχοῦ τὰς ἀμετρίας φεύγων ὁ Ἱπποκράτης χαίρει ταῖς συμμετρίαις. ταχυθάνατον γὰρ τὸ παχὺ σφόδρα σῶμα τῇ ἀμετρίᾳ τοῦ ὄγκου· ὅπερ γίνεται διὰ δύο αἰτίας, ὅτι τε ἀσθενές ἐστιν ἐν τοῖς τοιούτοις σώμασι τὸ ἔμφυτον θερμὸν καὶ ὅτι πλῆθος ὑπόκειται πιμελῆς καὶ περιττωματικὴ ὑγρότης καὶ πύκνωσις τῆς ἐπιφανείας. ἥστινος πεπυκνωμένης ἀδιαφόρητα γίνονται τὰ περιττώματα ταῦτα, μὴ διαφορούμενα, ἀλλ' ἀθροιζόμενα ἐν τῷ βάθει· ἐκεῖσε δὲ πλημυροῦντα πιλοῦσι τὰς ἀρτηρίας καὶ τὰς φλέβας· ὥντινων στενοχωρουμένων καταπνίγεται τὸ ἔμφυτον θερμόν, κἀντεῦθεν θάνατος ἐπακολουθεῖ τοῖς τοιούτοις.

Παχεῖς δὲ ἐνταῦθα τοὺς λίαν παχεῖς λέγει, ὅπερ ᾐνίξατο διὰ τοῦ σφόδρα· ἀλλὰ καὶ τοὺς ἐκ γενετῆς, τουτέστιν «ἐκ φύσεως», τὴν παχύτητα ἔχοντας. οὐδὲν γὰρ θαυμαστὸν ἐπίκτητον γενέσθαι ταύτην διά τε τροφὰς τοιαύτας καὶ βίον ἀργόν, τὰς δὲ ἀρτηρίας καὶ τὰς φλέβας ἔχειν τὸ ἐξ ἀρχῆς εὖρος καὶ μὴ στενοχωρεῖσθαι, ἐπειδὴ πρώην αὐτοῖς ἰσχνὸν ἦν τὸ σῶμα· τούτων δὲ εὐρυτέρων ὑπαρχουσῶν ἀνάγκη

3sq. μεμαθήκαμεν – πνεύμων] *cf.* Gal. De usu part. IV 15: I 235,14–17 Helmr. = III 320, 14–16 K.; VI 10: I 328,18–329,20 Helmr. = III 450,8–451,15 K. *infra*, vol. III, fol. 227v 6–8 ἀνάγεσθαι] *cf.* Gal. In Aphor. II 43: XVII B 544,17–545,6 K. 8 ἀλλὰ – 12] *cf.* Gal. In Aphor. II 43: XVII B 545,9–12 K. 22–29] *v.* Theoph. In Aphor.: II 336,3–13 Dietz 27 ἐκεῖσε – 29] *v.* Gal. In Aphor. II 44: XVII B 547,10–14 K. 30–234,2] *v.* Gal. In Aphor. II 44: XVII B 547,17–548,4 K.

1 αὐτῆς] αὐτη A 4 αἵματος *scripsi (cf. Gal.)*: πνεύματος α 7 οὐσίαν P 13 περὶ] ἐπὶ P 21 μᾶλλον *ante* γίνονται *colloc. infra, p. 234,4, Hipp. perpauci, ante* τῶν *Hipp. cett., Theoph.* 27 δὲ *om.* A 33 ἀρχῆς] αὐτῆς A 34 ὑπαρχουσῶν] οὐσῶν A

its substance is solid, but it assails the moister parts instead; and since the lungs are of this nature, it invades them and dissolves and decomposes their substance — as we saw already, the lungs are formed from airlike blood which feeds them — and by turning it into a thin film it produces the foam.

Some have said that the foamlike moisture is brought up from the belly and from the substance in the stomach. We must answer that if it were brought up from the stomach, it would be vomited. They in their turn retort that, if it were brought up through the chest, it should cause coughing. We can give them the following reason why it does not: coughing is a fight between moisture and gas; now what is brought up in this case does not have a sufficiently large component of moisture to cause coughing, but being more vaporous it can produce foam, but not coughing.

Thus, if in these cases we find foam about the mouth, we must predict death, because it indicates a radical breakdown and collapse of the innate heat; but if you find no foam, you may hope for survival, because this proves that the motion of the innate heat has not been very intense.

Cut down means "taken down after hanging".

Do not get up again, i.e., they cannot be brought back to life. Because life is up, and death is down, he uses the expression get up.

II 43. Those who are by nature very fat are closer to death than those who are thin.

Notice how in every respect Hippocrates fears excess and welcomes due measure. The cause that the very fat body is close to its death is its excessive bulk, and this for two reasons: first that the innate heat is weak in such bodies, second that there is a mass of fat, there is waste moisture and there is contraction of the surface. As a result of this contraction the waste matter cannot disperse, and instead of dispersing it collects deep within, where it overflows, thus compressing the arteries and veins; when these become too narrow, the innate heat is smothered, and the outcome is death.

By fat he means here the excessively fat, as implied by the word very; but he further intends their fatness to be congenital, "by nature". It is quite conceivable, indeed, that it may be adventitious, due to food of this type and a lazy life, while the arteries and veins retain their original width and do not become narrow, since their bodies were thin at the outset; and as long as these are wide

πλούσιον εἶναι καὶ τὸ ἔμφυτον θερμὸν καὶ μὴ ἑτοίμως ὑφίστασθαι πνιγμονὴν ἢ σβέσιν, ὅταν ἀποκλεισθῶσιν τοῦ σώματος τὰ περιττά.

Καλῶς ὁ Ἱπποκράτης εἰδὼς ταῦτα τοιούτοις ἐχρήσατο προ⟨σ⟩διορισμοῖς εἰρηκώς· Οἱ παχέες σφόδρα κατὰ φύσιν ταχυθάνατοι μᾶλλον γίνονται τῶν ἰσχνῶν. εἰπὼν δὲ μᾶλλον τῶν ἰσχνῶν διέβαλε καὶ τὴν ἰσχνότητα, ὅτι οὗτοι ἀποθνήσκουσι ταχέως, εἰ καὶ ἧττον ἐκείνων, ἐπειδὴ οὐκ ἔστιν ἐν αὐτοῖς τοσαῦτα περιττώματα ὥστε καταπνιγῆναι τὸ ἔμφυτον θερμόν· ἄλλῳ μέντοι τρόπῳ καὶ αὐτοὶ εὐάλωτοι γίνονται, τῷ λόγῳ τοῦ διαφορεῖσθαι τὸ ἔμφυτον αὐτῶν θερμὸν διὰ τὸ ἀβαθὲς καὶ κάτισχνον τοῦ σώματος. μεμαθήκαμεν γὰρ ἐν τῷ Περὶ τροφῆς, ὅτι οἱ εὐδιαφόρητοι ὑγιεινοὶ μὲν κατὰ τοῦτο, ἀσθενεῖς δὲ διὰ τὸ συνδιαφορεῖσθαι καὶ τὴν χρηστὴν ὕλην τῇ ἀχρήστῳ· οἱ δὲ δυσδιαφόρητοι εὐσθενεῖς μὲν μὴ διαφορουμένων τούτοις τῶν ἀναγκαίων ἑτοίμως, νοσεροὶ δὲ διὰ τὸ πλῆθος τῶν ἐπισωρευομένων αὐτοῖς περιττωμάτων.

Ταχυθανάτους γοῦν ἀκουστέον ἐνταῦθα τοὺς ταχέως γηρῶντας, ὅπερ συμβαίνει ἐπὶ τῇ ἀσθενείᾳ τοῦ ἐμφύτου θερμοῦ. οὐδὲν γὰρ ἕτερόν ἐστι γῆρας εἰ μὴ ἀσθένεια καὶ ὀλιγότης τοῦ ἐμφύτου θερμοῦ. ἐφ' ὧν ὀλίγον ἐστὶ τοῦτο, πᾶσα ἀνάγκη ἐπακολουθῆσαι τὸ γῆρας ταχέως.

Καὶ ἀποροῦσί τινες ὅτι· «Ἐὰν ἡ ἄμετρος παχύτης καὶ ἰσχνότης διαβέβληται, τί δήποτε ὁ Ἱπποκράτης τὴν μὲν παχύτητα διέβαλε, τὴν δὲ ἰσχνότητα οὐ διέβαλεν; ἔδει γὰρ αὐτὴν ὡς ἀμετρίαν διαβληθῆναι.» πρὸς ὅ φαμεν, ὅτι διὰ τοῦτο τὴν ἰσχνότητα οὐ πάνυ διαβάλλει, ἐπειδὴ ὁμογενὴς εἶναι δοκεῖ, κἂν ἐν ἀμετρίᾳ θεωρεῖται· θερμότητος γὰρ ἔκγονος ὑπάρχει, ἥτις φίλη ἡμῖν ἐστι καὶ προσηνής.

II 44 [II 45: IV 482,13–14 L.] Τῶν ἐπιληπτικῶν τοῖσι νέοισιν ἀπαλλαγὴν αἱ μεταβολαὶ μάλιστα τῆς ἡλικίης καὶ τῶν ὡρέων καὶ τῶν τόπων καὶ τῶν βίων ποιέουσιν.

Ἐπιληψία ἐστὶ σπασμώδης καὶ ἄτακτος κίνησις τοῦ παντὸς σώματος μετὰ βλάβης τῶν ἡγεμονικῶν ἐνεργειῶν. συγγενὴς δέ ἐστιν ἀποπληξίᾳ κατά τε τὸν τόπον καὶ τὸ εἶδος τῆς διαθέσεως καὶ κατὰ τὴν αἰτίαν τὴν ποιοῦσαν· καθ' ἑκατέραν γὰρ ἐγκέφαλος ὑπόκειται τὸ πεπονθός, ἡ δὲ διάθεσις ἔμφραξις, καὶ τὸ αἴτιον παχὺς καὶ γλίσχρος χυμός. καὶ αὕτη μὲν αὐτῶν ἡ συγγένεια· διαφέρει δὲ ἐπιληψία καὶ ἀποπληξία, καθὸ ἡ μὲν ἐπιληψία ἐν κινήσει ἔχει τὸ εἶναι, ἡ δὲ ἀποπληξία ἐν ἀκινησίᾳ καὶ ἀναισθησίᾳ· καὶ καθὸ ἡ μὲν ἀποπληξία παντελής ἐστιν ἔμφραξις τῶν κοιλιῶν τοῦ ἐγκεφάλου, ἡ δὲ ἐπιληψία ἀτελής, τόπος γάρ τις τῆς κοιλότητος ἐμφράττεται, διὸ καὶ ἐν κινήσει τὸ πάθος θεωρεῖται πλημμελῶς γινομένη· καὶ καθὸ ἡ μὲν ἀποπληξία

5 εἰπὼν – 9 σώματος] *v.* Gal. In Aphor. II 44: XVII B 547,14–17 K. Theoph. In Aphor.: II 336,13–18 Dietz 9 μεμαθήκαμεν – 13] *v.* Hipp. Alim. 28: CMG I 1, p. 82,5–8 26–34 γινομένη] *v.* Gal. In Aphor. II 45: XVII B 548,8–13 K. *cf.* De loc. aff. III 9: VIII 173,5–10 K. De sympt. diff. 3: VII 58,18–59,1 K. Steph. Ad Glauc.: I 316,28–29 Dietz 26–27 ἐνεργειῶν] *v.* Theoph. In Aphor.: II 336,30–337,1 Dietz

2 *ante* τοῦ *fort.* ἐν τῷ βάθει *addendum est* 3 προδιορισμοῖς α: *correxi* 5 διέλαβε α: *correxi* 11 ἀχρηστία P 16 *post* ὧν *fort.* οὖν *addendum est* 19 διέβαλλε A διέβαλλεν A 20 διὰ τοῦτο *om.* A 22 ὑπάρχει *scripsi*: ὑπάρχ *(ambig.)* A: ὑπάρχων P 24 μάλιστα *om. infra, p. 238,22* 24sq. καὶ τῶν τόπων] *item infra, p. 238,23, Hipp. quidam, Theoph.: non hab. Hipp.* C'MV

enough, the innate heat will also be abundant and it will not easily be smothered or extinguished, when the waste matter is trapped in the body.

Being well aware of this, Hippocrates made these restrictions: Those who are by nature very fat are closer to death than those who are thin. By saying closer than those who are thin he warned also against thinness: the thin, too, die soon, though less so than the others, because though in them there is not so much waste matter that it could smother the innate heat, yet they are exposed in another way, by the fact that their innate heat is dispersed owing to the spareness and meagerness of their bodies. We have seen in the On Nutriment that persons in whom dispersal proceeds quickly are healthy in this respect, but weak insofar as with the superfluous matter the useful matter is also dispersed, while those in whom it is slow are strong insofar as the necessary materials are not dispersed too readily, but threatened by disease by the mass of waste matter that accumulates inside them.

Close to death should be understood, then, as aging quickly, as a result of the weakness of the innate heat. This is exactly what old age means, weakness and scantiness of the innate heat. For those who have little of it, old age will necessarily come soon.

Some ask the question, "If excessive fatness and thinness are to be feared, why did Hippocrates warn against fatness, not against thinness, which should be branded as excess?" We answer that he is not too severe on thinness, because it seems to be kindred to us, even in its excessive form; for it is the offspring of heat, a friendly and congenial quality.

II 44. Youthful epileptics are cured mainly by changes in age, seasons, places, and ways of life.

Epilepsy is a convulsive and disorderly motion of the entire body with damage to the governing functions. It is related to apoplexy as regards the place, the nature of the condition and the cause that brings it about: in both, the brain is the organ affected, the condition is a stoppage, and the cause is a thick and sticky humor. In these respects they are related; but epilepsy and apoplexy differ in that epilepsy consists essentially in motion, apoplexy in immobility and insensibility; in that apoplexy is a total stoppage of the cavities of the brain, epilepsy an incomplete one, since only a particular point of the cavity is blocked, which results in an affection characterized by faulty motion; and in that apoplexy is

ὑπὸ γλίσχρου καὶ παχέος γίνεται χυμοῦ, ἡ δὲ ἐπιληψία ὡς ἐπὶ πᾶν μὲν καὶ αὕτη ἐπὶ τοιαύτῃ γίνεται ὕλῃ, οὐκ ἀεὶ δέ, ἀλλ' ἐνίοτε καὶ ὑπὸ μελαγχολικοῦ γίνεται χυμοῦ τὸ στόμα τῆς γαστρὸς καταλαμβάνοντος καὶ δάκνοντος αὐτὸ καὶ ἀνιῶντος, ὅπερ τῇ περιουσίᾳ τῶν νεύρων καὶ τῷ περιττῷ τῆς αἰσθήσεως ἀνιωμένων τῶν συγγενῶν νεύρων κραδαίνει καὶ ταράσσει τὸν ἐγκέφαλον, ὅπερ ἐστὶν ἐπιληψία.

Αὕτη τοίνυν ἡ ἐπιληψία πολυώνυμός ἐστι· λέγεται γὰρ ἐπιληψία, λέγεται καὶ παιδικόν, λέγεται καὶ ἱερὰ νόσος καὶ Ἡρακλεία νόσος· ἕκαστον δὲ τῶν ὀνομάτων κατά τινος εὐλόγου φέρεται σημαινομένου. ἐπιληψία μὲν γὰρ εἴρηται παρὰ τὸ ἐπιλαμβάνεσθαι ταύτην τοῦ ἐγκεφάλου καὶ μὴ συγχωρεῖν αὐτῷ τὰς οἰκείας προβάλλεσθαι ἐνεργείας. παιδικὸν δέ, ἐπειδὴ τοῖς παισὶ μάλιστα συμβαίνειν εἴωθε διὰ τὸ ἐξ ἀδηφαγίας καὶ ἀπεψιῶν ἀθροίζεσθαι ἐν αὐτοῖς ὠμὸν χυμόν. ἱερὰ δὲ νόσος καλεῖται, ὡς μέν τινες, διὰ τὸ ἱερὸν εἶναι τὸν πάσχοντα τόπον, λέγω δὴ τὸν ἐγκέφαλον, ὡς δὲ ἕτεροι, διὰ τὸ μέγεθος τοῦ νοσήματος· οὕτω γοῦν καὶ ἱερὸν ἰχθὺν τὸν μέγα⟨ν⟩ φαμέν. λέγεται καὶ Ἡρακλεία νόσος, οὐκ ἐπειδή τινες ὑπενόησαν ἐνεῖναι τὸ τοιοῦτον πάθος τῷ Ἡρακλεῖ, ἀλλ' ὅτι ὥσπερ ἐκεῖνος τῇ περιουσίᾳ τῆς δυνάμεως δυσκαταγώνιστος ὤφθη τοῖς πολεμίοις, οὕτω καὶ τὸ τοιοῦτον πάθος δυσκαταγώνιστον ὑπάρχει τοῖς θεραπεύουσιν. ἐπεὶ τοίνυν ταῦθ' οὕτως ἔχει, λοιπὸν ἐπὶ τὸ σπουδαζόμενον ἴωμεν.

Φησὶν ὁ Ἱπποκράτης τὰς ἐπιληψίας μάλιστα γίνεσθαι τοῖς νέοις· καὶ εἰ δοκεῖ, σαφηνείας χάριν τὸν λόγον γυμνάσωμεν. προσῆλθε γύναιον ἡμῖν φέρον ὑποτίτθιον παιδίον ἑαλωκὸς τῷ τῆς ἐπιληψίας πάθει. ἐπὶ τούτου ζητοῦμεν, μὴ ἀπὸ γονέων ἢ προγόνων τὸ τοιοῦτον πάθος κατὰ διαδοχήν ἐστιν ἐν τῷ παιδίῳ· καὶ ἐὰν τοῦτο ὁμολογηθῇ ὑπὸ τῆς μητρός, ἀποφαινόμεθα, ὡς οὐκ ἐνδέχεται θεραπευθῆναι διὰ τὸ τὴν καταβολὴν ὅλου τοῦ σπέρματος σύμφυτον ἐσχηκέναι τὸ πάθος. εἰ δὲ φαίη ἡ μήτηρ αὐτοῦ μηδένα ὅλως τῶν προγόνων αὐτοῦ τῷ τοιούτῳ συσχεθῆναι πάθει, ζητητέον πάλιν, μὴ τὸ γάλα, ὅπερ θηλάζει, μοχθηρόν ἐστι, ψυχρότερόν φημι καὶ φλεγματικώτερον ὑπάρχον· καὶ ἐὰν ταῦτα οὕτως ἔχῃ, κελεύομεν ἑτέρᾳ τροφῷ δοθῆναι τὸ παιδίον θερμότερον ἐχούσῃ τὸ γάλα, ὅπερ θηλάζον τὸ παιδίον θεραπευθήσεται. εἰ δέ γε μηδέτερον τούτων ὑποπέσοι τῇ ἐρωτήσει, δῆλον, ὅτι δι' ἑτέραν τινὰ αἰτίαν, ⟨τ⟩αὐτὸν δὲ εἰπεῖν διὰ φλεγματικὸν χυμὸν ὄντα ἐν τῷ ἐγκεφάλῳ, τὸ τῆς ἐπιληψίας αὐτῷ συμβέβηκε πάθημα· κἀντεῦθεν τρέπομαι ἐπὶ τὴν θεραπείαν καὶ κέχρημαι λεπτύνουσι βοηθήμασι καὶ θερμαίνουσι καὶ τροφαῖς ὡσαύτως. καὶ πολλὰ ποιήσας οὐδὲν τυχὸν ὤνησα· τί λοιπὸν ἐπὶ τούτῳ ἡ τέχνη φησίν, ἣν ὁ Ἱπποκράτης συνεστήσατο; ὅτι τὸ οὕτως πάσχον παιδίον τὸν τῆς ἥβης δεχόμενον καιρὸν ἡ κατὰ τὴν ἀκμὴν ἡλικία θεραπεύσει. δεῖ γὰρ εἰδέναι, ὅτι ἡ ἡμετέρα τέχνη ποτὲ μὲν ποιεῖ, ποτὲ δὲ τὴν ἐκ φύσεως καθ' ἡλικίαν ἐκδέχεται μεταβολήν· καὶ ποιεῖ μὲν λεπτύνουσα καὶ τέμνουσα καὶ θάλπουσα καὶ ὅσα τοιαῦτα, εἰ δὲ μηδὲν ἐπὶ τούτοις ἀνύσει, τότε τὴν ἐκ τῆς ἡλικίας ἐκδέχεται μεταβολήν. εἰ γὰρ ψυχρόν ἐστι τὸ πάθος, αὐτὴν τὴν ἀρχὴν τῶν νεύρων κατειληφός, χρεία δὲ τοῖς θερμαίνουσι χρήσασθαι, ὅπερ δὴ καὶ πράττομεν,

1sq. ἡ – ὕλῃ] *cf.* Theoph. In Aphor.: II 337,1–2 Dietz 10sq. παιδικὸν – χυμόν] *v.* Gal. In Aphor. III 29: XVII B 643,2–3 K. 13sq. οὕτω – φαμέν] *v.* Hom. Iliad. 16,407 Etym. magn. 468,20–23 c. adn. (ed. Th. Gaisford, Oxonii 1848 [Amstelodami 1962])

6 *post* γὰρ *add.* ἡ P λέγεται καὶ *om.* P 10 μάλιστα τοῖς παισὶ A 14 μέγα α: *correxi* νοῦσος P 15sq. δυσκαταγώνιστος τῇ περιουσίᾳ τῆς δυνάμεως A 16sq. ὤφθη – δυσκαταγώνιστον *om.* P 19 ἐπιλήψεις A 27 κελεύωμεν P 29 τινὸς α: *correxi* ταὐτὸν *scripsi*: αὐτὸν α 33 ὤνυσα P τοῦτο A 34 ἡ] ἢ P

caused by a sticky and thick humor, while epilepsy usually originates in that kind of matter, but not always: sometimes it also comes from an atrabiliar humor which settles in the orifice of the stomach, causing irritation and soreness in this part, and since, owing to its abundance of nerves and its hypersensitivity the related nerves are painfully affected, this leads to an agitation and disturbance of the brain, which is epilepsy.

This disease, epilepsy, has a variety of names: it is called epilepsy, it is also called children's evil, sacred disease and Herculean disease; each of these names expresses a meaningful conception. It is called epilepsy, because it takes possession (*epilambanesthai*) of the brain and does not permit it to exercise its own functions. "Children's evil", because it is especially common in children, in whom crude humor accumulates by greedy eating and indigestion. It is called the "sacred disease", according to some, because the affected organ, the brain, is sacred, according to others, because of the magnitude of the disease, just as we speak of a "sacred fish", meaning a big one. It is also called the Herculean disease, not because some have believed that Hercules suffered from this complaint, but because the disease is as difficult to overcome for physicians, as (Hercules) with his enormous strength was for his enemies. This being settled, let us now come to our subject.

Hippocrates says that epilepsy occurs especially in the young; if you agree, we will discuss some practical instances to illustrate this statement. A woman comes to see us with a sucking child that suffers from epilepsy. In this case we inquire whether the affection of the child is perhaps inherited from parents or grandparents; and if the mother confirms this, we declare that there is no cure, because the disease was inherent in the seed itself at the moment of conception. If, however, the mother says that not one of its ancestors has suffered from the disease, we must inquire further whether perhaps the milk with which it is fed is bad, i.e. too cold and phlegmatic; and if so, we tell her to give the child to another nurse with warmer milk; when the baby is fed with this, it will be cured. If neither question applies, it is evident that the epilepsy is due to another cause, in other words, to a phlegmatic humor present in the brain; so I now pass to treatment, applying comminuting and heating remedies and similar nutriment. Now suppose all my trouble is of no avail: what further solution has the art established by Hippocrates to offer? It tells that when the little patient reaches adolescence, the prime of life itself will provide the cure. We should remember that our art sometimes acts and sometimes awaits the natural change attending a particular age; it acts by comminuting, fragmentizing, heating, etc., but if these lead to nothing, it waits for the change that comes with age. If the disease is due to cold and has affected the very principle of the nerves, so that we must apply heating remedies, as we are doing, (and if we achieve nothing,) it is obvious that a

δῆλον, ὡς θερμοτέρας ἀγωγῆς καὶ καταστάσεως, ἧπερ ἡμεῖς χρώμεθα, πρὸς τὸ τοιοῦτον πάθος ἐστὶ χρεία· τί δὲ οὕτως θερμὸν τῷ οἰκείῳ καὶ ἐμφύτῳ θερμῷ ὡς ἡ ἀκμαστικὴ ἡλικία, ἥτις πυρωδέστερον αὐτὸ καὶ οἷον διακαὲς κέκτηται δραστήριον; διὸ καὶ πρὸς πᾶσαν πρᾶξιν τὸ τηνικαῦτα διεγείρεται τὸ ζῷον ὑπ' αὐτῆς κεντριζόμενον· ἥτις καὶ τὸ σπέρμα ποιεῖ αὔξειν. τὰ γὰρ βοηθήματα ἐνὶ τόπῳ προσφερόμενα, λέγω δὴ τῷ ἐγκεφάλῳ, οὐχ οὕτως διίασιν ὡς ἡ ἐπὶ τῆς ἀκμαστικῆς ἡλικίας μεταβολή· καθ' ὅλον γὰρ τὸ σῶμα τὸ τηνικαῦτα φοιτῶσα ἡ θερμασία ῥᾳδίως περιγίνεται τῆς ψύξεως.

Χρεία δὲ προπαρασκευάσαι καὶ τὴν τέχνην τὸ σῶμα ἐπιτήδειον πρὸς τὴν ἴασιν συμφώνοις βοηθήμασί τε καὶ διαιτήμασι τῇ ἀπὸ τῆς ἡλικίας ἐλπιζομένῃ μεταβολῇ καὶ θεραπείᾳ τοῦ πάθους. οὐδὲν γὰρ ἄτοπον τὴν μὲν ἡλικίαν διὰ τὴν οἰκείαν μεταβολὴν συνεπιλαμβάνειν εἰς βοήθειαν καὶ τὴν τέχνην τοῖς δέουσι προπαρασκευάζειν τὸ σῶμα, τὸν δὲ πάσχοντα ἀκολαστότερον καὶ ἀκρατέστερον ἀδηφαγίαις σχολάζοντα τὴν τοῦ φλέγματος αὔξειν γέννησιν καὶ ἀνίατον ἐντεῦθεν τὸ πάθος καταστῆσαι, ὡς ὑπερβῆναι αὐτὸν τὴν ἀκμαστικὴν ἡλικίαν μηδὲν ὠφεληθέντα. ἡνίκα καὶ προλέγειν δεῖ, ὡς ἀδύνατος ἐπὶ τούτου ἡ θεραπεία· εἰ γὰρ τὸ θερμὸν τῆς ἡλικίας, συνεπισχυσάσης καὶ τῆς τέχνης, οὐ κατηγωνίσατο τὸ αἴτιον, ποία ἐλπὶς ἀπαλλαγῆς ἐπὶ ψυχροτέραν λοιπὸν ἡλικίαν καὶ κρᾶσιν καὶ σύμφωνον τῷ νοσοποιῷ αἰτίῳ τοῦ πάσχοντος ἐρχομένου; καὶ γὰρ καὶ εἰ χειμῶνί τις συσχεθῇ τῷ πάθει, τὸ θέρος ἐπιλαμβάνον θεραπεύσει αὐτόν, ἐὰν σύμφωνος τῇ ὥρᾳ καὶ ἡ δίαιτα παραληφθείη, τουτέστιν ἐὰν καὶ τὴν ἐκ τῆς τέχνης σχοίη ἐπικουρίαν. καλῶς οὖν ἔφη ὁ Ἱπποκράτης· Τῶν ἐπιληπτικῶν τοῖσι νέοισιν ἀπαλλαγὴν αἱ μεταβολαὶ τῆς ἡλικίης καὶ τῶν ὡρέων καὶ τῶν τόπων καὶ τῶν βίων ποιέουσιν.

Ἰστέον δέ, ὅτι μάχεσθαι δοκεῖ ἡ ποιότης τῆς λέξεως τῇ διανοίᾳ τοῦ Ἱπποκράτους οὔσῃ τοιαύτῃ, φαμέν, ὅτι, ἐὰν ἐπιληψίᾳ τις ἐκ παίδων κρατηθῇ καὶ ταύτην ἡ τέχνη μὴ δυνηθῇ θεραπεῦσαι, τὴν ἡβητικὴν ἡλικίαν δεῖ ἐκδέχεσθαι ὡς γενησομένης αὐτῆς ἰατροῦ διὰ τὸ θερμὸν τῆς κράσεως. αὕτη μὲν ἡ διάνοια, δοκεῖ δὲ πρὸς αὐτὴν ἐναντίωσιν ἔχειν ἡ ποιότης τῆς λέξεως ἔχουσα οὕτως· τῶν ἐπιληπτικῶν τοῖσι νέοισι, τουτέστι τοὺς ἐν τῇ νέᾳ ἡλικίᾳ κρατουμένους ἐπιληψίᾳ ἡ νέα ἡλικία ἀπαλλάσσει, ἤγουν ἡ ἡβική· ἔξεστι γὰρ ἡμῖν ταὐτὸν νοῆσαι νέαν καὶ ἡβικὴν ἡλικίαν. ὡς ἐντεῦθεν ἀδιανόητον εἶναι τὸ λεγόμενον· ἐὰν γὰρ ἐν τῇ αὐτῇ ἡλικίᾳ γένηται τὸ πάθος, διὰ τὸ εἰπεῖν τοῖσι νέοισι, καὶ πάλιν ἡ αὐτὴ παύει αὐτό, φημὶ δὴ ἡ ἡβική, πῶς συμβαίη τοῖς λεγομένοις τὸ αἱ μεταβολαὶ τῆς ἡλικίας τῆς αὐτῆς ὑποτεθείσης; διὸ ἐνταῦθα γενόμενος ὁ Γαληνὸς «Δεῖ» φησὶ «προσυπακούειν τὸ παιδίοισιν εἰ ἐπιληψία γένηται, ταύτην ἡ κατὰ τὴν ἥβην ἤτοι νέαν ἡλικίαν μεταβολὴ παύει.» μήποτε δὲ καὶ ἄλλως ἔστιν ἑρμηνεῦσαι ἐκ τῶν Ἱπποκράτει εἰρημένων. ἰστέον τοίνυν, ὅτι τὸ ἐν μήτρᾳ δημιουργούμενον «κύημα» καὶ «ἔμβρυον» κυρίως λέγεται, τὸ δὲ ἀποτεχθὲν «παιδίον» ὀνομάζουσιν· ἔστι δ' ὅτε καταχρώμενος τοῖς ὀνόμασιν ὁ Ἱπποκράτης καὶ τὸ ἔτι κυοφορούμενον «παιδίον» ὀνομάζει, ὡς δηλοῖ ἡ ἐπιγραφὴ τοῦ Περὶ παιδίου φύσεως συγγράμματος. ἐκεῖσε γὰρ προθέμενος τὴν ἐκ τῆς μήτρας γινομένην δημιουργίαν τοῦ ἐμβρύου διεξελθεῖν οὐ «Περὶ κυήματος φύσεως» ἢ «ἐμ-

34sq. Δεῖ — παύει] *nihil tale apud Gal. h. l.*

3 *post* κέκτηται *fort.* καὶ *addendum est* 4 διὸ *om.* P 6 ἡ *om.* A 7 καθόλου P 9 τῇ τέχνῃ A² 18 σύμφωνα α: *correxi* 22 τοῖς A 29 νέᾳ *om.* A 31 τὸ^{II} *om.* A 32 δὴ *om.* P 36 Ἱπποκράτους α: *correxi*

hotter treatment and condition than we can supply is needed to overcome this affection; and what has as much natural and innate heat as the prime of life, in which it attains its most fiery, and one might say its most burning and effective stage? At that time the organism is stimulated and goaded by it to every kind of activity; it also causes the seed to develop. As for remedies, which are applied locally, i.e. to the brain, they cannot be as pervasive as the change that takes place in the prime of life, when the heat, spreading over the entire body, can easily overcome the cold.

But the art must also prepare the body for recovery by means of remedies and dieting concordant with the change and cure of the disease which is expected from the change of age. Indeed, even if the age by its characteristic change comes to the patient's aid and the art predisposes the body by appropriate measures, it may happen very well that the patient by indulging in undisciplined and uncontrolled overeating increases the production of phlegm and thus makes the disease incurable, so that presently he is past his prime without having improved at all. At that point our prognosis must be that recovery for this patient is impossible; for if the heat of youth, reinforced by the art, has not been able to overcome the cause, what hope is there of getting rid of it, now that the patient is reaching a colder age and temperament, which are in agreement with the cause that produces the disease? For that matter, if somebody contracts the disease in winter, the coming of summer will cure him, provided a diet agreeing with the season is also adopted, in other words, if medicine also comes to his aid. Hippocrates, therefore, is right when he says: Youthful epileptics are cured by changes in age, seasons, places, and ways of life.

It should be observed, however, that the actual wording seems to contradict the meaning intended by Hippocrates, which, as we believe, is this: If somebody suffers from epilepsy already in childhood, and the art cannot cure it, we must wait for adolescence to become his doctor thanks to its hot temperament. This is the meaning, but the actual wording seems to be in contradiction with it, when it says: youthful epileptics, in other words, those who suffer from epilepsy in their youth are freed from it by youth, i.e. by adolescence; for we may regard youth and adolescence as identical. The statement becomes senseless as a result; for if the affliction develops in the same age – youthful epileptics – which also puts an end to it, i.e. adolescence, how can the word changes fit in with such an interpretation, which takes the age to be the same? This is why Galen in his commentary on this passage says: "We must supply in thought, 'If children develop epilepsy' – then the change to adolescence, or youth, will cure it." Perhaps another interpretation is also possible on the ground of Hippocrates' own words. Remember that the offspring that is formed in the womb is properly called "fetus" and "embryo", while after birth it is called "child"; yet Hippocrates sometimes uses these terms loosely and applies the word "child" to what is still a fetus, as in the title of the treatise On the Nature of the Child. Though his subject there is the formation of the embryo from the womb, he did not give the book the title "On the Nature of the Fetus" or "of the Embryo", but "On the Nature of

βρύου», ἀλλὰ «Περὶ παιδίου φύσεως» τὸ βιβλίον ἐπέγραψε. μήποτε οὖν καὶ ἐνταῦθα κατεχρήσατο τῷ ὀνόματι, νέαν ἡλικίαν οὐ τὴν ἀκμαστικὴν κυρίως καλέσας, ἀλλὰ τὴν μειρακιώδη, ὡς εἶναι τοιοῦτον τὸ λεγόμενον· Ὅσοις ἐν νέᾳ ἡλικίᾳ, τουτέστι μειρακιώδει, γένηται ἐπιληψία, οὗτοι εἰς ἀκμαστικὴν ἡλικίαν ἐλθόντες θεραπεύονται.

Μεταβολὴν δὲ οὐ τὴν ἁπλῶς ἐφ' ὁπότερα ἂν γένηται λαμβανομένην νοητέον, ἀλλὰ τὴν ἀπὸ τοῦ χείρονος ἐπὶ τὸ κρεῖττον ἀλλοίωσιν. κατὰ κοινοῦ γὰρ τὸ τῆς ἀλλοιώσεως ὄνομα, ἐπί τε τῆς ἡλικίας καὶ τῆς ὥρας καὶ τοῦ βίου. καὶ ὥσπερ ἀπὸ τῆς χείρονος ἡλικίας, λέγω δὴ τῆς μὴ δυναμένης καταγωνίσασθαι τὸ πάθος, ἡ εἰς τὴν κρείττονα μεταβολὴ[ν] ἀπαλλαγὴν ποιεῖται, οὕτως καὶ κατὰ τὴν ὥραν τὴν ἀπὸ χειμῶνος καὶ φθινοπώρου καὶ ἔαρος, ἐν αἷς ἀκαταγώνιστον μένει τὸ πάθος, ἐπὶ τὸ θέρος μεταβολὴν νοητέον, πρὸς τὴν ἀκμαστικὴν ἡλικίαν συμφώνως κατὰ κρᾶσιν ἔχον. ὡσαύτως δὲ τῇ ὥρᾳ καὶ τὰ κατὰ τὴν χώραν νοητέον, ὥστε ἐὰν ἐν ψυχρῷ χωρίῳ ἢ ψυχρᾷ ὥρᾳ συσχεθῇ τις τῷ πάθει, τὴν εἰς θερμὴν ὥραν καὶ χώραν μεταβολὴν ἀπαλλαγὴν ἐλπιστέον. βίον δὲ τὴν δίαιταν ὑπακουστέον, ὥστε μηδὲ αὐτὴν συμφώνως ἔχειν τῷ νοσήματι, ἀλλ' ἀπὸ χείρονος ἐπὶ τὸ κρεῖττον μεταβεβλῆσθαι, οἷον ἀπὸ ἁδροτέρας καὶ παχυτέρας ἐπὶ λεπτοτέραν καὶ σύμμετρον, ἀπὸ δὲ ψυχροτέρας ἐπὶ λεπτύνουσαν καὶ τέμνουσαν. ταύτην οὖν καὶ τὴν τοιαύτην μεταβολὴν ἀπαλλάσσειν λέγει τοῦ πάθους τοὺς ὀχλουμένους. οὐδὲν δὲ θαυμαστὸν ἐπικρατέστερον γενέσθαι τὸ νόσημα καὶ δυσμετάβλητον καὶ δυσκαταγώνιστον, ὥστε μὴ ἐν τῇ ἀκμαστικῇ ἡλικίᾳ ἡττηθῆναι· καὶ οὐδὲν ἄτοπον ἐν παιδικῇ ἡλικίᾳ ἀποθανεῖν τὸν πάσχοντα καὶ μὴ φθάσαι τὴν ἀκμαστικὴν προσδοκωμένην ἴασιν.

II 45 [II 46: IV 482,15–16 L.] Δύο πόνων ἅμα γινομένων μὴ κατὰ τὸν αὐτὸν τόπον ὁ σφοδρότερος πόνος ἀμαυροῖ τὸν ἕτερον.

Φησίν, ὅτι, ἐὰν ἐν ἑνὶ τόπῳ, τουτέστι μορίῳ, δύο ὑποστῶσιν ὀδύναι, μία γίνεται. οἷον ὑπόκειται ὀδύνη ἐν ὤμῳ καὶ ἄλλη ἐν βραχίονι· αἵτινες διὰ τὴν γειτνίασιν τοῦ πάσχοντος τόπου συναπτόμεναι ἀλλήλαις μίαν συναίσθησιν παρέχουσι τῷ πάσχοντι. εἰ δὲ γένηται κατὰ διαφέροντα μόρια, οἷον ἐν χειρὶ καὶ ποδί, ἐνταῦθα ἡ σφοδροτέρα τὴν ἀμαυροτέραν ἀμαυροῖ καὶ ἐπικαλύπτει, οὐχ ὅτι καλύπτει αὐτήν, ἀλλ' ἐπισκιάζει, ὅλον τὸ κρῖνον εἰς ἑαυτὴν ἐφελκομένη. συμβαίνει οὖν τὸ τηνικαῦτα θατέρου μὲν τῶν πόνων αἰσθάνεσθαι τὸν πάσχοντα, τοῦ σφοδροτέρου λέγω, θατέρου δὲ μή, τοῦ ἀμυδροτέρου φημί. θαυμαστὸν δὲ πάνυ τὸ λεγόμενον καὶ καθολικὴν περιέχον ἔννοιαν, ὥστε μὴ μόνον ἐπὶ νοσημάτων οὕτως ἔχειν, ἀλλὰ καὶ ἐπὶ τῶν πολιτικῶν πραγμάτων, ταὐτὸν δὲ εἰπεῖν μὴ μόνον ἐπὶ σωματικῶν παθῶν, ἀλλὰ καὶ ἐπὶ ψυχικῶν.

2sq. νέαν – μειρακιώδη] *cf.* Theoph. In Aphor.: II 337,6–8 Dietz 7 καί^{III} – 14 ἐλπιστέον] *cf.* Gal. In Aphor. II 45: XVII B 548,13–549,2 K. 14 βίον – 17 τέμνουσαν] *v.* Gal. In Aphor. II 45: XVII B 549,5–8 K. βίον – ὑπακουστέον] *v.* Theoph. In Aphor.: II 338,3–4 Dietz 24–31 φημί] *v.* Gal. In Aphor. II 46: XVII B 549,12–550,5 K. 27 ἐνταῦθα – 29 ἐπισκιάζει] *v.* Theoph. In Aphor.: II 338,22–23 Dietz

4 μειρακιώδη α: *correxi* 9 μεταβολὴν α: *correxi* 22 γενομένων P 23 πόνος *om. supra, p. 142,28, non hab. Hipp.* 28 ἐπικαλύπτει] *fort.* ἐπικρύπτει *scribendum est* 32 περιέχων α: *correxi*

the Child". Here, we may have another instance of loose usage, youth being used, not in the strict sense of the prime of life, but in reference to older boys, so that the sense is as follows: Those who in youth, i.e. as older boys, develop epilepsy, are cured when they reach the prime of life.

Change should not be understood in its general sense, whichever direction it takes, but in the sense of a transformation from worse to better. This word transformation applies jointly to age, season and way of life. In the same way as the change from the worse age, i.e. the one that cannot overcome the disease, to the better age brings about recovery, so in terms of seasons the change (for the better) must be taken to be that from winter, autumn and spring, during which the disease remains unvanquished, to summer, the season that corresponds to the prime of life as regards its temperament. Place should be understood in the same way as season: if somebody contracts the disease in a cold region or in a cold season, we may hope that a change to a hot season and to a hot country will bring recovery. Way of life must be explained as the regime, which should not be allowed to have the same character as the disease either, but a worse one should be replaced by a better one, e.g. a heavier and coarser diet by a lighter and moderate one, a colder diet by a comminuting and fragmentizing one. This or a similar change, he says, will cure those who are troubled by this complaint. Yet it is nothing unusual if the disease is the stronger, and is difficult to change and to overcome, so that it is not defeated during the prime; further, the patient may conceivably die during childhood and not live to recover as expected on reaching the prime of life.

II 45. When there are two pains at the same time, but not in the same place, the more violent one obscures the other.

He means that if two pains occur in the same place, i.e. member, they become one. For example, someone has a pain in a shoulder and another in an arm; these pains, owing to the proximity of the affected place, unite and cause only one feeling in the patient. On the other hand, if they occur in different members, e.g. in a hand and a foot, the more violent pain obscures and veils the weaker one, which is not to say that it covers it up, but that it overshadows it by drawing the discerning faculty entirely to itself. The result is then that the patient is aware of one pain, the more violent one, but not of the other, the dimmer one. The saying is a most admirable one and it contains a universal idea, so that it holds good, not only for diseases, but for politics as well, in other words, not only in somatic afflictions, but in psychic ones too.

II 46 [II 47: IV 482,17–18 L.] Περὶ τὰς γενέσεις τοῦ πύου οἱ πόνοι καὶ οἱ πυρετοὶ συμβαίνουσι μᾶλλον ἢ γενομένου.

Ἰστέον, ὅτι ἡ πέψις ἢ ἀναγκαίων ἐστὶν ἀλλοίωσις ἢ περιττῶν ἀναγκαίων· καὶ ἢ κατὰ φύσιν ἐστὶν ἢ παρὰ φύσιν ἢ μικτή. ἀναγκαίων μὲν οὖν ἀλλοίωσίς ἐστιν ἡ ἐν γαστρὶ χυλοποίησις καὶ ἡ ἐν ἥπατι ἐξαιμάτωσις· περιττῶν δὲ ἀναγκαίων ἡ τῆς κόπρου καὶ τῶν οὔρων καὶ τῶν πτυσμάτων, ἐφ' ὧν καὶ κατὰ φύσιν ἡ πέψις ἐστί. παρὰ φύσιν δὲ πέψις ἡ λεγομένη σῆψις, ἐξ ἧς ἕλμινθες γίνονται καὶ ἀσκαρίδες καὶ πυρετοί. μικτὴ δὲ πέψις ἡ τοῦ πύου λέγεται ἀλλοίωσις· ἐνταῦθα γὰρ καὶ τὸ παρὰ φύσιν καὶ τὸ κατὰ φύσιν συνάγεται, τὸ μὲν παρὰ φύσιν, ὅτι σῆψις ἐγένετο μὴ δυνηθείσης τῆς φύσεως ὃν εἶχεν ἐξ ἀρχῆς διανύσαι σκοπὸν καὶ συμπέψαι τὴν ὕλην καὶ διαφορῆσαι, ἀλλ' ὃ δὴ λέγεται δευτέρου πλοῦ δεηθείσης· τὸ δὲ κατὰ φύσιν παρ' ὅσον τὸν οἰκεῖον κόσμον τῷ πύῳ ἐπέθηκε, λευκὸν καὶ λεῖον καὶ ὁμοιότερον καὶ ἥκιστα δυσῶδες αὐτὸ χαρισαμένη. ἐπεὶ τοίνυν ταῦτα καλῶς ἡμῖν εἴρηται, ἐπὶ τὸ σπουδαζόμενον ἔλθωμεν.

Δεῖ εἰδέναι, ὅτι ἐπιρρέει πολλάκις τινὶ μορίῳ χυμός, ὃς ἢ ἐν αὐτῷ ἀπεπτούμενος διὰ τὸ πλῆθος ἢ παχὺς κείμενος καὶ ἀδιάπνευστος ὢν ἐπὶ τῇ ⟨ἀ⟩διαπνευστίᾳ ἄρχεται σήπεσθαι. ἐνταῦθα οὖν ἐπεγείρεται ἡ φύσις καὶ τὸν ἐκεῖσε περιεχόμενον καὶ ἀκινητοῦντα τῇ ἀδιαπνευστίᾳ χυμὸν καὶ σήπεσθαι μέλλοντα πρῶτον διαχεῖ· οὗτος δὲ χεόμενος πλείονα τόπον καταλαμβάνει, καὶ πνεῦμα τῇ ἀναλύσει ὑφίσταται, ὡς ἐντεῦθεν διατείνεσθαι τὸ μόριον· ὅπερ διατεινόμενον εἰς ὄγκον αἴρεται καὶ τῷ κινδυνεύειν λυθῆναι τὴν συνέχειαν ὀδυνηράν τινα πάσχει συναίσθησιν, ἥτις ἐστὶν ὀδύνη. ἔτι γε μὴν καὶ αἱ παρακείμεναι ἀρτηρίαι μεταλαμβάνουσαι τῆς σηπεδόνος κατὰ τὸ συνεχὲς μεταδιδόασιν αὐτῆς τῇ καρδίᾳ, ὡς πυρετὸν τηνικαῦτα ὑφίστασθαι.

Ταῦτα τοίνυν θεωρήσας ὁ Ἱπποκράτης ἔφη περὶ τὰς γενέσιας τοῦ πύου οἱ μὲν πόνοι τῷ λόγῳ τοῦ τείνεσθαι τὸ τὴν ὕλην περιέχον μόριον διά τε τὴν χύσιν αὐτῆς καὶ τὴν τῶν πνευμάτων ἀνάλυσιν, πλείονα τόπον αὐτῶν περιέχειν δεομένων· οἱ δὲ πυρετοὶ διὰ τὴν μετάδοσιν τῆς σηπεδόνος τὴν διὰ τῶν παρακειμένων ἀρτηριῶν τῷ τὴν πυοποίησιν ἔχοντι μορίῳ ἐπὶ τὴν καρδίαν γενομένην. καὶ καλῶς ἔφη ἐν αὐτῷ τῷ γίνεσθαι τὸ πύον ταῦτα συμβαίνειν τῷ τε τῆς κινήσεως τῆς ὕλης λόγῳ καὶ τῷ τῆς φυσικῆς μεταβολῆς, μετὰ δὲ τὸ γενέσθαι τὸ πύον οὐκέτι πόνος, οὐκέτι πυρετός· ἤδη γὰρ ἐλεπτοποιήθη τὰ τῆς ὕλης καὶ ἐξητμίσθη τὰ πολλὰ τῶν πνευμάτων, πέπαυται δὲ καὶ τὰ τῆς σηπεδόνος τὸν φύσει κόσμον τοῦ πύου ἀπειληφότος. ὅσον γὰρ οὔπω καὶ ἐκρεῖν μέλλει τοῦ σώματος ἢ τεχνικῶς ἢ φυσικῶς τὸ πύον.

Καὶ μέμνησο τῶν αὐτῶν καὶ ἀνωτέρω σοι εἰρημένων ὅτι «Περὶ τὰς ἀρχὰς καὶ τὰ τέλη πάντα ἀσθενέστερα, περὶ δὲ τὰς ἀκμὰς ἰσχυρότερα.» ἐνταῦθα οὖν εἰ καὶ ἐν τῇ ἀκμῇ τοῦ πύου δοκεῖ σφοδρὸς εἶναι ὁ πυρετός, ἀλλὰ τῇ φαντασίᾳ ἐστὶ τοιοῦτος, οὐ

3–13 χαρισαμένη] *cf.* Gal. In Aphor. II 47: XVII B 550,14–551,5 K. 8 μικτὴ – 11 δεηθείσης] *cf. infra*, vol. III, fol. 178ᵛ 11 δευτέρου πλοῦ] *v.* Greg. Cypr. II 22: CPG I 359 τὸ – 13 χαρισαμένη] *cf.* Gal. De diff. febr. I 8: VII 301,1–4 K. 23–27 γενομένην] *cf.* Gal. In Aphor. II 47: XVII B 551,6–9 K. 24 οἱ – 31 ἀπειληφότος] *v.* Theoph. In Aphor.: II 338,27–339,6 Dietz 30 ἤδη – 32] *cf.* Gal. In Aphor. II 47: XVII B 551,11–14 K. 33sq. Περὶ – ἰσχυρότερα] Hipp. Aphor. II 30: IV 478,16–17 L.

2 γινομένου *infra, vol. II, fol. 124ʳ, Hipp. pauci* 9 τὸ] ποτὲ P 12 *fort.* ὁμαλώτερον *scribendum est* 15 διαπνευστίᾳ α: *correxi* 20 τὴν *om.* P 27 γινομένην *Theoph.* 30 ἐξετμήθη P

II 46. During the formation of pus pains and fevers occur, rather than once it has been formed.

Note that concoction is transformation either of necessary matter or of necessary waste matter; and that it is either normal or abnormal or mixed. Examples of transformation of necessary matter are conversion into chyle in the stomach and conversion into blood in the liver; of transformation of necessary waste matter, that of feces, urine and sputamen, in which cases concoction is normal. Abnormal concoction is so-called corruption, which produces worms, ascarids and fevers. The term "mixed concoction" is applied to the transformation of pus, in which the abnormal and the normal unite, the abnormal because there has been corruption due to Nature's inability to accomplish her original plan of concocting and dispersing the matter, so that she had to resort to her "second best plan"; the normal, insofar as she has imposed her own regular pattern on the pus, causing it to be white, smooth, even and free from any offensive odor. This having been settled to our satisfaction, let us come to our subject.

You must know that often a humor flows to any one part of the body, where, either because it remains unconcocted on account of its quantity, or because it lacks ventilation, having settled in a thick, unaerated mass, it begins to corrupt. Nature is now stirred to action and begins by diffusing the humor which is enclosed there, motionless for lack of ventilation, and which is going to be corrupted; when the humor is diffused, it takes up more room, and by its being dissolved gas is formed, with the result that the part in question is distended; thus distended, it swells to greater bulk, and owing to the danger of its continuity being disrupted, it is subject to a vexing sensation, called pain. Furthermore, the neighboring arteries, sharing in the corruption, pass it on to the heart by continuity, so that fever results.

Having observed this, Hippocrates says that during the formation of pus there are pains because the part containing the matter is distended owing to its diffusion and dissolution into gases, which need more room; and fevers through the passing on of the corruption to the heart by way of the arteries adjoining the part in which the pus is being formed. He rightly stated that these symptoms occur only in the course of the formation of pus, on account of the commotion in the matter and of the natural process of change, but that once the pus has been formed there is no more pain, no more fever; for by now the matter has been comminuted, most of the gases have evaporated, and the corruption also has come to an end now that the pus has reached its natural smooth condition. Very soon the pus will leave the body either by artificial or by natural means.

Remember you were told the same above, where it says: "About the beginning and the end everything is weaker, about the acme stronger." In the present case, though at the acme of the pus the fever seems to be violent, yet it is so only

μὴν τῇ δυνάμει· δηλοῖ γὰρ τὴν φύσιν κατακρατήσασαν τῆς ὕλης καὶ λεπτοποιήσασαν αὐτὴν κἀντεῦθεν σφοδρότερον, ἀλλὰ καὶ κουφότερον τὸν πυρετὸν ἐξάψασαν.

Μᾶλλον δέ φησιν ἐν τῷ γίνεσθαι τὸ πύον ταῦτα συμβαίνειν, οὐχ ὅτι μετὰ τὸ γενέσθαι αὐτὸ πάντῃ ἀνώδυνον καθίσταται τὸ μόριον καὶ ἀπύρετος ὁ ἄνθρωπος, ἀλλ' ἐπὶ μετρίοις τισὶ γίνεται· καὶ οὕτως βούλεται αὐτῷ μᾶλλον ἢ γενομένου. ταῦτα διὰ τούτων ἡμῖν παραδέδοται.

II 47 [II 48: IV 484,1–2 L.] Ἐν πάσῃ κινήσει τοῦ σώματος, ὁκόταν ἄρχηται πονέειν, τὸ διαναπαύειν εὐθὺς ἄκοπον.

Κίνησίν φησι πᾶν γυμνάσιον, εἴτε διὰ παλαίστρας εἴτε ἱππασίας εἴτε κωπηλασίας εἴτε δρόμου γινόμενον. νόμιζε οὖν ταῦτά σοι λέγειν τὸν Ἱπποκράτην· τὸ γυμνάσιον ἐπωφελές ἐστιν, ἐξάγει γάρ τινα τῶν ἐμφωλευόντων τῷ σώματι, πρὸς δὲ ἀναζωπυρεῖ τὸ ἔμφυτον θερμόν, ἀλλὰ καὶ ῥώννυσι πάσας τὰς ἐν ἡμῖν δυνάμεις, φυσικάς, ζωτικάς, ψυχικάς.

Τρία δὲ ταῦτα ἐπὶ τῶν γυμνασίων ζητοῦμεν· ποσόν, καιρὸν καὶ τρόπον χρήσεως. καὶ τὸν μὲν καιρὸν ζητοῦμεν, ὥστε πρὸ τροφῆς παραλαμβάνεσθαι τὸ γυμνάσιον. τὸν δὲ τῆς χρήσεως τρόπον, ἵνα ἕκαστος πρὸς τὸ οἰκεῖον ἔργον καὶ τὸ γυμνάσιον παραλαμβάνῃ, οἷον ὁ εἰθισμένος ἐν ὑγείᾳ παριππάζεσθαι, τοῦτο καὶ μετὰ νόσον μετερχέσθω τὸ γυμνάσιον. τὸ δὲ ποσὸν ζητητέον, ὥστε σύμμετρον εἶναι πρὸς τὸν τόνον τοῦ γυμναζομένου· τὸ γὰρ ἄμετρον καταλύει αὐτοῦ τὴν δύναμιν ἅμα τοῖς ἀχρήστοις καὶ τὰ χρηστὰ συνδιαφοροῦν καὶ τὸ ἔμφυτον θερμόν.

Ἀλλ' ἴσως ἐρεῖς ὅτι «Πόθεν τοῦτο ὁρίσαι δυνάμεθα;» αὐτὸς λέγει· ἐὰν τῷ δεομένῳ ἐπιτάξῃς γυμνάσιον καὶ βούλῃ συμμέτρως αὐτὸ παραληφθῆναι, πρόσεχε τῇ συναισθήσει τοῦ γυμναζομένου, εἰ ἐν αἰσθήσει κόπου ἄρξεται γίνεσθαι· κόπον δὲ ἀκουστέον τὴν ἀνιαρὰν καὶ ὀδυνώδη συναίσθησιν. παῦσον οὖν αὐτίκα τοῦ γυμνασίου αὐτὸν γινώσκων, ὅτι ὑπερέβαλε τὴν συμμετρίαν ἡ κίνησις, πλὴν εἰ μὴ διὰ βλακείαν ψυχῆς ἢ τὸ ἀσύνηθες ἐν τῇ ἀρχῇ τοῦ γυμνασίου ἄρξονται αἰσθάνεσθαι πόνου· τούτους γὰρ οὐ δεῖ παύειν εὐθέως. παυσάμενοι γὰρ τοῦ γυμνασίου οἱ συνήθως γυμναζόμενοι μετὰ τὸ αἰσθηθῆναι κόπου εὔκοποι παραχρῆμα γίνονται, ἀνακτᾶται γὰρ ἑαυτὴν ἡ δύναμις ἐν τῇ ἀνέσει.

Τὸ δὲ δεῖ ἀναπαύειν οὐ κατὰ τὴν παντελῆ ἐπίσχεσιν τοῦ γυμνασίου καὶ εἰς τὸν ἐφεξῆς χρόνον δεῖ νοεῖν, ἀλλ' ἐπὶ τοῦ παραχρῆμα· ἐς γὰρ αὔριον καὶ ἐφεξῆς, ἔστ' ἂν δεῖται τοῦ γυμνασίου, πάλιν αὐτὸν ἐπὶ τοῦτο προτρέπει.

II 48 [II 49: IV 484,3–5 L.] Οἱ εἰθισμένοι τοὺς ξυνήθεας πόνους φέρειν, κἂν ὦσιν ἀσθενέες ἢ γέροντες, τῶν ἀξυνηθέων ἰσχυρῶν τε καὶ νέων ῥᾷον φέρουσιν.

Ἀνωτέρω περὶ ποσοῦ διαλεχθεὶς τοῦ γυμνασίου ἐνταῦθα τὸν τρόπον τῆς

9–10 γινόμενον] *v.* Theoph. In Aphor.: II 339,14–15 Dietz 29 ἀνακτᾶται – ἀνέσει] *v.* Theoph. In Aphor.: II 339,20–21 Dietz 36 Ἀνωτέρω – γυμνασίου] *v.* Hipp. Aphor. II 48: IV 484,1–2 L.

5 *post* αὐτῷ *fort.* τὸ *addendum est* 7 ὁπόταν A 8 τὸ *om.* A 12 ἀναζωπυρὸν A 22 βούλει P αὐτῶ A 25 ὑπερέβαλλε A 28 αἰσθανθῆναι A κόπον A 30 δεῖ ἀναπαύειν] *immo* διαναπαύειν *(cf. supra, lin. 8)* 32 αὐτὸ A 34 ἀξυνήθεων *hic et infra, p. 246,10* α

in appearance, not, however, in effect: it proves that nature has gained mastery over the matter and has comminuted it, thus kindling a fever which, while more violent, is at the same time lighter.

(Hippocrates) says that these symptoms occur rather during the formation of pus, because he does not mean that after its formation the member is entirely free from pain and the patient free from fever, but that he is in better shape; this is the point of rather than once it has been formed. So much for this subject.

II 47. In any movement of the body, when fatigue sets in, stopping it immediately brings relief.

By movement he means any kind of sport, whether wrestling, horse-riding, rowing, or racing. So what Hippocrates is telling you is this: Sport is useful, for it expels certain kinds of matter lurking in the body, further it stirs up the innate heat, and finally it strengthens all our faculties, natural, vital and psychic.

There are these three questions to be raised with regard to exercise: the quantity, the moment and the form in which to take it. The moment is of interest insofar as we should take exercise before meals. The form is, in the sense that each should take exercise of a kind related to his own occupation; thus a man who used to ride on horseback while in good health, should take that kind of exercise also after an illness. The quantity is of interest, insofar as it should be adapted to the strength of the individual taking it; for immoderate exercise will destroy his resistance by dispersing the useful materials and the innate heat along with the useless matter.

You may ask: "How can we determine this?" (Hippocrates) himself tells you how: if you have prescribed exercise for a patient who needs it and you want it to be taken in due proportion, pay attention to the way the person in question feels, whether he begins to notice fatigue, fatigue being understood as a troublesome and painful sensation. Then make him stop the exercise at once, because you know that the motion has been excessive, unless you have to do with one of those people who out of indolence or from want of practice begin to feel pain right at the start of the exercise; such people should not be told to stop at once. As for those who take exercise regularly, if they stop the exercise when fatigue makes itself felt, there will be immediate relief, since their strength restores itself during relaxation.

Stopping it[1] should not be taken to mean complete termination of the exercise for good and all, but only for the moment; the next and following days, as long as (the patient) needs exercise, (Hippocrates) encourages him to take it again.

II 48. Those accustomed to regular exertion, even if weak or old, bear it more easily than the strong and young who do not have the habit.

Having discussed above the quantity of the exercise, (Hippocrates) now

[1] See the app. crit.

χρήσεως μεταχειρίζεται, καί φησιν οὕτως· τοὺς γυμναζομένους ἐπὶ τὰ συνήθη δεῖ φέρειν γυμνάσια καὶ μὴ ἐπὶ τὰ ἀσυνήθη, διὰ τὸ μὴ βαρέως μηδὲ ὀχληρῶς φέρειν τὰ συμπτώματα. εἰ γὰρ ὑποδείγματος χάριν παραλάβω γέροντα καὶ ἀκμάζοντα – ἴσμεν δὲ πάντες, ὡς οἱ γέροντες ἀδρανεῖς ὑπάρχουσιν, οἱ δὲ ἀκμάζοντες ἰσχυροί εἰσι – καὶ δοὺς ἀμφοτέροις τόξον ὥστε ἐντεῖναι καὶ τὸ βέλος ἀφεῖναι, καὶ εὕρω τὸν γέροντα τοξεύσαντα, τὸν δὲ ἀκμάζοντα μὴ δυνηθέντα καίτοι ἐρρωμενέστερον ὑπάρχοντα, ζητῶ τὴν αἰτίαν καὶ εὑρίσκω, ὅτι ὁ μὲν γέρων συνήθης ἦν τῷ κεχρῆσθαι τόξοις, ὁ δὲ ἀκμάζων ἀσυνήθης.

II 49 [II 50: IV 484,6–7 L.] Τὰ ἐκ πολλοῦ χρόνου ξυνήθεα, κἂν ᾖ χείρω τῶν ἀξυνηθέων, ἧσσον ἐνοχλεῖν εἴωθεν.

Καὶ οὗτος ὁ ἀφορισμὸς συνεχὴς τῷ πρὸ αὐτοῦ. ἀλλ' ἐκεῖνος μερικώτερος ὑπῆρχε, περὶ μόνων γὰρ γυμνασίων διελέγετο· οὗτος δὲ καθολικώτερος, καὶ γὰρ καὶ ἐπὶ λουτρῶν καὶ ἐπὶ τροφῆς στερεᾶς τε καὶ ὑγρᾶς καὶ ἐπὶ γυμνασίων ἁρμόζει. τοῦτο γὰρ βούλεται λέγειν ἐνταῦθα ὁ Ἱπποκράτης, ὅτι τὸ ἔθος μεγάλως συμβάλλεται τοῖς ἐθίζουσι πρεσβύτερον ὂν τῇ φύσει, καὶ διὰ τοῦτο οὐ δεῖ παραβαίνειν αὐτό.

Καὶ παραδείγματος χάριν ὑποκείσθωσαν δύο τινές, ὁ μὲν εἰθισμένος ἅπαξ λούεσθαι τῆς ἑβδομάδος, ὁ δὲ τετράκις, καὶ ταττέσθωσαν ἀμφότεροι ἐν ἀλουσίᾳ. τούτων ὁ μὲν ἀδικεῖται ἐκ τῆς ἀλουσίας, ὁ τετράκις εἰωθὼς λούεσθαι τῆς ἑβδομάδος, ὁ δὲ οὐ πάνυ τι ἀδικεῖται, εἴθιστο γὰρ τρόπον τινὰ ἄλουτος μένειν. ὑποκείσθω πάλιν ἕτερός τις καθεύδων ἐπὶ σκληρᾶς στρωμνῆς, τούτῳ δὲ δεξιᾶς τύχης ἐπιλαμψάσης συνέβη καθευδῆσαι εἰς ἁπαλὰ στρώματα· διὰ γοῦν τὸ ἀσύνηθες, μὴ εἰωθὼς εἰς μαλακὰ καθεύδειν, ἀλλ' εἰς σκληρά, μεταβαλὼν τὸ ἔθος ἐβλάβη. ἕτερος πάλιν εἴθιστο καθεύδειν ὑπαίθριος· οὗτος ὑπὸ στέγην ποτὲ καθευδήσας οὐκ ἠδυνήθη ὑπνῶσαι διὰ τὴν τοῦ ἔθους ἐναλλαγήν, κἀντεῦθεν ἠδικήθη.

Φησὶν οὖν τὰ ἐκ πολλοῦ χρόνου διὰ τὸ μηδὲν θαυμαστὸν εἶναι προσάπαξ τινὰ καὶ μὴ ἐν κατασχέσει μετελθόντα τόδε τὸ γυμνάσιον ἢ τήνδε τὴν τροφὴν ἐπὶ τὸ ἕτερον μεταβαλεῖν καὶ μηδὲν ἀδικηθῆναι διὰ τὸ μὴ ἐν συνεθισμῷ γενέσθαι τῶν προτέρων. διὰ τοῦτο οὖν φησι τὰ ἐκ πολλοῦ χρόνου· τὰ γὰρ τοιαῦτα εἴτε μοχθηρὰ εἶεν εἴτε μή, εἰ θελήσεις ἀπὸ τῶν τοιούτων μεταβαλεῖν τὸν εἰς ἕξιν ἐλθόντα τούτων, πάντως ἀδικήσεις. ⟨ὑποκείσθωσαν γὰρ δύο τινές, ὁ μὲν εἰθισμένος⟩ ἅπαξ λούεσθαι τῆς ἑβδομάδος, ἕτερος δὲ τετράκις· κελεύομεν ἀμφοτέροις ἀλουσίαν, καὶ ἑκάτερος βλάπτεται· ἀλλ' ὁ μὲν τετράκις εἰωθὼς λούεσθαι μεγάλως ἐβλάβη, ὁ δὲ ἅπαξ ὀλίγον.

Διττὸς δὲ ὑπάρχει οὗτος ὁ λόγος· ὁ μὲν γὰρ πρῶτος λόγος ἀποφαντικός ἐστιν ὅτι Τὰ ἐκ πολλοῦ χρόνου ξυνήθεα, κἂν ᾖ χείρω τῶν ἀσυνηθέων, ἧσσον ἐνοχλεῖν εἴωθε· τὸ δὲ ἑξῆς συμβουλευτικόν ἐστι, τὸ λέγον· [II 50: IV 484,7–8 L.]

3 εἰ – 8] *cf.* Theoph. In Aphor.: II 340,5–10 Dietz 11–13 ἁρμόζει] *cf.* Gal. In Aphor. II 50: XVII B 553,11–14 K. 11–12 διελέγετο] *v.* Theoph. In Aphor.: II 340,22–23 Dietz 34–248,1 μεταβάλλειν] *cf.* Gal. In Aphor. II 50: XVII B 555,9–13 K.

6 δυνηθέντες P: *corr.* P²: δυνηθέντ *(ambig.)* A 7 τὴν *om.* P τῷ] τὸ A τόξοις] τόποις P 9 συνήθεα A 11 τῷ *scripsi*: τῶν A: τὸν P 12 μόνον α: *correxi* καθολικώτερον α: *correxi* 19 ἄλουστος P 22 εἰς] εἰ P 30 ἀδικήσης P ὑποκείσθωσαν – εἰθισμένος *exempli gratia addidi* 35 συνήθεα A ἢ P

deals with the form in which it should be taken, and what he says is this: People should be made to take their familiar kind of exercise, not some unfamiliar kind, to avoid annoying and troublesome side-effects. If, for instance, I take an old man and a man in his prime – as we all know, old men are weak, men in their prime strong – and I hand a bow to each of them, to bend it and shoot the arrow, and if I find that the old man has shot, but the man in his prime, though stronger, has not been able to do so, I wonder what the reason is, and I find that the old man had the habit of handling a bow, while the man in his prime had not.

II 49. Things long familiar, even though worse than unfamiliar ones, will cause less trouble.

This aphorism, too, continues the one before it. The other one, however, was more special, since it dealt with sport alone, while this one is more general and applies to baths and to nutriment, solid and fluid, as well as to sport. What Hippocrates wants to say here is that habit, once acquired, plays an important part, for it has by nature the oldest rights; therefore we must not infringe upon it.

By way of example let us take two persons, one of whom has the habit of having a bath once a week, the other four times (a week), and let us suppose both are put on a regimen that forbids bathing. One of them suffers harm from the prohibition, the person who used to bathe four times a week, the other not at all, because in a way he was already used to being unwashed. Let us take another man who is accustomed to sleep on a hard mattress, but Fortune having smiled upon him things have turned out so that he now sleeps in a soft bed; now owing to the unfamiliarity, because he was not accustomed to sleep in a soft, but in a hard bed, the change of routine has done him harm. Another, again, had the habit of sleeping in the open air; this man, when for once he passed the night under a roof, could not get to sleep owing to this change from the customary, and this did him harm.

He says long familiar, because there is nothing to be surprised at, if a man, after taking this particular kind of exercise or this particular kind of food just for once and not regularly, then changes to another kind without any bad consequences, because he had not yet got accustomed to the first. This is why he speaks of habits long familiar; for whether such habits are bad or not, if you want to break a man of them after they have become a permanent condition with him, you will inevitably do him harm. Take two men, one of them accustomed to have a bath once a week, the other four times: we forbid bathing for both, and both suffer harm; but in the case of the man who used to bathe four times it is considerable, in the other case it is slight.

This aphorism is bipartite, the first part containing a statement: Things long familiar, even though worse than unfamiliar ones, will cause less trouble, the second a precept: so we must change even to unfamiliar

δεῖ οὖν καὶ εἰς τὰ ἀξυνήθεα μεταβάλλειν. τοῦτο φιλανθρώπως εἴρηκεν ὁ Ἱπποκράτης· ἀφορῶν γὰρ πρὸς τὴν τῶν ἀνθρώπων φύσιν καὶ γινώσκων τὰς τοῦ βίου περιστάσεις, αἵτινες οὐ συγχωροῦσιν ἡμῖν ἀεί τε ἑαυτῶν ἐξουσιάζειν καὶ ἃ βουλόμεθα διαπράττεσθαι, τοῦτο ἔφη. οἷον εἴθιστό τις πιοτέρᾳ τροφῇ κεχρῆσθαι· οὗτος ὤφειλεν ἑαυτὸν ἐπὶ ξηροτέραν μεταγαγεῖν καὶ σκληροτέραν καὶ προσεθισθῆναι καὶ τῇ τοιαύτῃ. πολλάκις γὰρ κατά τινα τυχηρὰν περίστασιν συνέβη αὐτῷ ἐν ἀποδημίᾳ γενομένῳ κατὰ τόπον γενέσθαι, ἔνθα τῶν συνήθων ἀπορήσειεν, ἢ μὴν πένητι καταστάντι μηκέτι τράπεζαν τρυφηλὴν ἔχειν. ἵν' οὖν μὴ ἐπὶ τὰ τοιαῦτα μεταβαλὼν ἀνάνδρως τις ἀποθνήσκῃ, δεῖ φησι καὶ ἐς τὰ ἀξυνήθεα μεταβάλλειν.

II 50 [II 51: IV 484,9–12 L.] Τὸ κατὰ πολὺ καὶ ἐξαπίνης πληροῦν ἢ κενοῦν, ἢ θερμαίνειν ἢ ψύχειν, ἢ ἄλλως ὁπωσοῦν τὸ σῶμα κινέειν, σφαλερόν· καὶ πᾶν τὸ πολὺ τῇ φύσει πολέμιον, τὸ δὲ κατὰ σμικρὸν ἀσφαλές, καὶ ἄλλως τὸ ἐξ ἑτέρου μεταβαίνειν ἐφ' ἕτερον.

Εἰπὼν ἀνωτέρω· «δεῖ οὖν καὶ εἰς τὰ ἀξυνήθεα μεταβαίνειν» καὶ τούτῳ ἑαυτὸν ἀνατρέπειν δοκῶν, τούτου χάριν φησὶν ὅτι οὐκ ἐπιλέλησμαι τοῦ οἰκείου κανόνος· καὶ γὰρ εἶπον ὅτι «δεῖ καὶ εἰς τὰ ἀσυνήθεα μεταβάλλειν». πρόσεχέ μοι τὸν νοῦν ἀκριβῶς. οἷον ἔστι χρεία πληρῶσαι τὸ σῶμα ἢ κενῶσαι, ἢ θερμᾶναι ἢ ψῦξαι· μὴ κατὰ πολὺ οὖν καὶ ἐξαπίνης, τουτέστι μὴ ἐξαίφνης, ποιήσῃς τὴν μεταβολὴν ταύτην, οἴδασι γὰρ αἱ ἀθρόαι κενώσεις ἀδικεῖν τὴν φύσιν. καὶ τὸ μὲν κατὰ πολὺ τὴν κατὰ πλῆθος δηλοῖ ἀμετρίαν, τὸ δὲ ἐξαπίνης τὸ ἀθρόως. οἶδε γάρ, ὅτι ἄμφω συνελθόντα τό τε αἰφνίδιον καὶ τὸ πολὺ νεωτερισμόν τινα καὶ ταραχὴν ἐμποιοῦσι τῇ φύσει. ὅρα δὲ τέχνην τοῦ παλαιοῦ· ἔφη γὰρ τὸ κατὰ πολὺ ἐπιστάμενος, ὅτι οὐδὲν θαυμαστὸν κατ' ὀλίγον χρήσασθαι ἢ τοῖς θερμαίνουσιν ἢ τοῖς ψύχουσιν, ἢ τῇ πληρώσει ἢ τῇ κενώσει, καὶ μὴ ἀδικῆσαι τὸν ἄνθρωπον, καὶ μάλιστα κατὰ μέρος καὶ ἐν πλείονι χρόνῳ τούτου γινομένου.

Εἶτά φησι καὶ ὁπωσοῦν ἄλλως τὸ σῶμα κινεῖν· ἐπὶ τὸ καθολικώτερον ἀνάγων ἑαυτὸν πᾶσαν κίνησιν διὰ τούτου τοῦ ῥησειδίου περιέλαβε, καὶ ἐπὶ πάσης ὡς εἰπεῖν ὁπωσοῦν ἐπιτελουμένης ὑφ' ἡμῶν κινήσεως κατὰ πολὺ καὶ ἀθρόως γινομένης ταραχὴν τῇ φύσει καὶ ἀγῶνα οὐ τὸν τυχόντα συμβαίνειν. ἵνα γὰρ μὴ ἀνεπιστήμων τις καὶ ἀμέθοδος εἶναι δόξῃ διὰ τῆς τῶν κατὰ μέρος ἀπαριθμήσεως συγκροτῶν τὸ καθόλου ἐν τῷ μεμνῆσθαι σκληρότητος καὶ μαλακότητος, πυκνώσεως καὶ ἀραιώσεως, ἰσχνότητος καὶ παχύτητος, φιλοσόφῳ ζήλῳ καθολικὴν ἐποιήσατο τὴν διδασκαλίαν. εἰπὼν γὰρ τὸ ὁπωσοῦν καὶ ἄλλως καθολικὴν περιέχον τὴν ἔννοιαν, τὸ ἔτι καθολικώτερον ἐπήγαγεν ἐν τῷ φάναι καὶ πᾶν τὸ πολὺ τῇ φύσει πολέμιον, τουτέστι πᾶν τὸ ὑπὲρ τὴν δύναμιν ὑπάρχον πολέμιόν ἐστι τῇ φύσει, τὸ δὲ ἐναντίον ὠφέλιμον, ὅπερ ἐστὶ τό τε σύμμετρον καὶ τὸ κατὰ μικρόν. ἔφη γὰρ τὸ δὲ κατὰ μικρὸν ἀσφαλές, δύο τούτου σημαίνοντος, τό τε ὀλίγον καὶ

14–19 φύσιν] *cf.* Theoph. In Aphor.: II 341,18–22 Dietz δεῖ – μεταβαίνειν] Hipp. Aphor. II 50: IV 484,7–8 L. *v.* Gal. In Aphor. II 51: XVII B 557,3–5 K. 16 δεῖ – μεταβάλλειν] Hipp. Aphor. II 50: IV 484,7–8 L.

1 οὖν] *item infra, lin. 14, Theoph.*: δὲ *Hipp.* C'MV *(?)* 9 ἀποθνήσκοι A 10sq. κενοῦν ἢ πληροῦν *Hipp.* 12 κατὰ μικρὸν *infra, lin. 37, Hipp.* C'V: κατ' ὀλίγον *Hipp. multi, Theoph.* 13 ἐφ'] πρὸς A ἕτερα *infra, p. 250,21* 17 ἢ κενῶσαι *om.* A 20 ἄμφω *scripsi*: ἄφνω α 33 περιέχων α: *correxi* 36 φύσει *scripsi*: κρίσει α

things. This latter is a kindness on Hippocrates' part: because he takes into consideration what human nature is like and knows the circumstances of life, which do not always permit us to be our own masters and to accomplish what we wish, he makes this addition. For instance, somebody has been accustomed to the richer kind of food; this man has been forced to pass to a drier and harder diet and to adapt himself to this. These things will come about by fortuitous circumstances: on a journey, he may come to a place where his usual fare is not available; or again, he may become poor and have to give up his gourmet table. Therefore, lest a man compelled to such a change should allow himself to die for lack of endurance, Hippocrates says: we must change even to unfamiliar things.

> **II 50.** Extreme and abrupt replenishment or evacuation, heating or cooling, or any other kind of interference with the body, are dangerous; and all excess is hostile to nature, while proceeding little by little is safe, and especially when changing from one treatment to another.

Because he has just said, "so we must change even to unfamiliar things", and thus has seemingly contradicted himself, he now goes on to say: I have not forgotten my own rule; I did say, "we must change even to unfamiliar things"; listen carefully. Suppose it is necessary to replenish or evacuate the body, or to heat or cool it: then do not bring about this change in an extreme degree nor abruptly, i.e. all at once, for sudden evacuations will harm the constitution. The word extreme denotes excessive quantity, and abrupt means "all at once". (Hippocrates) knows that the two together, suddenness and excessive quantity, cause a sort of tumult and turmoil in the constitution. Note the ancient author's skill: he uses the word extreme, because he is aware that it is quite possible to make a moderate use of heating or cooling remedies, or replenishment or evacuation, without doing harm to the patient, especially if it is done piecemeal and over a longer period of time.

He continues: any other kind of interference with the body; passing to a more general point of view, he comprised all possible interference by means of this phrase, and he says that practically any kind of interference by us, if it is extreme and sudden, will result in considerable disturbance and commotion for the constitution. As he does not want to make an unscientific and unmethodical impression by establishing the universal rule through enumeration of particular instances, such as hardness and softness, tightening and loosening, meagerness and fatness, he has, in imitation of philosophy, stated his doctrine in general terms. For after the expression any other kind, which is already general in purport, he proceeds to the even more general formulation, and all excess is hostile to nature, in other words, whatever exceeds the (patient's) strength is injurious to the constitution, and its opposite is beneficial, i.e. due proportion and application in small quantities. His words are, proceeding little by little is safe, which denotes two things, small quantity and due proportion; the former

τὸ σύμμετρον· κεφαλαιωδέστερον δὲ τὸ πρῶτον, δυνατὸν γὰρ τῷ συμμέτρῳ καὶ ἀθρόως χρήσασθαι μηδὲν βλαβέντας.

Ἐνταῦθά τινες ἀποροῦσιν· «Εἰ τὸ κατὰ πολὺ καὶ ἐξαπίνης πληροῦν ἢ κενοῦν ἢ θερμαίνειν ἢ ψύχειν σφαλερόν, τί δὴ ἐπὶ τῶν διακαῶς πυρεττόντων ὕδατος πολλοῦ πόσιν ἔστιν ὅτε καὶ ἀθρόως παραλαμβάνομεν, καὶ ὠφελοῦνται οἱ κάμνοντες ὑπὸ τοῦ ἐναντίου σβεννυμένης τῆς πυρεκτικῆς ζέσεως καὶ καύσεως;» πρὸς ὃ λέγομεν, ὅτι τῶν σπανίως γινομένων ἐστὶ τὸ τοιοῦτον· δεύτερον δέ, ὅτι πιότερόν ἐστι τοῦ ὕδατος οὐδὲν πρὸς τὴν ὑποκειμένην πυρεκτικὴν διάθεσιν. ἀλλ' ἔχει τις πρὸς τοῦτο εἰπεῖν ὅτι «Ἡ σηπεδὼν τοῦ πυρετοῦ ἐκπυρώσει αὐτὸ καὶ ὕλην ἑαυτῆς ποιήσεται, καὶ οὐδὲν ὁ κάμνων ὠφεληθήσεται ἐκ τῆς τοῦ ὕδατος πόσεως.» διὸ εἰπὲ τὴν ἀληθεστέραν αἰτίαν ἔχουσαν οὕτως· εἰ καὶ παρέχομεν πολὺ καὶ ἀθρόον ἐπὶ τῶν διακαῶς πυρεττόντων, ἀλλ' οὐχ ὡς ἔτυχε τοῦτο πράττομεν οὐδ' ἀπὸ τῆς φύσεως τοῦ νοσήματος καὶ μόνης τὴν ἔνδειξιν λαμβάνοντες, ἀλλὰ καὶ ἀπὸ τῶν συστοίχων καὶ ἀπὸ τῆς τῶν σπλάγχνων διαθέσεως. ἀπὸ μὲν οὖν τῶν συστοίχων οὕτως· σκοποῦμεν, εἰ θέρος ἐστίν, εἰ θερμὸν τὸ κατάστημα τοῦ ἀέρος, εἰ τὸ χωρίον θερμόν, εἰ ὁ ἄνθρωπος ἀκμάζων, εἰ ἔθος αὐτῷ τοῦ ἀβλαβῶς ἐν ὑγείᾳ μεταλαμβάνειν τοῦ ὕδατος. ἀπὸ δὲ τῆς τῶν σπλάγχνων διαθέσεως· ἐὰν ἀπαθὲς ἔχῃ τὸ ἧπαρ, ὡς δὲ καὶ τὸν στόμαχον ἐρρωμένον, μήτε φλεγμονῆς ἐν αὐτοῖς μήτε τάσεως οἱασοῦν ὑποκειμένης μήτε μὴν ἐμφράξεως ἑτοίμως γινομένης. καὶ ἡνίκα ταῦτα πάντα καθάπερ τις χορὸς σύμφωνος συσταίη, τότε κεχρήμεθα τῇ ἐπιδόσει τοῦ ψυχροῦ.

Εἶτά φησι· καὶ ἄλλως τὸ ἐξ ἑτέρου μεταβαίνειν ἐφ' ἕτερα. δεῖ γὰρ κἀνταῦθα ὑπομνῆσαι τῆς ἀκριβείας τοῦ Ἱπποκράτου⟨ς⟩· ὃ γὰρ βούλεται εἰπεῖν, τοιοῦτόν ἐστι. θέλει τινὰ ἴσως μὴ εἰθισμένον λουτρῷ κεχρῆσθαι ἐπὶ συνήθειαν λουτρῶν ἀγαγεῖν· τοῦτον οὖν, φησί, μὴ ἀθρόον καὶ κατὰ πολὺ πειραθῇς ἐπὶ ταῦτα ἀγαγεῖν λούων αὐτὸν καθ' ἑβδομάδα δεύτερον ἢ τρίτον, βλαβήσεται γὰρ τῷ ἀθρόῳ τῆς μεταβολῆς· ἀλλ' ἐν μὲν τῇ πρώτῃ ἑβδομάδι λοῦσον αὐτὸν ἅπαξ, ἐν δὲ τῇ δευτέρᾳ δίς, καὶ ἐν τῇ τρίτῃ τρίτον, καὶ οὕτως ἐν συνεθισμῷ γενόμενος ἀταράχως καὶ ἀβλαβῶς μεταβάλλει ἐπὶ τὸ λούεσθαι. ὁμοίως καὶ ἐπὶ πάντων.

II 51 [II 52: IV 484,13–14 L.] Πάντα κατὰ λόγον ποιέοντι μὴ γινομένων τῶν κατὰ λόγον μὴ μεταβαίνειν ἐφ' ἕτερα μένοντος τοῦ δόξαντος ἐξ ἀρχῆς.

Φησίν, ὅτι δεῖ σε διαγνωστικώτατον εἶναι τῶν αἰτίων καὶ τῶν νοσημάτων καὶ τῶν συμπτωμάτων καὶ ταῦτα ἀκριβῶς ἐπιστάμενον ἐπὶ τὴν θεραπείαν χωρεῖν. οἷον ὑπόκειται θερμὴ δυσκρασία ἐν τῷ σώματι· ταύτην διὰ μιᾶς καὶ δευτέρας περιόδου ἀκριβέστατα διαγνοὺς ἐπὶ τὴν θεραπείαν λοιπὸν τρέπου χρώμενος τοῖς ἐναντίοις, τουτέστι τοῖς ψύχουσι, καὶ τούτοις τοῖς κατὰ δύναμιν καὶ οὐ τοῖς κατὰ φαντασίαν, καὶ προσάγων τῷ σώματι ψυχρά τε βοηθήματα καὶ διαιτήματα· εἶτα τούτοις χρησάμενος καὶ μίαν καὶ δευτέραν τυχὸν ἡμέραν καὶ οὐδὲν κατὰ τὸ φαινόμενον ἀνύσας

19 καὶ – συσταίη] *cf. supra*, p. 116,17 36 καὶ – φαντασίαν] *cf. supra*, p. 118,4–5

4 δὴ] δεῖ A 7 πιότερόν] *fort.* ἠπιώτερόν *vel* ἐπιτηδειότερόν *scribendum est* οὐδέν ἐστι τοῦ ὕδατος A 17 ὡς α: *correxi* 21 ἐφ'] πρὸς A 22 Ἱπποκράτου α: *corr.* P[2] 23 εἰθισμένων A λουτρῷ] λουτρῶν α: *correxi* 28 μεταβάλλῃ α: *correxi* 30 ἕτερον *Hipp. (cf. infra, p. 252,31)* 32 δεῖ σε *om.* A 35 τρέπου *scripsi*: τρέπ *(ambig.)* P: τρέπει A 38 δεύτερον P

is more inclusive, since the proportionate can also be applied all at once without any harm.

To this some object: "If extreme and abrupt replenishment or evacuation, heating or cooling are dangerous, why do we sometimes administer large quantities of water at a time to patients in a burning fever, and with good results, too, as the seething, scorching heat of the fever is quenched by its opposite?" We can answer that such a case is exceptional; secondly, that nothing is more nourishing (?) than water to treat the existing feverish condition. Against this one can allege: "The corrupting force of the fever will inflame it and turn it into fuel for itself, so that the patient will derive no profit from the water he drinks." Therefore you will be nearer the truth if you give the following reason: though we give patients in a burning fever plenty of water at the same time, yet we do not do this at random, nor do we take our indication from the nature of the disease only, but also from the correlative factors and the condition of the inner organs. From the correlative factors as follows: we take into consideration whether it is summer, whether the atmospheric conditions are warm, whether the region is a hot one, whether the person is in his prime, whether he used to drink water without bad consequences while in good health. From the condition of the inner organs: we check if his liver is unaffected, similarly if his stomach is strong, both being free from inflammation and tension as well as from any tendency to obstruction. And when all these signs are, like a chorus, in perfect unison, then we proceed to administering the cold water.

Hippocrates adds: and especially when changing from one treatment to another. Once more, we must remind you of his scrupulosity; what he means is this. Somebody, let us say, is not accustomed to bathing, and he wants him to adopt the habit; now you must not try, he says, to make him do this all at once with great frequency by prescribing two or three baths a week, for the abrupt change would be harmful; rather, let him have one bath in the first week, two in the second, and a third in the third; in this way he will get accustomed to it and make the change to the bathing habit without distress or damage. This holds for everything else, too.

II 51. If you are doing everything according to rule and things do not come out according to rule, do not change the treatment, as long as things remain what they seemed at the outset.

He says that you must be able to make a careful diagnosis of causes, diseases and symptoms, and proceed to treatment when you know these exactly. For instance, we have to do with a hot distemper in the body: after diagnosing it accurately during a first and a second period, you can pass on to treatment by means of the opposite, i.e. that which cools – in effect and not merely in appearance – applying cold medication and a cold diet to the body; then, when you have used these for one or two days or so without any visible result, do not change to

μὴ μετέλθῃς ἐφ' ἕτερον βοήθημα, ὅπερ ἐστὶν ἰδεῖν τοὺς ἰδιώτας πάσχοντας· ἀλλὰ δεῖ σὲ τὸν ἐπιστήμονα τῇ αὐτῇ ἀγωγῇ ἐμμεῖναι, ἐξετάσαι δὲ τὰ προσαγόμενα βοηθήματα πρὸς τὸ ποσὸν τῆς ὑποκειμένης νοσοποιοῦ αἰτίας θεωρῆσαί τε, μήποτε τὸ μὲν αἴτιον δέκα μέτροις ὑπερβάλλει τὸ σύμμετρον κατὰ τὴν δυσκρασίαν, τὸ δὲ προσαγόμενον βοήθημα ἕβδομον ἢ ὄγδοον μέτρον ἀναλογεῖ καὶ διὰ τὴν ὀλιγότητα νικώμενον ὑπὸ τοῦ αἰτίου τὰ οἰκεῖα δρᾶν ἀδυνατεῖ. δεῖ οὖν μὴ μόνον τὴν κατὰ ποιότητα παρατροπὴν ἐξετάζειν, ἀλλὰ καὶ τὸ ποσὸν τῆς παρατροπῆς ἀκριβῶς διαγινώσκειν, ἵνα μὴ μόνον τοῖς ἐναντίοις κατὰ ποιότητα χρησώμεθα, ἀλλὰ καὶ πρὸς τὸ ποσὸν τῆς βλαπτούσης ἀμετρίας τὸ ποσὸν τοῦ παρεχομένου βοηθήματος ἁρμόσωμεν.

Εἰ δὲ καὶ τοῦτό σου πράξαντος, οὐ δίς, ἀλλὰ καὶ τρὶς καὶ τετράκις καὶ ἐφεξῆς, μηδὲν πρὸς τὴν ὑπαγωγὴν τῶν βοηθημάτων καθυπεῖκον φαίνεται τὸ νόσημα, μὴ ἀγανακτήσῃς μηδὲ ἐάσῃς τὸν καλῶς ἔχοντα τρόπον τῆς ἀγωγῆς, ἀλλὰ τοῖς αὐτοῖς ἐπίμεινον μέχρι πολλοῦ γινώσκων, ὅτι ἐπί τινων παθημάτων, ἐφ' ὧν παχεῖα τυχόν ἐστιν ἡ ὕλη καὶ ἐσφηνωμένη ἢ καὶ δυσκρασία καθ' ἕξιν τινὰ γινομένη, δρᾷ μὲν πάντως τὰ βοηθήματα ἐλάχιστόν τι καὶ κατ' ὀλίγον καὶ ἀνεπαισθήτως ἡμῖν ἐνεργοῦντα, χρόνῳ δὲ πλείονι αἰσθητὸν γίνεται καὶ κατάδηλον τὸ περὶ τὴν ὕλην συμβαῖνον πάθος.

Ἐνταῦθα διαλεκτικὴ ἡμᾶς ἀπορία διαδέχεται ὅτι· «Ἔστ' ἂν δρᾷ τὸ ποιοῦν, πάντως ἔστι τὸ πάσχον. ἀδύνατον γὰρ ἀνεπιτηδείως ἔχοντος τοῦ πάσχοντος ἐνεργεῖν τὸ ποιοῦν· οἷον καίει μὲν τὸ πῦρ, ἀλλ' οὐ σαλαμάνδραν ἢ ἀμίαντον ἢ ἀδάμαντα, διὰ τὸ ἀνεπιτηδείως ἔχειν ταῦτα πρὸς τὸ καυθῆναι. ὁμοίως καὶ τὸ ὕδωρ ψύχει, ἀλλ' ἐκεῖνα, ὅσα ἐπιτηδείως ἔχει τοῦ ψυχθῆναι, οὐδὲ γὰρ κρύσταλλον ψύχει ἢ χιόνα, ἀλλὰ σῶμα τυχὸν ζῴου. εἰ δὲ τοῦτο, πῶς ἐνδέχεται τὰ μὲν βοηθήματα δρᾶν, εἴ γε κατὰ λόγον αὐτοῖς χρώμεθα, τὰ δὲ νοσοποιὰ αἴτια ἐπιτηδείως πρὸς τὸ παθεῖν ἔχοντα μηδὲν ἐξ αὐτῶν ὑφίστασθαι;» πρὸς ὃ ῥητέον, ὅτι μιᾶς λέξεως τῷ ἀφορισμῷ προστεθημένης λυθήσεται τὸ ἄπορον· καὶ δεῖ προσθεῖναι «κατὰ τὸ φαινόμενον», τοῦτο γὰρ βούλεται ἡ ἔννοια τοῦ ἀφορισμοῦ.

Μένοντος τοῦ δόξαντος· τουτέστι τῆς ἐξ ἀρχῆς ὑποκειμένης διαθέσεως καλῶς διαγνωσθείσης, κἂν μὴ δοκεῖ ὑπακούειν ὡς πρὸς αἴσθησιν τὰ αἴτια, μὴ μετέλθῃς ἐπὶ ἕτερον βοήθημα. οὐδὲν γὰρ ἄτοπον ἐξ ἀρχῆς μὲν εἰσβαλεῖν τριταῖον, τελευταῖον δὲ μετάπτωσιν εἰς ἀμφημερινὸν γενέσθαι· καὶ δεῖ μετελθεῖν ἐφ' ἕτερον, οὐδὲ γὰρ ἔμεινε τὸ δόξαν, ἡ ἐξ ἀρχῆς διάθεσις, ὑπὲρ ἧς καὶ τὰ βοηθήματα ἡρμόσαμεν.

II 52 [II 53: IV 484,15–17 L.] Ὁκόσοι τὰς κοιλίας ὑγρὰς ἔχουσι νέοι μὲν ὄντες βέλτιον ἀπαλλάσσουσι ⟨τῶν⟩ τὰς ξηρὰς ἐχόντων, εἰς δὲ τὸ γῆρας χεῖρον ἀπαλλάσσουσι· ξηραίνονται γὰρ ὡς ἐπὶ τὸ πολὺ τοῖσιν ἀπογηράσκουσιν.

19 Ἐνταῦθα – ποιοῦν] *cf.* Gal. De fac. nat. III 7: Scr. min. III 217,18–23 Helmr. = II 161, 6–11 K. De temp. III 4: p. 103,13–104,20 Helmr. = I 674,9–676,7 K. Plat. Gorg. 476 b 3–d 4

2 σε α: *correxi* ἐπιμεῖναι A 5 ἀναλογῇ A 6 ἀδυνατοῖ A 8 χρησόμεθα P 9 ἁρμόσομεν P: *corr.* P² 17 πλεῖον α: *correxi* 21 καίει] καὶ εἰ P τὸ[II] *om.* A 35 τῶν *sec. Hipp. addidi* τὰς *Hipp. quidam, non hab. multi* (C')

another remedy, which is the way we see the amateurs react; you, as an expert, should stick to the same course of treatment, but check the remedies applied as regards their relation to the quantity of the underlying disease-producing cause, and consider if perhaps the cause in its distemper exceeds the normal measure by ten units, while the medication applied corresponds to seven or eight units, so that owing to its insufficient volume it is defeated by the cause and cannot achieve what it should. Therefore we should examine not only the qualitative deviation, but also carefully establish its quantity, in order that, besides applying remedies opposed to the cause in respect of quality, we can also adapt the quantity of the medication we administer, to the quantity of the harmful excess matter.

If, however, even after you have done this, not twice, but three, four and more times, the disease is found not to yield at all to the influence of the remedies, do not become impatient or abandon what is the correct mode of treatment, but adhere to the same plan for a long time, knowing that in certain affections, in which the matter is for example thick and closely packed, or in which there is a sort of constitutional distemper, the medication is working after all, though its effect is slight and gradual and imperceptible to us, but after a longer time the process enacted in the matter becomes perceptible and even manifest.

Here we come upon the following logical objection: "As long as the agent is working, there is necessarily something that undergoes the action. It is impossible, indeed, for the agent to work, if the object is unfit to undergo the action: thus fire burns, but it does not burn a salamander, or asbestos or diamond, because these are unfit for burning. Again, water cools, but only such things as are fit to be cooled: it does not cool ice or snow, but the animal body, for instance. If this is true, how is it possible for the remedies to work – since we are using them according to rule –, while the disease-producing causes, though fit to undergo the action, are not affected by them in any way?" Our reply must be that the problem will be solved if one word is added to the aphorism: we should add, "in appearance", which is what the sense of the aphorism requires.

As long as things remain what they seemed; i.e., if the (patient's) initial condition has been diagnosed correctly, do not pass on to a different remedy, even if the causes do not seem to respond to treatment in a perceptible degree. It is conceivable, after all, that at first there may have been an attack of tertian fever, which ended by turning into a quotidian; then we should change the treatment, for things have not remained what they seemed, i.e., the initial condition, in view of which we had chosen the remedies, is no longer there.

II 52. Those who have wet bowels are better off in youth than those who have them dry, but in old age they are worse off; for usually (the bowels) become drier as people grow older.

Οὗτος ὁ ἀφορισμὸς ἀνωτέρω ἡμῖν ἐξηγήϑη, ἐν οἷς φησιν· «Ὁκόσοισιν νέοι⟨ς⟩ ἐοῦσιν αἱ κοιλίαι ὑγραί εἰσι, τουτέοισιν ἀπογηράσκουσι ξηραίνονται» καὶ ἀνάπαλιν. οὐδὲν γὰρ ἐκείνου διαφέρει πλὴν τοῦ ὡς ἐπὶ τὸ πολὺ προσδιορισμοῦ. εἰρήκαμεν γὰρ ἐκεῖσε, ὅτι κατὰ πολλὰς αἰτίας ὑγρὰ ἐν νεότητι γίνεται ἡ γαστήρ· διά τε πλῆϑος σιτίων παρὰ φύσιν ἐπιτεταμένης γινομένης τῆς ὀρέξεως διά τε ἀσϑένειαν τῆς καϑεκτικῆς διά τε ῥώμην καὶ πρόωρον ἐπανάστασιν τῆς ἀποκριτικῆς καὶ δι' ἐνδεῆ ἀνάδοσιν, ἥτις γίνεται διχῶς ἢ ψυχροῦ ὄντος τοῦ ἥπατος ἢ χολῆς παρενοχλούσης τὰ ἔντερα καὶ συνεχῶς αὐτὰ πρὸς ἔκκρισιν ἐρεϑιζούσης. ξηραίνεσϑαι οὖν ἐπὶ τούτων συμβαίνει διὰ τὰς προφάσεις ταύτας ὑγρὰν ἐχόντων τὴν γαστέρα ἀπογηρασκόντων. ἀλλὰ τοῦτο ὡς ἐπὶ τὸ πολὺ γίνεται· τοῦτο οὖν εἰδὼς ὁ Ἱπποκράτης τῷ προσδιορισμῷ νῦν πρὸς ἀκρίβειαν ἐχρήσατο εἰρηκὼς τὸ ὡς ἐπὶ πολύ, ἵνα πάντῃ ἀληϑὴς ᾖ ὁ λόγος. ὅσοι οὖν ἐν νέᾳ ἡλικίᾳ ὑγρὰς ἔχουσι τὰς γαστέρας, ὠφελοῦνται, ἐπειδὴ ἐκεῖϑεν διεξέρχεται τὰ περιττώματα· ἐν δὲ τῷ γήρᾳ ξηραινομένοις αὐτοῖς ὡς ἐπὶ πολὺ δι' ἃς εἰρήκαμεν αἰτίας καὶ τῶν περιττωμάτων ἐπεχομένων συμβαίνει ἀδικεῖσϑαι, ὥσπερ οὖν καὶ τὸ ἀνάπαλιν.

II 53 [II 54: IV 486,1–2 L.] Μεγέϑει σώματος ἐννεάσαι μὲν ἐλευϑέριον καὶ οὐκ ἀηδές, ἐγγηρᾶσαι δὲ δύσχρηστον καὶ χεῖρον τῶν ἐλασσόνων.

Ἰστέον [δέ], ὅτι μία τῶν δέκα κατηγοριῶν ἐστι τὸ ποσόν, ὅπερ διαιρεῖται εἰς συνεχὲς καὶ διωρισμένον· καὶ τοῦ μὲν διωρισμένου εἴδη ἀριϑμὸς καὶ λόγος, τοῦ δὲ συνεχοῦς μέγεϑος – ταὐτὸν δὲ εἰπεῖν γραμμὴ ἐπιφάνεια σῶμα –, χρόνος καὶ τόπος. ἐπὶ τούτου οὖν πέφυκε τὸ τοῦ μεγέϑους ὄνομα φέρεσϑαι, καὶ κατὰ μικροῦ λαμβανόμενον καὶ κατὰ μεγάλου· μέγαν οὖν οἶκον τῷ μεγέϑει λαμβάνομεν καὶ πάλιν μικρὸν κατὰ τὸ μέγεϑος. ἓν μὲν οὖν τοῦτο σημαινόμενον τοῦ μεγέϑους· δεύτερον δὲ σημαινόμενον τοῦ μεγέϑους τὸ ἔχειν ηὐξημένας τὰς τρεῖς διαστάσεις, μῆκος πλάτος βάϑος· οὕτω γοῦν καὶ μέγαν λέγομεν σφυγμὸν τὸν πλεονεκτοῦντα κατὰ τὰς τρεῖς ταύτας διαστάσεις· ἀλλὰ μὴν καὶ ἄνϑρωπον κατὰ τοῦτον τοῦ σημαινομένου τὸν τρόπον μέγαν φαμέν. τρίτον σημαινόμενον τοῦ μεγέϑους τὸ ἐπὶ δυσὶ διαστάσεσι ϑεωρούμενον, πλάτει φημὶ καὶ βάϑει. ἔστι καὶ τέταρτον σημαινόμενον μεγέϑους, τὸ κατὰ μιᾶς διαστάσεως φερόμενον, φημὶ δὴ τοῦ μήκους. περὶ τοῦ τετάρτου τοίνυν ὁ λόγος τῷ Ἱπποκράτει.

Οὗτοι γοῦν οἱ ἄνϑρωποι, λέγω δὴ οἱ τὴν κατὰ μῆκος διάστασιν πλεονεκτοῦσαν ἔχοντες, ἐν νεότητι ἀξιάγαστοί εἰσι τῷ εἴδει καὶ εὐπρεπεῖς τοῖς ὁρῶσι καὶ περὶ πάντα ἄριστοι, περί τε τὰς κινήσεις καὶ τὰς πράξεις καὶ τὰ λοιπά· ὑπὸ δὲ τοῦ γήραος

1–3 προσδιορισμοῦ] *v.* Theoph. In Aphor.: II 343,5–8 Dietz 1sq. Ὁκόσοισιν – ξηραίνονται] Hipp. Aphor. II 20: IV 476,1–2 L. *v.* Gal. In Aphor. II 53: XVII B 558,11–14 K. 3 εἰρήκαμεν – 8 ἐρεϑιζούσης] *v. supra*, p. 178,7–27 14 δι' – αἰτίας] *v. supra*, p. 178, 28–37 19–21 τόπος] *v.* Aristot. Categ. 6: 4b 20–25 24 ἓν – 30] *v.* Theoph. In Aphor.: II 343,12–18 Dietz 24sq. δεύτερον – βάϑος] *v.* Gal. In Aphor. II 54: XVII B 559,5–6 K. De puls. ad tir. 2: VII 455,1–15 K. 29 ἔστι – 30] *v.* Gal. In Aphor. II 54: XVII B 559,7–9 K.

1 νέοι α: *corr.* A[2] 16 *post* Μεγέϑει *hab.* δὲ *Hipp. fere omnes* 19 δέ *delevi* 23 μέγαν] μέγα P 24sq. δεύτερον – μεγέϑους *om.* A 26 μέγαν *scripsi*: μέγ *(ambig.)* A: μέγα P 27 μέγα P 31 τὴν *om.* A 33 γήρως A

We already explained this aphorism above, under the one that runs, "In those who have wet cavities when young, they dry up as they grow old", and conversely. This one does not differ in any way from the other, except for the qualification usually. We told you there that there can be many reasons why the bowels are wet in youth: owing to the quantity of food, when there is an abnormally intense appetite, to weakness of the retentive faculty, to strength and premature activation of the secretory faculty, and to defective distribution, which can have a twofold origin, either a cold liver, or bile which upsets the intestines and continually stimulates them to excretion. So in the cases of those who have wet bowels for these reasons, they dry up as they grow old. But this is only generally true; and in view of this Hippocrates here, for the sake of accuracy, has added the qualification usually, so as to make the statement entirely correct. Those, then, who in their youth have wet bowels profit by it, for that is where the waste matter passes through; but in old age, when they usually dry up for the reasons stated and excretion is retarded, this is harmful to their health; the converse is equally true.

II 53. Magnitude of body in youth is noble and not unattractive, but in old age it is awkward and less good than a smaller stature.

Note that one of the ten categories is quantity, which is divided into continuous and discrete quantity; species of discrete quantity are number and ratio, of continuous quantity magnitude – i.e. line, surface and body –, time and space. This is the current meaning of the word magnitude, and it is used of the small as well as of the large: thus a "large house" is understood in terms of magnitude, and so is a "small house". This is one meaning of magnitude; a second is being extensive in three dimensions, length, width and depth: thus we call a pulse "big", if it is excessive in these three dimensions; and it is in this meaning, too, that we can call a man "big". In a third sense, magnitude exists in two dimensions, width and depth. Finally, there is a fourth meaning of magnitude, which applies to one dimension only, namely length. It is the fourth kind to which Hippocrates refers.

These people, then, that is to say, the excessively tall, are in their youth impressive by their stature, pleasing to look at, and superior in every respect, in their movements, their actions, etc.; but when old age overtakes them, they

καταληφθέντες δύσχρηστοι γίνονται καὶ ἀπρεπεῖς τοῖς ὁρῶσιν. εἴρηται γὰρ ἐν ταῖς Ἀνατομαῖς, ὅτι ῥαχῖται μύες εἰσὶν οἱ συνέχοντες τὴν ῥάχιν ἔσωθεν καὶ ἔξωθεν στηρίζοντες· ἐν δὲ τῷ γήρᾳ ἀποκάμνουσιν οἱ μύες καὶ ποιοῦσι τὴν κύφωσιν. ἐνταῦθα γενόμενος ὁ τρισευδαίμων σοφιστὴς Γέσιος καὶ τὸν ἀφορισμὸν τοῦτον ἐξηγούμενος, ἀστείως φερόμενος τοῖς ἀκροαταῖς ἔλεγεν· «Εἰ βούλεσθε ἀκριβῶσαι τὸ ὑφ' Ἱπποκράτους λεγόμενον ἐμὲ αὐτὸν ὑπόθεσιν τοῦ λόγου ποιήσασθε.» οὗτος γὰρ ἐν νεότητι μακρὸς ἦν καὶ εὐπρεπὴς τοῖς ὁρῶσιν, ἐν δὲ γήρᾳ κεκυφὼς ἐγένετο κατὰ τὴν εἰρημένην αἰτίαν.

1 εἴρηται – 3 κύφωσιν] *v.* Theoph. In Aphor.: II 343,20–24 Dietz 1sq. εἴρηται – στηρίζοντες] *v.* Gal. De anat. administr. V 10: II 529,11–531,7 K. De musc. diss.: XVIII B 991,6–992, 16 K. 4 ὁ – Γέσιος] *cf.* Ioann. In Epid.: 146 a 1–8; 150 Ba 48–54; *etiam* 143 d 37–40; 150 c 25–28 Pritchet

5 βούλεσθαι α: *corr.* P2 ἱπποκράτου P: *corr.* P2 6 ποιήσασθαι α: *correxi*

become awkward and unattractive to see. In discussing the Anatomies we mentioned the spinal muscles, which hold the spine in place by supporting it from the inside and from the outside; but in old age these muscles grow tired and cause bending of the back. At this point, when explaining the present aphorism, the highly revered professor Gesius used to tell his students by way of a joke: "If you want to know exactly what Hippocrates means, take me as a case in point." For he was tall and handsome to look at in his youth, but in old age his back became bent for the reason we mentioned.

Kolibri 360 GmbH
Ferdinand-Jühlke-Straße 7
99095 Erfurt, Deutschland
produktsicherheit@kolibri360.de